Therapeutic Voicework

also by Paul Newham

Using Voice and Song in Therapy
The Practical Application of Voice Movement Therapy
ISBN 1 85302 590 9

Using Voice and Movement in Therapy
The Practical Application of Voice Movement Therapy
ISBN 1 85302 592 5

Using Voice and Theatre in Therapy
The Practical Application of Voice Movement Therapy
ISBN 1 85302 591 7

of related interest

Self-Healing Through Visual and Verbal Art Therapy
R.M. Simon
Edited by S.A. Graham
ISBN 1 84310 344 3

Principles and Practice of Expressive Arts Therapy
Toward a Therapeutic Aesthetics
Paolo J. Knill, Ellen G. Levine and Stephen K. Levine
ISBN 1 84310 039 8

Songwriting
Methods, Techniques and Clinical Applications
for Music Therapy Clinicians, Educators and Students
Edited by Felicity Baker and Tony Wigram
Foreword by Even Ruud
ISBN 1 84310 356 7

Authentic Movement
Essays by Mary Starks Whitehouse, Janet Adler
and Joan Chodorow
Edited by Patrizia Pallaro
ISBN 1 85302 653 0

Therapeutic Voicework

Principles and Practice for the Use of Singing as a Therapy

Paul Newham

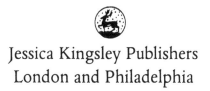

Jessica Kingsley Publishers
London and Philadelphia

First published in the United Kingdom in 1998 by
Jessica Kingsley Publishers
116 Pentonville Road
London N1 9JB, UK
and
400 Market Street, Suite 400
Philadelphia, PA 19106, USA

www.jkp.com

Printed digitally since 2005

Library of Congress Cataloging in Publication Data
A CIP catalog record for this book is available from the Library of Congress

British Library Cataloguing in Publication Data
Newham, Paul
Therapeutic Voicework: principles and practice for the use of singing as a therapy –
(Art therapies series)
1. Singing – Therapeutic use 2. Voice – Therapeutic use
I. Title
615.8'5154

ISBN-13: 978 1 85302 361 3
ISBN-10: 1 85302 361 2

Contents

This book is dedicated to my mother who taught me that all that is within can be voiced

Acknowledgements

I should like to begin by acknowledging the dedication, generosity, vision and support of all at Jessica Kingsley Publishers, especially Charles Catton. I have found their consistent belief in a project of this magnitude and their willingness to permit my work to be published unrestrained by impinging factors to be a rare experience in these present times. Indeed, I have not experienced such constant positive attitudes elsewhere in publishing.

In addition, I should like to express my extreme gratitude to the following people: Wendy Smith for contributing research and insight on the subject of voice and feminism; Mary Law for extensive research into the current practice of Voicework by contemporary practitioners; Brian Lee for lectures on harmonics; Barb Jungr for creating the notation system; Ian Hansum for computer font design; Melanie Harrold for working partnership, music and teaching assistance; Robert Freeburn and Laura Holland for making international accreditation possible; Andrew Samuels for supervision and advice; Penny Lewis, Shaun McNiff and Christina Shewell for support and encouragement; Anne Brownell for research and assistance in the USA; Jenni Roditi for first embodying the vision; Jane McDermott, Bernadette O'Brien, Paddy Holden, Sheri Kershaw and all of my students for making it happen; David Garfield-Davies for making video stroboscopic recordings; Nick Kershaw for recording and producing the CD; Peter Stoddart and Class Productions for directing and engineering the video; Dorothy Rosser for exquisite drawings; all at Fine Line Publishing Services for technical, editorial and design assistance; Jean McConnel for faith; Charlie, Mush and Barry for provisions and life beyond the computer; Patrick Pietroni for more than I could name; Martin for keeping Nipper in good shape; Duncan for accepting a writer's misery. Finally, and, without doubt, most significantly, Josephine for infinite and unwavering love.

About the Author and his Work

Before inviting the reader to explore the theoretical, historical and practical foundations of my research and application in the field of Therapeutic Voicework, it is apposite that I share the personal genesis of this work in my own history – for my life and my work have always been deeply connected.

I was born and raised in the middle of a working-class council housing estate about 20 miles north of London. My childhood was, on the whole, a time of anxiety.

My mother was of a mild and gentle nature who bonded with me as a confidant, companion, son and surrogate husband. My father was an angry and wrathful man who taught me how to rise early and work.

The relationship between my parents was both terrible and terrifying. My father was a very heavy drinker, had hands like dinner plates and a voice which was loud as a horn and rough as sandpaper. My mother, meanwhile, lived on instant coffee and cigarettes and raised her voice only in desperation.

Throughout my young years my immediate environment was a stage upon which my mother and father repeatedly enacted the same savage opera. Regularly my father would return to the house, often in the middle of the night, call for my mother to descend from the bedroom where she was praying for respite and begin shouting and hollering. These thunderous baritonal yells of rage and frustration blended with the high, moaning sobs of my mother, producing an orchestral duet with a dark and bleak ambience.

My sister and I, persistently keen to ascertain the story behind the sounds, would creep into the bathroom and take the toothbrush cup from the sink, place it upside down on my bedroom floor and take turns to listen, hoping to discover what all the shouting was about. Alas, we could never hear the words that were being uttered, only the ferocious and intense passion with which the voices resounded.

It was not until I was an adult that I learned of the suffering that my father and mother both endured as children and was able to understand the roots of his rage and her timidity. It was not until I was an adult that I understood my father as something more than the hungry wolf and my mother as something more than the angel at his table. I lay no blame at their door and to both of them I owe a large portion of what it is I know and teach.

For some reason, which to this day I have not understood, I wanted to be an actor. So, as soon as I could, I left home, auditioned, lied about my age and was accepted as a student at the Drama Centre, London's school for those wishing to train in the methodological approach to acting instigated by the Russian theatre practitioner Constantin Stanislavski and appropriated by the American Lee Strassberg.

The two most important classes to me at Drama Centre were Movement Psychology and Voice. In the first Yat Malmgren subjected each individual to an analysis based on his own idiosyncratic combination of Rudolf Laban's dance notation system and Jung's Psychological Typology. In the latter we stretched out on the floor and listened to ourselves breathe.

In the Movement Psychology sessions my appetite for psychological issues was stimulated. In the voice sessions, meanwhile, I was deeply moved by the process of breathing but desired to know more about the way the respiratory process could access emotional material.

The work at Drama Centre was extremely provocative and demanded a high level of public exposure of intimate personal details but was an inappropriate place for someone as vulnerable and as volatile as I was then. In addition, during my time there, I smoked a great deal of cannabis, took large quantities of LSD and became quite ill.

After drama school I needed somewhere to cool off, dry out and simmer down. So, by some mysterious set of circumstances, I took a job which comprised both practical work and training in the operating theatre of a general hospital. The post was called 'Operating Department Assistant' and consisted, primarily, of helping the anaesthetist. For a year I drew drugs from glass phials into syringes, wheeled patient trolleys, changed oxygen cylinders and, above all, watched hundreds of people have tubes placed down their throats. During some operations, patients who could not, for medical reasons, withstand a general anaesthetic would be given an epidural injection, which would nullify any pain but leave them fully awake during surgery. When this happened, I was often asked to sit by the patient and talk to them. This was my first experience of 'holding' someone during a disturbing situation – other than my mother, who, in a certain way, I had held for many years.

Meanwhile, in the lectures and seminars which were provided, I learned an enormous amount about breathing, the function and disease of the larynx and lungs and the effect of respiratory processes on the body. It seemed remarkable to me that I was many miles away from the dramatic theatre where I had expected to work, yet in this medical theatre I found at least some access to the knowledge of breath and voice which I was seeking. It was also at this hospital that I met the woman who is now my wife.

During this time my mother imparted news to me which radically altered the way I perceived myself: my father was in fact not my father; I had been conceived by artificial insemination by an anonymous donor. The only information available about the man who had spawned me was that he had been a medical doctor at the hospital where I was conceived at a time when such practice was couched in stigma and a certain amount of secrecy.

After a year of the operating theatre, I left and took a job as a trainee psychiatric nurse at Shenley Hospital. In these lectures I learned about neurosis and psychosis, the history of mental illness and what can go wrong with the mind. On the ward, far from silent, the patients gabbled and babbled and spun stories about John the Baptist and the reason why the earth was round and moved with a choreographic sensibility which made Laban's dance forms seem tame. It was here that I was befriended by a senior psychiatrist who recommended that I apply to study at Dartington College of Arts where, he said, they taught performance combined with a study of psychological and psychotherapeutic principles of analysis.

So, having dried out, cooled off and simmered down, I went to Dartington where I enjoyed four years of the most fruitful and rewarding study. Among the staff was Tavistock psychotherapist Anne Kilcoyne who became my mentor and, later, my friend. Whilst at Dartington I also had the opportunity to work with some prolific contemporary performance artists and teachers, including Mary Fulkerson and Steve Paxton. Yet, at Dartington, just as at Drama Centre, little attention was paid to the voice. Then, in the final year of my studies, I began to take workshops outside of the college with a number of contemporary leaders, including Enrique Pardo of the Roy Hart Theatre, which catapulted me into committed investigation of the human voice.

Whilst working with Enrique, he told me the story of Alfred Wolfsohn, a German Jew who cured himself of a mental illness through vocalising his aural hallucinations. Wolfsohn had escaped Nazi persecution and set up an experimental singing studio in London where he worked, with a small group of pupils over a period of fifteen years, to investigate ways in which the contents of the psyche could be given formal expression in sound. When Wolfsohn died, one of his pupils, Roy Hart, took the leadership of those students who remained and formed the Roy Hart Theatre, of which Pardo was a part.

I became fascinated with the story of Wolfsohn, particularly when I discovered he had died a few weeks before I was born, so I set about the task of locating each pupil who had worked with Wolfsohn but who had dispersed to different quarters of the globe upon his death. With an obsessional determination, as though Wolfsohn was in some way my lost and unobtainable father, I located each pupil and interviewed them to discover how Wolfsohn had worked, what had been effective and what had not. This culminated in the publication of his official biography *The Prophet of Song*.[1]

On graduating from Dartington I received a grant from the British Academy and registered as a doctoral student with the intention of researching the use of vocal sound in the ancient Greek theatre. To further subsidise myself I took work offering drama and movement workshops in institutions caring for people with a variety of so-called handicaps and disabilities.

One of the most familiar things about this environment was the volume, diversity and magnitude of the vocal sounds which my clientele made – many of whom were unable to speak. Whilst to many of the staff this was one of the most daunting aspects of the environment, to me it was an opportunity to put the experience of my childhood to use. All those years of the toothbrush cup, of being presented with vocal sounds in the absence of the verbal content, seemed to be revisiting me in the presence of the handicapped men and women who screeched and screamed, bellowed and wailed.

With a certain amount of knowledge, and a lot of nerve, I began searching for ways of utilising these sounds artistically, attempting to make original performance pieces devised from the natural sound and movement patterns produced by the participants. To this end I was appointed as Director of Libra Theatre Company, which was composed of both able and so-called disabled and handicapped people and with whom I devised many performances that were full of vocal sound – yet often not a word was uttered.

During this period of working with those who had been labelled handicapped I was struggling to find ways of contextualising unusual vocal sounds in a framework that would alter people's perception of them as ugly and meaningless. The way that I discovered such a means was quite extraordinary.

At a time of some stress, I took a holiday in Turkey during the festival of Ramadan. On a hot and dusty evening when the town was deserted, I took a walk and, as I turned a corner to buy some water, I heard a sound which grabbed my attention: a moaning, pleading, yearning sound which had a pump-like pulse to it. I could not understand the words uttered but the sound was neither despairing nor euphoric, it was neither melodic nor was it lacking in musical form. Was he crying? Was he singing? Was he praying? I could not answer any of these questions but could only imagine that the ambiguity and unclassifiable nature of this vocal dance was somehow an important part of why it moved me so much.

After this holiday, when working in a centre for mentally handicapped adults, I went around the circle one by one, each member calling out a sound which the group called back. When it came to Jonathan's turn something happened that caused me to experience a deep sense of awe. He called out a sound which I had not heard since the time I had stood on that hot dusty street corner in Turkey and I thought only one thing: if we had taken Jonathan to Turkey and placed him in a room with blinded windows and asked him to call out his sound, passers by may have asked all kinds of questions. Is he praying? Is he chanting? Is he singing? But they would not for a moment have thought to ask: is he handicapped? Jonathan's sound was not handicapped, it was full of religiosity, yearning, needing, pleading and worship. It was also full of music, but it was a music of a different cultural ethos to the classical European tradition.

This experience radically influenced the way I worked, for I now realised that I could treat so-called handicapped sounds as a form of music and arrange the utterances of such people to produce beautiful and original artistic forms. It simply required a broader understanding of the meaning of music and of singing.

However, through this work I also realised that in order to communicate with someone, you have to speak their language; in the case of Jonathan, this consisted of the music of his voice. Thus, in order to pursue my work, I had to train my own voice to acquire the malleability with which to mirror back to Jonathan and others like him a broad range of sounds without damaging my vocal instrument. Fortunately, in the following years, I received a number of grants which enabled me to research vocal training techniques in service of this objective from organisations which included *The Wates Foundation, Shell UK Ltd, The Baring Foundation, The Sobell Foundation* and *The Sir Jules Thorn Charitable Trust.*

In the process of training my own voice, the first discovery which I made was that it was extremely easy for me to sing high-pitched falsetto sounds, whilst low-pitched sounds were somehow out of my reach. It dawned on me rapidly that this was in some way connected to a negative identification with my father, whose deep voice had plagued me, and a positive identification with my mother, whose high voice had attracted my sympathy. As a result of this dawning, I realised that to discover a positive relationship to the depths of my voice I had to look deep into myself and find a positive relationship to the man I knew as my father. In addition, I also felt propelled to explore the deep feelings which I had regarding my 'artificial origins'. It thus became obvious that the process of excavating the full expressive potential of my voice would require significant psychological investigation of my inner core. In response to these recognitions, I began my own psychoanalysis.

Parallel to this, I began to learn how to use my voice to its fullest potential by observing the muscular action which occurred in response to the vocalisation of extreme emotion – such as that which I mirrored back to the handicapped people with whom I was working. In my practical work I would allow my body to move and my voice to spontaneously improvise in response to images, emotions and characters which would pass fleetingly through my imagination. I would then seek to facilitate the same malleability in my clients. At this stage, the name I gave to my work was 'Voicedance'.

In order to understand in more detail the physiological process of vocalisation I needed to observe the internal workings of my larynx whilst vocalising. I was, therefore, honoured and grateful when David Garfield-Davies, at that time consultant laryngologist at the Middlesex Hospital, London, offered to make a video stroboscopic recording of my working larynx by threading a fibre optic camera through my nasal passages.[2] This confirmed that the techniques I was forging not only enabled the vocal instrument to radically increase timbral malleability but that they did so in a way entirely synonymous with healthy methods of voice production. Excerpts of this film footage of my larynx made by Garfield-Davies can be seen on the video which accompanies this book. So it was that as I trained my own voice, underwent my own analysis, researched the academic background of vocal training techniques and facilitated creative voice workshops – primarily for disabled and handicapped people – it became apparent that I was indeed forging a systematic method for liberating voices from constriction. I thus began to publish articles about my work in a number of publications, which have included *The Journal of Analytical Psychology*[3], *Voice: Journal of the British Voice Association*[4], *The British Journal of Dramatherapy*[5], *Human Communication*[6] and *New Theatre Quarterly*[7]. The written results of my research culminated in my first book, *The Singing Cure.*[8] A full list of my previous publications can be found in the Bibliography.

As my approach began to be recognised, a number of professional staff members at various institutions asked me to teach them how to impart the work with their own clientele and, in response to such requests, I began to offer one-to-one sessions of an hour in duration to fee-paying people. The purpose was to allow the client to experience the approach to vocal work which I was developing so that they could begin to pass it on to those in their care. However, I now began to recognise that such a clientele presents a completely different set of problematics.

Whereas with the so-called handicapped people the impediments hindering liberated vocal expression were primarily of a neuromuscular nature, with my new clientele the obstacles were also of a psychological kind. Embarrassment, self-criticism, fear, unexpressed anger or grief and lack of self-confidence often stood between their expressive impulse and their voice. Furthermore, when the voice did release itself from constriction it often provoked extremely powerful emotional reactions in the vocalist. Whilst my artistic and physiological understanding had been the foundation of my work until now, it seemed that my own psychoanalysis provided the most appropriate model for this new aspect of the work that I was beginning to explore.

During the individual voice sessions which I was conducting, people would often experience sensations which they described as not being part of them, as though there was an aspect of their psyche being expressed which appeared to have no history in their own life. People made sounds which they described as 'moving through them' and which made them cry or laugh, feel intense grief, joy, rage and other unnamed passions for which they could offer no personal explanation. As a result of my own experience of encountering parts of myself which I could not trace because I had no knowledge of my genetic father, I understood such people not only intellectually but also experientially. This influenced my work quite considerably.

As my private practice of one-to-one voice sessions grew, I had the opportunity to apply the system of vocal work to a broad range of clients – some of whom came in the hope of alleviating physical problems such as constriction, asthma and stammering, whilst others came for psychological reasons such as shyness, debilitating grief or repressed anger. The systematic approach which I had forged from my work with mentally and physically handicapped people was equally effective with this clientele and the added dimension of acknowledging the psychological significance of the process deepened the work with both client groups.

Over the next period I began to withdraw from working in institutions with primarily handicapped people and concentrated my attentions on running a private practice for a vast range of adults. In addition, my own voice was, by now, highly developed and I was fortunate to receive a number of commissions to compose and sing original vocal music using the extended range of my voice – including the score for Motionhouse Dance Theatre's *House of Bones*, which was supported by the Arts Council of Great Britain and won the Digital Prize in 1990.

My primary focus, however, was on my client practice, with the result that I had more clients and more work than I could possibly handle. Therefore, I considered that I could actually reach more clients by training others to impart the work as facilitators, teachers, therapists and community workers and began running short courses in the techniques and methodologies which I had forged. At this stage in the development of the work I called my approach 'Voice Movement Therapy'. I had altered the label which I used from the original 'Voicedance' because the effects of the work which I was pursuing were clearly based in a therapeutic model and most of the support and assistance which I received came from physiotherapists, psychotherapists, occupational therapists and remedial teachers.

In the summer following the first series of short courses I became unable to work due to exhaustion and an exceptionally talented graduate of one of my training courses, Jenni Roditi, offered to take over my client practice. Jenni did this with extraordinary proficiency and skill and, in so doing, verified that the techniques were indeed solid enough to be passed on.

On returning to teaching the courses which I was developing, and as I observed graduates apply the work in various settings, I began to be convinced that there was a need for trained and qualified practitioners who could use voice to facilitate liberated expression in others. For, many of the people who attended my short courses subsequently, upon graduation, utilised the work in an educational context as teachers, in workshops as group leaders and within artistic projects as performers and composers, as well as in therapeutic settings.

In 1994 I began conducting sessions in collaboration with Melanie Harrold, who had been a singer, singing teacher and song-writer for many years before training with me. On graduating, Melanie began using her improvisational musicianship to accompany individual sessions which I conducted with a range of clients. In addition, she would offer instruction to the client, which enabled them to develop their singing voice towards greater formal virtuosity. The combination of her insight into the artistic and technical process of singing and my ability to facilitate an authentic expression of emotion, sensation and experience provided the framework within which we continue to develop a working partnership. In response to the artistic as well as therapeutic results of our practice, reflected in the psychological and creative development of our students and clients, I developed the short courses which I had been teaching into a full professional training leading to the Royal Society of Arts Examinations Board Diploma in Voice Movement Therapy – which I now direct in London, UK and Boston, USA and on which both Jenni and Melanie are co-teachers.

In order to gain a more global perspective on the current state of vocal work, I undertook a lecture and workshop tour in 1995 – during which time I presented my work in Europe, Australia and the USA. It was during this time that I was honoured to have an opportunity to meet some of the major practitioners whose work I had both studied and admired. Among these senior pioneers was Penny Lewis, innovator in the field of dance movement therapy. Until meeting her and sharing with her some of my work, I was unaware that Penny was investigating the therapeutic application of movement, breath and sound. I remain extremely honoured to receive her support and encouragement. Another key practitioner whose work has inspired me is Shaun McNiff, a key initiator in the development of an integrated model of arts therapy and with whom I have also been honoured to share the complex struggle of what he calls the 'artist therapist' and to whom I am also grateful for support.

In England, meanwhile, Andrew Samuels, author and training analyst for the Society for Analytical Psychology, David Garfield-Davies, consultant laryngologist, and Jane Comins, speech and language therapist, have provided invaluable support and insight which has enabled original work to remain grounded in the existing professional arena.

The major focus of my work now is directing the professional training in Voice Movement Therapy. This course provides a thorough practical, experiential and technical education in an approach to Therapeutic Voicework which synthesises the physiological, artistic, psychological and educational aspects of vocal work in a single strategy. Because of its broad, but integrated, nature, it has attracted students from many backgrounds from all over the world – including Italy, France, Switzerland, Sweden, Germany, Hungary, Canada, USA and Brazil. Trainees include musicians or performing artists seeking to develop their vocal and compositional skills, psychotherapists seeking to incorporate vocal work into their strategy, speech and language therapists seeking an integrated and experiential model to compliment their allopathic training, freelance peripatetic group leaders who run workshops and offer sessional work for a variety of client groups, those seeking to offer Voice Movement Therapy to clients in one-to-one sessions and many others whose professional intention is unclear but who seek a personal vocational training which unites exploration of the self with the acquisition of technical skills.

The diverse student fraternity provides a particularly fertile environment and graduates utilise the work in very different ways. For example, some graduates practice Therapeutic Voicework, working with clients or patients in clinical institutions or in private one-to-one sessions; some engage in creative Therapeutic Voicework, devising performances and leading experiential workshops; some impart educational Therapeutic Voicework, offering vocal training in drama schools and in individual client practice; and others work in a way that combines a number of different models.

Although the designing and teaching of this course in many ways provided a culmination to my intentions, there was still a missing link for, on graduating from the training course, practitioners encounter many complex issues relating to the practice of Therapeutic Voicework for which they need and deserve further support and a sense of being part of a team. Therefore, I formed the *International Association for Voice Movement Therapy*, governed by a code of ethics and a constitution, to which qualified graduate practitioners of Voice Movement Therapy could belong. This Association is in its early days but provides an entirely necessary forum for supervision and investigation of Therapeutic Voicework practice.

In my search to develop a consolidated body of vocal work which meets a broad spectrum of predicaments, I was confronted with the need to synthesise the practical application of principles drawn from a range of disciplines including psychotherapy, massage, remedial voice training, stress management, singing, music, ethnomusicology and special needs education. It is the diverse spectrum of sources from which I have drawn, the way in which they can be synthesised and the methodological manner in which an integrated model of Therapeutic Voicework can be employed in a range of contexts that I impart to my trainees, which they, in turn, utilise in their work and which I shall attempt to explain in this book.

Notes

1   Newham, P. (1997) *The Prophet of Song: The Life and Work of Alfred Wolfsohn*. London: Tigers Eye.

2   Newham, P. (1997) *Shouting for Jericho: The Work of Paul Newham on the Human Voice*. London: Tigers Eye Press/Class Productions.

3   Newham, P. (1992) 'Jung and Alfred Wolfsohn: analytical psychology and the singing voice.' *Journal of Analytical Psychology,* 37, pp.323-336.

4   Newham, P. (1992) 'Singing and psyche: towards voice movement therapy'. *Voice: Journal of the British Voice Association.* 1, pp.75-102.

5   Newham, P. (1994) 'Voice movement therapy: towards an arts therapy for voice'. *Dramatherapy* 16, no. 2 & 3, pp. 28-33.

6   Newham, P. (1993) 'The singing cure: how voice movement therapy has evolved'. *Human Communication* 2, no. 2, February 1993 pp.6-8.

7   Newham, P. (1993) 'The psychology of voice and the founding of the Roy Hart Theatre'. *New Theatre Quarterly,* IX, no. 33, February 1993, pp.59-65.

8   Newham, P. (1993) *The Singing Cure: An Introduction to Voice Movement Therapy*. Boston: Shambhala.

Preface

The purpose of this book is to introduce the reader to a field of work which uses the non-verbal and sung sounds of the human voice as a means to investigate the self and generate creative activity. It is, to my knowledge, the first book to explain an integrated and holistic methodology for working with the voice which synthesises physiological, psychological and creative principles and strategies. It is also, I believe, the first book which attempts to acknowledge the vast breadth and diversity of work within the field of vocal expression as represented by the major pioneers and practitioners of the nineteenth and twentieth centuries who have, knowingly or not, provided the impetus for a new discipline which I have named 'Therapeutic Voicework' and from which I have distilled the components of a specific methodological approach to Therapeutic Voicework called Voice Movement Therapy.

In this book I have thus tried to explain the system of enquiry which I have forged and, at the same time, locate it in the historical and theoretical context of work initiated by many other practitioners and researchers who have contributed theory and technique to the process of working with the human voice. In so doing I have had extreme difficulty in finding a balance between offering practical insight into my own working methodology and giving due space to the acknowledgement of others. The present book has been composed from over fifteen years of research and has been the most difficult task I have attempted. Following the publication of my first book, *The Singing Cure*,[1] I was honoured to receive communication from many who had been inspired, including a number of leading clinicians, who suggested that I write further and in more detail about my practical approach. However, I have always been sceptical of books which speak of practice without being contextualised in preceding models of action and theory. At the same time, a massing together of diverse approaches to working with the voice from the annals of recorded history is of little use without an introduction to current technique. Thus in writing this book I attempted to combine both and unwittingly engaged myself in a daunting and relentless task.

Therefore, to those who feel there are relevant figures whom I have not honoured, or that I have seemingly passed off with a cursory gesture, as well as to those who feel I have included too much description of other approaches at the expense of explaining my own work, I apologise. I had only so much space and I have arranged that space to the best of my abilities, which have been surely tested by the process of writing. Readers who, having read this book, wish to gain more insight into the practical application of my work are referred to the three forthcoming volumes *The Therapeutic Use of Singing and Vocal Sound*, which will provide ample case study material and description of techniques.

Throughout this book my continuous thread of proposition is that although the history of vocal investigation in various delineated areas provides stimulus for a number of different ways of working with the voice, there is, nonetheless, an obvious lack of and need for an integrated and holistic approach to Therapeutic Voicework which synthesises theory and practice from multifarious sources into a single framework. Central to my research is an attempt to make a modest contribution to this dearth by introducing to teaching, therapeutic and artistic practice a systematic methodology of Therapeutic Voicework which I have founded. This book is part of that project and seeks to explain my research to the reader who is unfamiliar with it.

To begin, in Chapter 1, I describe clearly and concisely the physiology and mechanics of voice production and extract from this what I have found to be a reliable system of vocal analysis. In Chapter 2 I use this system as the basis to explore some of the key psychological elements which are expressed through the voice. In addition, I apply the system to an analysis of the voices of known singers. Having laid this foundation, I offer the reader a series of chapters which locate the use of vocal expression in distinct models of enquiry, delineated by the particular subject of each chapter. In Chapter 3, the first of these, I describe the application of Therapeutic Voicework within a developmental approach rooted in the infant experience of vocalisation, suited to investigating early personal experiences. In Chapter 4 I describe the use of non-verbal vocal sound within an instinctual model of Therapeutic Voicework suited to the exploration of deep feelings and experiences of a collective nature. In Chapter 5 I describe the work of those who have paid particular attention to the therapeutic relevance of non-verbal sounds within the discipline of psychoanalysis, founded by Sigmund Freud, and intimate a psychoanalytic approach to Therapeutic Voicework. In Chapter 6 I explore the way that certain principles of the psychoanalytic 'talking cure' can be applied to the act of singing, song-writing and the use of the singing lesson.

In addition, I show how the methodological approach to Therapeutic Voicework which I have developed can, through the singing lesson modality, provide the basis for a thorough vocal training for performers. In Chapter 7 I focus on the healing use of voice and singing in ancient indigenous practices and the way this use has been revived by those currently working as teachers, healers and workshop leaders. In Chapter 8 I explore the way non-verbal vocal expression has been investigated within the field of Analytical Psychology, as founded by Carl Jung, and intimate an archetypal approach to Therapeutic Voicework. In Chapter 9 I explore the rich history of vocal investigation within the field of theatre and drama, pointing out the performance-orientated nature of Therapeutic Voicework. In Chapter 10 I look for the fusion of psychological and artistic approaches to vocal expression within the fields of music therapy, dance movement therapy and dramatherapy. Then, in Chapter 11, I return to the physical and physiological nature of the voice and look at Therapeutic Voicework as a form of body work, focusing on the breathing process and the relationship between vocal and physical expression. That completes the series of chapters on delineated models for Therapeutic Voicework.

Throughout Chapters 3 to 11 I concisely describe units of the methodology of Therapeutic Voicework which I have developed and which is taught on the training programme leading to the RSA Diploma in Voice Movement Therapy, the first and only acredited training in a holistic and integrated approach to Therapeutic Voicework which I designed and which I direct. These descriptions are thereby interwoven with historical and theoretical precedents for my work. In addition, at the end of each of these chapters I provide a case study from my own Therapeutic Voicework client practice which in some way relates to the field elucidated by the focus of the chapter. I am grateful to my clients for permission to publish these cases. However, names and some events have been changed to maintain certain confidentiality.

Finally, in Chapter 12 I outline some of the complex contentions which emanate from the integrated and multifaceted paradigm which I have called Therapeutic Voicework, investigating the relationship between art, science, mind and body within the process as well as analysing the relationship between subjectivity and objectivity within the working strategy. In the first of the Appendices, 'Ethics and Guidelines', I briefly outline some of the ethical and logistic issues pertinent to the practice of Therapeutic Voicework.

I have created a number of audio visual resources which provide further insight into the methodology of Voice Movement Therapy, its technique and its application, which though produced independently of Jessica Kingsley Publishers, provide useful compliments to this book by bringing the practical side of work alive through the medium of the voice – something which is obviously difficult to achieve through the written word. First, a video film, *Shouting for Jericho: The Work of Paul Newham on the Human Voice*,[1] combines video stroboscopic analysis of my working larynx and vocal folds during the utilisation of the techniques described in this book with interviews, demonstration of client work and extracts from vocal presentations. Second, a set of audio cassettes, *The Singing Cure: Liberating Self Expression through Voice Movement Therapy*,[2] which offers a systematic introduction to the sound of each vocal component of vocal expression and their various combinations as outlined in this book. Finally, on the CD, *Prayers and Prophecies*,[3] I sing a series of original compositions which demonstrate the use of Voice Movement Therapy techniques to reflect the transformative journey of the psyche through a series of original compositions, sung with the extended vocal range which arises from the use of such techniques.

Information on how to obtain these and other available supporting resources, a training prospectus for the Diploma in Voice Movement Therapy and a list of qualified practitioners offering one-to-one work is included in Appendix 3: 'Further Information'.

Throughout the book the therapist has been given a male gender, and the client a female gender, to reduce possible confusion. This is simply a means of clarifying the text, and no adverse conclusions should be drawn from it.

Notes

1   Newham, P. (1997) *Shouting for Jericho: The Work of Paul Newham on the Human Voice*. London: Tigers Eye Press/Class Productions.

2   Newham, P. (1998) *The Singing Cure: Liberating Self Expression through Voice Movement Therapy*. Boulder: Sounds True.

3   Newham, P. (1997) *Prayers and Prophecies*. London: Tigers Eye Press.

On Voice and Voicework

The human voice is a primary medium of communication in human beings. It is an expression of who we are and how we feel. In the timbre of a person's voice you can hear the subtle music of feeling and thought. The ever shifting collage of emotions which we experience infiltrate the voice with tones of happiness, excitement, depression and grief. The human voice is also one way in which we preserve our identity and the voice and the psychological state of an individual mutually influence each other. The physical condition of the body is also reflected in the vitality of vocal expression: illness, physical debilitation and habitual muscular patterns all take their toll on the way we sound.

The voice is both an expression of psychological state, a physiological operation and the means by which a person asserts his or her rights within the social order. But many people find themselves negatively affected by psychological dynamics such as stress, anxiety and depression, by physical factors resulting from congenital conditions, illness, injury or bodily misuse and by socially enforced inhibitions. If these effects continue unabated, they often begin to reduce the agility and vitality of body and voice and thereby deplete the capacity for unencumbered expression.

Because the voice is composed of such a complex set of dimensions, the condition of vocal inhibition, restraint or depleted function – from which so many people suffer – leads to an expressive impairment on a psychological, physiological and social level. To reverse the process and revive vocal function, therefore, necessitates attention to both psychological, physical and social processes. Providing these processes are properly understood, working with the voice can be an enlivening way of helping people overcome difficulties which hinder the acoustic and kinetic expression of the Self. Such work may be called 'Voicework'.

Voicework may, perhaps, best be described as a generic term which includes any work with or on the voice. Within this definition a singing teacher could be said to practise Voicework in developing the vocal skills of her pupils; a bereavement counsellor could be said to practise Voicework in helping a client feel safe and comfortable in giving voice to grief; a speech and language therapist conducts Voicework in helping a patient to be relieved of pathological conditions which threaten the health of the voice; a choir leader may be said to practise Voicework in enabling a mass of disparate voices to synthesise into a harmonious whole; a gestalt psychotherapist may draw upon Voicework in assisting a client to give vent to rage through shouts and yells; a repétiteur conducts Voicework when helping an anxious opera singer with the task of sustaining the demands of the music whilst articulating the poetic text; a music therapist uses Voicework when helping a young child create a song from a simple rhyme; a priest employs Voicework when using the tonal contours of his voice to communicate to the congregation; a politician uses Voicework when deliberately employing specific vocal timbres to convince and persuade.

All of these people are using the voice as a channel through which to express or 'push out' something from the inside; the voice is indeed a major bridge between the inner world of mood, emotion, image, thought and experience and the outer world of relationship, discourse and interaction.

Because the voice is so intimately connected to the expression of feelings and ideas and is a primary channel through which we communicate who we are, Voicework is innately therapeutic. However, it has been said with a tone of healthy cynicism that 'it would be hard to think of an approach to human life' that has not been called 'therapeutic'.[1] Yet a properly researched introduction to an integrated approach to Voicework which acknowledges this therapeutic dimension and draws on the rich and diverse history of vocal investigation is still seriously lacking and it is such a dearth to which this book seeks to respond.

A sign of the growing interest in the use of singing and non-verbal vocal expression as a means to explore the Self is the inclusion of a chapter on the subject in the 1994 handbook of *Innovative Therapy in Britain* written by Melinda Moore Meigs.[2] In fact, Meigs was, perhaps, the first to identify Voicework as a specific dimension to the healing use of sound and music in the UK.[3]

Meigs defines Voicework as a process of 'using the medium of your voice to find and develop aspects of yourself which may be new to you and to understand what these aspects mean for you'. Meigs says that the term 'Voicework' is used 'to cover singing, overtone chanting, improvisation, breathing techniques, bodywork, visualisation and ear training when they are used to expand the expressive range of your voice and, through this, to explore your Self'. This, she says, 'involves a search for emotional understanding and integration'.[4] In my view, such an exploration of the Self through the voice turns Voicework into Therapeutic Voicework.

However, the term 'Therapeutic Voicework' is not synonymous with 'voice therapy'. Voice therapy denotes a clinical allopathic field of work conducted by 'voice therapists', that is speech and language therapists who alleviate a wide range of disorders, some of whom specialise in voice problems. Though such practitioners approach the voice as a somatic phenomenon, increasing numbers of speech and language therapists are beginning to incorporate attendance to the influence of emotional and psychological factors upon the voice. In addition, medical doctors who have specialised in ear, nose and throat dysfunction and disease (ENT consultants) with a special focus on laryngological problems may provide treatment which has a therapeutic effect on the voice as well as giving advice with regard to care of the voice; but such clinicians do not call themselves voice therapists or name their work voice therapy.

Although, strictly speaking, the term 'voice therapy' designates the aforementioned field within speech and language therapy, in recent years an increasing number of people working in the broad area of 'complementary', 'alternative' or 'holistic' medicine have utilised the term 'voice therapy' to denote the process by which vocalisation through speech, song and non-verbal sound is used as a means through which to express and explore aspects of the psyche. These practitioners utilise the term 'therapy' for its psychic rather than its somatic implication, inviting comparison with the work of psychotherapists rather than speech and language therapists or ENT consultants. However, few of these practitioners are trained in psychotherapy or counselling – which adds further confusion to the vernacular meaning and signification of the term 'voice therapy'. There are also many artistic practitioners, some of long-standing excellence, particularly within the field of the theatre, who describe their teaching as being, in part, a therapy. This invites the work of theatre practitioners who impart or facilitate vocal work, such as directors, actors and workshop leaders, to be compared to that of a dramatherapist. Yet few of these artists are trained or qualified in dramatherapy. There are also many individuals working in community centres with so-called handicapped children, in mental health wings of hospitals, in special schools and in the voluntary sector who are helping others towards positive change. Those who utilise vocal expression as part of their approach may be understandably perceived as disseminating 'voice therapy', yet few of these people have a therapeutic training or qualification.

The widespread use of the word 'therapy' is, therefore, beginning to denote a broad style of work and a particular kind of outcome rather than identifying someone who is trained and qualified in a therapeutic discipline. Furthermore, the word 'therapy', particularly in the current political climate is subject to so much scrutiny and currently designates such a broad field that it is, for many, time to consider carefully the variety of meanings which the term has.

One useful precept is to conceive of therapy as involving the alleviation of pathology. Voice therapy would, therefore, involve attendance to vocal pathology. A modality which is therapeutic in outcome rather than a form of therapy, meanwhile, may have results which assist in improving the condition of the mind or body but does not aim to heal pathology. Whilst medical practitioners and speech and language therapists heal physical pathology with some attendance to psychogenic factors, there is no existing professional practitioner whose role is the exclusive and singular investigation of the psychological influences upon vocal expression.

My assertion is that Voicework can most certainly be therapeutic. Moreover, its therapeutic effects can be somatic as well as psychological. This does not, however, necessarily make a Therapeutic Voicework practitioner a therapist – which depends on the breadth and nature of his or her training and qualification – for a Therapeutic Voiceworker may be concerned with developing the health of the voice, not with ministering to pathology. Of course, there is a thin and ever movable line between alleviating pathology and facilitating the development of health; illness is spectral and exists by degrees.

In my view, Therapeutic Voicework can help people whose expressive activity has been detrimentally influenced by emotional problems, trauma and mental illness, those whose lives have been turned around by the effects of severe injury or the development of diseases such as Multiple Sclerosis, those with congenital conditions such as Cerebral Palsy and Down's Syndrome and those who have been discouraged from asserting or expressing themselves by overpowering and infertile environmental influences. In addition, Therapeutic Voicework can respond to the needs of those whose social or professional predicament places exceptional demands upon the voice and who often find themselves ill equipped to preserve the health and longevity of their vocal instrument and therefore require education and rehabilitation. No less important are those who, whilst healthy and not overtly impeded, can nonetheless discover an increased potential for expression and creativity through singing and sound making.

If not conducted with skill and expertise, Therapeutic Voicework can also be threatening to the health of mind and body and there are some people for whom Therapeutic Voicework may not be expedient to the maintenance of health no matter how proficient the practitioner. Consequently, someone practising Therapeutic Voicework needs to be competent in understanding the psychophysical nature of vocal expression and, in addition, must learn to recognise those for whom Therapeutic Voicework is an inappropriate medium through which to work for physical or psychological reasons.

In my view, someone who utilises Therapeutic Voicework should be trained and practitioners who graduate from the RSA professional training in Voice Movement Therapy and join the International Association for Voice Movement Therapy facilitate vocal development in a vast range of clients.

All students of the professional training which I direct undergo a thorough physical and psychological journey in order to facilitate the same in others. In addition, all trainees study both creative, allopathic and psychological models of intervention and analysis. They are thereby trained to be Therapeutic Voiceworkers who can deal effectively with the psychological and physical aspects of vocal expression and who, in suspecting serious pathology of mind or body, will refer the client to an appropriate trained and qualified practitioner.

Although, as Meigs points out, the term 'Voicework', and perhaps I might add the term 'Therapeutic Voicework', is generic and covers a broad field of investigation, the approach to working with the voice which I have developed consists of a specific systematic synthesis of a number of creative, psychological and physical components to form a methodology which can be disseminated and applied in a number of contexts.

The approach to Therapeutic Voicework which I have developed and which I have named Voice Movement Therapy can be conducted with individuals and with groups. The clients begin by making their most effortless natural sound whilst the acoustic tones of the voice and the muscle tone of the body are heard and observed. In response to an informed analysis of breathing, sound and movement, the practitioner massages and manipulates the client's body, gives instruction in ways of moving and suggests moods and images which the client allows to effect and infiltrate the vocal timbre. The voice is thereby sculptured and animated through a graphic and authentic expression of the Self. In order to facilitate this process, the Voice Movement Therapy practitioner also offers pedagogic technical training by which the voice develops in range and malleability. This helps the client find access to sounds which give expression to hitherto dormant aspects of the Self. The result of such Therapeutic Voicework is psychologically uplifting, physically invigorating, creatively rejuvenating and serves to release vocal function from constriction.

In this book I will introduce the reader to the historical background, the practical application, the underlying principles and case study examples of this work. In so doing I hope that it will inspire ideas, consolidate intuitions and inform thoughts. Moreover, I hope it will draw attention to the profound power of the human voice to move, stimulate, uncover, express and, perhaps, to heal.

Voice Movement Therapy is a specific approach to the general field of Therapeutic Voicework; it is a new discipline and seeks to occupy a collaborative and co-operative relationship with other serious approaches to vocal therapeutics. However, throughout the book, I rarely refer to the term Voice Movement Therapy but frequently speak of Therapeutic Voicework. My reason for this is that, although one purpose of this book is to introduce the reader to the specific methodological approach which I am developing, my deeper intention is to locate my own inquiry in the broader field of Therapeutic Voicework in the hope that those outside the specific modality of Voice Movement Therapy might find aspects of my research and practice useful and applicable within their own paradigm. When introducing a particular exercise or strategy, I therefore refer to 'Therapeutic Voicework Methodology'. By avoiding a zealous and repetitive reference to Voice Movement Therapy, I hope that the book will maintain as its primary focus the general field of Therapeutic Voicework, acknowledge the rich diversity of this area and avoid claiming a grandiose position for the specific contribution which I seek to make to this field through the practice of Voice Movement Therapy.

Notes

1   Kovel, J. (1991) *A Complete Guide to Therapy: From Psychoanalysis to Behaviour Modification.* London: Penguin p.215.

2   Moore Meigs, M. (1994) 'Therapeutic Voicework.' In David Jones (ed) *Innovative Therapy: A Handbook*. Buckingham: Open University Press, pp.174–188.

3   Moore Meigs, M. (1992) 'Therapeutic Voicework.' *Self and Society*, XX, 1, pp.18–19.

4   Moore Meigs, M. (1994) 'Therapeutic Voicework.' In David Jones (ed) *Innovative Therapy: A Handbook*. Buckingham: Open University Press, pp.174–188.

CHAPTER I

Vocal Function and Structure
Physiological Basis for a Systematic Methodology of Therapeutic Voicework

Introduction: To Begin with Mechanics

Most readers of this book will, I assume, be eager and excited to gain some insight into the way the human voice reveals, disguises, sublimates and presents the subtle and awesome contours of the inner self, psyche or soul and it is my wish that such readers will be satisfied as far as my knowledge and experience can provide. However, one of the reasons that a practicable model for Therapeutic Voicework is so lacking in contemporary therapeutic and educational practice is that such a modality implicitly and necessarily begs for a fundamental understanding of the plain mechanical principles of voice production which, at one level, are composed not of psyche but of soma; the voice may be an emissary for the intangible fabric of feeling and thought but it is also a vehicle made of muscle, blood, tissue and bone.

Consequently, in order to comprehend my presentation in this book of the way in which the voice may be a window to the soul, the reader will require a rudimentary sense of the physiological, anatomical and acoustic principles of voice production. Naturally, this is a complex subject and it will be my intention to make the processes by which the voice works accessible without allowing simplification to merge with inaccuracy. Because the information presented in this chapter is a simplification of complexity aimed at those with a creative and psychotherapeutic interest or background, the reader is referred to the currently available seminal texts on the science of voice function, singing and musical sound for more sophisticated insight. These include detailed yet readable scientific explanations by Bunch[1], Sundberg,[2] Appleman,[3] Miller,[4] Pierce,[5] Fry[6] and Ladefoged.[7]

Unlike the writers of these aforementioned texts, I shall attempt only to provide a modest level of physiological and acoustic understanding with the aim of making plain and apparent the various components or parameters which subtly weave together to produce that complex and often unfathomable fabric which is the sound of the human voice. I will then present a system of components which are present in each person's voice and provide the platform upon which to build a viable model of therapeutic, creative and pedagogic Voicework.

The Internal Terrain of Tubes

The internal terrain of the human body is composed of an array of tubes or cylinders: cylindrical or tubular veins and arteries which transport blood, tubular intestines which transport digested food matter and tubular nerves which transport neurochemical liquids.[8]

At various junctures this complex network of cylinders distends and swells up into curved and curvilinear, semi-spherical organs such as the heart, the stomach and the womb. The result is an inner maze with outlets at the base and top of the body (Figure 1.1).

The infant experiences the inner somatic landscape as such a set of tubes which connect with the outside world and our early life is consumed with learning to control what enters in and what passes out of these tubes.

One of these tubes or cylinders of crucial importance to our study is that which begins at the lips and through the nostrils and nasal passages before branching into a labyrinth of conduits, ducts and channels which permeate into the lungs. When we breathe in, air passes through the lips and along this continuous tube or cylinder – which, for convenience, may be divided into named sections consisting of the mouth, the pharynx, the oro-pharynx, the larynx and the trachea. Here it branches into two separate tubes known as the bronchi, each of which enters a lung. When we breathe out, air passes from the lungs and along the same passage in the opposite direction. This tubular passage of cylinders through which air passes is generally referred to as the respiratory tract (Figure 1.2).

When we eat, the food substance which we ingest shares the same tube or passage as inspired and expired air for the first part of its journey, passing through mouth and pharynx, but taking a different route down through the oesophagus into the stomach. The direction of food away from the trachea and into the oesophagus, and the direction of air away from the oesophagus into the trachea, is controlled by a flap of tissue called the epiglottis, which

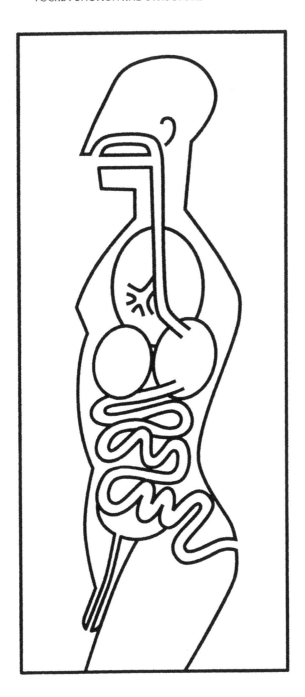

Figure 1.1

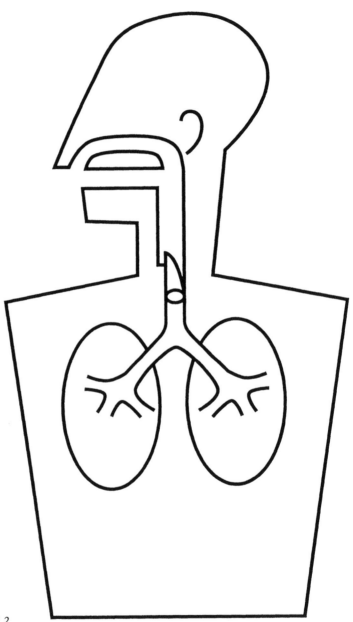

Figure 1.2

descends like a cover or trap door over the top of the trachea when we swallow food. The tubular passage of cylinders through which food substances pass towards the stomach is generally referred to as the digestive tract. The network of cylindrical pathways which further carry digested and semi-digested substances through the intestines of the abdominal cavity and expel feacal matter through the anal orifice is generally referred to as the gastrointestinal tract.

Because both eating and breathing are core elementary experiences and processes, the first portions of this tube which host the passage of both breath and food is the locus for a pantheon of psychosomatic phenomena. This is further compounded and intensified by the fact that vocal sound is also emitted through this tube – in relation to which it is called the vocal tract.

The initial sound which emerges from the lips as a vocal signal is made by the vibration of the vocal cords, more appropriately called the vocal folds, which are housed by the larynx and which create a sound-wave out of the air particles expelled from the lungs during expiration which is then amplified by the pharynx, oro-pharynx and mouth through which the wave passes. The sound-wave of air particles does not exit completely from the mouth; some air in breathing and in vocalisation passes up above the roof of the mouth and through the nasal passages, finding an outlet through the nose.

The Voice Tube

The vocal tract begins at the lips, runs more or less horizontally to form the mouth, or oral cavity, curves downwards and narrows slightly to become the oro-pharynx, then curves to a further degree and opens out again forming the pharynx, at which point, if the head is facing forwards, the tube is now almost at right angles to where it begins at the lips. Below the pharynx the tube hosts a cylindrical segment known as the larynx (Figure 1.3).

The Vocal Folds

Lying stretched out in the larynx are two flaps of tissue called the vocal folds. At the front they are attached to the Adam's apple or thyroid cartilage and at the back they are connected to two movable cartilages called the arytenoids.

These two pieces of tissue are further attached to the trachea and the surrounding inner walls of the larynx by a complex set of muscles known collectively as the intrinsic laryngeal musculature. During normal breathing the vocal folds lie at rest, one each side of the larynx, like an open pair of

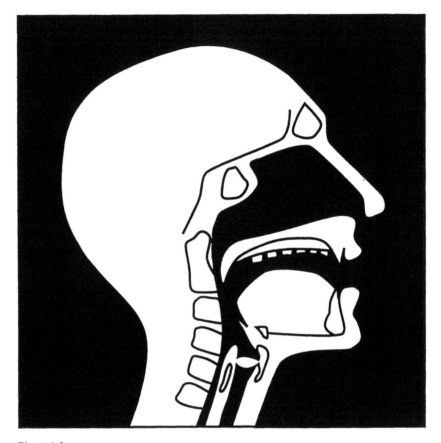

Figure 1.3

curtains allowing air to pass freely through a window. The hole between the vocal folds through which air passes is called the glottis (Figure 1.4a).

However, adjustments in the distribution of tension in the laryngeal musculature can cause the vocal folds to close, preventing air from entering or leaving the trachea, like a thick pair of curtains drawn tightly shut across a window (Figure 1.4b).

The sound of the human voice is generated by the rapid and successive opening and closing of the vocal folds hundreds of times per second and it is to this process that people refer when they speak of the vibration of the vocal folds. The opening of the folds is called abduction and the closing is called adduction.

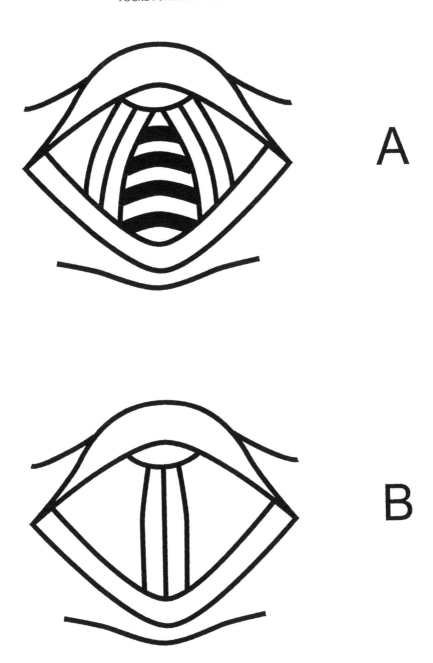

A

B

Figure 1.4

This rapid abduction and adduction of the vocal folds causes the expelled air from the lungs to be released through the glottis in a series of infinitesimal puffs which create a wave which, between certain frequencies or vibrational cycles, is heard as the sound of the human voice. This process is called phonation.

One of the criteria for a wave of air to be heard as an acoustic sound is that the constituting air puffs must be released at a rate of between approximately 20 per second and 20,000 per second. This means that the vocal folds must be opening and closing, or phonating, between 20 and 20,000 times per second. Naturally, the ear can hear a wider range than the voice can sing and the vocal folds cannot vibrate as slowly or as fast as the extremes of this range. Singing the lowest C on the piano would require the vocal folds to phonate about 32 times per second and singing the highest C on the piano would demand them to phonate around 4,186 times per second. There is no one who can do either. As a useful point of reference, singing middle C on the piano requires vocal fold phonation to be at a frequency of about 263 times per second.

The puffs of air released through the glottis create a push and shove, or compression and rarefaction. The folds open and the pressure of the released breath causes air molecules to compress, pushing into one another in the manner of a domino effect so that the molecules next to the ear drum push the thin membrane in. Then the folds close, the pressure is depleted and the compressed air molecules fall back, or rarefy, such that the molecules next to the ear drum ease off and allow the thin membrane to bend outwards (Figure 1.5).

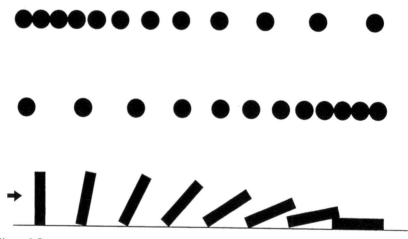

Figure 1.5

When this happens at high speeds, the rapid vibrational in and out movement of the ear drum registers a sound. Indeed, any vibrating object is capable of effecting the ear drum in this way so long as it vibrates between 20 and 20,000 times per second and providing that the pressure of the air is great enough to move the ear drum so that the sound is loud enough to be heard. Waves caused by extremely low frequencies generally cannot be heard and those which are extremely high may actually be painful.

To picture the process of air compression and rarefaction as caused by vocal fold vibration or phonation, it might be helpful to imagine a contraption which we will call the air puff machine (Figure 1.6).

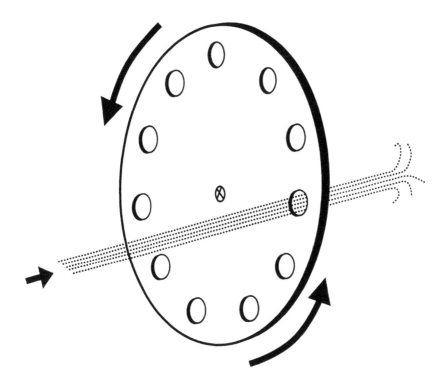

Figure 1.6

First, there is a jet of air – this compares to the airstream released from a pair of lungs. The air molecules which are released under pressure then meet a plate with holes drilled in it which is spinning on a metal rod. When the air hits the solid metal between the holes it can not pass through; when the airflow is level with a hole in the metal plate it passes through to the other side. This compares to the air molecules travelling from the lungs and meeting the larynx. When the vocal folds are closed, as in Figure 1.4b, they cannot pass through; when they are open, as in Figure 1.4a, they can.

If the plate is kept spinning at a constant speed, the airstream is released through the plate in a series of puffs. If the speed of the plate is very slow, we do not register a pitch. However, if the rotational speed of the plate is increased, so long as the jet of air is travelling with enough force to create necessary loudness, we hear a sound which is higher in pitch the faster the plate is rotated. Once a certain speed is reached, the air-wave would pass beyond and above the threshold of hearing and, if loud enough, may actually be hurtful. The air puff machine thereby creates a sound-wave composed of a string of air molecules and produces a pitch in a manner comparable to the way that sound is created by the puffs of air released through the glottis between the vocal folds.

Because the vocal folds are attached front and back to the thyroid and arytenoid cartilages, which are in turn connected to muscle tissue, they can be stretched out by tensile adjustment in the laryngeal musculature making them longer, thinner and more tense. When this happens, like all elastic objects which are tightened, they vibrate at a higher frequency so that, consequently, an increased number of air puffs are released per second, causing the domino effect or compression and rarefaction to occur with greater speed. This makes the ear drum vibrate more quickly, which, therefore, registers a higher sound or pitch. Conversely, an alternative adjustment of the laryngeal musculature causes the vocal folds to slacken, so that they become shorter, thicker and more lax. When this happens, like all elastic objects which are relaxed, they vibrate at a lower frequency and release less puffs of air per second. Consequently, we hear the sound of the voice as being deeper in pitch.

In establishing a component system of intuitive vocal analysis, the first physiologically-generated component parameter of perceivable acoustic sound which we can identify as being present in a person's voice is, therefore, the pitch – also referred to as the note or the tone.

COMPONENT ONE: PITCH

Each vocal sound is perceived to have a certain pitch, note or fundamental tone determined by the frequency of vocal fold vibration or phonation. This is perceived within the metaphor of high to low, though, in fact, does not relate to spatial dimensions but to speed of vibration in time.

Interval, Pitch Fluctuation and Vibrato

During phonation, the vocal folds may not remain absolutely constant in their speed of vibration or phonation over a given time. For example, they may phonate at 440 times per second for three-quarters of a second and then phonate at 445 times per second for a further half of a second.

There are two components to this pitch fluctuation: interval distance and time. Interval distance is the magnitude of the pitch jump. For example, a voice which jumps from a vibrational frequency of 440 to 450 times per second makes only a tiny pitch jump from the A above middle C on a piano to a sound not even high enough to sound the B flat above it. Meanwhile, a voice which jumps from 440 to 493 times per second makes an interval jump equivalent to going from the A above middle C on the piano to the B above it. The term 'interval' thereby denotes the size of the frequency jump between two specific notes or pitches.

The next factor, time, is the speed with which the jumps are made. A very slow alternation between 440 times per second – which is the A above middle C on the piano – and 450 times per second – which does not have a note on the piano – may well sound 'out of tune' to a listener. But if the same inconsistency is quickened, it may sound like a very professional singing voice. Indeed, very fast alternations in vocal fold vibration over a very small pitch interval constitutes what is known as vibrato, that deliberate flutter which is heard in the classical European voice. If a singer produces such pitch fluctuations too slowly, or takes them across too great a pitch interval, the skill of the vibrato turns into what we hear as untuneful singing.

The second vocal component parameter which we can identify within the human voice then is pitch fluctuation, which, under certain conditions, would be referred to as vibrato and, under others, may be called inconsistency or untunefulness. Furthermore, each culture uses different intervals and permits different degrees of fluctuation, within different time parameters.

COMPONENT TWO: PITCH FLUCTUATION

The pitch of the voice sustains more or less constancy or fluctuation in a given time across a given range of tones, often called vibrato and sometimes perceived as an inability to remain attuned. This is determined by the shifting frequencies of vocal fold phonation.

Frequency

In order to picture more clearly the relationship between tension and speed of vibration, imagine a piece of string stretched taught between two

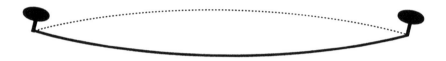

Figure 1.7

stationary pins. If you take hold of the piece of string at its centre and pluck it, the string will vibrate from side to side, passing through its rest position many times before coming to rest again (Figure 1.7).

Now, if we made a slow motion film of this action, we would discover that the string makes a definite number of side-to-side vibrations per second. This number is called the string's fundamental frequency and is measured in Cycles Per Second (c.p.s.) or Hertz (Hz). It is the frequency of vibration that determines the musical note or pitch that an object gives off. The same holds true for the human voice. The amount of times that the vocal folds adduct and abduct or phonate per second is called the frequency of vibration or the frequency of phonatory cycles, and this determines the musical pitch that the voice emits. The lower the frequency the deeper the pitch.

To clarify this it may be useful to return to the air puff machine and imagine that the plate, which has 11 holes, spins at 40 c.p.s. (see Figure 1.6). It will, consequently, release 440 puffs of air per second. A person blessed with optimal hearing will, therefore, hear the pitch designated as the A above middle C. If, however, we were to speed it up so that it spins at 80 c.p.s., it would release 880 puffs of air per second and we would hear the note A an octave higher for doubling frequency is equal to jumping or transposing upwards by one octave.

Loudness

If we were to leave the plate of the air puff machine spinning at 40 c.p.s. but increase the pressure or force with which the air was directed towards the plate, the resulting pitch would remain constant but the sound would be louder. This compares to the function of the human voice, which gets louder when we use the contractile power of the torso's musculature and the compressive force of the diaphragm to increase the pressure of the air expelled from the lungs. Increased force of muscle contraction creates an increase in sub-glottal air pressure, that is the amount of force with which air expelled from the lungs presses against the adducted vocal folds. When the folds open during phonation, the puffs of damned up air are released under greater pressure which, when the wave which they create hits the ear drum, creates more intense or louder sounds than waves stimulated by puffs of vibrating air under low pressure.

The third vocal component parameter which we can identify in a human voice then is loudness, often equated with what physicists call intensity and which results from increased air pressure.

COMPONENT THREE: LOUDNESS

The sound of the voice is perceived on a spectrum from loud to quiet, determined primarily by the pressure of breath released from the lungs.

Force of Vocal Fold Adduction

Increased pressure of breath expelled from the lungs draws the vocal folds together with a greater force, causing them to hit each other with higher impact. Decreased air pressure, meanwhile, draws the folds together with less force, causing them to hit each other with low impact. The impact with which the vocal folds come together, or adduct, during vocalisation is, therefore, partly determined by the sub-glottal air pressure – which also governs the loudness of the voice. However, the impact with which the vocal folds adduct is to some degree independent of the pressure of the emitted breath and determines an acoustic quality which, though it can often be mistaken for loudness, is, in fact, a different dimension. This quality is referred to as glottal attack.

Because the sub-glottal air pressure is a primary contributory factor to the impact of vocal fold adduction, both glottal attack and loudness are intimately related and an increase in sub-glottal air pressure often yields an increased impact of adduction. We witness this concept when watching or listening to a pair of drawn curtains flap together during a high wind. As the pressure of the wind against the curtains increases, so they flap together with greater impact, giving off a louder sound. Conversely, as the wind dies down, the curtains hit one another more gently, making the sound softer. However, unlike the curtains, the vocal folds are not only reliant upon the wind from the lungs for their movement as they are connected to muscles which are fed by nerves. It is, therefore, possible to vary the impact of vocal fold adduction without major changes in air pressure by increasing and decreasing vocal fold impact and creating sounds with varying degrees of glottal attack whilst maintaining a constant loudness.

The fourth component parameter of vocal sound which we can identify is, therefore, glottal attack, determined by the impact of vocal fold adduction.

COMPONENT FOUR: GLOTTAL ATTACK

The voice is perceived as having greater or lesser attack determined by the impact under which the vocal folds come together or adduct during phonation.

Tension and Mass

To further understand the nature of voice production it will be useful to again imagine a piece of string attached at both ends to two stationary pins.

If we wanted the string to vibrate faster, thereby sounding a higher pitch, we could achieve this by tightening and stretching the string. If, conversely, we wanted the string to sound a deeper pitch, we would loosen it, causing it to become lax and thus vibrate at a lower fundamental frequency. However, we could also change the frequency and pitch of the string by altering its mass.

A thick, dense string made of ten grams of fibre will vibrate at a slower frequency and, therefore, give off a lower pitch to the ear than a thin string made of only five grams of fibre even when both are stretched to the same degree, that is under the same tension. This principle applies also to the human voice. Someone with thick dense vocal folds will tend to speak within a lower pitch range than someone with thinner, lighter folds. Moreover, a person with thick dense folds will have to stretch them and place them under much greater tension to achieve a frequency of 440 c.p.s., producing the pitch A just above middle C, than a person with thinner lighter folds.

The guitar acts as a useful metaphor. To get a high pitch from the thin tight string, usually made of nylon or gut, closest to the player's lap on a guitar does not require it to be tightened a great amount because it is so thin and has a small mass. To get an equally high pitch from the thickest guitar string, usually over-woven with metal, furthest away from the player's lap, however, would require much greater tightening because, by comparison, it is so thick and dense and has greater mass. The same piece of ten gram string will vibrate at a higher frequency the tighter it is stretched and a twenty gram piece of string will have to be stretched and tightened more than a ten gram piece of string to achieve the same frequency.

This relationship between mass, fundamental frequency and pitch is pertinent to the vocal folds and is best illustrated by the pitch range difference between men and women. The morphology of the male body is such that tissue structures like the vocal folds are thicker, heavier and more dense than women's whilst, conversely, much of the tissue of women's bodies has less mass than men's. Consequently, for a man to sing as high as a woman, the natural tendency is to stretch and tense the vocal folds to a much greater extent than is necessary for a female. By the same token, the thick, dense vocal folds of men yield more easily to slow fundamental frequencies which produce low notes than do the thin, less dense folds of women which yield more easily to the production of higher notes. However, the vocal folds of both men and women do not, like a guitar string, maintain constant mass but, as a result of complex chemical and physical changes deep inside the constituting tissue, alter their density and thickness with resulting alterations in pitch.

Length

To return to a string, the frequency of vibration – and, therefore, the pitch – is also determined by its length. A piece of string will vibrate faster the shorter it is made. This concept is observable on a guitar when we move a finger up and down the frets, lengthening and shortening the vibrating portion of the string and producing lower and higher notes respectively. The same principle is used in voice production in that one way of creating faster fundamental frequencies of phonation and sounding higher notes, rather than stretching and tensing the entire length of the vocal folds or decreasing the mass of the constituting tissue, is to hold a portion of the fold's length squeezed shut, or adducted, and allow only a short portion to phonate.

In Figure 1.8a. the entire length of the vocal folds is phonating, producing, let us imagine, a fundamental frequency of 110 c.p.s. and thus sounding the A one octave and a half below middle C.

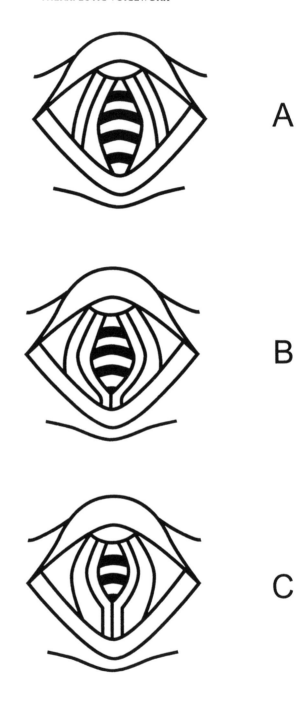

Figure 1.8

In Figure 1.8b. a small portion of the vocal folds is kept pushed together during phonation whilst the remaining lengths phonate. This would produce a higher note if all other factors were kept constant, let us say Middle C with the folds vibrating at 263 c.p.s.

Finally, in Figure 1.8c. only a little more than half of the folds are phonating, which, using the principle of a shorter string vibrating more quickly, produces a faster frequency and sounds a higher note, let us say 880 c.p.s. sounding the A an octave and a half above middle C.

The lengthening and shortening of the phonating portion of the vocal folds, which is initiated in order to assist in changes of fundamental frequency and consequent pitch, inevitably alters the shape and size of the glottis, which is created between the folds and through which the air puffs escape, as we can see from Figure 1.8. To understand more completely the mechanics of voice production it is necessary to realise that this change in glottic size and shape also effects the quality of the voice , that is, not its pitch but its timbre.

Glottic Size and Shape

Changing the size of the glottis is comparable to changing the size of the holes in the metal plate of the air puff machine. Let us imagine again that the jet of air is directed towards the plate under a consistent pressure and that the plate spins at 40 c.p.s. so that a listener hears the note A just above middle C. Then, imagine that a person swiftly replaces the spinning plate with one that is absolutely identical, and spinning at exactly the same speed, except that the holes in the plate are a different size and shape. The listener, as a result of this exchange, would still hear the same pitch of A but it would have a different quality or timbre.

Timbre denotes the particular properties which a sound has independent of the pitch and we very often use imagistic and metaphorical words rather than acoustic terms to describe timbre. For example, we may say that the timbre of a flute is 'brighter' compared to the 'darker' sound of a clarinet; we may say that a voice sounds 'bitter' or 'sweet', 'twangy' or 'wispy'. To utilise such metaphorical language we might say that one of the aspects of timbre is its 'airiness'. A pipe organ, for example, sounds more airy than a piano. With regard to the human voice, we may be more likely to use the word 'breathy' than 'airy' but we would be referring to the same dimension of a sound.

This airiness would be one of the timbral aspects we could expect to change if the original air puff machine was replaced for one with larger holes.

Providing the speed was kept constant, the pitch would remain that of A but the sound would sound more airy. This compares to one of the effects resulting from an increased glottis size. The larger the glottis, the more air passes out per opening and, often, the more 'breathy' the sound will be.

To produce a sound from the second large-holed air puff machine would actually require a larger quantity of air as more would be escaping through the large holes, causing the puffs to be bigger. This principle applies also to the human voice in that the more breath released per glottal opening the more quickly the lungs' contents empty and the more rapidly they need to be replenished. This passage of air is called transglottal airflow and the higher the transglottal airflow the more breathy the timbre. But there is another way of increasing the transglottal airflow in addition to enlarging the size of the glottis.

To understand the second way that breathiness can be manufactured it is necessary to understand that there are two ways of causing the vocal folds to phonate at a given frequency. One is where the folds have their rest moment when they are open and another is when they rest while closed. One can experience this through clapping hands together, say 25 times per minute, first so that the hands remain closed between claps and second where they are held open between claps.

Returning from hands to vocal folds, one of the major differences in voice production between these two methods of phonation is that if the vocal folds rest during their open phase, the sound of the audible contact between the folds can resonate in the spaces below the glottis, such as the trachea and the lungs, whereas if they rest while closed, all these lower portions of the body are closed off and the voice resonates only in the spaces above the glottis. The second difference is that if they rest while closed, no air can escape through the glottis whereas if they rest while open, air can pass through with the effect of increasing transglottal airflow, potentially making the sound appear to the ear more breathy.

Of course, if the vocal folds are closed, but are not kept pushed together tightly, then even during their closed phase, air can pass through the folds in the form of a trickle or a seepage. This, again, could cause the voice timbre to have a certain breathiness.

The fifth component parameter to the sound of a human voice which we can identify is, therefore, the degree of audible transglottal air or the level of breathiness, a component which, within the model of Therapeutic Voicework which I have developed, is referred to as 'free air'.

The quality of the voice is perceived as being more or less breathy or airy, determined by the volume or quantity of transglottal airflow.

Vocal Fold Friction

We have so far assumed that during vocalisation the vocal folds are drawn together so as to meet flush and smooth along their phonating edge, preventing air from escaping other than during their rhythmic opening and thereby producing a clear tone. However, as I have just intimated, if they are not brought together firmly then air continues to seep through. In addition, under certain circumstances, not only may the vocal folds not meet under enough pressure to prevent air escaping but the vocal folds may crash together unevenly, their edges being corrugated and unmatched, rubbing against each other and producing a sound which sounds broken, frictional, rough and discontinuous. These broken sounds are referred to as disrupted and the sixth vocal component parameter which we can identify within the human voice is, therefore, disruption.

COMPONENT SIX: DISRUPTION

The human voice may or may not be to some degree disrupted, that is broken or sporadically interrupted by noise or air which appears to interfere with the continuity of the tone. This can be caused by friction or uneven contact between the vocal folds.

Voice Register

If a person begins to sing the lowest note possible and rises one note at a time up to the highest he or she can sing, it will be possible to discern alterations in the timbre at certain points as though the person has 'changed voices'. Among the changes which a listener would observe would be a shift of 'register'.

Most voices have two main registers in singing, known as modal and falsetto. The most familiar and easily recognisable changes between the modal and falsetto registers occurs when a man or a woman ascends upwards from a deep pitch towards higher ones – during which, at a certain point, a 'register break' occurs where the voice 'breaks' out of modal and into falsetto. It is this register break which is exaggerated and musicalised in the yodelling style of singing which is often associated with the Alps of Switzerland and the Cowboys of the Prairies.

Although the same transition can be heard in the voices of men and women, in the tradition of Western classical singing teaching the two main registers in a female voice are generally referred to as chest register, which is comparable to a man's modal, and head register, which is comparable to man's falsetto. These terms originate in the idea that the falsetto quality stimulates increased acoustic vibration in the head area whilst modal resonates in the chest region. In fact, this is very misleading as the changes in voice production which give rise to register changes do not have any relationship to shifts of vibration in these parts of the body.[9] Scientific instrumentational investigation has not yet been able to explain exactly what does cause the audible shifts in timbre which give rise to particular registers[10] and some clinicians propose that no scientific instrumentation or process will ever fully account for the particular characteristics of a voice which we readily recognise as belonging to a particular person.[11]

However, we do know that the alterations in the size of the glottis are instrumental in effecting change in what is known as voice register. When the vocal folds are phonating using the majority of their length, the voice register produced is usually modal – that is the quality of voice which most people use to speak. When the vocal folds decrease the length of their vibrating portion there is usually a perceivable change in register from modal to falsetto. Both modal and falsetto register can be produced on low and high pitches, though the higher the voice in pitch the more natural and easier it is to produce falsetto and the lower the pitch of the voice the more natural and easier it is produce modal. In addition, through precise control of the laryngeal musculature, a vocal sound can be produced which blends together the two registers into a single quality.

If the vocal folds remain closed along the majority of their length so that only a minimal portion is vibrating, making a tiny glottis, the voice quality produced is like a piercing scream and is known as the whistle register.[12] Because this requires extreme tension in the vocal folds, the pitch of the whistle register is always very high. If, in contradistinction, the vocal folds are very lax and their entire length is phonating then the quality of voice often produced is like a low, airy grumble known as the vocal fry register, or alternatively as vocal creak, which, due to the lack of tension in the folds, is always produced on low notes.[13]

The seventh component to vocal sound which we can identify, therefore, is vocal register – of which the two main ones are modal and falsetto with two less frequently heard registers named whistle and vocal fry.

COMPONENT SEVEN: REGISTER

The voice is produced within what is perceived as a certain register, either modal, falsetto, whistle or vocal fry. The voice can also be perceived as being composed of a blended combination of modal and falsetto.

The Resonating Tubes

Some of the air released in puffs through the vocal folds may also pass through the nasal passages which run from the oro-pharynx up above the roof of the mouth and out through the nose. The amount of air which passes through this tract influences the vocal quality. The passage of air through the nasal tube can be controlled by the raising and lowering of the velum, also known as the soft palate, which closes and opens the port of entry to the nasal tract respectively (see Figure 1.3). At one extreme, the movement of air through this passage can be completely prevented and, at the other, the maximum amount of air capable of passing through this port can travel through the nasal passages and out of the nose. Between these two extremes an entire spectrum of nasal airflow is possible. The inhibition of this nasal passage as a resonating chamber, such as when blocked with mucus during influenza, gives the voice a certain sound, which we often call nasal but, in fact, we should call lack of nasal resonance because it is indeed a vocal quality which is produced by preventing the sound-wave passing through and resonating in the nasal passages. When the nasal passages are open and clear, the voice has full nasal resonance – though because this is the usual vocal sound for most people, we tend not to notice nasal resonance until it is missing.

The eighth vocal component which we can identify is, therefore, the degree of nasal resonance. Maximum nasal resonance is called hypernasality whilst depleted nasal resonance is called hyponasality. By controlling the velum, or soft palate, nasal resonance can be radically increased, infusing the voice with a particular quality of sound used in many singing styles. In the model of Voicework which I have developed that particular quality of voice which arises from a radical increase of nasal resonance is given the instrumental and metaphorical name of violin. Increased violin in the vocal timbre is, therefore, directly proportional to increased nasal resonance.

COMPONENT EIGHT: VIOLIN

The human voice may be heard as possessing a spectral degree of nasal resonance. When nasal resonance is radically increased, the sound may metaphorically be described as possessing a high degree of violin; when nasal resonance is minimal, the voice may be heard as lacking in violin.

Harmonic Resonance

The most significant tube for the refined operations of voice and speech is not the nasal passage but the vocal tract which runs from the larynx, becomes the pharynx, turns into the oro-pharynx and curls round to become the mouth. It is the shape and movement of this tube which governs so much of the specific quality of a voice which we hear, regardless of the degree and combination of the eight component parameters hitherto identified.

To understand how the movement and configuration of this tube effects vocal quality it will be useful to imagine three crude tubes, closed at the

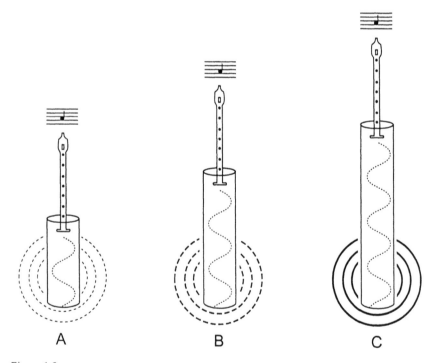

Figure 1.9

bottom but open at the top, all made of exactly the same substance and constructed to the same diameter but to different lengths. The first is short, like a flute; the second is relatively longer, like a clarinet; and the third is much longer again, like a saxophone but without the bend. Imagine that we hold the air puff machine, a metaphor for the vocal folds, spinning at a constant speed of 440 c.p.s., and thus producing a constant pitch of A, over the top of each tube in turn and listen to the sound of the note echoing or resonating inside the tubes. In moving from listening to the sound inside the first tube to the same note echoing or resonating in the second and then the third, the listener would hear a change of timbre. Perhaps the sound in the first tube would sound 'bright', 'twangy', 'shiny' and 'shimmery'; perhaps the sound resonating in the second tube, by comparison, would sound 'thicker', more 'solemn' or 'fruitier'; and perhaps the sound resonating in the third tube would sound 'full', 'moaning', 'rounded' and 'dark'. Probably, the first tube would sound more comparable to a flute, the second tube would sound more comparable to the clarinet, and the sound produced by the third

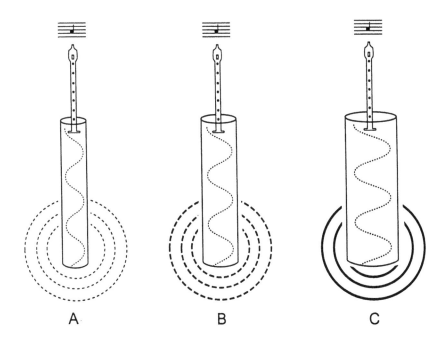

Figure 1.10

tube would sound more akin to the saxophone; they would all, however, produce the note A. This change in timbre would occur whatever constant sound source was held inside or over the top of the tubes. For example, one could play a penny whistle, keeping the note the same, whilst pointing it into each of the tubes and the result would be a change in timbre from one tube to the next (Figure 1.9).

In this experiment the tubes act as resonators which amplify the sound source and, when using a tube as a resonator, it is not only the length but also the diameter which effects the timbre. To exemplify this it will be useful to imagine another three crude tubes, closed at the bottom but open at the top, like a bottle, again all made of exactly the same substance but this time constructed to the same length but to different diameters. Again, if a penny whistle or any other object that produced a constant note was played inside or over the top of each of the tubes in turn, the timbre would change (Figure 1.10).

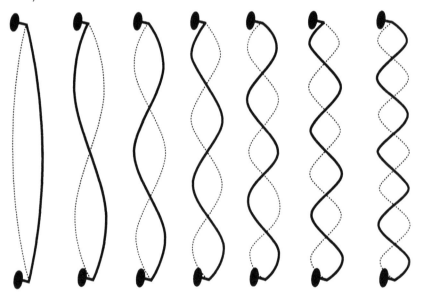

Figure 1.11

One of the major laws of sound-making is that the size and shape of a resonator such as a tube, or indeed of any cavity in which air vibrates at a frequency within the threshold of hearing, influences the timbre. The way that different timbres can be accentuated within the same pitch occurs as a result of a concept known as harmonics.

Harmonics

A string of wire, or of air molecules, vibrates in a wave of segments sounding not only one pitch determined by its fundamental frequency but simultaneously emitting a number of other higher pitches which are determined by the frequency of the segments. A vibrating string is, therefore, behaving in a way that we could conceive of if all the pictures in Figure 1.11 were placed on top of one another.

The series of upper faint pitches which a sound-wave gives off are called overtones, upper partials or harmonics which, considered together, make what is called a harmonic series. Of course, it is very difficult to hear these overtones or harmonics independently because they exist only in combination with the fundamental frequency which is bolder or more intense and, therefore, masks out the upper partials in most situations. However, what they do is blend in with the pitch produced by the fundamental frequency giving it a particular harmonic resonance.

With regard to voice production, both the length and the diameter of the vocal tube or tract can alter, producing a variety of timbres, yet the pitch can be held constant by an unchanging frequency of vocal fold phonation. Now imagine that instead of an air puff machine or penny whistle at the top of three crude tubes, you have vibrating vocal folds at the bottom of one tube which can change its length and diameter to assume the relative dimensions of all three tubes. This gives some idea of how harmonic resonance is created by the vocal instrument (Figure 1.12).

The vocal tract which runs from the lips down to the larynx is an elastic tube which can be increased or decreased in size by three options. We can expand the walls outwards, lower the floor downwards or raise the top upwards. In the case of the vocal tract, the lips mark the top of the tube, the vocal folds in the larynx form the floor and the roof and sides of the mouth, along with the curved surfaces of oro-pharynx, pharynx and larynx, form the tubular walls.

The part of the tract where movement of increasing and decreasing diameter can be felt most easily is, of course, the mouth, which can open wide – as in a yawn – and close down to very narrow dimensions – as in whistling. But this opening and closing, or sphinctral changes, in the diameter of the mouth mirrors the potential movements along the entire length of the vocal

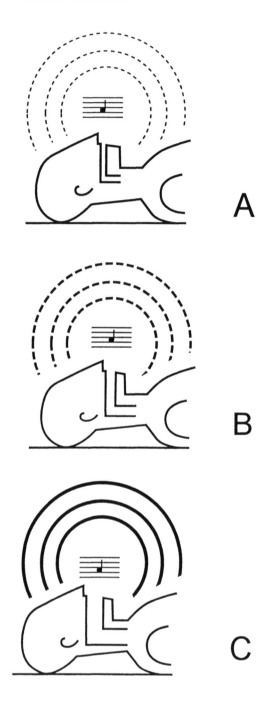

Figure 1.12

tract as well as within the larynx itself. In fact, if we allow ourselves to fully yawn, the complete length of the vocal tract, including the larynx, dilates. Conversely, this tract can be made to constrict.

The vocal tract can also lengthen and shorten. The first means of achieving this is to protrude and retrieve the lips and jaw, making the resonating tube longer and shorter respectively. The second means of achieving this is to lower and raise the floor by causing the larynx to descend and ascend in the neck. If you place your finger and thumb around your Adam's apple and yawn, you may feel your larynx naturally descend in the neck. If you now stop yawning and whistle, you will probably feel it rise. As the vocal tract is that tube which runs from the lips to the larynx, the descending of the larynx in the neck actually makes the vocal resonating tube longer while the rising of the larynx in the neck makes it shorter, increasing and decreasing its dimensions respectively.

In fact, the lengthening of the vocal tract by lowering the larynx also tends to widen or increase its diameter. This operates according to the same principle as a collapsing telescope. When the larynx descends, it pulls or stretches the tissue walls of the pharynx down with it, decreasing the thickness of the wall and causing the pharyngeal space to dilate. Conversely, to shorten the vocal tract by raising the larynx causes a simultaneous narrowing or decrease in diameter of the tract because when the larynx raises, the tissue of the pharyngeal wall piles up and thickens.

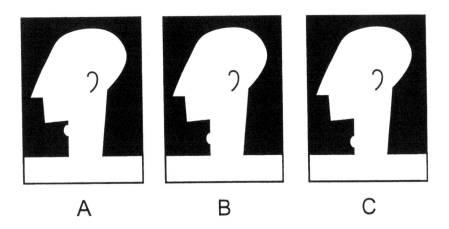

Figure 1.13

According to the acoustical laws which I have described, these alterations in length and diameter of the vocal tract have the effect of changing the harmonics of the fundamental frequency, which are accentuated, creating voice qualities with different harmonic resonances.

Three Vocal Harmonic Resonances

In place of the three crude tubes, therefore, we can now pin-point three arbitrary degrees of dilation and lengthening along the path of the vocal tract. The first compares to a flute-like tube whereby the larynx is high in the neck, creating a short tube, as shown in Figure 1.13a, which is quite narrowly constricted, as shown in Figure 1.14a, such as when we blow a kiss or whistle. The second configuration, which compares to the clarinet-like tube, is characterised by a lower position of the larynx in the neck, creating a longer tube as shown in Figure 1.13b, which is more dilated, as shown in Figure 1.14b, such as when we steam up a pair of glasses. The third configuration, which compares to the saxophone-like tube, is characterised by a complete descent of the larynx in the neck, creating a long tube, as shown in Figure 1.13c, with a simultaneous maximum dilation of the vocal tract, as shown in Figure 1.14c, such as when we yawn.

If the vibratory frequency of vocal fold phonation is maintained at a constant, say at 440 c.p.s. producing the note A, whilst the vocal tract moves from flute configuration through clarinet to saxophone configuration, the effect will be to sing the same note with three very distinct timbres, comparable to that achieved when playing the note A on a sound source held inside or over the top of the three separate crude tubes imagined earlier.

Therefore, we can now identify the ninth component of vocal sound which is its harmonic resonance governed by the shape and dimension of the vocal tract. Because the harmonic resonance is infinitely variable, we can, for the sake of systematic convenience, isolate three harmonic resonances: the flute timbre, produced by a short narrow vocal tract (Figure 1.14a); the clarinet timbre, produced by a moderate length and diameter (Figure 1.14b); and the saxophone timbre, produced by a vocal tract of maximum length and diameter (Figure 1.14c).

However, the vocal tract does not maintain a consistency of tubular dimension throughout its entire length. One portion or section may be narrow, another lengthened but dilated and another constricted. Just as the degree of lengthening and dilation or shortening and constriction is infinite, so are the portions into which the length of the vocal tract can be divided,

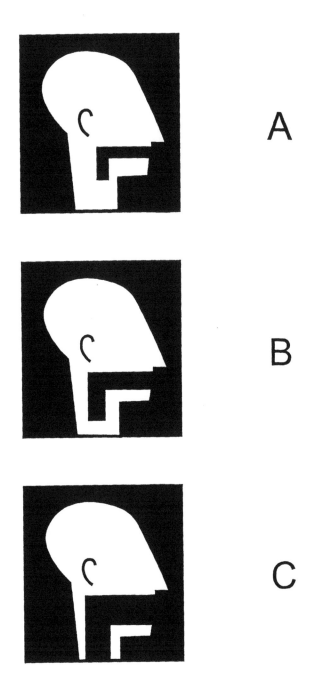

Figure 1.14

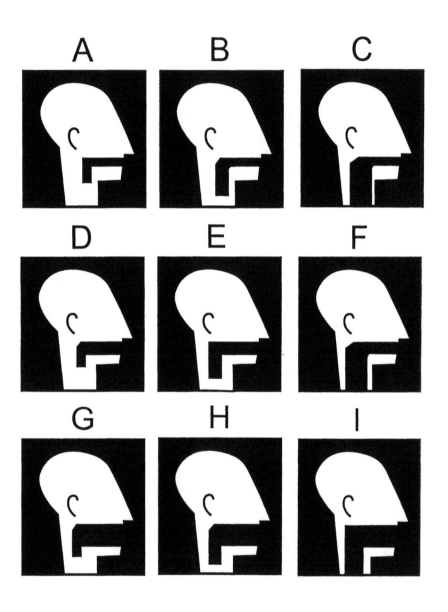

Figure 1.15

and each portion behaves with some degree of independence. In order to keep the system of harmonic resonance analysis simple and within the bounds of what it is possible for the human ear to detect in a voice, the Therapeutic Voicework Methodology which I have founded incorporates attention to the voice in a way that ascertains the likely dimensions of two halves of the vocal tract. One is the shape and dimension of the mouth and oro-pharynx, that is the oral tube, and the other is based on sensing the shape and size of the pharynx and supra-glottal spaces, that is the sub-oral tube.

This means that in listening to voices, we can perceive the shape and dimensions of the oral cavity and the shape and dimensions of the sub-oral cavity as close to one of the three configurations of flute, clarinet and saxophone, giving nine combinations in all – as illustrated in Figure 1.15.

COMPONENT NINE: HARMONIC RESONANCE

This is the most dominant component of the voice which gives it a particular character and arises from the configuration of the vocal tract. Harmonic resonance may be arbitrarily divided into three qualities arising from a short narrow tract, a medium length and diameter tract and a fully lengthened and dilated tract. Within the model of Therapeutic Voicework which I have founded, these are given the names flute, clarinet and saxophone respectively.

Vowels

It is the harmonic embellishment of a pitch caused by changing dimensions of the vocal tract which gives rise to specific timbres which we call vowels and which are born from very specific shapes of the vocal tract. Each vowel is produced by a particular degree of accentuation of specific harmonics.

The fact that vowels and harmonic resonance are the same, resulting as they do from the process of harmonic amplification, presents a major problematic for singers who have to make a compromise between the demands of vowel articulation on the one hand and voice quality on the other. Often, when we listen to a song, we hear the singer make adjustments which give rise to interesting vowel approximations, such as 'I lerv you' rather than 'I luv you', because the singer is compromising the vowel in order not to forgo the quality with which she wishes to sing.

The tenth and last vocal component or parameter is, therefore, vowel, which, technically speaking, however, is the same as harmonic resonance.

The Ten Vocal Parameters or Components

From the rudimentary physiological and mechanical operation of voice production it is possible to deduce the ten ingredients or component parameters which are, in degree, more or less present in the sound of the human voice, whether singing, speaking or vocalising instinctively and spontaneously. For the purposes of recapitulation, these components are as follows.

PITCH

Each vocal sound is perceived to have a certain pitch, note or fundamental tone determined by the frequency of vocal fold vibration or phonation. This is perceived within the metaphor of high to low, though does not, in fact, relate to spatial dimensions but to speed of vibration in time.

PITCH FLUCTUATION

This pitch sustains more or less constancy or fluctuation in a given time across a given range of tones, often called vibrato and sometimes perceived as an inability to remain attuned. This is determined by the shifting frequencies of vocal fold vibration or phonation.

LOUDNESS

The sound of the voice is perceived on a spectrum from loud to quiet, determined, in the main, by the pressure of breath released from the lungs.

GLOTTAL ATTACK

The voice is perceived as having greater or lesser attack, determined by the force under which the vocal folds come together during phonation.

FREE AIR

The quality of the voice is perceived as being more or less breathy or airy, determined by the volume or quantity of transglottal airflow.

DISRUPTION

The human voice may or may not be to some degree disrupted, that is broken or sporadically interrupted by noise or air which appears to interfere with the continuity of the tone. This can be caused by friction or uneven contact between the vocal folds.

REGISTER

The voice is produced within what is perceived as a certain register, either modal, falsetto, whistle or vocal fry. The voice can also be perceived as being composed of a blended combination of modal and falsetto.

VIOLIN

The human voice may be heard as possessing a spectral degree of nasal resonance. When nasal resonance is radically increased, the sound may metaphorically be described as possessing a high degree of violin; when nasal resonance is minimal, the voice may be heard as lacking in violin.

HARMONIC RESONANCE

The most dominant component of the voice which gives it a particular character arises from the configuration of the vocal tract. Harmonic resonance may be arbitrarily divided into three qualities arising from a short narrow tract, a medium length and diameter tract and a fully lengthened and dilated tract. These are given the names flute, clarinet and saxophone respectively.

VOWEL

The human voice may be perceived as producing sounds which appear close to a sound usable within the spoken language of a particular culture and which are produced by the shapes of the vocal tract in combination with the movements of tongue and lips.

COMPONENT TEN: VOWEL

The human voice may be perceived as producing sounds which appear close to a sound usable within the spoken language of a particular culture and which are produced by the shapes of the vocal tract in combination with the movements of tongue and lips.

The Component Parameters of Voice

From a simple understanding of vocal physiology it is, therefore, possible to deduce ten elements which combine to form the sound of the human voice. When listening to a person vocalising, whether in song or speech in a therapeutic or creative context, a Therapeutic Voiceworker can be trained to listen to the voice in terms of these manageable units which provide the basis for interpretation, analysis and training. These component parameters of vocal expression form the core of a system of Therapeutic Voicework which I have called Voice Movement Therapy which is both an analytic profile for interpreting voices, a psychotherapeutic means by which to investigate the way psychological material is communicated through specific vocal qualities, a training system for developing the expressivity of voices and a physiotherapeutic means by which to release the voice from functional misuse.

The Newham/Jungr Voice Movement Therapy Notation System

These vocal components which constitute an integrated system have, for the purposes of notation, been translated into a graphic alphabet of signs by Barb Jungr as part of a research programme at Goldsmith's University, London. Jungr's work involves using the component system to plot the vocal characteristics which are identifiable in individual vocalists drawn from a multicultural context and representative of a spectrum of world singing styles.[14] The system is known as the Newham/Jungr Voice Movement Therapy Notation System.

In the Newham/Jungr system the three arbitrary vocal tract configurations and consequent timbres are given graphic harmonic resonance signs: the flute configuration and timbre is denoted by two horizontal inwardly pointed arrow heads > <, the clarinet configuration and timbre is denoted by two horizontal outwardly pointing arrow heads <>, and the saxophone configuration and timbre is denoted by two horizontal half circles ( ).

To indicate whether the oral or sub-oral part of the tube or vocal tract is being denoted, the letter signs **O** or **SO** respectively are placed to the left of the harmonic resonance signs. Thus **O** >< denotes an oral tract in flute configuration, **O** <> denotes an oral tract in clarinet configuration and **O** () denotes an oral tract in saxophone configuration. Meanwhile, **SO** >< denotes a sub-oral tract in flute configuration, **SO** <> denotes a sub-oral tract in clarinet configuration and **SO** () denotes a sub-oral tract in saxophone configuration.

The voice registers are also indicated by letter signs which are placed to the right of the harmonic resonance sign. The letter sign **M** stands for modal, **F** stands for falsetto, **W** stands for whistle and **VF** for vocal fry.

The degree of free air is indicated by placing a vertical line between the two symmetrical shapes which form the harmonic resonance sign. To indicate the amount of free air which is heard in a sound, the line is placed either in the centre, to the left or the right. A vertical line placed in the centre indicates a moderate amount of free air, a vertical line placed to the right indicates a maximum amount of free air and a vertical line placed to the left indicates just a minimal amount of free air. Thus >|< denotes a voice in flute timbre with a moderate amount of free air, <|> denotes a voice in clarinet timbre with a moderate amount of free air and (|) denotes a voice in saxophone timbre with a moderate amount of free air. Meanwhile, >|< denotes a voice in flute timbre with a maximum amount of free air, <▷ denotes a voice in clarinet timbre with a maximum amount of free air and (▷ denotes a voice in saxophone timbre with a maximum amount of free air. Finally, >|< denotes a voice in flute timbre with a minimum amount of free air, ◁> denotes a voice in clarinet timbre with a minimum amount of free air and ◁) denotes a voice in saxophone timbre with a minimum amount of free air.

The pitch of the voice is denoted by a sign composed of two adjacent vertical lines, II, across which a horizontal line is placed to indicate height or depth of pitch. The higher the horizontal line is placed, the higher the pitch it designates. Thus ⊞ indicates a voice produced in a middle-pitch range, ⊤⊤ indicates a high-pitched voice and ⊥⊥ indicates a low-pitched voice.

A voice perceived to be loud is indicated by placing a vertical, upwardly pointing arrow head ⌢ at the top of the pitch sign whilst a voice perceived to be quiet is indicated by placing a vertical, downwardly pointing arrow head ⌣ at the bottom of the pitch sign. Thus ⊤̂⊤ indicates a loud voice high in pitch, ⊤⊤̣ indicates a quiet voice high in pitch, ⊞̂ indicates a loud middle-pitched voice, ⊬ indicates a quiet middle-pitched voice, ⒤ indicates a loud voice low in pitch and ⒰ indicates a quiet voice low in pitch.

The pitch fluctuation is denoted by zigzag wave lines. The interval distance between the notes is denoted by the height of the points; the higher the point, the larger the interval distance. The speed of pitch fluctuation is denoted by the breadth between the points; the wider the breadth, the slower the speed. Thus ⋀⋀ indicates a pitch fluctuation between widely-spaced notes, that is across a large interval, vocalised very quickly, ⋀⋀⋀ indicates the same large pitch interval but vocalised very slowly, ⋀⋀ indicates a pitch fluctuation between closely related notes, that is across a narrow interval, vocalised very quickly, ⋀⋀⋀ indicates the same small pitch interval but vocalised very slowly. The sign for glottal attack is comprised of a double-curve, Ƨ, which is placed in relation to a vertical line, |, so that the line placed to the right of the double curve, Ƨ|, indicates a voice with hard glottal attack and the line placed to the left of the double curve, |Ƨ, indicates soft glottal attack.

The presence of disruption is indicated by a series of corrugated lines, with more lines indicating greater degree of disruption. Thus ≋ indicates a mildly disrupted voice whilst ≋≋ indicates a more extreme disruption.

Finally, the quality of violin is indicated by an inverted triangle, ▽, and a vertical line, |, which, when placed to the right of the triangle, ▽|, indicates a voice with maximum violin whilst the line placed to the left of the triangle, |▽, indicates a voice with minimal violin.

Through the use of this systematic notation, the vocal sounds emitted by all voices, in song, speech and other kinds of vocal release, can be recorded. Because a voice is constantly changing its timbral components during vocal expression, a cluster of signs will denote a specific moment in time – at which point a particular vocal picture is presented. At a moment where a voice changes from one set of vocal parameters to another, a separation sign, /, is entered before a new cluster of signs is recorded.

For example, imagine a handicapped young woman with extreme muscular tension with her mouth wide open as she tries to indicate her needs but whose larynx is tight and constricted. Her voice is extremely loud, in a high pitch range and, because she is crying, has a very fast pitch fluctuation between widely-spaced notes. In addition, her voice is mildly disrupted. Such a vocal profile would be indicated by the following cluster of signs: O () SO >< ⒯ ⋀⋀ ≋. Imagine then that a Therapeutic Voiceworker helps the young woman expand the sub-oral cavities and alleviate the disruption, during which the voice softens and quietens, drops to a mid-pitch range and is now comprised of clarinet configuration both orally and sub-orally with a lot of free air and a moderate amount of violin. In addition, as she stops crying, the pitch fluctuation slows down and covers a lesser interval. This new vocal profile would be indicated by the cluster of signs ++ <▷ |▽ ∧∧∧. In making a profile notation of this major transformation, a Therapeutic Voiceworker would record the clusters divided by the separation sign: O ⟨⟩ SO >< π̄ ∧∧∧ ≋ / ++ <▷ |▽ ∧∧∧.

The Newham/Jungr system of notation has a number of uses. First, for Therapeutic Voiceworkers, it provides a quick and convenient way of recording the major vocal transformations which occur in a session – which can be consulted as a reminder of what happened when discussing a case in supervision or in other professional contexts. Second, for ethnomusicologists and researchers working in the field, it provides an expedient way of recording the predominant vocal singing styles used in various cultures – enabling analytic work to be initiated by comparing the spectrum of sign clusters recorded.

Other Systems of Voice Description

The attempt to organise an interpretative system of vocal analysis which could locate and plot the nature of various cultural vocal styles was first initiated by Alan Lomax, who perceived singing 'as a specialised and easily identifiable kind of vocal behaviour.'[15] Lomax proposed that there are distinctive features within singing styles that we immediately associate with particular cultural groups and claimed that 'once a listener has heard Negro African, Indian, Oriental, Australian, or Polynesian songs he will seldom fail to recognise the style on a second encounter.'[16] The goal of Lomax's research was to 'devise a descriptive technique' that would isolate the components which underlie the vocal patterns specific to named cultures throughout the world, one of which was the shape of the vocal tract.[17]

Lomax discovered that one of the features which the listener responds to in identifying the cultural, emotional and musical origination of a song is the dimensions of the mouth and throat and that all singing, by physiological necessity, involves certain choices regarding these dimensions which influence the timbral quality of the voice. The contributions of Alan Lomax to the notion of a relationship between singing style and physical voice production are indispensable to an understanding of any kind of analytic Therapeutic Voicework. However, Lomax had limited comprehension of vocal physiology and resorted often to descriptive terms which confused his aim. Key researchers of recent years have, therefore, pointed out that 'the problem is to find more precise terminology' which can be used in place of Lomax's 'subjective terms' such as 'tense', 'raspy', 'throaty' and 'husky'.[18]

Another voice researcher of significance is Alfred Wolfsohn, who discovered that each note within a singer's pitch range could be produced with a number of identifiable timbral qualities to which he gave the instrumental names of violin, cello and viola. It is from his idea of naming vocal timbres after instruments that I have taken the terms flute, clarinet, saxophone and violin. However, Wolfsohn also ignored physiology and focused primarily on the individual subjective experience of singing with little concern for systematic analysis. The system of voice analysis which I have distilled from the physiological operation, and which is being used by Jungr to analyse world singing styles, seeks to take the work of Lomax and of Wolfsohn a step further.

A further researcher of comparable significance is the phonetician Laver, who, with more precision than Lomax, breaks the voice down into a number of what he calls 'articulatory settings' – a term first used by Honikman[19] in 1964. Laver describes these settings as the particular muscular adjustments underlying voice production which a person has acquired and tends to use consistently.[20]

Laver is a key figure because, with more detailed scrutiny than any other, he has attempted to create a 'phonetic description of voice quality'[21] – that is a way of labelling and describing vocal sounds by identifying the muscular use of the vocal apparatus which generates them, in the same way that verbal sounds are described according to movements of the articulatory apparatus including the tongue, lips and jaw in the field of phonetics.

One of Laver's intentions has been to overcome the long history of 'impressionistic labelling of voice types that are not related to physical mechanisms, and the proliferation of confusing terminology'.[22] Among Laver's 'settings' are 'raised larynx' and 'lowered larynx', modal and falsetto register, 'open lip rounding' and 'closed lip rounding' and 'nasal voice' and 'denasal voice'. Laver also places significant emphasis on the degree of muscular tension within the component structures of the vocal mechanism and the influence this has on vocal quality.

Laver sought to utilise his phonetic description of voice quality to design a systematic voice profile which has been employed by some speech and language therapists to identify the mechanical and muscular misuse of the vocal apparatus which gives rise to pathological conditions and their consequent acoustic qualities.[23]

The limitations to Laver's work do not negate its importance but need to be acknowledged. First, Laver's system is not related to a methodology of enabling a vocalist to acquire certain settings. Furthermore, it is based on the perception of the vocal or paralinguistic aspects of the spoken voice and does not emanate from an exploration of sung tones.

A contemporary researcher who overcomes both of these limitations, however, is Jo Estill, a singing coach and voice researcher who created what she calls 'voice craft'. Estill is a pioneering figure in the field of vocal physiology with the unique disposition of having begun her career as a lieder and opera singer before investigating voice through scientific measurements. Her special focus is concerned with discovering the precise physiological and mechanical processes which give rise to specific singing styles and vocal qualities such as 'nasal twang',[24] 'the 'belting' style used in musical theatre[25] and what she calls the 'ringing'[26] quality, all of which she has compared to the classical operatic style. By taking precise measurements of various physiological components using highly sophisticated measuring equipment, Estill has been able to observe and analyse the different methods of voice production which singers with different stylistic approaches utilise. However, unlike other investigators, she has applied her understanding to developing a method of teaching singers to produce voice qualities hitherto considered threatening to the health of the voice, such as the big Broadway belting sound. Her technique consists of teaching the student to locate sensation in, and independently articulate, eight structures within the vocal apparatus. These are the vocal folds, which may be made thick, thin or stiff; the soft palate, which may be totally open, half open or totally closed; the tongue, which can be relaxed or compressed; the pharynx, which can be widened and made short or long; the laryngeal cartilages, which can be tilted or levelled; the extrinsic laryngeal musculature, which can assume a number of configurations; and the band of muscle around the vocal folds, which can be relaxed or constricted.

Estill's practical application of physiological analysis has found its most receptive use amongst voice teachers and speech and language therapists, who are enabled to connect physical sensation and voice quality. There are, however, apparent limitations and problems with Estill's approach, some of which have been identified by Comins.[27] First, Estill's teaching method does not accommodate attendance to emotional and figurative expression and the influence this has on the muscle use. Students are, therefore, implicitly required to treat the voice purely mechanically, many of whom find this uncomfortable and inexpedient. Second, the various combinations of movements which Estill attempts to teach are incredibly subtle, often requiring students to effect minute adjustments of very precisely localised anatomical parts. For many, such localised anatomical articulation further compounds the technical and non-emotive dimension to the work, which, for singers, can be frustrating.

It would be audacious and counterfeit to claim that my work within the field of vocal analysis compares in any degree to the sophisticated studies of either Laver or Estill. In comparison, my system of vocal profile is simplistic and incomplete. However, such simplicity has been necessitated by the genesis of my work first with handicapped people and latterly with novice vocalists, both of whom could respond immediately to simple mechanical concepts but were further ostracised from expression by complexity. Second, my work attempts to synthesise emotional movement with physical movement and this has meant sculpturing a language of compromise which can walk the middle road between somatic mechanics and emotional transformation.

Conclusion: Making Use of Mechanics

Part of the step which I have taken in identifying ten component parameters of vocal expression is to offer a framework within which all voices can be analysed and notated. However, the most significant use of this system is not simply to analyse what one hears but to enable a single human voice to acquire the dexterity with which to manifest manifold combinations of vocal qualities. When this is achieved, the voice is able to serve both artistic procedures by bringing greater vocal flexibility to the process of singing and is also able to express a greater range of emotional and psychological experience. The work which I have augmented is, therefore, predicated upon a synthesis of analytic, artistic and therapeutic principles and it is these principles that I will outline in this book.

To begin, in the following chapter I will offer the reader an opportunity to understand how these components of vocal sound make themselves apparent in the expression of psychological material through spontaneous vocalisation and in the vocal qualities of various singing voices.

Notes

1   Bunch, M. (1993) *Dynamics of the Singing Voice*. New York: Springer-verlag Wien.

2   Sundberg, J. (1987) *The Science of the Singing Voice*. Illinois: Northern Illinois University Press.

3   Appleman, R. (1986) *The Science of Vocal Pedagogy*. Indiana: Indiana University Press.

4   Miller, R. (1986) *The Structure of Singing: System and Arts in Vocal Technique*. New York: Schirmer.

5   Pierce, J. (1992) *The Science of Musical Sound*. New York: Freeman and Co.

6   Fry, D. (1991) *The Physics of Speech*. Cambridge: Cambridge University Press.

7   Ladefoged, P. (1996) *Elements of Acoustic Phonetics*. Chicago: University of Chicago Press.

8   Keleman, S. (1985) *Emotional Anatomy*. Berkeley: Center Press.

9   Lindsley, C.F. (1934) 'The psycho-physical determinants of voice quality.' *Speech Monograph*, 1, pp.79–116.

10   Sundberg, J. (1987) *The Science of the Singing Voice*. Illinois: Northern Illinois University Press, p.50.

11   Greene, M. and Mathieson, L. (1989) *The Voice and its Disorders*, 5th edn. London: Whurr, p.57.

12   Moolenaar-Bijl, A. (1957) 'The laryngeal whistle.' *Folia Phoniatrica*, 9, pp.164–68.

13   H. Hollien et al. (1966) 'On the nature of vocal fry.' *Journal of Speech and Hearing Research*, 9, pp.245–47.

14   Jungr, B. (1997) 'Three singers in London.' Unpublished Masters thesis, Goldsmiths College, London.

15   Lomax, A. (1978) *Folk Song Style and Culture*. New Jersey: Transaction Books, p.3.

16   Lomax, A. (1978) *Folk Song Style and Culture*. New Jersey: Transaction Books, p.13.

17   Lomax, A. (1978) *Folk Song Style and Culture*. New Jersey: Transaction Books, p.71.

18   Merriam, A. (1980) *The Anthropology of Music*. Illinois: Northwestern University Press, p.105.

19   Honikman, B. (1964) 'Articulatory settings.' In D. Abercrombie, D. Fry, P. MacCarthy, N. Scott and J. Trim (eds) *In Honour of Daniel Jones*. London: Longman, pp.73-84.

20   Laver, J. (1978) 'The concept of articulatory settings: an historical survey.' *Historiographia Linguistica*, 5, pp.1–14.

21   Laver, J. (1980) *The Phonetic Description of Voice*. Cambridge: Cambridge University Press.

22   Pittam, J. (1994) 'Voice in social interaction: an interdisciplinary approach.' *Language and Language Behaviours*, vol.5. London: Sage, p.31.

23   Laver, J., Wirz, S., MacKenzie, J. and Hiller, S. (1981) 'A perceptual protocol for the analysis of vocal profiles.' *Work in Progress, Department of Linguistics, University of Edinburgh*, 14, pp.139–155.

24   Estill, J. (1986) 'An EMG study of two voice qualities: nasal twang and opera with squillo.' In M. Hirano and S. Hibi (eds) *Proceedings of the International Conference on Voice*, Karume, Japan, pp.74–82.

25   Estill, J. (1988) 'Belting and classic voice quality: some physiological differences.' *Medical Problems of Performing Artists*, 3, pp.37–43.

26   Estill, J., Yanagisawa, E., Kmucha, S. and Leder, S. (1989) 'The contribution of aryepiglotic
       constriction to 'ringing' voice quality: a video laryngoscopy study with acoustic analysis.'
       Journal of Voice, 4, 3.

27   Comins, J. (1996) 'Voice clinic: let's get physical.' *The Singer*, September/October.

CHAPTER 2

Sound and Psyche
An Applied System of Interpretation for Vocal Sound

Introduction: A Methodology For Training, Therapy and Analysis

The set of vocal component parameters which I have distilled from physiological function offers a framework of analysis within which voice production can be analysed perceptually in the absence of objective measuring equipment. For, with training, it is possible for an attentive listener to sense the composite combination of the ten components which may be present in a voice at any given time. Those who train in Therapeutic Voicework can, therefore, learn to hear the voice as comprising a set of vocal tract dimensions and their consequent acoustic timbres – known as flute, clarinet and saxophone – which can be produced on certain vowels across a range of pitches, each of which can fluctuate to some degree. These sounds can all be vocalised with degrees of loudness, with a greater or lesser amount of glottal attack and with a spectrum of more or less free air, creating a sound which may be to some degree disrupted and produced in a certain vocal register with a greater or lesser amount of violin.

The various combinations of these components are obviously manifold, each giving specific vocal qualities expressive of distinctive artistic styles and with particular psychological connotations. Because these vocal components are rooted in the elementary physiological and mechanical operation of the voice, they can be applied with equal efficacy whether analysing vocal expression in a therapeutic or educational setting or vocal styles in an artistic context.

Because a Therapeutic Voiceworker is approaching the voice subjectively, intuitively drawing upon his or her own responses in the absence of empirical measuring procedures, the system which I have constructed provides a non-judgmental, non-affective framework in which to locate such responses. It is always tempting to analyse the voice by labelling sounds according to emotional, figurative or attitudinal constructs which emanate from the Therapeutic Voiceworker's own associations. This gives rise to descriptive terms such as 'whiny', 'depressive', 'bubbly', 'childlike', 'aggressive' or 'weak'. In contradistinction to this approach, the provision of measuring devices and the clinical language of allopathic systems describes the voice with terms based in physiological pathology, such as 'hyperkinetic' and 'whispered aphonia'. Whilst the former acknowledges the emotionality and imaginative capacity of the voice, it risks a dangerous disconnection from the mechanics of voice production and can potentially perpetuate a prejudicial reinforcement of vocal stereotyping. The latter, meanwhile, has the advantage of being grounded in an objective understanding of mechanical and physiological voice production and avoids preconceived interpretative conclusions but, on the other hand, relies on scientific procedures and equipment and locates the voice in a language of medical pathology which has little to do with the creative and psychological function of vocal expression. The system of voice profile and analysis which I have augmented offers an opportunity to walk the middle way between these two approaches.

The analytic and interpretive use of the system requires the Therapeutic Voiceworker to translate associative subjective responses to the vocalist into a profile based on the component parameters. With training, this is possible with some ease because it is these components to which we attend unconsciously when interpreting voices. We may believe someone to be angry because their voice becomes disrupted and the speed of their pitch fluctuation increases, as the sound becomes loud and deep in pitch. We may believe someone is joyous and excited because their voice breaks out of modal into falsetto as it rises in pitch and the quantity of free air increases as the vocal tract lengthens and dilates into saxophone configuration. We may think someone is frightened because their voice has a rapid pitch fluctuation and is very quiet with little glottal attack. We may believe someone to be pessimistic and despondent because their voice is infused with violin and free air within a very small pitch range and is produced with the narrow and shortened vocal tract of flute configuration. This system enables the

Therapeutic Voiceworker to suspend supposition regarding the emotional experience or personality characteristics allegedly expressed and ascertain the component parameters.

We also listen unconsciously to these components when we hear different singers. Some vocalists utilise free air whilst others have very disrupted voices. Some types of song are well suited to the expanded saxophone dimensions of the vocal tract whilst others require the contained nature of the flute configuration. Furthermore, the singing styles and voice production techniques indigenous to a specific culture tend to favour certain parameter combinations. This component system of perceptual analysis, therefore, also aims to provide a framework within which various cultural and artistic styles of singing can be located.

The pedagogical use of the system requires the Therapeutic Voiceworker to teach clients how to attain sufficient malleability of the vocal instrument to be able to combine all vocal components, thereby having at their disposal the broadest possible vocal palette for professional, artistic and personal use. In order to facilitate this in others it is absolutely essential for Therapeutic Voiceworkers to possess such malleability themselves. A significant aspect of the Voice Movement Therapy training is, therefore, focused upon training the student's own voice to manifest a broad range of component parameter combinations. Subsequent to the acquisition of this ability, trainees learn the strategies by which to facilitate maximum vocal expressivity in others.

The process of administering any kind of thorough Therapeutic Voicework naturally involves investigating both the physical and the psychological reasons for the particular limitations to a client's voice. The application of this system, therefore, involves a certain therapeutic process on a somatic and psychological level which requires of the Therapeutic Voiceworker a compassionate, humanitarian and empathic response to the vocal process at all times.

Naturally, both the application of the work by professionals and the experience of the work by clients is an idiosyncratic phenomenon and generalisations serve only to dilute and demean. However, in order to clarify my propositions I will present some of the elementary psychological and artistic aspects of the work, locating the system in both behavioural and musical expression. Taking each of the component parameters in turn, I will describe some of the related psychological connotations as well as giving examples of singers who make overt use of those component parameters. Naturally, a singer will, in the course of a single song, often change combinations to achieve certain effects. Thus when giving examples of singers, I have chosen those who tend to exemplify certain component parameters quite consistently.

I have tried to choose a range of known singers from which it is hoped most readers will recognise enough to be able to acquire a sense of the system in action. I have also chosen examples which can be obtained currently on CD or cassette, details of which are given in the Bibliography. I have deliberately confined myself mainly to Western singers as it is assumed most readers will be less familiar with multi-cultural music. However, I have included reference to a small number of singers from non-Western traditions by way of token example.

Each of the components and various combinations thereof are also systematically presented with technical voice production explanations on the set of audio cassettes, *The Singing Cure: Liberating Self Expression through Voice Movement Therapy*,[1] which accompanies this book. In addition, I have demonstrated how the various components can be combined to produce a range of tonal and timbral singing styles on the accompanying CD, *Prayers and Prophecies*.[2] Finally, the internal workings of the larynx and surrounding tissue structures during the vocalisation of these parameters can be seen on the accompanying video, *Shouting for Jericho*.[3]

PARAMETER ONE: PITCH ⧀ ⧁ ⧂

For clients of Therapeutic Voicework there are frequently occurring images of universal significance which are provoked by vocalising in a pitch range which is higher or lower than that used in daily speaking. Consequently, the Therapeutic Voicework process can be aimed at extending the vocal pitch range, which for men usually means developing a higher voice and for women a lower one, with a view to investigating the psychological significance of those images associated with height and depth in the voice.

For men there are, of course, innate physiological restrictions which make it difficult to access the extremely high tones due to the length and density of vocal fold tissue. By the same token, the shorter, less dense folds of a woman make it hard to establish lower notes. However, the limitations to male heights and female depths are by no means as immovable as classical training procedures have led us to believe.

In seeking to contemplate the psychology of height it is useful to note that, beyond a certain threshold, high sounds can be physically and mentally damaging and frequencies above 20,000 c.p.s. can be experienced as penetrating and destructive. Furthermore, each sound is composed of a harmonic series of overtones or partials which may give the sound an appearance of height or sharpness creating penetrating sensations. Usually, such sounds which are considered to be acoustically 'sharp' may consequently be perceived as piercing objects. The client who gains access to the high voice may, therefore, feel that she is penetrating others as well as herself, which can stimulate sensations of shame or of extreme power and may stimulate sadistic or masochistic instincts. In addition, access to high tones may mobilise the verve necessary to emerge from suppression or disempowerment.

Naturally, the high voice can be exhilarating both to listen to and produce and, because it is conceived within the metaphor of vertical space, it can feel as though the vocalist has 'ascended' and is moving through the clouds. Indeed, most clients will instinctively move towards the high voice in singing when a more rousing affect is desired.[4] Moreover, clients will usually elevate their body upwards as they try to reach high notes. The shadow to this is the difficulty which a client may have in feeling grounded and stable during heightened experience for the high voice seems to facilitate a certain psychological lift which can stimulate elation at the expense of stability. The popular cultural promotion of a higher consciousness which tempts many to search for a higher self can often be symbolised in the client's desire to reach ever higher notes. In addition, the sense of achievement which many feel when they have vocalised in a high pitch range further endorses the sociological notion of elevation towards higher positions of success.

In the opera, high female voices are as commonplace as the depths of the male baritone and bass; within the tradition of Western popular music, however, the crystal heights of the 'top end' are less familiar and are usually used only momentarily to embellish a song. One well-known popular example of such use of high pitch is Minnie Riperton's rendition of 'Loving You', where she utilises a vocal tract configuration which oscillates between flute and clarinet with a moderate amount of free air in modal and falsetto, **>|< M /<|> F**, then withdraws free air and jumps up into the whistle register, **<> W**.[5] Riperton's technique of utilising the whistle register is rare, but use of high pitch range **ᴨ** is also exemplified by the voice of Kate Bush.[6]

At the other end of the pitch scale is the deep voice, **ᴜ**, which, in opera, is reserved for men and is called 'bass'. The notion of a bass voice has its psychological equivalent in the 'base' aspects of the personality. To sing bass is to confront all that is base in us and this notion has two aspects. First, base is the foundation, the bedrock, that which underpins and forms the very foundation of our character. We speak of the base of things as the ground upon which the thing is built. Thus, with the deep voice, there is a sense of deep-rootedness, of contact with the earth, of strength and support. Second, 'base' means crude, unrefined, flagrant, obscene and coarse and, as such, it represents our animal instinct. Singing bass may, therefore, require the vocalist to contact and express a certain primeval core of sensation, which may include the animalistic libido.

The base is also the depths and, within the metaphor of vertical space, low sounds are conceived as being low to the ground. Moreover, when singing low sounds there is a sense of going down into the deeps, a descent not only in musical scale and physical space but in the emotional scale also. The base voice feels down in the same way that we feel down in the dumps, in the pits, in the doldrums and this can feel depressing.

The sense of descent can also be experienced in relation to the body and singing low sounds can feel as though there is stimulation of the abdominal quarters, which can animate experiences connected to the intestines, stomach and womb.

It is unfortunate that the notion of 'deep' also refers to depth of integrity, authenticity and substance and, within the process of stereotypical judgment of voices, a high-pitched voice can, therefore, often be associated with superficiality, surface and lack of depth. Because the morphology of the female tissue tends to yield a higher pitch range in speaking than in men, this also contributes to the sexist component to vocal perception. Women can, therefore, feel pressurised to lower the pitch range of the speaking voice to compete with men in a sociological framework which mistakenly associates low sounds with psychological depth and high sounds with psychological surface.

Perhaps one of the more renowned classically trained yet popular male singers with a deep pitch range was Paul Robeson, who traversed a number of song style traditions.[7] More recently and currently, within the rock genre, a number of contemporary male singers utilise a deep pitch range; among them are Brad Roberts, lead singer with the *Crash Test Dummies*,[8] Eddie Vedder, lead singer with *Pearl Jam*[9] and Barry White.[10]

Whilst in opera and the European classical tradition the deep pitch range is reserved for men, in other singing styles women utilise this range also. For example, access to deep pitch ranges are a hallmark of many jazz singers including Sarah Vaughan,[11] Etta James[12] and Nina Simone.[13] Also, Odetta[14] and Tracy Chapman[15] sing lower than the classical female voice.

In addition to those singers who utilise a pitch range at one of the extremes, there are those who have specialised in the acrobatic ability to move across an extremely wide range, often within a single song. One of the more renowned singers who utilised a range which extended from extremely high to very low was Yma Sumac, whose voice travels across about four octaves.[16] Kate Bush also makes obvious leaps and forays from high to low pitches within a single song.[17] Other singers who use a wide pitch range include Mariah Carey[18] and the modern gospel performer Ellen Baylor.[19] Outside of the West, wide pitch ranges can be heard displayed by one one of the most revered Hindustani singers, Pandit Jasraj, who moves from a grumbling bass in saxophone **Ⅱ ()** up to a tenor range in flute **H > <**, yet never utilises falsetto.[20] It is interesting to note that Jasraj, along with many other Indian singers, does not consider it negating of the performance to cough in order to clear a disturbing sensation in the throat following the singing of a particular phrase.

Through careful and informed application of integrated methodology, Therapeutic Voicework can assist a client in extending the pitch range, facilitating access to the psychological and emotional material contained within certain frequency bands.

PARAMETER TWO: PITCH FLUCTUATION ᴡᴡ ᴡᴡ ᴧᴧ ᴧᴧᴧ

Pitch fluctuation is the kind of wavering or shaking which occurs when we are extremely anxious or nervous and, often, the subtle muscular changes of tension which causes the inconsistency of the vocal fold vibration tingles all down our body at such times. In music such fluctuation can be perceived as incompetent tunelessness if it is too slow, if it covers too wide a pitch range or if the extreme points between which it fluctuates are not kept stable. However, if it is fast, within a narrow band and consistent, it is often adored. Naturally, operatic singers utilise vibrato a great deal. However outside of this tradition there are other singers, mostly female, whose voice is identified, in part, by use of vibrato. These include Barbra Streisand,[21] Shirley Bassey,[22] Liza Minnelli[23] and Sarah Vaughan.[24] It is also used a lot by the great gospel singers, such as Mahalia Jackson,[25] and it was one of the identifying features of Edith Piaf, who used a lot of violin and sang entirely in modal **<> M ▽| ᴡ**.[26]

A particularly unique form of vibrato was developed by Buffy Sainte-Marie, whose voice employs very specific use of glottal attack and pitch fluctuation. In addition, she moves back and forth between modal and falsetto, as is typical of the North American folk style.[27] Vibrato was also used consistently by Joan Baez.[28] Outside of the West there are many styles which utilise dramatic frequency fluctuations, either as embellishment or as an integral part of the melodic intervals – for example within the Quaqwaali singing form as exemplified by Nusrat Fateh Ali Kahn,[29] within the Dhrupad Hindustani classical tradition, the Zairean style exemplified by music of Grand Maœtre Franco Luambo Makiadi[30] and within the classical Persian style.

In Therapeutic Voicework the client's experience of uncontrollable pitch fluctuation can often create the sensation of not being able to maintain any stability, consistency or calm. It is as though everything is shaking and the sound of pitch fluctuation, particularly when it is combined with free air, reinforces a self-image of uncertainty, reticence and lack of surety. Through Therapeutic Voicework, however, such pitch fluctuation can be amplified and enhanced, leading to a voice with the kind of passionate vibrato associated with the opera. Such a radical transformation from a negative experience of pitch fluctuation to a positive one, what Jung called an enantiodromia, can be very inspiring for a client. Alternatively, Therapeutic Voicework can enable a cathartic release of the energetic core of nervousness and anxiety, removing some of the fluctuation in the tones.

PARAMETER THREE: LOUDNESS

Producing a loud voice can stimulate feelings of extreme power, strength and forcefulness in the vocalist, which, to a listener, can be experienced as both marvellous and terrifying. For many audients the loud voice can be experienced as an assault and a number of clients themselves have been affronted and, in some cases, abused by the loud voices of a parent, partner or other individual. In fact, the biological reality of noise is that levels of intensity above 80 decibels are potentially destructive to physical tissue and mental processes and, at a certain point beyond this limit, it becomes an 'immaterial weapon of death'.[31] Since noise is a threat of death, it is associated with primal power, as though it is the wrath of God made audible. Thus 'in most cultures, the theme of noise' is 'at the origin of the religious idea'.[32] Before the world was ordained by the divine, there was chaos. Then, with the divine idea for the world comes form – which compares to the transition from noise to music. To move backwards from music to noise, therefore, is to move from life to death and, in this way, noise is murder.[33]

Some of those clients who have difficulty in generating loud sounds are restrained not by physical inability but by negative associations with loudness, many of which are cultural rather than personal. In many contexts acoustic loudness is associated with certain personality traits equivalent with being 'loudmouthed' and which are given negative connotations, such as being brash, impudent, audacious, belligerent and pugnacious. This is, of course, only one side to the loudness complex, which is also woven with celebration, delight, joviality, rhapsody and rapture but which, for many, have been spoiled or defused by the emphasis on negative aspects of loudness. Loudness is also a means by which a person fills, and thereby claims, space, the shadow of which is that it takes space from others. Loudness thus has a territorial dimension. In addition, loud noise wards of approaching danger, stops an aggressor in their tracks and thus protects.

At the other end of the loudness scale is extreme quiet, the soft voice which can appear to express a personality which is timid, recalcitrant, disinclined, afraid, frail, unassertive and shy. Of course, the quiet voice also has another side which is mellow, gentle, tender and sensitive. Quietude is also often synonymous with the expression of intimacy and delineates a small contained space within which closeness may be explored. The loud voice can, sometimes, mask a fear of such intimacy and enabling a client to safely reduce loudness can facilitate the expression of hitherto defended vulnerability.

The quiet voice is equivalent to a soft touch and those with quiet voices may often maintain a voice which touches gently because that is how they wish to be touched. Such persons may be bruised or sore and in vocalising quietly may be asking for a soft voice to bandage and tend to them.

In recorded music it is difficult to exemplify the quiet end of the loudness spectrum because levels are adjusted by the engineering of the microphone receptivity. However, the Brazilian singer Astrud Gilberto[34] sang noticeably quietly.

The loud singing voice, meanwhile, has been most consistently utilised in the genres of Punk Rock, as exemplified in the yelling style of Sid Vicious;[35] in Heavy Metal, as exemplified in the singing of Ozzy Osbourne;[36] and in the 'big rock' sound, as exemplified in the singing of Meat Loaf[37] as well as Bonnie Tyler.[38]

It should be pointed out that the pejorative use of words such as 'loud', 'shouting' and 'screaming' to describe certain singing styles is culturally based. In contexts where sung music has arisen from outdoor activity – such as hunting, rail-road building or nomadic travelling – the method of voice production is always one which uses high sub-glottal air pressure, creating a sound loud enough to be heard across distances in the outside air – a fundamental precept of the rural shouting blues or the 'blues holler'. This quality characterises a great deal of non-Western music and gives it a style comparable to spontaneous calling rather than a singing style which has been trained within the élite quarters of a room. The jubilational and spirited calling style can be heard, for example, in the singing of the Bengali Purna Das Baul[39] and the Bulgarian 'open throat' style of choral singing.[40]

There are also singers whose excellence is, in part, revealed in exceedingly precise and manipulative control of a spectrum which runs from very quiet to very loud crescendos. Perhaps the most renowned Western example of such a technique is Barbara Streisand.[41] Outside of the West, exquisite control of the loudness spectrum is utilised by the Pakistani singer Nusrat Fateh Ali Khan, who has become more renowned through his contribution to the score of the film *Dead Man Walking*.[42]

Some people use their usual speaking voice in a manner that alternates rapidly between quiet and loud, with little acoustic expression in between. Such a voice settles momentarily in a quiet quality of ease and contemplation but is frequently disturbed by eruptions into increased intensity. These volcanic outbursts followed by soft reprises can stimulate in the listener associations with someone who is snappy, irate, unpredictable and effervescent with irritability. The vocalist, however, may be suffering from the torture of mood fluctuation and may be struggling for consistency. In Therapeutic Voicework such a quality can be amplified and used to artistic end through the process of applying it to singing styles which technically suit and provide a psychological container for such intensity fluctuations.

For many people opening the mouth and making sounds can be unfamiliar, frightening, embarrassing and difficult for it can feel as though 'others might penetrate' them and destroy their self-defence,[43] and this is often revealed in the very quiet voice which does not ever seem to be fully expressed. Indeed, the most common factor which prevents the liberation of the voice is a fundamental expressive inhibition, a reticence, a lack of confidence or shyness in letting the voice out. In vocal terms we might call this state 'phonophobia', a fear of voicing.

Phonophobia, or extreme shyness, manifests in an extremely quiet voice and is both a psychological and a vocal problem, the one feeding the other in a cyclical syndrome from which the person suffering from it feels they cannot escape. Phonophobia is the means by which a person denies herself the right to express and those who experience it are usually found to be suffering from the repercussions of having been continually silenced by a dominating individual or by a series of suffocating circumstances which have stifled the right to express and which have thus silenced the voice. Phonophobia is the result of a quashing of confidence and is often achieved by inhibiting the voice of the child through consistent prohibitions: 'don't whine', 'don't whimper', 'don't pester, 'don't be cheeky', 'don't be rude', 'don't give me any lip'. All these are the phrases by which the child's right to voice is subdued and all of them represent the vestiges of the abominable Victorian dictum that 'children should be seen and not heard'.

Later in life the oppressor becomes introjected as an inner critical voice which inhibits and censors the outward voice of the adult self. The shy person thus sits in silence while those around them speak. However, people who are shy almost exclusively complain not of an inner silence, as one might expect, but of an internal mindscape of unbearable noise – the noise of their own reactions which they dare not and do not vocalise but instead retain in their heads.

The phonophobic often knows exactly what they think and feel, but between the conception and the word falls their shadow, the sum of all those parts of themselves which they hide and which they do not want to associate themselves with. The shy person's shadow is the critical judge, the bombastic extrovert who dominates the stage of the unconscious and prevents the words of the shy ego from coming out. The phonophobic's internal world of noise is populated with silent verdicts and this inner critical nature combined with the shy person's outward silence can lead her to being wrongly perceived as arrogant.

Through Therapeutic Voicework, the personal and archetypal implications of the loudness spectrum can be explored and the client's voice can be trained to overcome its confinement to a single part of the spectrum, which may have occurred as a result of psychological and physical factors.

PARAMETER FOUR: GLOTTAL ATTACK ʔ ʔ

Glottal attack is heard in the speaking voice when someone is making a series of points; it is like a vocalised full stop. We also tend to increase the force of vocal fold adduction when we are angry but controlled enough to drive our point home. Naturally, forceful glottal attack is usually combined with the lack of free air, whilst soft glottal attack is often heard as a voice high in free air.

For many people there is not enough force of adduction to create a sound of any solidity or strength and such clients, who produce a sound high in free air and of low intensity, may feel that their voice is weak and without substance. Conversely, for others, force of adduction may be so strong that such clients, who produce a sound without free air and of high intensity, may feel their voice to be intimidating and without gentility. Between these two extremes is an infinite spectrum of possibilities and by drawing on exercises and careful guidance, the Therapeutic Voiceworker can assist the client in discovering the potential for variation and diversity in the manipulation of air pressure and force of adduction in all three elementary harmonic timbres of flute, clarinet and saxophone.

Glottal attack tends to produce a voice which is punctuated rhythmically with quick staccato sounds of intensity, rather than a voice which is consistently loud. In singing styles, therefore, glottal attack is used to create rhythmic composition and is exemplified most familiarly in the scats jazz style, used, for example, by Cleo Laine[44] and Ella Fitzgerald.[45] It is also used in singing styles which serve the kind of song which makes a point, such as the protest song. A British singer who uses the punctuational quality of hard glottal attack is Billy Bragg, many of whose songs have a protest quality which is aided by the abrupt nature of glottal attack.[46] Such strong glottal attack is indigenous to the London cockney dialect, in which Bragg sings, and the same combination of dialect and glottal attack can be heard in the singing style of Tom Robinson's early protest-orientated singing.[47] The use of sudden 'glottal stop' sounds proliferate throughout non-Western music, where they provide a sense of percussive accompaniment.

The antithesis of the confrontational aspect to hard glottal attack commonly used in the protest song is exemplified in the vocal delivery style of Leonard Cohen,[48] who is renowned for his introverted depressiveness. Lack of glottal attack is also used in singing styles which are predicated on constancy and lack of rhythm, such as the Gregorian and other forms of chant.

PARAMETER FIVE: FREE AIR |

Glottal attack relates to free air because high sub-glottal air pressure and forceful vocal fold adduction tends to produce a voice with minimum free air. Conversely, voices with a high degree of free air generally lack sub-glottal air pressure and strong adduction. There are some exceptions to this, such as in the flamenco deep song where both men and women maintain high sub-glottal air pressure and forceful fold adduction yet also imbue the sound with high degrees of free air.[49]

Increasing free air is something which many people do subconsciously when they wish to appear gentle, empathic and receptive. It is also a natural tendency to imbue the voice with free air when we wish to speak softly or when we are feeling despondent. The withdrawal of free air, meanwhile, gives the acoustic signal of the voice the appearance of firmness and is, perhaps, more often used to communicate authority.

Singing with free air is like singing on a whisper and it is hard to produce with loudness because the necessary sub-glottal air pressure is absent. Singing with no free air is a lot more efficient for maintaining intensity, yet the absence of free air often leaves the sound devoid of the contour of tenderness, acoustic and emotional.

For many people sustained non-verbal vocalisation with a high degree of free air is experienced during sexual activity, particularly the period culminating in orgasm. This climactic experience of orgasm has been musicalised by Irene Papas, who, utilising a voice with a high degree of free air, created a vocal song with the simple text 'I am to come I was' – which vocalises the journey towards orgasmic climax accompanied by minimal percussion.[50] Perhaps it is due to the instinctive use of free air during orgasmic expression that male heterosexual listeners have associated the 'breathy' voice in women with magnanimous sexual appetite.

Sexuality is always latently present in the act of singing, which is essentially a libidinous process that indulges the ability of the mouth, tongue and lips to stimulate and exhilarate.[51] However, there are a number of performers within the contemporary rock music genre who have utilised a voice high in free air to sexualise and sensualise their performance, exaggerating this libidinous dimension to the singing process. Marilyn Monroe is probably the most familiar modern precedent to such a style, whose gentle, coy and coquettish vocal quality was infused with free air as can be heard, for example, in her rendition of 'I Wanna to be Loved by You'.[52] The renowned rock performer Madonna, who amplifies the sexual component of the singing process to great proportion, also uses free air in many of her songs.[53]

The variety of sexual issues which can arise when working with a client on free air sounds are numerous. Among some client groups with poor super-ego defences, delayed socialisation or other difficulties, genital erections among the men and seminal secretions among the women can occur and a mood of orgiastic excitement can develop. The work can, therefore, be extremely challenging, yet can provide an excellent forum for investigating the interface between sexual stimulation and personal containment. In groups of able-bodied people with emotional or psychological difficulties, previous instances of abuse can be recapitulated and fears of boundaries being disrespected can come to the foreground. As with all Therapeutic Voicework, therefore, the process requires extreme maturity and insight on the part of the practitioner.

Free air is, however, not innately sexual. For example, free air seems to find its way into the acoustic signal when extreme exasperation is experienced. At such times, the voice continually sighs both during and in between speaking. It is also a component parameter which can bring to the voice a quality of lament, melancholy and quietude. During the 1950s this vocal quality was used by Julie London, whose mellow airy quality is particularly evident in her rendition of 'Cry me a River'.[54] More recently, one of the most innovative uses of a free air voice is the singing and compositional style of Elizabeth Fraser, lead singer with the *Cocteau Twins*.[55] Use of free air to create a melancholy sound has been used by Suzanne Vega, which can be heard very clearly in her singing of the song 'Night Vision'[56], and by Margo Timmins, lead singer with the band *The Cowboy Junkies*, whose version of 'I'm so Lonesome I Could Cry' demonstrates an exquisite use of free air.[57] Whilst most singers tend to use free air consistently throughout their singing career, others have deliberately employed it for specific purposes. For example, Sinead O'Connor radically changed her singing timbre, infusing her voice with lots of free air, to sing the songs for her album 'Am I Not Your Girl?'[58] – which was a definite departure from the vocal qualities which she had hitherto utilised. Other singers, meanwhile, use free air in certain pitch ranges. For example, Joni Mitchell tends to increase the amount of free air when she rises in pitch and simultaneously moves from modal to falsetto register ++ >|< M ⫶ π >|< F.[59] The Irish singer Enya also moves in and out of free air, bringing the sensation of an interchange between lightness and density to her vocal quality.[60] One of the most stimulating uses of the free air parameter is that of Delores O'Riordan, the singer with the band *The Cranberries*, who yodels from a modal register without free air to a falsetto register with free air throughout all of her songs **<> M¡<▷ F**.[61]

For some reason, use of free air is less common in contemporary male singers. Exceptions to this include J. J. Cale, who uses a high degree of free air to create a vocal style which is languid, soporific and sensual.[62] Art Garfunkel also uses a lot of free air, as can be heard particularly in his rendition of the song 'Bright Eyes', which, like most of his songs, are sung in flute and clarinet **>K¡<▷**.[63] Randy Newman also uses free air but lower down the pitch scale;[64] as does Seal.[65] Outside of the West, an exquisite use of free air can be heard in the singing of west Kenyan Ayab Ogada, who has the same audible transglottal airflow as Garfunkel but a vocal tract primarily in saxophone configuration **⟨▷**.[66] Ogada's free air style typifies the soft gentility of many male East African voices.

In Therapeutic Voicework a client with a high degree of free air in the voice can be both trained to decrease it and simultaneously enabled to use it to express underlying psychological and emotional connotations through song and non-verbal sound-making.

PARAMETER SIX: DISRUPTION 〰 〰

Disruption is a disturbance, a dishevelment. We often use such sounds when we growl in order to scold an animal or a small child or when we screech, shout or holler. Disruption can also reveal an inner distress and anguish. The frictional disrupted voice in singing is widespread both within and outside of the West. Like free air, however, it is not permitted in the opera.

Within Western popular music, well-known frictionally disrupted male singers include Louis Armstrong,[67] Rod Stewart, Jo Cocker[68] and Tom Waits.[69] Given that disruption is employed to express anger and aggressive instincts, it is interesting that there are fewer female singers who use the quality in Western singing. Though it is true that the female vocal folds are less dense and thus more prone to damage as a result of friction and pressure, the reasons for this dearth are primarily cultural. For, in the West, women are less permitted to vocalise anger and aggressive instincts. There are, however, a number of female singers whose voice is identified, in part, by the use of frictional disruption including Bonnie Tyler[70] and Tina Turner.[71] Outside of the West, frictional Disruption can be heard alongside other remarkably extreme vocal techniques in the style of singing indigenous to Tuva, just north of the Mongolian border.[72]

Disruption does not always denote friction. It can also refer to other kinds of tonal and timbral inconsistency. For example, Janis Joplin used a disruption which 'broke up' the very high notes by alternating sound with silence very quickly.[73]

In Therapeutic Voicework disruption can be an excellent means of reclaiming assertive, retaliatory and aggressive feelings and their expression. It can also bring deeply buried anguish to the surface, facilitating acknowledgment, integration or catharsis. However, the Therapeutic Voiceworker needs to be aware that some singers have caused severe tissue damage through the use of disrupted sounds whilst others have enjoyed a pathology-free life and career. There are safe and unsafe ways of using the sound and proficiency in imparting healthy ways of using disruption should be an essential part of any Therapeutic Voiceworker's training.

PARAMETER SEVEN: VOCAL REGISTER M F VF W

Whilst in Swiss yodelling singers seek to exaggerate and amplify the register break, in Western classical singing the aim is to sing in only one of the registers – such as the falsetto soprano or the modal baritone – or to blend the qualities of modal and falsetto – eradicating any perceivable break, as in the contralto.

There are contemporary male singers who sing exclusively in the falsetto register – such as Jimmy Somerville, whose consistent register use can be heard particularly in his version of 'Don't Leave Me this Way'.[74] This singing style was precedented by singers such as Eddie Holman, whose version of 'Hey There Lonely Girl'[75] is sang in falsetto. *The Beach Boys*, meanwhile, created harmonies by combining male falsetto with modal registers.[76] Other male singers have sung predominantly in modal register with occasional breaks into falsetto. Of course, the classic demonstration of this musical form of register transition is the rendition of 'Great Balls of Fire' by Jerry Lee Lewis.[77] This sudden register break was slowed down and extended by Elvis Presley, particularly in his love songs,[78] and by Roy Orbison.[79] This style has been amplified and perfected contemporaneously by Chris Isaak, who travels a wide pitch range as well as moving from vocal fry through modal into falsetto; this can be heard particularly clearly during his song 'Wicked Game'.[80] Bono, lead singer with the band *U2*, also makes forays into falsetto at the top of his pitch range[81] whilst both Michael Jackson[82] and Prince[83] constrict the vocal tract into flute, creating a sound which passes in and out of falsetto.

The smooth but exaggerated passage from modal to falsetto in the male voice can also be heard in the so-called 'singing cowboys', such as Jimmie Rodgers,[84] and the renowned disseminator of the American yodel, Eddy Arnold, whose version of 'The Cattle Call' demonstrates a deliciously relaxed singing voice in both registers.[85] Many of these American men had incredibly wide pitch ranges – as can be heard in Tex Ritter,[86] who sings in the region of the baritone and bass yet still manages to create occasional falsetto breaks high in the pitch range, and Tennessee Ernie Ford, who not only moves between modal and falsetto but jumps from the baritone and tenor range up into extremely high pitches.[87] The same transitions are also heard in the yodelling style originating in Switzerland and Austria where both men and women swing between registers.[88]

A common term for the sudden change from modal to falsetto or vice versa is the 'break', for indeed it can feel as if something is breaking. The vocal changes which occur to the pubescent boy involve a transition from the childlike falsetto to the mature modal and this change is often described as the 'voice breaking'.

This breaking occurs naturally to the adult speaking voice during moments of excitement, such as when we laugh or express surprise. In Therapeutic Voicework the break between the two registers can, therefore, be used as an acoustic doorway into exploring tumultuous emotions. The modal voice also breaks into falsetto when we cry and, by gently guiding the voice repeatedly over the modal-falsetto interface, sorrowful emotions can be excavated.

Whilst some male singers have confined themselves to the falsetto range reserved for women in opera, some female singers have cultivated a voice which uses only the modal register. Grace Jones,[89] for example, sings only in modal, as does the American singer Odetta.[90] Coming further up the pitch scale, Siouxsie, from the band *Siouxsie and the Banshees* also sings exclusively in modal.[91]

Earlier in history, Mae West[92] sang almost exclusively in modal, as did Ava Gardner,[93] whilst Gloria Swanson[94] ventured into falsetto and gave the high pitch range a very fast vibrato. Rita Hayworth,[95] meanwhile, used both modal and falsetto as well as using a blended quality.

In listening to the great mid-century female cinema performers, one is reminded that modal is the usual speaking register whilst the falsetto is a quality especially employed for singing. In the cinematic musical, particularly, one can hear performers such as Joan Crawford, Judy Garland

and Jean Harlow go from speaking their text in modal to singing in falsetto. The men, meanwhile, would both speak and sing in modal and, therefore, one can sometimes barely hear the join between the speaking and the singing voice. This stylistic drift in and out of singing and speaking in modal register is exemplified in the cinematic performances of Tyrone Power, Bob Hope and Bing Crosby.

There is indeed something in the falsetto sound which is unnatural, unreal, a facet woven into the root meaning of the word itself: *falsetto* from the Latin for false.

Because falsetto is usually produced in the region of a high pitch range which, in turn, is normally associated with a woman, there is also something apparently feminine about the falsetto voice. During the Baroque and the Renaissance, some boys were castrated – which prevented the hormonal voice changes at puberty, removing the seat of male virility, and preserved a high falsetto voice comparable to a female soprano in a man's body. Because the high voice has its roots in the pre-pubescent stage of our development, it is naturally associated with the child in us and the ability of a man to sing in this register often requires contacting the inner child and giving it expression.

The overt masculinity shown in the castrati's face and body combined with a high-pitched and falsetto voice created not so much the image of a woman but of an androgyne or hermaphrodite, a perfect blend of male and female. This androgynous character appears widely in the mythology of many cultures as an expression of the unity of male and female in every human being. For, just as biologically the male possesses female genes and the woman male, so too, psychologically speaking, we possess elements of the other sex. Jung named the male part of a woman the animus and the female part of a man the anima, both of which are dormant and unconscious, rising up out of the sleeping soul in our dreams. Accepting qualities normally associated with the other sex is often a difficult process and meets with greater resistance the more we consciously stress our given gender. In men the usual difficulty encountered when attempting to sing in falsetto high in pitch has much to do not with a lack of physical proficiency but with this psychological resistance against contacting and expressing the feminine.

The androgynous figure is not only a synthesis of male and female but is also connected to the spirit and to God, which gives the sound its mythical and spiritual dimension. God, in transcending the world, transcends all opposites and is neither male nor female but both. Behind the Christian patriarchy which worships an all-male God there is a wealth of mythology which stresses the androgynous aspects of God and all of these mythologies tell that the world was created by a sexless being who was heaven and earth, fire and water, male and female. Plato proposed that it was from such an androgynous original God that human beings descended and he believed that in earlier times all people were androgynous and only later became divided into opposite sexes. Thus for a man to sing falsetto he has to unite his masculinity with the dormant anima, to rise above the conscious one-sidedness of his male gender and enter a fusion of opposites which creates an audible symbol for the spirit.

In the female voice, meanwhile, developing the modal register, its richness and viscosity, can assist in animating the animus, bringing a strength and power to the voice and the personality which is not related to force and pressure.

A particular technique, which is one of the identifying features of North American country music initially popularised by Patsy Cline[96] and exemplified in the singing styles of Billie Jo Spears[97] and Dolly Parton,[98] consists of sustaining the point of transition between modal and falsetto. This produces a suspended sound – neither modal, falsetto or blended – like a gentle sob.

Vocal fry usually occurs in the speaking voice at the end of sentences, where the voice feels as though it evaporates and disappears. However, neither the vocal fry nor the whistle register is heard very much in Western music other than as a brief excursive embellishment. In the Tuvanese style, however, the whistle register is sustained and amplified with specific shapes of the vocal tract to produce sustained piercing sounds.[99] Vocal fry, meanwhile, is central to the singing style of the Inuit peoples.

PARAMETER EIGHT: VIOLIN |ᐁ ᐁ|

Children and actors tend to increase nasal resonance, producing a voice with lots of violin when they play someone wicked, like a witch. Evil or wicked characters, such as Shakespeare's Richard III, are often given voices with lots of violin by actors. In singing the use of the violin component combined with extreme loudness to portray evil is used by Diamanda Galas in her vocal performance 'The Divine Punishment'.[100] Violin is also the sound which many people instinctively produce when impersonating both a baby and a very old person.

Each individual has differently sized and shaped nasal passages and there are certain races whose skeletal structure is composed of particular nasal shapes. Chinese, Afro-Caribbean and Anglo-Saxon people, for example, all have nasal passages with a fundamentally different shape, which gives rise to certain core sounds which are often recognisable as the vocal identity of a particular culture. Outside of the West, singing styles which utilise a high amount of violin include that indigenous to South Africa, exemplified in the singing style of Miriam Makeba, who also utilises a very mild disruption ⊽| ⌇⌇⌇.[101] The use of violin with saxophone configuration is also indicative of the singing style used in the Gambia.[102]

Violin is also the quality which English and American children automatically use when impersonating a Chinese or Japanese person. Indeed, the violin quality is evident in a number of oriental song styles – such as, for example, that used by the Cantonese opera,[103] the women singers of the Shanghai Opera of China[104] and those of the Hát Chéo, the traditional folk theatre of Vietnam.[105] Unlike the West African style, the oriental form of singing seems to favour more narrow vocal tract configurations.

The quality of violin is also a feature of the belting style of singing used in Broadway musicals, epitomised in the singing of Ethel Merman.[106] It was also distinctly audible in the singing of Gene Pitney,[107] Neil Sedaka[108] and, to a lesser extent and lower down the pitch range, in the singing of Johnie Ray.[109] Violin was also a strong feature in the voice of Billie Holiday,[110] the early singing of Bob Dylan[111] and of Mick Jagger[112] and it still characterises the voice of Neil Young[113] and the later work of Marianne Faithfull.[114]

It is interesting that many Afro-Caribbean singers have increased nasal resonance and in the West it was the violin quality, combined with vibrato, which characterised the voice of Al Jolson, who used make-up to give him the appearance of a black minstrel.[115] A similar use of violin and vibrato is heard in the voice of Marlene Dietrich.[116]

Violin, combined with the flute configurtion and the use of a lot of free air, >|< ⊽|, was used consistently by the 1960s singer Melanie, who created the image of the archetypal child, born to be free, and who made popular fame with her song 'I've Got a Brand New Pair of Roller Skates'.[117] Outside of the West, this combination of violin with free air is used by the women of Eastern Java, as typified in the voice of Gandrung Temu.[118]

PARAMETER NINE: HARMONIC RESONANCE AND VOCAL TRACT CONFIGURATIONS

The vocal tract behaves in compartments, which, for the sake of simplification, can be divided into two: the oral and the sub-oral.

For example, a classical baritone may be singing in saxophone at the sub-oral level, utilising the fully expanded pharyngeal space to amplify the harmonic spectrum which gives rise to the richness of tone necessitated by the opera. Simultaneously, however, the oral cavity may be in flute, utilising the narrowness of the mouth to enable the articulation of the words **O >< SO ()** (See Figure 1.15c, p.60). On the other hand, someone with a neuromuscular handicap may vocalise in saxophone at the the level of the oral cavity, the mouth wide and gaping. However, the sub-oral tract may simultaneously be very tightly constricted and narrow, that is in the flute configuration **O () SO ><** (see Figure 1.15g, p.60).

In observing clients in Therapeutic Voicework it is useful to keep this in mind. However, given that most singing requires articulation of a text, the mouth is usually used to create the configurative dimensions necessary to articulate vowels and consonants. The vocal timbre which identifies the singing style is, therefore, usually determined by the dimensions of the sub-oral tube, particularly the pharyngeal space. In using exemplifying singers it is thus this part of the vocal tract to which I refer.

THE FLUTE CONFIGURATION AND TIMBRE ><

Flute is a very narrow vocal tract configuration with the larynx held high in the neck with the result that the air expelled from the lungs and the sound-wave generated by the vocal folds is driven through a very confined space. As one might expect, voice use in flute can consequently create sensations of 'squeeze', 'tightness' and 'compression,' particularly where the sub-glottal air pressure is extremely high. Whilst this can often cause pathology, there are healthy ways of using the flute configuration combined with high air pressure and extreme loudness to produce moving singing styles.

One of the few Western singers to sing consistently in flute using modal register is Demis Roussos, who combines it with a warbling vibrato comparable to that used by Buffy Sainte-Marie;[119] another rare male flute is Charles Aznavour.[120] There is, however, an abundant non-Western use of flute configuration with high sub-glottal air pressure. When accompanied by soft glottal attack and low sub-glottal air pressure, the vocal timbre produced from this configuration can often sound 'thin' as it is resonating in a lean and slender space. This thin quality can conjure images of insubstantiality, weakness and lack of magnitude. Indeed, many of those who describe their own voice as sounding weak tend to make habitual use of the flute. Often, such persons feel that their voice is tenuous because they think that it is high in pitch and very quiet, when, in fact, it has more to do with the vocal tract dimensions. By enabling the tube to expand, such persons feel their voice to be stronger and more substantial, often mistakenly thinking it has become louder and deeper.

The breath arising from the flute configuration is cool and it is the configuration which we spontaneously make when we want to cool down hot food by blowing air from the mouth. Moreover, the resulting vocal timbre can often feel to the vocalist and sound to the listener as though it expresses a cool disposition. The experience of vocalising in flute is often one of feeling frosty, passionless and stoic. It is also, of course, the configuration which the mouth assumes during speech and it is the flute timbre which characterises the voices of many singers who have epitomised the highly enunciated form of singing, such as Julie Andrews.[121] This highly articulate, yet, therefore, controlled, form of vocalisation is naturally threatened by the lengthening and dilating of the vocal tract. To allow the flute configuration to increase dimensions and assume the clarinet and saxophone shapes often creates the feeling of letting one's heart be seen. And this can be intimidating, exposing and terrifying.

THE CLARINET CONFIGURATION AND TIMBRE <>

Clarinet is the basic configuration from which many trained or accomplished singers work; known Western singers who sing or have sung in clarinet include Matt Monroe,[122] Joe Jackson,[123] Joan Armatrading,[124] k. d. Lang and Karen Carpenter.[125] Vera Lynn sang in clarinet and used free air to soften the romantic and melancholy lyrics and vibrato to enhance crescendo whilst concentrating on the enunciation of the text. She also hardly ever used falsetto.[126] This technique was used by Doris Day, who also sang in clarinet.[127]

Marc Cohn displays extreme virtuosity in combining varying amounts of free air with a light glottal attack and a very mild frictional disruption in clarinet, <|> 〜〜 M ++ |2, with just enough loudness to be strong without compromising the emotional vulnerability engendered by the other components.[128] The same use of mild frictional disruption, but with greater force of glottal attack and loudness in clarinet, can be heard in the big rock singing style of Bryan Adams[129] as well as in the voice of Jon Bon Jovi, who also uses violin for certain phrases – particularly when high in pitch.[130] Of course, the great forerunner of the big rock style is Bruce Springsteen, who sings in clarinet with consistent mild frictional disruption but uses a spectrum of loudness from very quiet to very loud depending on the song.[131] In the blues genre the relaxed clarinet configuration with a mild frictional disruption is also typified by the singing of B. B. King,[132] and the same combination of components was also used by James Brown.[133]

The clarinet timbre is used as a container within which to combine an number of components by Michael Bolton, who uses disruption from mild to strong, moves from loud to quiet and also produces remarkable register changes from modal to falsetto, exemplified most clearly in his rendition of 'Said I loved you...but I lied'.[134]

THE SAXOPHONE CONFIGURATION AND TIMBRE ()

The most common everyday reasons for opening the vocal tract this wide are to yawn, belch or vomit. Therefore, when a client is approaching the full opening of the pharyngeal space, issues associated with digestion, regurgitation and illness connected to the digestive and gastrointestinal tract are often animated. Also, because the vomiting carries with it taboo or disturbing associations, pharyngeal opening into saxophone often instigates resistance, fear and shame.

Because of the connection between this vocal process and digestive tract sensations, clients will almost always place their hands upon the abdominal wall during saxophone work and describe the sensation of the sound being rooted there. The stomach and the guts are consequently present by implication and other sensations or sensory memories located in the abdominal region are often animated by saxophone work. A common sensation is that something palpable and ugly, such as semi-digested food, is going to 'come up', which causes the client to cease attempts at vocalisation and become captivated by a kind of shameful silence. It is as though the only safeguard against regurgitation is to close down the channel of oral expression and expulsion completely and become mute.

The process of extreme pharyngeal opening is further emotionally charged by the fact that, often, the acoustic timbre generated by the client who does vocalise in saxophone is rich in harmonics and is regularly described by vocalists and listeners as 'gaping', 'wide open' or 'booming'. Consequently, many clients are actually very surprised that they are able to produce the saxophone timbre without vomiting. However, the vomit which is expected often gets psychically located in the perception of the acoustic timbre. Clients find the sound indelicate, disgusting, raw and crude – as if they are regurgitating something which ought to remain within. They feel as though their voice is like vomit.

Because of the crude nature of the saxophone timbre on its first appearance, some women describe the sensation of vocalising menstrual blood or the placental fluid. Issues, difficulties or tragedies associated with pregnancy and child birth are, therefore, by implication, often provoked by the saxophone work. In addition, the crude nature of the sounds which are often initially produced may, to the client, 'sound like shit' in two ways. First, the client may feel that the sounds are undesirable, unmusical and, therefore, 'shitty'. Second, they may sound like an acoustic expression of faeces. One psychoanalytic interpretation of speech is that as spontaneous and uncontrolled urination and defecation become subjected to management and command through the process of toilet training, the act of speaking provides an alternative outlet for free-flowing and unrestricted discharge. Consequently, where vocalisation becomes subject to impedance and is over-tempered by outside demand, it cannot serve the function of expressing such discharge, causing retention and anxiety.[135] Therapeutic Voicework can, therefore, offer a contained framework for cathartic discharge of pent-up energetic sensations.

Because of the inevitability of provoking abdominal sensations or sensory memories through vocal work, it is vital to remember that working in saxophone is not a simple matter of getting the client to 'open up the throat'. Opening the pharyngeal space to its widest gauge carries with it a complex of implications which require delicate and committed attention and understanding. One of these issues is the nature of sexuality and sexual abuse. The shape of the vocal folds compares to that of the vagina and the opening of the laryngeal interior can feel equatable with the opening of the pelvic region. In fact, it is common for the pelvis to mirror the movement of the vocal tract during physicalised Therapeutic Voicework. This is intensified by the fact that opening the vocal tract makes one vulnerable to oral penetration; memories of such penetration, vaginal or oral, are thus almost inevitably provoked by Therapeutic Voicework.

The opening of the vocal tract to saxophone position is rarely necessitated by grown adults in everyday life. It is, however, a common experience in certain handicaps where depleted muscular control of the speech apparatus is accompanied by sporadic vocalisation emitted and amplified though a dilated tract. Often, such people simultaneously drool, for the open mouth makes it more difficult to retain the saliva and, if this is coupled with a neuromuscular dysfunction in the swallowing mechanism, the saliva has nowhere to go but outwards. So-called able-bodied people who experience this opening into saxophone often report identification with an image of someone handicapped. Others find that their voice characterises a figure whom they conceive to be stupid. The great archetypal figures of literature, such as Hugo's Quasimodo, Shelley's Frankenstein and Steinbeck's Lenny, are, in the theatre, often portrayed by actors who utilise maximum expansion of the sub-oral cavity to produce a saxophone timbre. It is also the natural vocal tendency of children when they want to impersonate someone they have identified as an idiot. The saxophone timbre is also that which is heard during both deep sobbing and guttural 'belly laughter'.

Western singers who have sung or do sing in saxophone include Heather Small, lead singer with *M People*,[136] Dean Martin,[137] who managed to sustain precise textual annunciation whilst maintaining expanded pharyngeal dimensions; Van Morrison, who in his early days used a lot of violin but in his more recent work has decreased his nasal resonance with the effect of maturing the sound;[138] and Bill Withers.[139] Saxophone timbre combined with use of disruption and vibrato at extremely high loudness was used by Screamin' Jay Hawkins, whose power and dexterity can be heard most splendidly on his rendition of 'I Put a Spell on You'.[140] However, probably two of the most expanded vocal tract dimensions are those used by Cleo Laine[141] and Nina Simone,[142] in both of whom the enormous acoustic vessel can be heard very clearly.

Conclusion: From the System to its Origins

The physiological operation of certain tissue structures, which I have reduced to a set of components, therefore actually combines to produce something elliptical, sonorous, liquid, transient and magnificent which we call the sound of the human voice. Furthermore, the expression of our self through this palate of components is rooted in the most elemental primary experience: birth and early life.

It is, therefore, to the very early experience of the infant and the relevance of vocal expression to infantile life that I shall now turn my attention.

Notes

1   Newham, P. (1998) *The Singing Cure: Liberating Self Expression through Voice Movement Therapy*. Boulder: Sounds True.

2   Newham, P. (1997) *Prayers and Prophecies*. London: Tigers Eye Press.

3   Newham, P. (1997) *Shouting for Jericho: The Work of Paul Newham on the Human Voice*. London: Tigers Eye Press/Class Productions.

4   Robbins, A. (1986) *Expressive Therapy: A Creative Arts Approach to Depth-Orientated Treatment*. New York: Human Sciences Press, p.245.

5   Minnie Riperton, 'Loving You', on *The Best of Minnie Riperton*, track 5. CD. (Capitol Records).

6   Kate Bush, *The Whole Story*. Cassette. (EMI Music).

7   Paul Robeson, *Live Concert from Tchaikovsky Hall, Moscow*. CD. (Fenix Entertainment).

8   Crash Test Dummies, *God Shuffled His Feet*. CD. (BMG Music).

9   Pearl Jam, *Pearl Jam*. CD. (Sony Music).

10   Barry White, *The Collection*. Cassette. (Polygram Records).

11   Sarah Vaughan, *The Best*. CD. (BMG Music).

12   Etta James, *Etta James*. CD. (BMG Music).

13   Nina Simone, *Lady Blue*. CD. (Charly Popular).

14   Odetta, *The Essential Odetta*. CD. (Vanguard Records).

15   Tracy Chapman, *Tracy Chapman*. CD. (Elektra Records).

16   Yma Sumac, *Fuego del Ande*. CD. (The Right Stuff).

17   Kate Bush, *The Whole Story*. Cassette. (EMI Music).

18   Mariah Carey, *Music Box*. CD. (Columbia Records).

19   Ellen Baylor, *The Live Experience*. CD. (World Records).

20   Pandit Jasraj, *Ragas: Triveni and Multani*. CD. (Navras Records).

21   Barbra Streisand, *Greatest Hits Vol. 1 & 2*. CD. (CBS)

22   Shirley Bassey, *Four Decades of Song*. CD. (EMI Records).

23   Liza Minnelli, *Maybe this Time*. CD. (Capitol Records).

24   Sarah Vaughn, *The Best*. CD. (BMG Music)

25   Mahalia Jackson, *21 Songs of Faith and Inspiration*. CD. (Music Collection International).

26   Edith Piaf, *The Legendary Edith Piaf*. CD. (EMI Records).

27   Buffy Sainte-Marie, *I'm Gonna Be a Country Girl Again*. CD. (Vanguard Records).

28   Joan Baez, *Hits/Greatest and Others*. CD. (Vanguard Records).

29   Nusrat Fateh Ali Kahn, *Shahen-Shah* CD (Real World Music).

30   Franco Luambo Makiadi, *Azda*. CD. (Sonodisc).

31   Attali, J. (1989) *Noise: The Political Economy of Music*. Trans. by B Massumi. Minneapolis: University of Minneapolis Press, p.27.

32   Attali, J. (1989) *Noise: The Political Economy of Music*. Trans. by B Massumi. Minneapolis: University of Minneapolis Press, p.27.

33   Attali, J. (1989) *Noise: The Political Economy of Music*. Trans. by B Massumi. Minneapolis: University of Minneapolis Press.

34   Astrud Gilberto, 'Love for Sale' on *Unchained Melody*. CD. track 13 (Temptation).

35   Various Artists, *Punk: The Worst of Total Anarchy*. (Disky Records).

36   Ozzy Osbourne, *Bark at the Moon*. CD. (Sony Music).

37   Meat Loaf, *Bat out of Hell*. Cassette. (Sony Music).

38   Bonnie Tyler, *The Collection*. Cassette. (Sony Music).

39   Purna Das Baul, *Songs of Love and Ecstasy*. CD. (Real World).

40   Bulgarian Women's Choir, *Le Mystère des voix Bulgares*, Vol. 1. CD (4AD).

41   Barbra Streisand, *Greatest Hits* vol. 2 & 2 CD (CBS).

42   Eddie Vedder and Nusrat Fateh Ali Khan, *The Long Road*, track 12. CD. (Sony Music).

43   Lebrun, Y. (1990) *Mutism*. London: Whurr, p.38.

44   Cleo Laine, *Solitude* CD (BMG Records).

45   Ella Fitzgerald, *Live in Berlin*. CD. (Verve Records).

46   Billy Bragg, *Workers Playtime*. Cassette. (Warner Communications).

47   Tom Robinson Band, *Power in the Darkness*. CD. (EMI Records).

48   Leonard Cohen, *Songs of Leonard Cohen*. CD. (CBS).

49   Various, *Cante Flamenco*. CD. (Nimbus).

50   Irene Papas, 'I am to Come I Was' on Aphrodite's Child, *666*, disc 2, track 5. CD. (Polygram Records).

51   Lebrun, Y. (1990) *Mutism*. London: Whurr.

52   Marilyn Monroe, 'I Wanna be Loved by You' on *Melodies of Love: Timeless Love Songs*, tape 1, track 10. Cassette. (GTV).

53   Madonna, *Something to Remember*. CD. (Warner Communications).

54   Julie London, 'Cry me a River' on *Melodies of Love: Timeless Love Songs*, tape 1, side 1, track 8. Cassette. (GTV).

55   Cocteau Twins, *Milk and Kisses*. CD. (Capitol Records).

56   Suzanne Vega, 'Night Vision' on *Solitude Standing*, side 1, track 5. Cassette. (A & M Records).

57   Margo Timmins, 'I'm so Lonesome I Could Cry', on The Cowboy Junkies, *The Trinity Session*, track 5, side 1. Cassette. (BMG Music).

58   Sinead O'Connor, *Am I not Your Girl?* Cassette. (Ensign Records).

59   Joni Mitchell, *Reprise*. CD. (Warner Communications).

60   Enya, *Watermark*. CD. (WEA Records).

61   The Cranberries, *Everybody Else is Doing it, So Why Can't We?* CD. (Island Records).

62   J J Cale, *Naturally*. Cassette. (Phonogram International).

63   Art Garfunkel, 'Bright Eyes', on *Scissors Cut*, track 6. CD. (Columbia Records).

64   Randy Newman, *Lonely at the Top*. CD. (Warner Communications).

65   Seal, *Seal*. CD. (ZTT Records).

66   Ayab Ogada, on *African Voices: Songs of Life*, tracks 1-3. CD. (Narada Media).

67   Louis Armstrong, 'What a Wonderful World', on Various Artists, *The All Time Greatest Love Songs*. CD. (Columbia Records).

68   Rod Stewart, *The Best of Rod Stewart*. Cassette. (Warner Communications).

69   Tom Waits, *Rain Dogs*. CD. (Island Records).

70   Bonnie Tyler, *The Collection*. Cassette. (Sony Music).

71   Tina Turner, *Simply the Best*. Cassette. (Capitol Records).

72   Shu-De, *Voices from the Distant Steppe*. CD. (Real World Music).

73   Janis Joplin, *Greatest Hits*. Cassette. (Columbia Records).

74   Jimmy Somerville, 'Don't Leave Me This Way', CD.

75   Eddie Holman, 'Hey There Lonely Girl', on *Unchained Melodies*, disc three, track 11. CD. (Star Direct).

76   The Beach Boys, *Twenty Golden Greats*. CD. (EMI Records).

77   Jerry Lee Lewis, 'Great Balls of Fire', on *The EP Collection*, track 1. CD. (See for Miles Records).

78   Elvis Presley, *From the Heart: His Greatest Love Songs*. Cassette. (BMG Music).

79   Roy Orbison, *All-time Greatest Hits*. Cassette. (Skyline Records).

80   Chris Isaak, 'Wicked Game', on *Wicked Game*, track 1. CD. (WEA Records).

81   U2, *The Joshua Tree*. CD. (Island).

82   Michael Jackson, *Thriller*. CD. (Sony Music).

83   Prince, *Greatest Hits*, vol. 1 & 2. CD. (Warner Communications).

84   Jimmie Rodgers, *20 of the Best*. Cassette. (RCA).

85   Eddy Arnold, 'The Cattle Call', on *The Singing Cowboys*, track 3. CD. (K-Tel).

86   Tex Ritter, 'High Noon (Do not Forsake me)', on *The Singing Cowboys*, track 9. CD. (K-Tel).

87   Tennessee Ernie Ford, 'Mule Train', on *The Singing Cowboys*, track 8. CD. (K-Tel).

88   Various Artists, *Yodelling Songs of the Alps*. CD. (Legacy International).

89   Grace Jones, *Warm Leatherette*. CD. (Island Records).

90   Odetta, *The Essential Odetta*. CD. (Vanguard Records).

91   Siouxsie and the Banshees, *Once Upon A Time and Twice Upon A Time*. CD. (Polydor/Geffen).

92   Mae West, *One Hundred Years of Cinema*. CD. (IREC).

93   Ava Gardner, *One Hundred Years of Cinema*. CD. (IREC).

94   Gloria Swanson, *One Hundred Years of Cinema*. CD. (IREC).

95   Rita Hayworth, *One Hundred Years of Cinema*. CD. (IREC).

96   Patsy Cline, *Twelve Greatest Hits*. CD. (MCA Records).

97   Country Collection, vols. 1-3. CD. (Hallmark).

98   Dolly Parton, *Dolly Parton: Her Greatest Hits*. CD. (Woodford Music).

99   Shu-De, *Voices from the Distant Steppe*. CD. (Real World Music).

100 Diamanda Galas, *The Divine Punishment*. CD. (Mute Records).

101 Miriam Makeba, *Welela*. CD. (Polygram Records).

102 Tiramakhan Ensemble, *Songs from the Gambia*. CD. (Sounds of the World).

103 Cantonese Opera, *Red Mansion Dream*. (Sound Factory).

104 Shanghai Opera, *An Introduction to Chinese Opera*, vol. 4. CD. (Marco Polo).

105 Hát Chéo, *Traditional Folk Theatre of Vietnam*. CD. (Unesco Collection).

106 Ethel Merman, *I Get a Kick Out of You*. CD. (Pavilion Records).

107 Gene Pitney, *Greatest Hits*. Cassette. (MAMC Music).

108 Neil Sedaka, *Oh Carol: His Greatest Hits*. CD. (Woodford Music).

109 Johnie Ray, *Remember Johnie Ray*. CD. (Document Records).

110 Holiday, Billie, *The Lady Sings The Blues*. CD. (Verve)

111 Bob Dylan, *Bob Dylan*. CD. (CBS Records).

112 Rolling Stones, *Rolled Gold: The Very Best of the Rolling Stones*. Cassette. (Decca).

113 Neil Young, *After the Gold Rush*. CD. (Warner Communications).

114 Marianne Faithfull, *Strange Weather*. CD. (BMG Records).

115 Al Jolson, *The Very Best of Al Jolson*. CD. (MCA Records).

116 Marlene Dietrich, *The Great Marlene Dietrich*. CD. (Intermusic).

117 Melanie, *The Four Sides of Melanie*. CD. (Unidisc Productions).

118 Gandrung Banyuwangi, *Songs Before Dawn*. CD. (Smithsonian/Folkways).

119 Demis Roussos, *The Story of Demis Roussos*. CD. (BR Music).

120 Charles Aznavour, *Greatest Golden Hits*. CD. (EMI Music).

121 Julie Andrews, *Broadway: The Music of Richard Rodgers*. CD. (Philips).

122 Matt Monroe, *Born Free: Greatest Hits*. CD. (EMI Records).

123 Joe Jackson, *Stepping Out*. CD. (A&M Records).

124 Joan Armatrading, *Joan Armatrading*. CD. (A& M Records).

125 The Carpenters, *25th Anniversary Celebration*. CD. (A & M Records).

126 Vera Lynn, *We'll Meet Again: Her Greatest Hits*. CD. (Woodford Music).

127 Doris Day, *Doris Day*. CD. (Telstar Records).

128 Marc Cohn, *The Rainy Season*. CD. (Atlantic Records).

129 Bryan Adams, *So Far So Good*. Cassette. (A & M Records).

130 Bon Jovi, *These Days*. CD. (Polygram Records).

131 Bruce Springsteen, *Greatest Hits*. Cassette. (Sony Music).

132 BB King, *Ain't Nobody Home: The Best of BB King*. Cassette. (MCA Records).

133 James Brown, *20 All Time Greatest Hits*. CD. (Polygram Records).

134 Michael Bolton, 'Said I Loved You…But I Lied', on *The One Thing*, track 1, side 1. Cassette. (Sony Music).

135 Sharpe, E. (1940) 'Psychophysical Problems Revealed in Language.' *International Journal of Psychoanalysis*, 21, pp.201–213.

136 M People, *Bizarre Fruit*. CD. (BMG Records).

137 Dean Martin, *The Best of Dean Martin*. CD. (EMI Music).

138 Van Morrison, *Days Like This*. CD. (Vanguard Records).

139 Bill Withers, *Greatest Hits*. CD. (Sony Music).

140 Screamin' Jay Hawkins, *Voodoo Jive*. CD. (CBS Records).

141 Cleo Laine, *Solitude*. CD. (BMG Music).

142 Nina Simone, *Lady Blue*. CD. (Charly Popular).

CHAPTER 3

The Infant Voice
A Developmental Approach to Therapeutic Voicework

Introduction: Recovering Lost Years

For many, Therapeutic Voicework can be a useful modality by which to work through and resolve early difficulties, trauma and injury of a very personal nature – for there are many whose adult voice has been thwarted, constricted, stifled and silenced by the negative results of infant and childhood experience. Consequently, the innate malleability and variability of the vocal instrument and its propensity for fluid expressivity through manifold combinations of vocal parameters becomes hindered: pitch range becomes restricted, harmonic resonance becomes limited and all other acoustic components of the voice assume the rigidity of a single compositional pattern.

It is thus extremely important that a methodology of Therapeutic Voicework is founded upon an understanding of the developmental psychological and physiological history of vocalisation in early infantile life. However, such an understanding is of use only if we can utilise it to design and implement physical exercises, educational strategies and compassionate procedures which enable the voice to find release from the developmental obstacles, problems and hindrances which few people are fortunate to escape.

Having outlined the rudimentary psychophysical components for an analytic system of creative, pedagogic and therapeutic Voicework, I shall begin, in this chapter, to place the system in the context of child development and introduce the reader to some of the methodological techniques which I have developed in response to my research into the progressive development of vocal expression in the child.

Dancing in the Womb

A healthy foetus moves inside the womb with a unique choreographic pattern of daily activity which is entirely self-motivated and does not correlate to external environmental circumstances such as the time of day or to whether the mother is awake or asleep.[1] This movement increases in magnitude and complexity during gestation so that the foetus 'has already the full repertoire of movements' which will be found in the new born baby.[2] This includes the movements which facilitate and accompany breathing and, consequently, vocalisation. The foetus is, therefore, artistically speaking, an improvising solo dancer rehearsing for the impending performance of life.

Visible movement appears at about seven and a half weeks with slow flexing and extension of the vertebral column and passive displacement of arms and legs. Then, at ten weeks, yawns, jaw opening and tongue movements begin to occur regularly as well as sporadic hiccups, which reach maximum frequency and magnitude at thirteen weeks.[3] Until this point in time during gestation, the tissue cylinder which will become the vocal tract is in clarinet configuration, that is to say that it is neither actively shortened and narrowed nor lengthened and dilated. Rather, it is passively positioned in a shape which, as adults, we experience only in rare moments of stillness, self-absorption and contemplation. With the occurrence of yawning and hiccups, however, the cylinder acquires the ability to actively increase length and diameter assuming the saxophone configuration, that is to say that through motor action of the laryngeal and physiognomical musculature, the elastic tube which will become the vocal tract is able to lengthen and dilate.

By twelve weeks, sucking and swallowing are present and are combined with more magnanimous breathing movements which are consistently rehearsed and which reach maximum magnitude at about thirty weeks. Despite this intricate expressive emergence of physiological process and skeletal muscular movement, the foetus remains mute without any acoustic self-accompaniment. Although the foetus is capable of registering and reacting to a range of sounds in the external environment,[4] the voice is released from silence only with the passage from womb to world. Whilst in the womb, where the foetus is completely surrounded by supportive fluid, enclosed, enveloped and enwrapped in an environment that is dark, wet and sonorous, the ears receive but the voice cannot react. Viewed from an adult perspective, there is, therefore, a shadow side to this container which stimulates a foetus who is unable to respond; it reminds us of the dual nature of water which is at once soothing and containing but at the same time drowning and suffocating. Later, this ambivalence will be experienced towards the mother, who will also be perceived as both nurturer and stifler. Furthermore, sound too is experienced by the adult as being dual in nature. Sound can bathe us, soothe us and surround us with a calm and undulating ambience but it can also penetrate, overwhelm and drown us out.

Despite its shadow, this womb is the safest place the impending infant will ever know – and in later life he/she will almost certainly attempt to recreate such a safe haven through every means possible.

Therapeutic Voicework Methodology: Establishing a Safe Spherical Space

At the core of every person's self-seeking is a pilgrimage to find a place of safety which will be strong enough yet flexible enough to contain the rampant and intemperate tide of their expressions and, as embryonic little people, our first experience of such a container is the womb which holds the physical body. Therefore, the experience of being safely contained can be rediscovered through activities which create for the body a sense of being held without restriction of movement.

The preliminary stage to the systematic methodology of Therapeutic Voicework which I have developed provides a matrix of physical movements and explorations called Spherical Space, which seeks to offer the body an opportunity to experience such sensations. The aim of the process, like the objective of all therapeutic strategies, is to facilitate the client's own self-containment. To this end, therefore, the Spherical Space work seeks to facilitate in the client the sensation that the space which surrounds the body itself is wombful, fluid, sonorous, all encompassing and, above all, spherical in shape.

The initial and persistent obstacle to this is the misconception that space is cubicle in nature, a notion reinforced by the fact that most adults live inside cubist constructions. In fact, however, all space, from the microcosm to the macrocosm, is spherical and curved. To reinstate a sensation which honours this physical fact, clients are introduced to the first stage of Spherical Space work known as 'Establishing the Sphere'.

Clients are asked to go to a part of the studio where they feel comfortable. Standing still, with arms hanging loosely by their sides, they are then asked to imagine themselves to be in the centre of a sphere. The studio is usually dimly lit and the practitioner or assistant provides vocal music. Clients are then asked to venture forwards and backwards, side to side and up and down,

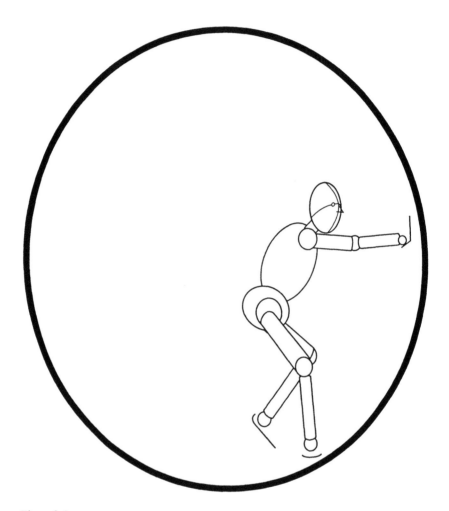

Figure 3.1

making hands-on contact with the imagined internal curved surfaces of the surrounding spherical space (Figure 3.1).

The first aspect which is immediately highlighted in this exercise is the diversity of magnitude between the spheres of different clients. Whilst some create for themselves a sphere which occupies half the studio, others create one so small that they barely need to leave the centre to make contact with the extremities. Moreover, the size of the sphere created by clients in ongoing work changes each time the exercise is pursued. It is as though we live in a transient process where the amount of space which is truly ours and in which we can move alters in connection with the transitional flux of our psychic operations. There are times when we are hemmed in, compressed and stifled and other times when we experience the spaciousness of our personality and self. There are also times when we seem to deliberately limit the size of our sphere, as though pulling in the boundaries and the limits of our self for protection and control. This is allegorised in the experience of having more or less room to be heard and in sensations of needing 'room to breathe'. As clients create for themselves a sphere, the practitioner observes its magnitude – which often reflects how much space the client feels there is in which to express herself.

It is useful for clients to imagine that the sphere contains their moods, preoccupations, desires, fears and sensations and that their selfhood does not end at the skin but also surrounds them. By offering clients this opportunity, the area of psychological reality which is experienced as being around, rather than within, the somatic container is made palpable.

As clients move through their sphere, it is usual for specific places within it to arouse particular affects – even though the relationship between identifiable geometric points within the sphere and the feelings, moods and sensations aroused by them is different for each person. For example, most clients experience a radical difference in mood when they are close to the back of the sphere compared to that which is provoked by being up against the front surface. For many, the back of the sphere instigates sensations of withdrawal, depression, introversion and fear whilst for others, meanwhile, it offers security, protection and a sense of confident stability. The front of the sphere for some is unnerving, exposing and feels dangerously unprotected whilst for others it is experienced as liberating and a place from which they can be seen and heard.

Spherical Space physicalises the sense of Self. This is not surprising given that so much of our self-language is geometrical. We speak of a damaged Self as being 'spaced out' and 'in orbit'; mental anxiety creates a feeling of being 'on the edge'; in depression we feel 'down' and in elation we feel 'up'; our minds go round in circles, we misplace our memories, shelve ideas and bury our desires; we conceive of the unconscious as being located in space beneath consciousness and the spiritual aspirations of the higher Self as being vertically above the conscious psyche. In fact, the concept of Self remains verbally inarticulate without recourse to a spatial metaphor or what Bachelard has called the 'poetics of space'.[5] The pitch parameter of sound is also experienced within the metaphor of physical space on a spectrum from high to low. Furthermore, sound is experienced as surrounding the listener 360 degrees, that is spherically. Establishing a spherical space thus prepares the ground for acoustic exploration.

The Body Mass of Spheres and Cylinders

The foetus, when fully grown at approximately 36 weeks, is a terrain of spheres and the human body remains spherical for the duration of its mortal existence before decomposing into the spherical atoms and molecules of ashes and dust.

On the outside, the human body is composed of spherical and semi-spherical surfaces which, at points of protrusion, are convex and at points of indentation are concave. The eye sockets, the navel and the mouth, the arch of the foot, the crest of the neck beneath the chin, the palms of the hands, the pits of the arms, the backs of the knees and the small of the back – all these are concave. And their nature is mirrored by the protruding ankles, the balls of the feet, the shins, thighs and buttocks, the belly, breasts and brows – all of which are convex (Figure 3.2). This concave and convex nature of the body is choreographically scored deep into the structure of the tissue during the gestating period when the foetus is curled in a position which, at the front of the body, is concave with an indentation at the bottom of the sternum and where the back of the body mirrors this with a convex arch of the spinal column. The inner environment of the body is also modelled on the sphere where a vital network of spherically-walled cylinders transports the elemental liquids and gases to and from the curvilinear organs in order to maintain the life force. Air passes through the cylindrical trachea and bronchi into the semi-spherical lungs whilst blood flows through the cylindrical veins and arteries, pumped through the semi-spherical heart. The body contains no cubes and no planes, only curves and cylinders.

Therapeutic Voicework Methodology: Convex–Concave Interchange

Having established and explored the imaginal sphere primarily with the hands, clients find it a logical step to revisit the inner surfaces of the sphere once again – this time allowing the convex curves of the body to lean into, and be received and supported by, the imagined concave surfaces of the sphere. This soon turns naturally into a dance as the convex head, shoulders,

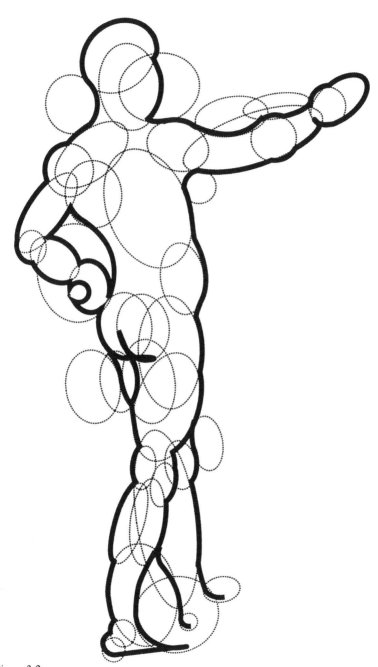

Figure 3.2

abdomen, hips and other protruding body surfaces are cradled by the imaginal inner concave surfaces of the sphere.

I have found that all clients, including those with muscular rigidities or congenital disability, find this process extremely liberating. Perhaps the notion of spherical space is so indigenous to the psyche's experience of spatial dimensions that the imagination is powerful enough to allow an imaginary spherical surface to offer actual physical support to the body's motion. Furthermore, spherical space allows the curvature of limbs, digits and spine commonly found amongst those with congenital neuromuscular disabilities to be amplified and stretched within their natural predisposition for movement, amplifying the artistic choreographic expression inherent in the kinetics of the disability itself.

It is during this dance through spherical space that it is useful to point out that while clients exaggerate a convex protrusion which is supported by the inner surface of the sphere, they are also inevitably creating an increased concave geometry on the opposite surface. In order to prevent these resulting concaves from causing vertebral compression or undue muscular fatigue, the client is asked to imagine that the grand sphere in which they move is populated with a variety of differently sized spheres which fit snugly into all the concave spherical indents made by the body. For example, as the arms stretch up, the hips drop down and the left side of the torso creates a convex curve resting into the concave wall of the grand sphere, so, meanwhile, the concave implosion created on the right side of the torso rests over the imagined convex surface of a sphere which gives further support. As the back protrudes and the spine curves over, making a convex arch which leans against the concave wall of the grand sphere, the concave curve simultaneously made at the front of the body lies over the imagined convex surface of another sphere. As the head leans over to the right, clients conceive of a small sphere fitting snugly into the concave curve running down the side of the face and across the shoulder. In other words, everywhere there is a concave indentation created in the body, so it is imagined that this is supported by the convex surface of a sphere of equal magnitude. Meanwhile, the client moves so as to lean all convex surfaces into the receptive concave wall, floor and ceiling of the grand sphere which contains their movement (Figure 3.3).

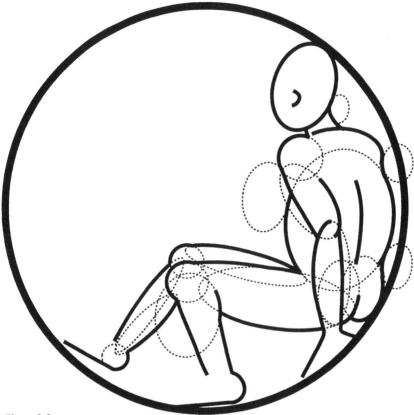

Figure 3.3

Therapeutic Voicework Methodology: The Personal Developmental Postural Cycle

Having established a sense of containing spherical space, clients are introduced to a simple, yet profoundly effecting, series of postures and movements which, throughout my methodology of Therapeutic Voicework, are varied to form a matrix of physical processes which I have called the Developmental Postural Cycle.

The first of this matrix is the Personal Developmental Postural Cycle. To begin, clients stand erect, with arms hanging loosely by the sides of the torso, the vocal tract shortened and narrowed into flute configuration and the lips, tongue and jaw held as though ready to speak. From this posture, clients move around the sphere in what I have called Walking Position (Figure 3.4a).

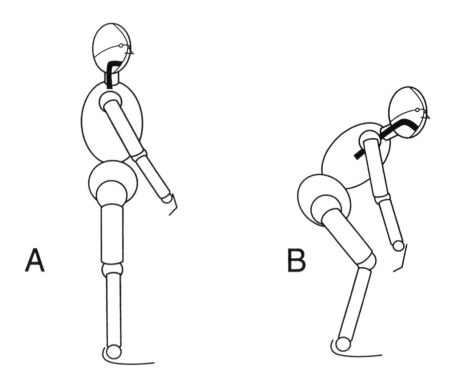

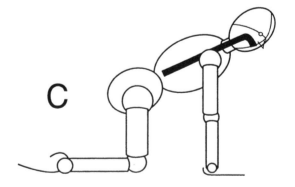

Figure 3.4

Second, clients allow the legs to bend at the knees, the torso to implode into a concave curve at the front, the pelvis to tilt forward and descend towards the floor and the head to hang over so that the eyes are focused downwards. This mirrors the concave curl of the foetus. As clients move into what I have called the Squatting Position (Figure 3.4b), they travel around their spherical space and allow the vocal tract to open and lengthen into clarinet configuration, as though they were going to drool, babble and coo.

Third, clients fall forwards, place the hands on the floor before them, bring their knees into contact with the ground and assume the Crawling Position (Figure 3.4c). As they do this they allow the vocal tract to fully dilate and lengthen into the saxophone configuration, as though belching, yawning or regurgitating. Clients then roll over onto their sides into a foetal position, onto their back and through onto all fours again before coming up through the Crawling Position into the Walking Position with simultaneous shortening and constricting of the vocal tract. They then begin the cycle again.

This choreographic journey provides a framework within which to experience a degree of regression to an infantile form of movement and vocal tract behaviour. As clients become familiar with the cycle, they begin travelling through the sphere, walking, crawling, squatting, rhythmically pushing themselves along on their buttocks and rolling. Through this process, clients experience the degree of muscular tension which is required to hold the vocal tract in flute configuration in preparation for speech and begin to relinquish such necessity, focusing on the acquisition of expanded vocal tract dimensions which will later serve increased non-verbal vocal malleability of expression.

Therapeutic Voicework Methodology: Orbit and Gravity

Working in a group situation, the sensation of spherical space is changed by the interelationship between participants. This means that sensations aroused at different points within the sphere depend, to some extent, on proximity between the various spherical spaces of participants.

During the work, the practitioner leading the exploration frequently asks the client to return to the centre of the sphere and then make a fresh departure. Thus as clients move and explore the Convex-Concave Interchange and the Personal Developmental Postural Cycle which is contained by Spherical Space, they regularly return to, and depart from, the centre of the sphere, thereby creating what is called Orbital Spherical

Movement. When at the extremities in a group situation, there is often a sense of being away from the centre – which can instigate a sensation of insecurity, of being without the stability of a home base or a place to come from. When pursued in a group, as other clients move into and out of each others spheres, participants can feel as though they are being caught off guard, psychically intruded upon or even penetrated.

To return a sense of personal boundary and self-protection to the exploration, it is, therefore, useful to introduce an alternative experience of moving. Instead of travelling in such a way as to be away from a centre to which it is possible to return, the client now moves in such a way that wherever they go the sphere moves with them in exact proportion and direction, as though they were gravitationally rooted to the centre of the sphere. This is generally referred to as Gravitationally Rooted Spherical Movement.

By interchanging between this sense of Gravity and sense of Orbit, a group of clients can explore the full range of possible relationships between sphere and body which appear to somatise and spatialise various experiences of the self in relation to others. This work then usually highlights a further psychosomatic phenomenon.

The degree to which another client or participant is experienced as 'close' has less to do with their actual spatial proximity and results more from where each one experiences themselves in relation to their own sphere. Two people can, to the outside eye, be millimetres from face-to-face contact. Yet if both are conceiving themselves as at the dead centre of their respective spheres, psychic proximity may not be particularly intense. By the same token, two people may appear to be separated by a considerable distance yet if both happen to be close to the edge of their respective grand spheres, the vulnerability may create the sensation of intense psychic proximity.

When explored in group work, it is during this stage of the spherical work that participants report a shift of sensation in response to proximity, real or psychological, to different members of the group; they become effected by what they sense of another person as they pass through or around their sphere.

This work, therefore, tends to bring into sharp focus the universally impending issue of how to balance the maintenance of a personal emotional continuity and contained boundary on the one hand with a receptivity to the influence of other people's expressions on the other.

The Architecture of the Cradle

Because our physique is spherical, it is most comfortably contained and supported by objects which mirror its convex or concave surfaces.

The convex curves of the body's shape rest with ease in concave receptacles, like the buttocks in a well-worn indented chair seat or the convex spherical surfaces of the head lying in the concave indent of a pillow. By the same token, the concave implosions of the body receive comfortably convex spheres, like a tennis ball in the palm of the hand or the convex inner sole of a shoe in the concave arch of the foot.

This natural tendency of the body to fit with itself and with other objects according to spherical geometry is epitomised in the two primary developmental architectures: suckling and cradling. In suckling, the protruding convex nipple rests in the receiving concave sphere of the mouth (Figure 3.5).

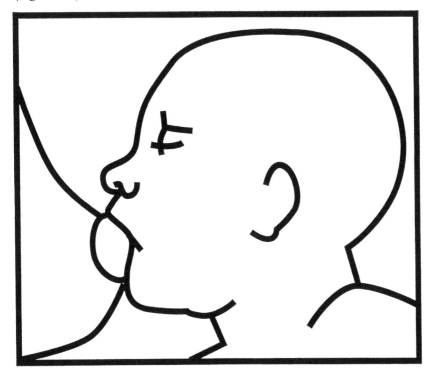

Figure 3.5

In cradling, the mother or primary care-giver creates a set of concave surfaces with arms, hands and torso which mirror, receive and contain the convex curves of the infant. As the baby's tiny body gyrates and wriggles, kicks and undulates, so the mother responds to the neonatal choreography with the kinetics of mirrored opposites, increasing degrees of concave receptivity where the baby's body becomes more convex and becoming more convex to

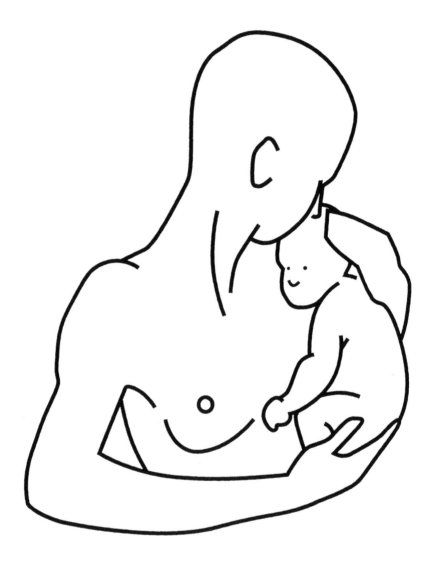

Figure 3.6

fit snugly in the crevasses created where the baby's body becomes concave (Figure 3.6).

Therapeutic Voicework Methodology: Relational Spherical Movement

The next stage of Spherical Space work, ideally suitable for group process, uses the symbiotic exchange of spherical choreography between mother and neonate as the foundation for an improvised dance called 'Relational Spherical Movement'.

With careful and methodical attention to one another's affective ambience, two people bring isolated body parts together in a concave-convex relationship. For example, the spherical head rests in the concave curve of the partner's shoulder and neck, then the partner becomes an initiator and bends forward creating a concave implosion of the torso which is supported by the other who creates a convex spine on all fours. This crouched position naturally creates a concave implosion of the abdomen and so the partner lying over the convex back now slides off and curls underneath, snugly fitting the torso into the abdominal concave. As clients relax and increase their sense of trust, couples begin rolling over one another and a dance is created from the simplest and most archetypal somatic design, simultaneously listening for the rhythm and pattern of breathing and allowing the mechanical turn-taking to slip into a more fluid dance where it is possible for each partner to remain in constant contact with the other. By this process, the other's body begins to play the same role as the imaginary spheres in the earlier individual work. The other body becomes a womb and a cradle yet, at the same time, separate and distinct. In this work each partner becomes a kind of substitute for the good mother who contains and cradles whilst, at the same time, in alternation, each partner becomes the child contained by that mother.

During this process, libidinous issues and concerns related to sexuality often arise for it is a highly sensual activity to move in physical contact with another person with an exaggerated focus of attention on the respiratory process whilst simultaneously exploring points of contact around a convex-concave interaction which, naturally, simulates eroticised physical contact. This work can thus provide a forum for the reclaiming of open, affectionate sensuality which need not connect with sexual consummation. However, due to the lack of differentiation in our culture between sensuality and sexual activity, the Relational Spherical Movement, which, for some, reflects the architecture of convex genital penetration of a concave orifice, can provoke attention to libidinous issues. The work therefore demands an extreme professional maturity of the practitioner, to which I refer in Appendix I under the subject of 'Ethics and Guidelines'.

The Waterlogged Ear

The passage of the babe from the liquid environment of the womb to the solid environment of the cradle is accompanied by a change in acoustic perception. The outer, middle and inner ear of the foetus functions in a liquid environment and is adapted to perceive acoustic frequencies through amniotic fluid. For about ten days after birth, the middle ear, particularly the eustachian tube, retains some of this fluid but then empties itself, causing the infant to lose its perception of high frequencies. At this point, only the inner ear remains full of liquid whilst the middle and outer ear are evacuated and have to adapt themselves to the impedance of air. The infant then spends some weeks adapting to hearing things in air and regaining the full frequency spectrum.

It is the work of Alfred Tomatis, a French doctor who began his career as an ENT specialist in the 1940s and who pursued years of detailed research into the connection between the voice and the ear, from which we can understand the therapeutic significance of this acoustic passage from womb to world.

Tomatis constructed experiments which simulate the sonorous aspects of foetal birth by electronically generating sounds played through a piece of equipment called the Electronic Ear. This device is able to filter sounds so that only certain frequency ranges or timbres are heard; it can, therefore, be used to take a person slowly through the acoustic changes which occur to the neonate as it passes from a liquid to a gaseous environment. Through this process, Tomatis says, it is possible 'to bring about reactions which touch the depths of the psyche' by enabling the ear to retrace the steps of birth.[6]

The psychotherapeutic use of Tomatis' work is exemplified in an example offered by Joshua Leeds regarding his own experience of treatment. Leeds came 'from a household with a controlling, angry, verbally abusive father' who shouted at him consistently, causing Leeds to 'tune him out', thereby minimising 'the impact of his verbal assaults'. When Leeds was subjected to a Tomatis Listening Test it showed depleted sensitivity to frequencies in the range which Leeds claims corresponds to that of an adult male voice. Thus, says Leeds, 'not only did I lock my father out, but I shut down my ability to clearly hear anyone or anything in that range'. The Tomatis programme used the Electronic Ear to retrain Leeds to hear frequencies in this range. As a result, says Leeds, 'I find relating to my elderly father no longer a problem', 'for the first time, I can hear what he is saying when he speaks'. Furthermore, 'I notice that I now crave male friend contact' and 'am also hearing myself more clearly than ever'.[7]

In his work with vocalists, Tomatis discovered that singers who had difficulty in producing constant tones in a certain pitch range were revealed to be deaf to that pitch range also. His suspicion was that there was nothing wrong with the larynx but with the sensitivity of the ear. So, rather than retraining the singers' voices, he retrained their ears and when singers were enabled to hear frequencies in a range hitherto unavailable, the ability of the voice to sing them followed. From this work, Tomatis concluded that a person can only produce vocally what he is capable of hearing.

The implications of Tomatis' work for a practical model of Therapeutic Voicework cannot be overestimated for expressive use of the voice requires what Gemma Fiumara has called an intense listening to oneself and others.[8]

The First Cry

Not only does noise in air sound very different to sounds filtered through the amniotic fluid but the newly born infant can now contribute to this acoustic environment. Indeed, it is the sound of the voice which marks the birth of every healthy neonate and, in the absence of crying, there was a time when a baby was induced to do so by the proverbial slap on the posterior. The life and soul of the baby depends upon its capacity to breathe and the voice consists of nothing but this breath made audible by the puffs of air rhythmically released by the vibrational opening and closing of the vocal folds.

Within moments of being born, the mucous clears from the baby's throat and soon after it cries. This cry of birth is the first mark which a human being makes upon the world. Moreover, healthy neonates will compose melodic structures of rising and descending pitch using the full vocal range available to them from the moment they are born.[9]

At fourteen days old, a baby's vocal folds are only about 3mm long and the lungs are so small that he or she has to breathe at a rate of around 90 cycles per minute in order to inspire sufficient oxygen to remain alive. But, despite the size of its tiny body, the baby is able to make an incredible volume of sound by maintaining a high sub-glottal pressure of air from the lungs against the vocal folds. Sometimes the baby sustains this intense sound-making for periods of such duration that it continues to amaze scientists that damage resulting from misuse of the laryngeal apparatus in neonates is almost unheard of. The sound of a baby's crying is one of the great acoustic archetypes and there are few people who do not respond to it with a definite reaction, be it positive or negative. This sound is loud, high in pitch, often with lots of free air. However, its main definitive feature is that it is so rich in violin, or nasality. This explains why adults instinctively utilise the violin quality by increasing nasal resonance when they impersonate a babyish or infantile sound. It also offers some insight into why adults who, for psycho-physical reasons, have a high amount of violin in their vocal timbre are often identified, labelled and sometimes ridiculed as being of an infantile disposition.

For the first three months the baby cries only as an expression of hunger and distress, the melody of which rises and falls like a siren. To midwives and paediatricians world-wide, each of these new-born cries is much like any other. However, within weeks, a mother will be able to distinguish her child's cry from that of many others without face-to-face contact. The mother has an innate aptitude, an in-built ability, to detect the idiosyncratic cadences, the unique quality of rhythm and melody, which her baby alone possesses. In addition to these tonal cries, the baby also makes what are called vegetative sounds: coughs, dribbles, hiccups, lip-smacking, burps and wheezes which result from physiological processes. It is this orchestra of vegetative sound, so instinctive and necessary to the infant, that is rarely tolerated in an adult within many cultures.

Many clients coming to work on their voice have a very fixed idea of the vocal sounds which are acceptable and those which are not. For many, the idea of making vegetative primitive sounds of little etiquette are abhorrent. Yet it is so necessary that such acoustic prejudices be overcome and that the voice be permitted to give free reign to the complete canvass of potential emissions, as it is in early infancy, if the original and primal malleability of the voice is to be rescued from the constriction of social priority.

At around three months old a new quality of crying emerges, which also has a rising and falling melody but which usually has a slightly higher pitch range than the melody of distress. This is identified as the emergence of the first pleasure cry. We observe this basic developmental acoustic principle as adults when pleasurable experiences instigate an instinctive rise in the pitch of the voice. From the issue of the so-called pleasure cry, the mother is able to differentiate between cries of hunger and cries of tiredness, between cries of physical discomfort and those of emotional irritability, between cries of distress and those of pleasure. In short, the mother has the capacity to perceive in the infant's melodic arrangement of pitch a language which is as sophisticated as the baby's needs.

The emerging pleasure sounds contain acoustic properties which act as the precursor for the vowels that will later be used in words and the differentiation between the melody of distress and that of pleasure is the baby's first step towards the acquisition of speech.[10] However, whereas the verbal infant will later organise such sounds according to the rules of the dictionary, the baby, not yet familiar with such a scheme, arranges them according to an intuitive, creative and innate sense of pitch, melody and rhythm in a fashion akin to the composition of music. This inborn natal musical aptitude which a baby has was the subject of some remarkable research conducted in the early 1960s in which the melodic patterns of pitch sung by a number of babies were plotted and their compositions published on vinyl gramophone by Folkways Records, an organisation now absorbed by the Smithsonian Institute.[11] The results of ongoing subsequent research in this area point to a meaningful relationship between the breadth and complexity of a baby's melodious and musical crying and its proficiency in the later acquisition of speech. It seems that a limited pitch range in pre-verbal singing often occurs in children who subsequently manifest delayed functioning in the proficient employment of speech.[12] There are also a number of impending developmental or congenital conditions, such as Down syndrome and Chromosome 5 deficiency, which can be detected in the melodic nature of early crying. More surprising than this is the evidence to suggest that the cry of a baby at risk from Sudden Infant Death Syndrome (SIDS) – more commonly referred to as 'cot death' – has certain acoustic characteristics, such as radical shifts of pitch, which may be recognisable enough to assist in its prevention.[13]

This instinctive musical arrangement of spontaneous vocal sounds in which are recognisable the raw material for vowels, and in which emotional predicament and perhaps even certain dysfunctional conditions can be detected, is known as 'cooing' and, in addition to the presence of the violin timbre, there is generally a high degree of free air in the sound. Again, it is this mixture of free air and violin in an adult voice which can give it an infantile appearance.

Between the ages of about 3 and 6 months a new kind of sound called 'babbling' issues forth. Babbling is identified as the emergence of sounds which form the raw material for consonants. The first to occur are those known as 'back consonants', in which the air flow from the larynx is interrupted at the rear of the oral cavity – such as 'k' and 'g'. This is followed by the production of what are called 'labial consonants', in which the air flow is interrupted at the front of the mouth – such as 'b' and 'm'. The ultimate achievement·of the babbling stage is the ability to combine these new staccato percussive sounds, which are akin to consonants, with the earlier sustained tonal sounds, which are like vowels. This gives rise to a stage in the child's communicative development which rewards parents, researchers, linguists and paediatricians with the utmost pleasure and fascination. The child talks in its own language, in which the attentive listener can hear, or so he thinks, words from his own language, words from foreign languages and words which are pure ingenious invention. This babbling continues until around 12 months, by which time the vocal folds in a healthy infant will have developed from their original 3mm to around 5.5mm. These continue to grow and by fifteen years old they are about 9.5 mm. Simultaneously, the original rapid rate of breathing slows down as the lungs grow in size.

Up to about 12 months the acoustic utterances of the baby – the crying, cooing and babbling – emerge purely instinctively and not as a result of any instruction from the mother or care-giver. Deaf babies cry, coo and babble just as hearing babies do.[14] The vocalisation is phylogenetically inherited in the same way as the instinct to suckle at the breast – it is one of the biological patterns of behaviour which the human species universally possesses – and, despite the unique quality to each baby's voice, there is a ubiquitous similarity to the crying, cooing and babbling of all babies that is recognisable world-wide. It is this innate universal attribute that gives it a specific quality of humanity and which may be described as the universal acoustics of primal vocalisation.

Hargreaves has shown how this innate aptitude for spontaneous babbling and melodic utterance in infants plays a pre-eminent role in the unfolding of musical awareness.[15] In addition, the pioneering developmental psychologist Howard Gardner has identified this pre-verbal ability to coo and babble as the inherent neurologically encoded capacity to compose and sing music, referring to the infant's first acoustic expressions as 'spontaneous song'.[16] Gardner reminds us that singing precedes speech and that 'the musical component drops out of speech after a year or so, and the child's singing and talking can be readily distinguished'.[17] For Gardner and many other researchers, as I shall later show, the acquisition of speech often involves the simultaneous loss of song.

Artistically speaking, prior to the acquisition of language the solo improvising dancer emerges from the womb to become their own accompanying vocalist, weaving the original and eternal song and dance routine that celebrates life without need for translator, director, conductor or choreographer. It is during this stage, before the rules of speech have been demanded of the infant, that the rudiments of songful composition and performance are explored and are often impeded by the overwhelming demands of language.

The next stage to the matrix of work which I have named Spherical Space involves facilitating an opportunity for clients to explore the sphere whilst accompanying themselves with spontaneous vocalisation, reanimating the early infantile experience of pre-verbal composition. This is called 'Sounding Spherical Space'.

Therapeutic Voicework Methodology: Sounding Spherical Space

In this exploration clients leave their partners and return to working alone where they re-explore the components of Spherical Space which they have, hitherto, experienced mute, accompanied by their own vocal utterances. Now, as they roll and turn, rise and fall, investigating the Convex-Concave Interchange and passing through the Personal Developmental Postural Cycle, they gently phonate. Clients are encouraged to allow a high quantity of free air to be present in the sound to let the vocalisation be gentle, vulnerable and towards the upper end of the pitch scale in falsetto register. The vocal tract is allowed to relax into the clarinet configuration and the mouth is left open, through which breath passes in and out. As clients enter deeper into the work, they are encouraged to begin allowing the lips and the tongue to momentarily stop the airflow, creating consonants and weaving a compositional babble which accompanies the choreographic gyration of their body. As the clients vocalise, they are encouraged to infuse the sound with a high quantity of violin and to allow the voice to trace out the melody of a siren.

The atmosphere provoked by this work is usually one of exquisite gentility and introverted awareness of very primary emotions. It is not uncommon for clients to weep as they work whilst others in the group may be smiling or laughing. It is important that all concerned are permitted the space to continue working physically and vocally as they experience and express such emotions. This prepares the ground for later Therapeutic Voicework where, like the greatest singers, clients will continue vocalising at their moments of most intense affect.

The Mother and Baby Duet

Just as the infantile capacity for the creation of spontaneous song is an innate phylogenetic predisposition utilised in the pre-verbal stage of infancy, so too, if the mother bonds with the infant according to ideal propensity, her perceptive faculty enables her to recognise the content of these songs in response to a pre-programmed instinct. That is to say that the mother has the potential to comprehend the emotion or need communicated by her baby's crying as an integral aspect of her genetic predisposition. Thus we might say that during the pre-verbal stage there exists between mother and baby a phylogenetic and symbiotic communication in which the mother associates the various qualities of the baby's crying, cooing and babbling with certain needs, ideas and references. It is by way of her positive response to them that the baby receives affirmation of the communicative efficacy of the sounds which it makes and the babbling eventually leads to mock conversations with the mother or care-giver which further serve to comfort and arouse.

Assuming adequate relational bonding does take place through the acoustic dialogue, the child absorbs a pleasure from making these audible emissions – a pleasure that is thereafter forever craven for, a pleasure that is entirely oral. The mouth thus becomes the seat of sensory stimulation on two counts: it is the locus of contact with the nourishing breast and the centre of operation in the production of sound. Furthermore, as Tomatis says, 'the vocal nourishment that the mother provides to her child' through her voice 'is just as important to the child's development as her milk'.[18] Indeed, we may go so far as to say that the mother's voice is a kind of substitute milk which flows out of the mother's mouth and into the baby's ears as the milk flows out the mother's breast or from the bottle in her hand and into the baby's mouth. Descriptions of sound making based on digestive metaphors such as 'chewing things over' or ' bringing things up' remind us of the fundamental connection between eating and vocalising and this elementary developmental fact provides a useful starting point in an attempt to understand why Therapeutic Voicework can often provoke reactions in connection with issues concerning eating and digestion, to which I shall refer in more detail later.

The mouth is not only one of the first centres of pleasure, it is also the original means by which a sense of power or control is achieved. The infant learns quickly that his needs are met in consequence to sound making and the positive response to his crying is the first experience an infant has of command and influence.

The vocal rapport between infant and mother is crucial to the former's development. When the infant vocalises and the mother or primary care-giver offers responsive vocal replies in return, the infant is likely to vocalise again.[19] However, this is only the case when the stimulating sound source is a human voice; the same response is not obtained when other noises are presented in answer to the infant's vocalising.[20]

There are other signals or clues which the baby observes or senses from the mother and, assuming that the baby is sighted, one of the most significant is the mother's facial expression which provides visual reinforcement of the acoustic message.[21] According to a theory concerning the 'roots of fascination' developed by Siegfried Bernfeld as part of his 'Sprachtheorie' and further developed by Paul Moses, the child will seek to 'imitate what is perceived' in order to 'master intense stimuli'.[22] Though the sounds which the mother makes do not require facial expression, the baby will nonetheless assume them in order to 'master' their effect upon her. However, where the mother's face is inexpressive, the baby may find it hard to mobilise its own physiognomy. This close developmental relationship between facial expression and vocalisation is remembered in many cases of selective mutism where physiognomical stasis and immobility accompanies the vocal silence.[23] Moreover, a number of electively mute children have also been reported to have minimal eye contact.[24]

The notion of imitation and fascination can be seen at work in the singing lesson where the teacher will often 'make faces' which correspond to the sound required and the student reflects the visual appearance of the face with a particular vocal quality. It is almost impossible to give a singing lesson without recourse to such an engagement and teachers who become overly tied to the piano, or who find active facial demonstration difficult, deny themselves and their students of this precious relational dynamic which is rooted in the earliest experience of life.

The optical relationship between mother and infant seems to contribute to the development of vocal rapport independently of facial expression. The vocabulary and variation of the 'gaze' between mother and infant was first described by Catherine Bateson as 'proto-conversation'[25] and visual acknowledgement between mother and infant seems to contribute substantially to the experience of attachment and bonding.[26] For example, five-month-old babies are more successful in discriminating happy, angry and sad vocal expressions when given the appropriate accompanying visual facial expression as an added cue.[27] When the eyes of an adult talking to a three-month-old infant are hidden behind opaque glasses, the baby is much less likely to vocalise[28] and blindness in either party effects the development of vocal and verbal rapport and conversance.[29] However, the visual field is considerably restricted when compared to the acoustic field of the baby's hearing. The baby, infant and adult can see less than 180 degrees and when a significant object, such as the mother, leaves this field, the baby can experience considerable anxiety. The sound of the mother's voice, however, like all sounds, surrounds the baby 360 degrees and the mother can maintain vocal contact with the baby at a greater physical distance from her. Sound, consequently, provides a more substantial source of sustenance and security than visuals.

The intonational patterns, prosodic composition, melodies and pitch contours which parents use to communicate non-verbally to their infant are the same in languages which, in all other respects, are entirely different in phonetic and annunciate form – such as Japanese, German, Italian and English.[30] Co-ordinated patterns of looking and vocalising, however, are not universal and in some non-Western cultures it is taboo for the mother to gaze directly into the baby's eyes. For example, in Papua New Guinea mothers hold their babies facing outward and talk in a high-pitched voice from behind the infant to make it seem as though the baby speaks.[31] The fact that healthy children in all cultures with differing codes of behaviour with regard to optical rapport acquire verbal language at roughly the same time would seem to imply that face-to-face co-ordinated optical and vocal rapport is not a prerequisite for the acquisition of verbal language.

Although for sighted individuals the voice quality of a speaker is only part of a complex multitude of signals which combines with visual and kinetic messages of face and body, for the visually impaired infant the acoustic messages of the mother's voice are elevated to a position of predominant importance and it is primarily from them that the blind and minimally sighted listener makes sense of what is said.

Whether sighted or not, for the hearing baby the sensitivity to sound which the foetus possesses is further developed after birth where, for example, babies of only a few days old will suckle more actively during feeding with music than without.[32] Moreover, babies respond in the same way to two entirely different verbal sentences if the pitch contour, prosody or melody underpinning the speech is identical. All hearing infants, sighted and non-sighted, respond to the emotional element of the mother's vocalisation contained in this melodic pattern, which has moderating effects on the baby and influences her emotional state.[33] In the early life of the neonate there is, therefore, a communication in which the baby recognises certain affective contents in the acoustic features of the mother's voice,[34] particularly in the pitch contours of different intonational patterns.[35]

The Sonorous Envelope

The maternal voice does much more than provide a conversant partner for the baby's acoustic emissions. It also acts as a container, an acoustic equivalent to a safe, delineated and boundaried spatial area in which to experiment with the actions which facilitate growth, the crucial necessity for which has been consistently described by the influential Bion.[36] The musical and acoustic dimension of this container, formed from the emissions of the mother's voice, has been named a 'sonorous envelope' which 'surrounds, sustains, and cherishes the child'[37] and a number of psychoanalytically-orientated thinkers have drawn attention to its significance. Julia Kristeva conceives of this acoustic container as a 'mobile receptacle'[38] whilst Claude Bailbé, acknowledges it as a primary exemplification of the quality of containment inherent in music.[39] Didier Anzieu has suggested that this envelope of sound created between the voice of mother and infant creates a 'bath of sounds'[40] forming an 'audio-phonic skin' which contains the emerging ego of the infant in the same way as the epidermal skin. Anzieu has also proposed that in cases where the mother's voice is abrupt it can prevent such a skin being formed, leading to later problems in ego development.[41] Silverman, meanwhile, says that the maternal voice provides the 'acoustic mirror' in which 'the child first hears itself' reflected.[42] Thus the vocal and physical relationship between mother and child reflects and moulds the child's developing identity and, indeed, it has been suggested that where the mother's vocal input is absent or too penetrative, resultant problems in identity may occur.[43] Also, a sense of insecurity experienced by the mother can be communicated to the baby through specific vocal timbres, which may give the baby the impression of a container which is unstable, undefined and frail, impeding the baby's own sense of security. This significance of the maternal voice as such a reflector is, according to Silverman, evident in the tradition of oral storytelling where the 'acoustic mirror' is held up not only by mothers but by grandmothers and nurses too who reflect the voice of childhood through fairy-tales, rhymes and songs. Silverman also shows how it has become commonplace to theoretically·characterise the maternal voice as a 'blanket of sound' and points out the negative implication of such a proposition.[44] This shadow side of the glorious and cherishing acoustic container provided by the maternal voice, which can also act not as a nurturing envelope but as an enclosure, constricting and suffocating, has been identified with particular incisiveness by Michel Chion, who states that the voice of the mother is 'woven around the child' and 'originates from all points in space as her form enters and leaves the visual field' which he is 'tempted' to name an 'umbilical net' and which he admittedly calls 'a horrifying expression, since it evokes a cobweb'. However, he claims that the 'original vocal tie will remain ambivalent'.[45] Silverman characterises Chion's descriptions as a vision of 'complete engulfment' and panic, comparing it to the visions of the other theorists to whom the maternal voice is 'a sonorous envelope', 'a mobile receptacle', 'a bath of sounds' or simply 'music'. Silverman observes in Chion's negative images 'an astonishing amount of negative affect around the maternal voice'. Trapped within the suffocating confinement of the mother's voice, the newborn child resembles a prisoner or prey. She concludes from the images and metaphors of enclosure that this view of the maternal voice facilitates the alignment of femininity with a negative and threatening conception of inner space.[46]

The French psychoanalyst, philosopher and feminist Julia Kristeva, influenced by the psychoanalytic theories of Sigmund Freud and Jacques Lacan, privileges the close contact between the child and its mother's body during the pre-verbal stage of the infant's life, concurrent with what Freud called the pre-Oedipal phase of development. Kristeva terms the disposition between mother and child during this stage as 'semiotic', a state of being where distinctions between subject and object are not yet formed. During this stage of development the infant is said to live in 'symbiotic' union with its mother in a non-verbal world of plenitude and fullness. However, when the father enters the scene of this asocial mother-child diad, as he is predestined to, he disrupts and separates the child from its mother's body.[47]

However, if the mother has little faith in the ability to contain, expressed in a voice which lacks certainty, the child is not so much a prisoner of over-containment or entrapment but an orphan without an acoustic home, wandering without a sense of being held. For such babies the relationship and rapport with the father may offer an opportunity to establish such containment.

The sonorous envelope of sound is potentially a perfect replacement for the watery container of the womb which supported the spherical convex and concave surfaces of the gestating body. Sound and water behave in similar ways, they travel multidirectionally, filling every crevice and passing through every chink. Unlike the optical field of the infant's vision, which is limited by the angle of the eyes' receptivity to light, the aural field is 360 degrees and sound stimulus can be heard from all directions. For the infant, containing sound replaces the containing womb, which can be both nurturing or suffocating and which can be over-present or not present enough.

Therapeutic Voicework Methodology: Relational Sounding and Movement

The next stage to the methodological exploration of Spherical Space is to bring clients together into pairs to re-explore relational movement in combination with sound making. As couples allow convex and concave surfaces to meet and depart, investigating the sensations stimulated by physical contact and withdrawal, so they simultaneously coo and babble, allowing themselves to hold and be held physically and vocally. In addition, combinations of looking and hearing are explored by working sometimes with eyes open and during other periods with eyes closed. This process of investigation creates, for many, a sense of wonderful sonorous containment, whilst for others it is a cacophonous cobweb. For everybody, however, it offers an opportunity to explore the artistic relationship between sound, sight and movement as rooted in the developmental psychology of early mother-infant relationship.

The Song as a Comfort Blanket

This work on Spherical Space provides the client of Therapeutic Voicework with a doorway leading to the powers of self containment, that is a sense of being held supportively within a private and boundaried field of experience. The essential necessity of such containment for the infant was central to the work of the renowned D. W. Winnicott, who started his career as a paediatrician and who stressed that the infant's psychic and physical relationship to the mother is established through a continuity of care, or what he called 'good-enough mothering'. For Winnicott, the continuation and development of physiology and psyche is thus dependent on the quality and reliability of maternal care;[48] 'good enough' mothering is natural, the mother must simply 'hold' the infant's environment so that the self can emerge and the infant only becomes aware of 'holding' when it fails or is dissonant. One example of the mother's holding is the act of rocking, during which what Winnicott calls 'the crude evidences of life' are signalled to the mother and include 'the heartbeat', 'breathing movements', 'warmth of the breath' and motions 'that indicate a need for change of position'.[49] In response to these signals, 'a mother may synchronise her rocking and walking with the baby's breathing. She might sing or hum a song that fits with the rocking rhythm' and she might find 'just the right moment' to 'put her baby down' in a way that is 'non-interruptive'.[50] This level of attention 'might seem like hard work or seem idealised, but Winnicott's point is that most mothers make these minute adjustments all the time without much thought'.[51]

In Winnicott's terms, the mother must actively adapt to the needs of the infant and, according to him, 'this active adaption demands an easy and unresented preoccupation with one infant; in fact, success in infant care depends upon the act of devotion, not on cleverness or intellectual enlightenment'.[52] The Winnicott infant is always 'good enough', thus, 'it is only the mother who is culpable'.[53] Winnicott 'effectively reduces woman's pleasure to pleasure in her baby, confining her to what is natural, keeping her from dangerous knowledge'.[54] It has been proposed that in his writing and broadcasts Winnicott assumes 'the voice of nature'[55] and that his wish is to act as a mirror for mothers, reflecting back at them what they already naturally know about infant care. He desires to play 'good mother' to his readers and patients, who are themselves like infants. This ventriloquizing of the mother's voice is, allegedly, effectively a surreptitious means to silence and control her.[56] Doane and Hodges propose that Winnicott is blind to the strains put upon a 'good enough' mother which, they say, 'calls for people who are relatively powerless', who are prepared to identify their interests with those of an infant, 'who are selfless' and who are 'always aware of another's needs' and willing to make them a priority.[57]

Given these extraordinary demands, Chodorow asks why women want to mother at all, rejecting the two typical explanations that it is women's natural destiny to mother and that women are conditioned by society to be mothers. Chodorow proposes dual parenting as a solution to the problem of destructive gender roles, believing that it would allow women and men to cultivate the underdeveloped parts of their psyches, thus enabling the next generation of males and females to raise children equally. Chodorow holds the conviction that the oppression of women originates in maternal omnipotence and the 'female monopoly' of mothering[58] and she has been criticised for her seeming lack of consideration for external influences as a source of women's oppression and for her use of the paradigm of a white, middle-class, heterosexual, nuclear family. However, she does provide for a serious consideration of how the notion of mothering as a gender-specific function might be substituted for the notion of caring as a trans-gender act.

Reframing for the Good Enough Dialogue

The work of Relational Movement and Sounding Spherical Space, in which couples move and sound together, reframes the traditional assumption that it is the mother's responsibility to provide 'good enough' care for an infallible infant. In the Spherical Space work emphasis is on the relationship and shared responsibility for holding and containing, rocking and nurturing between two equal persons.

During the exploration, as is often revealed through participants' discussion after the work, both partners experience positive and negative feelings in response to the other's provision. There are times when both parties feel held too tightly or not firmly enough, times when both parties feel abandoned and left for too long and times when both feel a synchronistic and symbiotic care which is just fast enough, just firm enough and which lasts just long enough before the bodies are released into their own space.

Furthermore, the work on Relational Movement in Spherical Space transcends the traditional gender setting of the female care-giver and the male or female infant. In this work men and women may work together in same-gender and different-gender partners. Furthermore, the age, sexual orientation, cultural origin or degree of parental experience is not a prerequisite for entering into the work. The capacity to give and receive good enough mothering becomes the capacity to enter into a good enough dialogue of exchange between holding and being held.

Holding One's Self and Remembering Being Held

It was Winnicott who also identified the function of what he called 'transitional objects'. This is the child's ability to invest an inanimate object with the feelings attached to a primary loved one, often the mother. The feelings projected onto the object give it the power to represent the mother and provide a substitute for her love and affection and, in particular, to continue providing a sense of containment in her absence. Winnicott said that the sounds produced by the infant's singing themselves become a transitional object and that singing is 'vitally important to the infant for use at the time of going to sleep', where it substitutes the mother's calming tones and creates 'a defence against anxiety'.[59] Subsequent researchers have also proposed that the infant's solo concertos which continue in the absence of the mother act as a transitional object. Gardner, for example, has pointed out that young children often give names to compositions and treat them as if they refer to particular events and persons.[60] The developmental psychologist Susan Engel has also proposed that a story, invented and repeated verbally by a child, can act as a transitional object by which it provides a container and receptacle for a complex web of ideas, thoughts and feelings associated with a primary person, thereby offering a comfort similar to that which they might find in fondling a teddy bear.[61] What Engels has proposed in relation to the story is surely even more true of children's songs, which, given the increased emotionality of musical utterance, provide an even more potent container for emotions.

Therapeutic Voicework Methodology: The Lullaby

Having explored relational activity in pairs, the next stage of Spherical Space work is to allow each client to return once more to a private sphere alone, where they are encouraged to explore moving and sounding in such a way as to recapture the sense of relationship with the partner whilst working alone. Through curling and turning, rolling and crawling, rocking and cradling, clients find the means to hold themselves by using one part of the body to take hold of another. Curling and rolling over onto one side, the head may rest in the concave implosion where forearm meets upperarm like a young child sleeping or the hands may take hold of the tummy as though aching or hungry. Combined with this self-caring and self-holding, clients recapture the sense of spheres, allowing the inner concave surfaces of the grand sphere to receive the convex protrusions of the body and allowing the convex surfaces of free-floating spheres to support the concave implosions of the body.

As clients develop their work, they are encouraged to vocalise in such a way as to compose a simple lullaby, without words or a conscious tune but with the natural self-absorbed sounds of a babe in arms. Contentment, safety and placidity is encouraged of the client as he or she moves and vocalises, creating a sonorous envelope and a kinetic cradle which holds the vulnerability of the tissue and bone, the soul and the mind in a protected, cherished and nurtured way.

After experiencing this self-holding in sound and movement, clients are asked to record their experiences of this journey through a short piece of spontaneous writing in the form of a simple lullaby. Usually, approximately four lines are enough to encapsulate the experience and the words are very simple. The client is then given an opportunity to gently sing the lullaby, witnessed by the practitioner and the group where appropriate. In the singing the client is encouraged to sing in a voice with free air and violin in falsetto register quite high in pitch. In addition, the client allows the prosody of the words to reveal the melody without any conscious attempt at musicalisation.

Intimacy and Bonding

The acoustic relationship between mother and baby is highly pertinent to the practice of psychotherapy, which is an entirely verbal and vocal relationship, often without face-to-face contact. One psychoanalyst who focuses particularly on the intonational component of this relationship is Riccardo Steiner, who says that because 'intonation belongs to the earliest moments of the communicative interaction between the baby, the mother and the father' it is, therefore, 'of paramount importance in helping to understand the characteristics' of how this relationship is re-enacted through the relationship between patient and therapist during psychoanalytic treatment.[62] But what Steiner says of psychoanalytic treatment is even more apposite to other forms of professional relationship, such as that between singing teacher and pupil. For many people entering into singing lessons, it is the first time since infancy that they have opened their mouths and expressed pure non-verbal sounds to another human being. There need be little wonder then why so many pupils find themselves experiencing intense emotions of all kinds towards their singing teachers and why the teachers can often feel overwhelmed by a dimension of the educative process for which there is little recognition and even less training.

One of the ways in which Therapeutic Voicework, as I conceive it, differs from the traditional process of singing training is its acknowledgement of the way that the intimate and primal rapport between parent and baby, which is predicated upon the exchange of non-verbal sounds, can be recaptured and re-enacted in the relationship between Therapeutic Voiceworker and client. Consequently, in Therapeutic Voicework the practitioner must understand that, at a certain level and at certain moments, the client will behave towards him or her with the same set of precepts, grievances, attachments and ambiguous feelings as are held towards the parent. In fact, at times the Therapeutic Voiceworker attracts a transference of the client's relational issues from the parents to the practitioner so that, in a certain way, the Therapeutic Voiceworker is perceived as the parents.

It is, in my view, this relationship between client and practitioner and the Therapeutic Voiceworker's willingness to receive the client's intensified sensations through the singing process that can make Therapeutic Voicework generally, and Voice Movement Therapy specifically, such a profound vehicle for change, for it offers a palpable and overt recapitulation of the most primary experience: the act of vocalising rudimentary feelings which exist before words.

Therapeutic Voicework Case Study: A Case of Gagging and Stammering

Martin was thirty-six. He was married with two children and had driven a taxi for twelve years. His reason for attending work with me was that he had what he described as a 'stutter', which no previous endeavour had succeeded to alleviate. He found it difficult to remember exactly when he developed a stammer but he felt that it was around the age of eight. I noticed at first that his stammer was irregular and vowels were as equally affected as consonants. However, the most striking thing about Martin's speech pattern was the involuntary jerking movements of his head and neck which accompanied vocalisation and which were particularly exaggerated during his 'stammering'. His eyes closed, his head tilted backwards and to one side, his neck stiffened and his facial muscles contorted. His head would then jerk rhythmically and spasmodically for the duration of the stammered sound. The look upon his face during such episodes was, to my personal eyes, one of tremendous fear. Then, on further listening to the so-called stammered sounds, I noticed that what was happening was more adequately described as a kind of contorted gagging of the larynx. The sounds which occurred during this balking were flute-like, strained and contracted and he described that it felt as though 'air could not get out'. I therefore became convinced that the majority of Martin's speech difficulties originated not in a stammered 'trip over words' but in a constriction of the pharynx and larynx. The number of times he stumbled over consonants made with tongue or lips were actually very few but the gagging occurred with all vowels as well as with certain consonants, particularly 'k', during which he would extend the sound into a gurgling noise which, if I refrained from witnessing the fearful expression on Martin's face, reminded me of a baby regurgitating or expelling unwanted milk.

Martin could not locate any single incident in his life which he could describe as severely traumatic. However, he spoke about his relationship to his father as having been a source of ongoing trauma. His father was a devout and extremely strict Catholic and a professor of chemistry; his other two sons were both doctors. It had been clear from quite an early age that Martin was not going to reveal the same predisposition to academic activity as the rest of his family. Another significant memory for Martin was that he had been the brunt of jokes made by his peers at school and by his brothers at home, who called him 'bunny' because he had an involuntary twitch in his cheek. And, though Martin could not locate any single traumatic event, it became obvious over the period of our work together that his entire childhood had been a very unhappy one. Not only did he grow up in the shadow of his brothers' achievements, but he also had a mother who showed him little attention and no physical affection. He could not remember ever being held or cuddled or kissed by his mother. Furthermore, he never saw his parents hold hands or show any physical signs of love to one another. The picture of his family life that emerged was an incredibly sterile one: dry academic conversations, competitive brothers, meals at regular times – often with guests who would parade their expert intellectual preoccupations – and a mother with a cool and distant relationship to her sons and her husband.

When, in the first session, I had asked Martin if he had any other illnesses or difficulties apart from his stammer, he said that he had for many years suffered periodically from extreme headaches. He dealt with them by taking a variety of analgesics but they rarely alleviated what he described as the 'sensation of pressure between his temples'. On investigating further the genesis of these headaches, it was revealed that they worsened during times of extended verbal activity; the more he stammered the more his head ached.

Martin liked his job as a taxi driver because 'on a bad day' he could 'get away' without talking to anyone. However, on a good day he would enjoy chatting to his customers and was frustrated intensely because he felt the stammer was preventing him from partaking of the social activities which he enjoyed. Martin was also keen to point out that as a taxi driver he frequently escorted customers of some importance: 'scientists', 'writers', 'actors' and others whom he described as having 'made it'. When asked to describe how he thought such people perceived him when he stammered, Martin was categorical that he appeared 'stupid'. The words he used to describe the way he thought that he was perceived included 'daft', 'idiotic', 'a moron' and 'a dim-wit'. These were all words which his brothers had used against him.

It emerged gradually that Martin had associated verbal proficiency with intelligence. The fact that he had not lived up to the academic standing of his father and brothers had made him feel stupid and his stammer further compounded this feeling and, in many ways, became a symbol for it. It was also clear that Martin wanted sympathy for his condition and he responded very eagerly to a sympathetic attitude. In this respect he had very clear memories of his grandmother, who had been a very important figure in his life as a child and a single source of comfort, understanding and physical affection and who had been been very kind about his stammer. It was also his grandmother who had told him that when he was born the doctors had told his mother that he was 'much too small and light' and that she should rectify this by feeding him twelve bottles of milk per day. Martin had, therefore, been awakened from sleep continually as an infant and force-fed with milk.

As I asked Martin to articulate different sounds and listened to his gagging, I could not help but see him still as a helpless baby being force-fed, desperately trying to spit out unwanted milk, screaming and crying and not knowing whether to swallow or spew. On asking Martin to speak of his defecating habits, he admitted that he suffered from both constipation and diarrhoea and rarely had prolonged periods of normal bowel activity. With this information in mind, I heard in Martin's vocalisations the strained, contracted sounds which we all make when trying to defecate during constipated periods.

I therefore asked Martin to extend all the sounds on which his pharynx constricted and simulate the sounds of a baby being forced to swallow milk which it preferred to expel. Naturally, this provoked some resistance in the

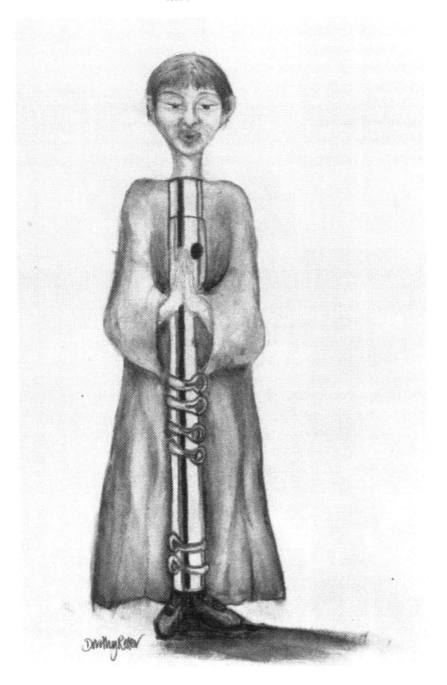

Figure 3.7

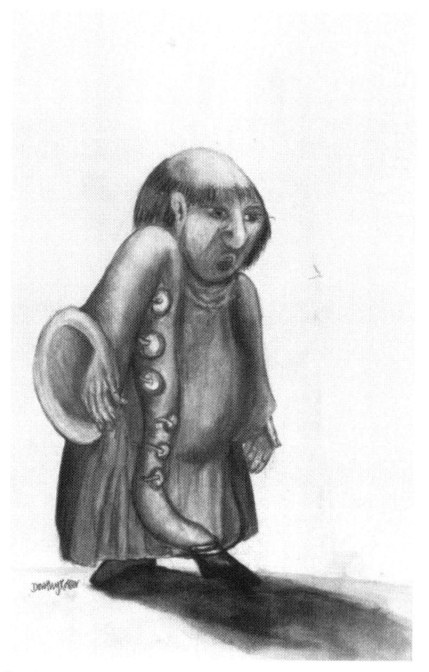

Figure 3.8

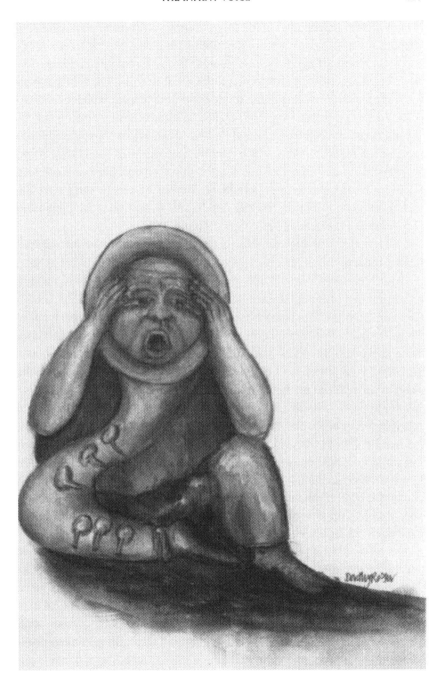

Figure 3.9

form of embarrassment and irritability. However, with gentle persistence he began to compose a very authentic symphony of baby-like babbling sounds made up entirely of the noises which arose from his inability to speak. The entire vocalisation was produced with the vocal tract in flute configuration > < and I found the quality of the sound moved me to tears, which stimulated in me a desire to rescue him. As I listened to him vocalise, I noticed that he had his hands clasped together and that his voice, when I listened through musicians ears, had a quality which reminded me of a Gregorian chant. It had lots of free air with very little force of adduction with no vibrato and was very quiet in a middle pitch range > ⟨ ⊨ ⊢⊢. I asked Martin to exaggerate the posture and the voice by raising his hands as in prayer and focusing imaginatively on the image of a monk (Figure 3.7).

Though this was easy for Martin, it also caused him some resistance because my suggestion reminded him of the religious demands of his father.

I knew that Martin would only overcome his gagging if he could vocalise with expanded pharyngeal dimensions and so I began to encourage him to open and lengthen the vocal tract. I asked him to stay with the Monk image but to imagine the figure to be fatter with a protruding abdomen and encouraged him to allow the vocal tract to lengthen and dilate into saxophone configuration ⟨⟩ (Figure 3.8). Although Martin was able to make progress with this, he became extremely agitated at this work, expressing fear and worry about 'what might come out' if he 'opened it all up'. He described feeling insecure when his 'throat expanded' as though he was going to vomit and not be able to 'control the spillage'. He also said that the work was beginning to cause him to be flatulent. I therefore began to teach Martin the Personal Developmental Postural Cycle, enabling him to pass from the constricted flute configuration and timbre of the Standing Position through more dilated and lengthened dimensions of the vocal tract towards the saxophone configuration and timbre in the Crawling Position.

The act of crawling and vocalising became very appealing to Martin as he crouched on all fours and cooed and spat, opening the pharyngeal space to resonate a gentle sound yet one rich in harmonic resonance. As his voice discovered the saxophone timbre, we realised that he had a beautiful bass voice and that he could sing the most complex linguistic phrases with complete fluidity, not stammering or gagging on a single sound. At one point during the exploration, Martin made a quality of sound which was more raucous than I had heard from him before and he sat on the floor and placed his hands on his head explaining that he felt a 'weird sensation' going from his temples down through to his anus (Figure 3.9). As Martin practised the vocal and physical work over a period of time, he reported two developments: first, his defecating habits normalised and, second, the frequency of his headaches substantially reduced.

It seemed that Martin's infancy had been couched in some confusion with regard to what should come out and what should stay in. First, he was forced to take in more milk than he desired and his natural instinct to expel it had been quashed by a mother who had been told to force it into him. Second, his parents had placed great pressure on all of the children to 'express' or 'push out' intelligent language and 'digest', 'swallow' or keep in anything that was not the material for academic progression. Martin, in realising he was not as 'bright' or as 'clever' as his siblings, had therefore kept quiet and when he did say something was simultaneously aware that it would not be welcomed or received with any respect or affirmation. Martin's thoughts and words were, like his milk had been, all stored up inside him, desperate to get out yet forced to stay in. This had led to a build-up of pressure, causing headaches and constipation which frequently transformed into unstoppable diarrhoea when he could not hold any more inside him. When we began working through the Personal Developmental Postural Cycle, his fear was that the equivalent to diarrhoea would come flowing uncontrollably out of his mouth. So the constriction of the vocal tract served to prevent this from happening.

Indeed, when we did dilate and lengthen the vocal tract, Martin experienced a feeling of endless fluidity with the bass and baritone quality of his voice flowing like a deep dark river. In fact, the first song we worked on with this newly discovered voice was 'Ol' Man River'. But, in time, Martin was able to shape and sculpture this voice in speaking and singing, articulating language without any gagging or stammering and without the ambivalent feelings of fear which originated in an infantile confusion about what should be taken in and what should be expressed.

Conclusion: From the Babble to the Word

Through the work presented in this chapter I have argued that use of the non-verbal human voice is, in the very first instance, connected to the elementary processes and experiences of early life and inseparable from the emerging relationship with the mother or primary care-giver. However, the infant soon passes out of the period of non-verbal vocalisation and simultaneously separates out from the intimate union and rapport with the mother to acquire a language with a cultural context.

In the next chapter I shall attempt to focus on the effect of this development into language, not only in the infant but in the species as a whole. In so doing I will try to show how Therapeutic Voicework can excavate the deeper strata of human experience which are beyond or beneath language, locating vocal expression in the instinctual and primitive experience of the human species.

Notes

1   Rayburn, W. (1982) 'Clinical applications of monitoring fetal activity.' *American Journal of Obstetrics and Gynaecology*, 144, pp.967–80.

2   Piontelli, A. (1992) *From Fetus to Child: An Observational and Psychoanalytic Study*. London: Tavistock/Routledge, p.30.

3   Piontelli, A. (1992) *From Fetus to Child: An Observational and Psychoanalytic Study*. London: Tavistock/Routledge, pp.29–30.

4   Herbenet, E. & Busnel, M. (Eds.) (1982) *L'Aube du Sens*. Paris: Stock.

5   Bachelard, G. (1994) *The Poetics of Space*. Boston: Beacon Press.

6   Tomatis, A. (1991) *The Conscious Ear: My Life of Transformation Through Listening*. New York: Station Hill Press, p.132.

7   Leeds, J. (1995) 'Revising the map of the musician's odyssey.' *Open Ear*, 3, pp.15–22, (p.17).

8   Fiumara, G. (1990) *The Other Side of Language: A Philosophy of Listening*. London: Routledge, p.162.

9   Ostwald, P. (1973) 'Musical behaviour in early childhood.' *Developmental Medicine and Child Neurology*, 15, pp.367–75.

10   Lewis, M.M. (1936) *Early Response to Speech and Babbling in Infant Speech*. London: Kegan Paul.

11   Greene, M. and Conway, J. (1963) *Learning to Talk: A Study in Sound of Infant Speech Development*. New York: Folkways Records, FX 6271.

12   Greene, M. and Mathieson, L. (1989) *The Voice and its Disorders*, 5th edn. London: Whurr, pp.62–65.

13   Stark, R.E. and Nathanson, S. (1975) 'Unusual features of crying in an infant dying suddenly and unexpectedly.' In J. Bosma and J. Showacre (ed) *Development of Upper Respiratory Anatomy and Function: Implications for SID*. Washington: U.S. Department of Health Education.

14   Greene, M. and Mathieson, L. (1989) *The Voice and its Disorders*, 5th edn. London: Whurr, p.64.

15   Hargreaves, D. (1992) *The Developmental Psychology of Music*. Cambridge: Cambridge University Press.

16   Gardner, H. (1982) *Art, Mind and Brain: A Cognitive Approach to Creativity*. New York: Basic Books, p.150.

17   Gardner, H. (1994) *The Arts and Human Development*. New York: Basic Books, p.190.

18   Tomatis, A. (1991) *The Conscious Ear: My Life of Transformation Through Listening*. New York: Station Hill Press, p.132.

19   Rheingold, H., Gerwirtz, J. and Ross, H. (1959) 'Social conditioning of vocalisations in the infant.' *Journal of Comparative Physiological Psychology*, 52, pp.68–73.

20 Weisberg, P. (1963) 'Social and non-social conditioning of infant vocalization.' *Child Development*, 34, pp.377–88.

21 Hortaçsu, N. and Ekinci, B. (1992) 'Children's reliance on situational and vocal expression of emotions: consistent and conflicting cues.' *Journal of Non-Verbal Behaviour*, 16, pp.231–48.

22 Bernfeld, S. (1954) cited in P. Moses, *The Voice of Neurosis*. New York: Grune & Stratton, p.11.

23 Ruzicka, B. and Sackin, D. (1974) 'Elective mutism.' *Journal of the American Academy of Child Psychiatry*, 13, pp.551–61.

24 Lebrun, Y. (1990) *Mutism*. London:Whurr, p.18.

25 Bateson, C. (1975) 'Mother-infant exchanges: the epigenesis of conversational interaction.' In D. Aronson and R. Rieber (eds) *Developmental Psycholinguistics and Communication Disorders*, Annals of the New York Academy of Sciences, vol. 263. New York: New York Academy of Sciences.

26 Wright, K. (1991) *Vision and Separation Between Mother and Baby*. London: Free Association Press.

27 Walker-Andrews, A. and Lennon, E. (1991) 'Infants' discrimination of vocal expressions: contributions of auditory and visual information.' *Infant Behaviour and Development*, 14, pp.131–42.

28 Bloom, K. (1974) 'Eye contact as a setting event for infant learning.' *Journal of Experimental Child Psychology*, 17, pp.250–63.
   Bloom, K. (1990) 'Selectivity and early infant vocalisation.' In J. Enns (ed) *The Development of Attention: Research and Theory*. New York: Elsevier.

29 Fraiberg, S. (1977) *Insights from the Blind*. New York: Basic Books.

30 Fernald, A., Taeschner, T., Dunn, J., Papousek, M.D., De Boysson-Bardies B. and Ikuko, F. (1989) 'A cross-language study of prosodic modifications in mothers' and fathers' speech to preverbal infants.' *Journal of Child Language*, 16, pp.477–501.

31 Schieffelin, B. (1990) *The Give and Take of Everyday Life: Language Socialization of Kaluli Children*. New York: Cambridge University Press.

32 Butterfield, S. (1968) *An Extended Version of Modification of Sucking with Auditory Feedback*, Bureau of Child Research Laboratory, Children's Rehabilitation, M.I.T. Medical Centre. Working Paper no 43.

33 Lewis, M. (1936) *How Children Learn to Speak*. New York: Harcourt Brace.

34 This, B. (1982) 'Foetologie.' In E. Herbenet and M. Busne (ed) *L'Aube de Sens*. Paris: Stock, pp.275–283.

35 Stern, D. et al. (1982) 'Intonation contours as signal in maternal speech to pre-linguistic infants.' *Developmental Psychology*, 18, pp.727–735.

36 Bion, W. (1962) 'A theory of thinking.' *International Journal of Psychoanalysis*, 43, pp.306–310.

37 Rosolato, G. (1974) 'La voix: entre corps et langage.' *Revue Francaise de Psychanalyse*, 37, no 1, 81.

38 Kristeva, J. (1978) *Desire in Language: A Semiotic Approach to Literature and Art*. New York: Columbia University Press, p.282.

39 Bailbé, C. (1978) 'Programmation de l'ecoute (1).' *Cahiers du Cinema*, 293, pp.53–4.

40 Anzieu, D. (1976) 'L'enveloppe sonore du soi.' *Nouvelle Revue de Psychanalyse*, 13, p.173.

41 Anzieu, D. (1979) 'The sound image of the self.' *Int. Review of Psychoanalysis*, pp.23–36.

42 Silverman, K. (1988) *The Acoustc Mirror: The Female Voice in Psychoanalysis and Cinema* (Bloomington and Indianapolis: Indiana University Press, p.100.

43 Anzieu, D. (1979) 'The sound image of the self', *Int. Rev. Psycho-Analysis*, 6, pp.23–36.

44 Silverman, K. (1988) *The Acoustic Mirror: the Female Voice in Psychoanalysis and Cinema*. Bloomington and Indianapolis: Indiana University Press.

45 Chion, M. (1982) *La Voix au Cinéma*. Paris: Editions de L'Etoile, p.57.

46 Silverman, K. (1988) *The Acoustc Mirror: The Female Voice in Psychoanalysis and Cinema*. (Bloomington and Indianapolis: Indiana University Press.

47 Moi, T. (ed) (1986) *The Kristeva Reader*. Oxford: Blackwell.

48 Winnicott, D. (1970) 'The mother-infant experience of mutuality.' In E. J. Anthony and T. Benedek (eds) *Parenthood*. Boston: Little, Brown and Co., p.253.

49 Winnicott, D. (1970) 'The mother-infant experience of mutuality.' In E. J. Anthony and T. Benedek (eds) *Parenthood*. Boston: Little, Brown and Co., p.253.

50 Hamilton, V. (1982) *Narcissus and Oedipus: The Children of Psychoanalysis*. London: Karnac, p.95.

51 Hamilton, V. (1982) *Narcissus and Oedipus: The Children of Psychoanalysis*. London: Karnac, p.96.

52 Winnicott, D. (1991) *Playing and Reality*. London: Routledge, p.10.

53 Smith, W. (1996) 'Voice, psychotherapy and feminism.' Paper Presented to the International Association for Voice Movement Therapy. London: October 1996.

54 Smith, W. (1996) 'Voice, psychotherapy and feminism.' Paper Presented to the International Association for Voice Movement Therapy. London, October 1996.

55 Doane, J.J. and Hodges, D. (1992) *From Klein to Kristeva: Psychoanalytic Feminism and the Search for the 'Good Enough' Mother*. Michigan: University of Michigan Press, p.22.

56 Smith, W. (1996) 'Voice, psychotherapy and feminism.' Paper Presented to the International Association for Voice Movement Therapy. London, October 1996.

57 Doane, J.J. and Hodges, D. (1992) *From Klein to Kristeva: Psychoanalytic Feminism and the Search for the 'Good Enough' Mother*. Michigan: University of Michigan Press, p.40.

58 Tong, R. (1989) *Feminist Thought: A Comprehensive Introduction*. London: Routledge, p.156.

59 Winnicott, D. W. (1991) *Playing and Reality*. London: Routledge, p. 4.

60 Gardner, H. (1994) *The Arts and Human Development*. New York: Basic Books.

61 Engel, S. (1995) *The Stories Children Tell: Making Sense of the Narratives of Childhood*. New York: W. H. Freeman, pp.38-39.

62 Steiner, R. (1987) 'Some thoughts on *"La Vive Voix"* by Ivan Fónagy.' *International Review of Psycho-Analysis*, 14, pp.265–272 (p.271).

CHAPTER 4

The Primitive Voice
An Instinctual Approach to Therapeutic Voicework

Introduction: On the Infancy of the Species

The development of the infant and the significance of vocalisation to this process is accessible through direct observation, both of infantile behaviour and of the adult repercussions of early experience. The development of the species as a whole and the potential role of voice in primitive forms of communication, meanwhile, remain the subject of speculation.

Nonetheless, throughout my experience of working professionally with people through non-verbal vocalisation, I have encountered a consistently recurring experience in the client. There is, in many, a general feeling that they possess a realm of experience, highly charged with feeling yet unnamed and beyond labelling, a realm which is at some times aggressive and at other times sorrowful, a realm which is desperate, urgent, vital and volatile. Dissatisfied with the ability of verbal modalities to provide a safe containing framework for the investigation of this realm, these people have found themselves pursuing Therapeutic Voicework in the hope that they can gain an opportunity to give voice to the deeply primitive feelings, moods and attitudes which words seem too refined and abstracted to express.

Through this vocal process there often seems to be a regression to an earlier period of human experience which makes palpable the idea that, perhaps, the species, like the infant, originated from a preverbal mode of perception and expression. During the work the client often appears to vivify and reanimate an earlier time in our history and evolution as sounds emerge which seem of mythical proportion: piercing screeches, bellowing sobs, spirited cries, beauteous and angelic melodies of glee as well as crude implorings of despair. Moreover, the client is often driven by a desire to reclaim, uncover or get back in touch with something which they feel has been buried.

Perhaps such a drive is not always the sign of an early personal trauma which begs for a cathartic release or objective analysis but rather a desire to reconnect with the power and the passion of experience which is too vivid for words to describe and which was once released through non-verbal vocalisation in the dim and distant primitive past.

The Dawn of Language

In the early part of the babbling stage of development the infant combines consonants and vowels to make his or her own language according only to the music of emotion and instinct. The smallest units of this spontaneous 'jumble-talk' that are usable for speech are known as phonemes, which are the acoustic differences in sound formations 'employed within a language to distinguish different words.'[1] For example, the sounds 'p' and 'b' are classified as distinct phonemes because words which are differentiated only by substituting these sounds will be decoded to signify different meanings – such as: pop/bop, big/pig and fop/fob. However, phonemes are not identical with the written letters of the alphabet as many require more than one letter to signify their sound, for example the sound 'oy' as in the word 'boy' and the sound 'ow' as in 'cow' are both phonemes. When listening to a child combine these phonemes in the preverbal stage, we are aware of his or her predicament – not from 'what' is uttered but by the 'way in which' it is vocalised. Likewise, the child responds not to the linguistic content of a parent's voice but to its pitch and quality.

This babbling is uttered instinctively according to a musical or tonal spontaneity in which 'vowels and phonemes are all just various ways of singing the world'.[2] However, the child's success as a potential adult with full communicative faculty depends upon his ability to bring vocal sound making into line with an order which is structured according to laws by which the phonemes are combined to formulate words which society understands as the language particular to its culture. The ability to use this code of language efficiently in differing social contexts has been called 'communicative competence'[3] and a prerequisite for this competence is the successful acquisition of an ability to combine phonemes into morphemes.

Although phonemes are the smallest units of sound formations which constitute language, they have to be further combined into larger units to disclose a linguistically meaningful message. The smallest units of sound formations capable of such conveyance are called morphemes. For example, in the words 'the foxes were frightened and ran for cover', the unit 'es' is a morpheme because it conveys the meaning that there was more than one fox.

The transition from a universal musical tonality of babbling to the acquisition of the language specific to the child's culture is achieved by a process of education. The care-giver, in responding to the child, repeats, encourages and 'rewards' those morphemes and combinations thereof which have a place in the words of her language and ignores, discourages or 'punishes' those which her particular language does not utilise, so that the unusable ones become 'extinct'.[4] The rules of this acquired verbal communication change from one context to another and from country to country and some sounds are accepted in one place and not in another. In German, for example, many words end with 'unf', a sound which is not accepted in English; the spoken language of Arabic as well as that of German makes use of the sound 'ach' – as in the name of the musical composer Bach – yet, again, this sound is not used English. Evidence arising from the most recent linguistic research seems to reveal that the human neurology is innately predisposed to organise articulate sounds into words and sentences according to grammatical laws. Though children are dependent on the 'punishment' and 'reward' responses of a care-giver to enter into a specific language, they also appear to make appropriate grammatical choices which have not been taught.[5] However, what remains certain is that the infant's original acoustic tapestry of spontaneous phonemic emissions, the jumble-talk and gobbledygook which utilises the entire range of semi-articulate sounds available to a human voice is, through the process of training, reduced until the only remaining sounds are those which are of linguistic use in the particular cultural context. This process, though on the one hand representing a development, also necessitates a cessation. For the English infant, for example, it means death to the 'unf' and the 'ach'.

Therapeutic Voicework Methodology: Free Phonetic Improvisation

Therapeutic Voicework can provide an opportunity to rediscover the ability to compose and sing one's own melodies, expressing emotion, mood, nuance and idea through spontaneous improvisation, without the impending necessity to make verbal sense. Free Phonetic Improvisation is a process which liberates instinctive musicality by returning to the client the complete canvass of semi-articulatory sounds corresponding to the entire palette of potential phonemes, which infants of all cultures possess prior to the acquisition of culture specific language.

The client is asked to vocalise, sometimes accompanied by a supportive sonorous instrumental drone, in such a way as to pretend to take a journey through every conceivable language of the world, real and imaginary. The Therapeutic Voiceworker, using images and technical instruction, thus inspires the client to locate the phonetic sense of Portuguese, Spanish, Russian, Arabic, Swedish and a host of languages. This stimulates a very primary infantile enjoyment, for many children pretend to speak a foreign language and emulate sounds which they have associated with a particular country.

One of the outcomes of this process is that clients usually find a magnificent musicality, as though being set free from cognition of linguistic meaning releases them into an experience of the underlying music and emotion. I have demonstrated this method on the audio-visual resources which offer further insight into the principles presented in this book.

The Language of the Father

In recent years an increasing amount of fresh psychological insight, knowledge and interpretative paradigms have emanated from feminist and post-feminist studies which have focused on two primary phenomena: first, the infant experience of the maternal body and voice and, second, the acquisition of language and its shaping of human development. Given these two subjects, 'it is apparent that psychoanalytic feminism holds particular relevance for the arts therapies where work is carried out at the interface of non-verbal and verbal experience'.[6]

Central to the tenets proliferated by feminist thinkers is recognition of the dominating significance of the infant's passage from a non-verbal stage of vocal rapport with the mother to the acquisition of verbally articulate language. Furthermore, a considerable proportion of feminist theory proposes that the acquisition of this language is coincident and simultaneous with the father's intervening in the hitherto exclusive duet between mother and baby. Thus the father is said to occupy the same position as language. Furthermore, 'because language is a substitute for the object it signifies, the child comes to understand that language is a sign of absence'.[7] In other words, in the preverbal or semiotic phase, vocal sounds act as a direct expression of experience. With the advent of language, however, the words serve to describe this experience. The word 'sad' replaces the sound of sadness. The word 'joy' replaces the sound of joy. As a result, the experience of sadness or joy is no longer necessary to the communication of their meaning and the nature of such emotions, therefore, to some extent evaporates.

As the infant enters the cognitive process of acquiring and repeating culturally specific sound signals according to an arbitrary linguistic order, the verbal language which is formed comes to replace the instinctive semiotic language of sound making which is hitherto endorsed, encouraged and understood by the mother. The instinctive, musical, semiotic 'other language' is at this time lost and its disappearance creates a sensation of absence or lack. There is no progression without bereavement.

For the French psychoanalyst Jacques Lacan and for feminist writer and psychoanalyst Julia Kristeva, this lack or absence is in direct contrast and opposition to the plenitude and fullness of symbiotic vocal discourse between mother and baby. Kristeva points out that, classically, this tonal language which accompanies the preverbal or 'semiotic phase' of infant development unfolds in an enclosed world of unity with the mother to whom 'the first affections, the first imitations, and the first vocalisations as well are directed'.[8] Borrowing the term 'chora' from Plato, she uses it to denote the mother's voice, which she proposes is the centre of the maternal container – what she calls a 'mobile receptacle' for the infant. However, the child's close contact with its mother through this voice is soon replaced by verbal language, which then acts as a medium through which the child can make contact with other persons in the social order, particularly the father.[9] Silverman, meanwhile, accuses Kristeva of underestimating the tutorial role which the mother classically assumes with respect to the child's linguistic education.[10]

Underneath and within the façade of verbal language, Kristeva hears 'a pattern or play of forces' which represents a residue of the early preverbal, semiotic phase during which the infant 'does not yet have access to language'. During this phase the infant's body is 'criss-crossed by a flow of urges, needs, feelings and desires'.[11] However, once the child enters the symbolic world of language, this flow becomes organised and articulated and, in consequence, the semiotic process is repressed and appears to be 'made prisoner of language'.[12] However, the crucial point with regard to Therapeutic Voicework is that this semiotic, preverbal world of need and experience may still be heard through the timbral and melodic undertones of language contained in the musicality of the voice.[13] Therapeutic Voicework, therefore, has the potential to reclaim the semiotic. Underneath the linguistic signification of verbal language is the musical realm of prosody, that is the melodic intonation with which words are uttered and this can occasionally change the meaning of sentences. For example, the sentence 'Susan kissed her mother and then Phillip kissed her' can indicate that Phillip kissed Susan or that he kissed Susan's mother, depending on the prosody. To indicate that he kissed Susan, we would probably sing a musical slide down the pitch scale on the last word: 'Susan kissed her mother and then Philip kissed *her*'. To indicate that Philip kissed Susan's mother we would be more likely to vocalise the '*her*' on a single note. This musical variation of linguistic content to change the messages which language encodes is called 'prosodic phonology'.[14]

Marius Schneider proposes that in ancient and primitive 'sound languages' the meaning of a sound or syllable may have depended upon the pitch on which it was 'sung' and may have formed the common source for both speech and song.[15] Today, this concept can be seen most abundantly in the language of Chinese where the tone or pitch upon which a syllable is uttered can completely change its meaning. Consequently, the melody of many Chinese songs is but an exaggeration of the tonal accents of the spoken lyrics.[16]

In most other languages, however, with the exception of sentence prosody, the relationship between sung melody and meaning is made redundant by verbal dexterity.

Piaget's Progress or the Loss of Instinct

Acquired verbal language has evolved to meet the demands of particular problems and forms of expression but is very poorly adapted to communicating information in certain areas. For example, verbal language is far less adequate at describing how to tie a knot than the language of a pencil diagram; it is also 'bad at conveying pain or emotion'.[17] Despite this, there is a widespread assumption that because speech supersedes song chronologically in infant development it therefore represents progression to a more advanced level of functioning. The predominant source of such an assumption descends from the work of Piaget.

In Piaget's model of development the qualities which differentiate the later and so-called higher stages of infant growth from those accompanying the earlier years pertain to the child's ability to construct and combine abstract symbols and comprehend their relationship to the phenomena therein represented. Language is one of these abstract symbol systems, numerical figures constitute another. Piaget's view of the child's aging is one which perceives a goal-directed movement towards ever increasing sophistication in the cognitive assimilation of logical ideas and relations through the manipulation of abstract symbols. In the early stages of development a child is unable to conceive that an object exists when it is out of sight or hearing or when it cannot be touched, tasted or smelled. The child's knowledge derives from the senses. However, it gradually realises that objects continue to exist and exert an influence upon the world even when the child cannot experience their presence sensately and it is this mental dawning which facilitates the linguistic process of naming things. By giving objects names, they acquire a permanence and the child is then able to process relationships between these linguistic symbols without ever having to come into sensory contact with the objects which they signify. The names become abstracted from the things and come to stand in their place. Language represents the missing object; it signifies a lack.

The most comprehensive critique and criticism of this overly logical aspect to Piaget's schema comes from Howard Gardner, who points out that Piaget has 'paid little heed to adult forms of cognition removed from the logic of science', has given 'scant consideration' to 'the thought processes used by artists, writers, musicians, athletes' and offered 'equally little information about processes of intuition, creativity or novel thinking'.[18] Gardner points out that an adult's ability to comprehend, appreciate and 'know' a phenomenon does not depend on the degree to which he cognitively understands the systematic logic of the underlying structures.[19] A composer or a deeply insightful music buff may have as highly developed faculties relevant to the production and perception of music as an expert in score notation but the former's approach is intuitive, creative and non-logical. In Kristeva's terms, perhaps, this intuitive approach is semiotic.

The implications of Gardner's thesis for childrens' education reminds us how little attention has been paid to the significance of this non-cognitive apprehension and perception in schools. This is as apparent in music as it is in any other subject, where the emphasis, the criteria for future development and the accessibility of higher education and training has been linked more to the individual's cerebral understanding of the logical operations around which music supposedly coheres and by which its virtuosity of execution is supposedly preserved than on his or her artistic perception of the extra-logical aspects of the human condition which music was, in the first instance, born to express. Fortunately, this situation is slowly being dismantled as a result of contemporary research.

Much of this research has emanated from Project Zero, an interdisciplinary programme based at Harvard University, of which Gardner is part and which provides a long-overdue antidote to the logical legacy of Piaget.[20] A key figure in this research is Jeanne Bamberger, who discovered that the more proficient children became in musical notation the less able they were to demonstrate the creative ability to sense and describe its moods and affects or recreate them through improvisation. Bamberger calls this the 'wipe out effect'[21] and her plea is for an increased respect for natural, non-formal, playful and spontaneous music-making in the school classroom. Research contemporaneous with Bamberger's, carried out by Moog,[22] Dowling[23] and Davidson,[24] has shown a widespread innate tendency to create music through the organisation of repetitive pitch patterns amongst very young infants. The increased ability in cognitive comprehension, such as in the reading and reproduction of musical notation, may, therefore, be seen as much as a process of extinguishing a natural skill as the acquisition of a new one.

In the schooling of children the emphasis is slowly shifting towards an appreciation of children's non-formal capabilities in music lessons. The recommendations for music in the UK National Curriculum now acknowledge the need for 'intuitive' alongside 'formal' musical activity and creative music making may already be overcoming the 'wipe out effect' in some school classrooms.[25] This is helped by a number of independent projects, such as The Voices Foundation, which, with the patronage of Lord Yehudi Menuin and in affiliation with a pan-European project called M-USE, aims to transform music in schools by working through the use of singing games.[26] Moreover, many teachers are recognising that the demands of the National Curriculum can be met through the use of singing and do not require pupils to be instrumentally competent or musically literate.[27]

Other workshop leaders who work with children through singing in the UK include Mary McLaughlin, who also works with children who have 'special needs';[28] David Oliver, education officer for the 1996 Folkworks Festival at the London Barbican;[29] Carolyn Robson, a trained teacher and, at one time, Education Officer for the English Folk Dance and Song Society;[30] Paul Schofield, who teaches singing games to both children and group leaders in the playgroup setting;[31] Leon Rosselson, who, in collaboration with Sandra Kerr, runs children's singing workshops;[32] and Margaret

Kenyon, who runs singing groups and instrument-making sessions for people of all ages as well as offering training for teachers and play scheme leaders.[33]

Projects such as the Voices Foundation and practitioners such as those aforementioned draw on the recent history of pioneering challenges to traditional music education mobilised by a number of key pioneers. These include the Swiss pedagogue Émile Jaques-Dalcroze, who capitalised on children's capacity for physical rhythm through movement to teach music;[34] the Hungarian teacher and composer Zoltán Kodály, who remodelled musical education in Hungarian schools bringing the singing of traditional folk songs to the centre of the teaching process;[35] and Rudolf Steiner, whose body of work known as Eurythmy is taught in schools based on his philosophy throughout Europe.[36]

The Non-Language of Voice

A strategy of communication which uses messages which are non-cognitive, non-symbolic and non-linguistic but intuitive, semiotic and musical draws on what Gardner terms an artistic 'intelligence' which suits those who cannot or do not want to transform their inner mental schemas and ideas into understandable verbal patterns.[37] Perhaps, then, rather than perceiving the relationship between preverbal and verbal forms of expression as a developmental progress from one to the other, we would create a truer and less prejudicial picture of the human condition by considering them as two equally important aspects of our expressive potential. We know that music is processed by neurological operations quite separate from those serving language formation because brain-damaged patients who lose verbal capacity are often left with musical ability intact. From an extensive study of patients with brain damage, Gardner has proposed that human beings comprise distinct neurologically-localised intelligences, seven in total, of which musical intelligence is one. Gardner argues that these intelligences have their own language, their own symbol systems and need to be treated distinctly with equal respect.[38]

One of the most influential and significant contributions to an understanding of the underestimated importance of non-logical and intuitive expression has come from the research of an American philosopher, Susanne Langer, who, in response to Ernst Cassirer's delineation between artistic and scientific forms of thinking,[39] proposed that human beings have the capacity to utilise two distinct types of language: one is intuitive, instinctive and creative – such as the natural music of the infant voice – the other, meanwhile, is logical, cognitive and learned – such as the verbal language of a culture. Langer's hypothesis, which has subsequently been expanded by Nelson Goodman,[40] points out that the realm of human experience is wider than that which linguistic verbal language is capable of representing. She proposes that within the field of 'our experience there are things which do not fit the grammatical scheme of expression', things 'which require to be conceived through some symbolistic schema other than discursive language'.[41] Langer refers to the units of this other symbolistic schema as 'non-discursive symbols', the aspects of human communication which are the vital expression of an individual's subjective experience and which can only be understood by way of an intuitive interpretation. The non-verbal sounds of the human voice – sighs, grunts, gasps, the subtle variations of pitch, quality and volume and the idiosyncratic application of prosody – are, she proposes, non-discursive symbols. Langer asserts that, historically, it has been the special role of the artist to deal primarily in non-discursive symbols which are 'untranslatable' and 'cannot be explicated by any interpretation'.[42]

For Langer the oldest and most primal example of non-discursive artistic expression is music, which she describes as 'a tonal analogue of emotive life'[43] and an expression of 'the greatness and brevity and eternal passing of everything vitally felt',[44] the origins of which she traces to the preverbal vocal utterances not of the individual infant but of early humankind.

Langer believes that spontaneous sounds arising from 'work rhythms, dance measures, choric utterance' and other instinctive expressions 'formed music out of the sounds that are natural to man' and which 'he utters at work, or in festival excitement, or in imitation of the world's sounds – the cuckoo's cry, the owl's hoot, the beat of hooves, feet, drums, or hammers'. For Langer such noises 'are transformed into characteristic motifs', which are the constituting intervals, rhythms and melodies of sung music. That is to say that 'all the actual ingredients of song' are 'inspired by sounds heard in nature'.[45]

The universality of the non-verbal but highly vocal period of neonatal expression has led a vast battery of speculating minds, including Langer, to postulate that the infancy and development of the human species as a whole also evolved from a period in which primitive peoples did not speak with words but voiced with sounds. According to this conjecture, before the acquisition of language in the development of the human species, communication took the form of a combination of vocal sound and bodily movement, an acoustic gesture, a vocal dance, an act of singing. Allegedly, to communicate anger, fear, sadness or revenge, people had to both vocalise and physicalise the essence of these emotions, which involved a spontaneous translation of affective experience into a synthesis of acoustic and kinetic expression.

From what we can observe in neonatal behaviour, we might reasonably posit that the composition and choreography of this historically imagined primeval song and dance was not an abstract representation of emotions but a direct expression of affect and instinct through muscular action. We may expect the communication of fear to have involved the combination of increased breathing rate and loud panting, a raised vocal pitch punctuated by a flickering vibrato and accompanied by a defensive bodily pose, perhaps crouched with arms covering the head.

Because such communication would have necessitated the total involvement of body and voice in the enactment of affect, it would also have been necessary to experience emotions even when describing them in retrospect. A preverbal expression and communication of the fear and retaliation provoked by an encounter with a raging bull would have required the same physical and vocal animation whether experienced in the present or many moons ago. Moreover, perhaps, this principle of a communicative song and dance, based upon the reproduction of experience, was applied not only to the expression of emotions but also to objects, animals, the climate and, in fact, to all subjects of communication. To describe the danger of an approaching bear, perhaps it was necessary to enact and emulate the essential nature of the animal with the body and the voice, to growl and grunt in deep, booming and thunderous tones accompanied by bodily movements which mimicked the rearing and careening of the approaching beast. Indeed, the origin of expressive movement may well derive from such communicative emulations and it has been argued that animal movements constitute the origin of dance as we know it.[46]

In the absence of words, the body and the voice probably had to assume a thousand different shapes in the course of describing a single day's events. These presupposed people of preverbal cultures therefore had to be great performers, sculpturing and orchestrating their bodies and their voices like singing acrobats, embodying a child, an animal, performing fire and rain, expressing triumph and defeat. And, perhaps, it is from these essential and primal vocal utterances that the act of singing and songwriting originates.

Early Song

In the early 1920s Otto Jesperson asserted that human beings 'sang out their feelings long before they were able to speak their thoughts' and that both 'our comparatively monotonous spoken language and our highly developed vocal music are differentiations of primitive utterances' which compare to 'the singing of birds', 'the roaring of many animals and the crying and crooning of babies'. For Jesperson such sounds are 'exclamative, not communicative', arising 'from an inner craving of the individual'.[47] Jesperson had been influenced by a famous essay on the origin of music by Herbert Spencer, which proposed that the function of 'singing' in these postulated preverbal cultures was to release emotional energy, ventilating and dispensing the psychological excitation generated by the vital experiences of life. That is to say it was equivalent with what Freud described as 'abreactive catharsis', the discharging of pent-up energy absorbed as a result of negative or traumatic experience. It is such emotionalised sounds of release that Jesperson thought provided the raw material out of which the earliest songs were born.[48] Ernst Kurth, in his famous text *Musikpsychologie*, written in the late nineteen twenties, also points out that the 'thematic roots of folksong' actually stem from the 'psychological roots' of the human condition revealed in the songs of all races through 'certain recurrent, simple idioms' such as 'calls, chimes, cradle-rhythms, work rhythms', 'shouts' and 'hunting-calls' which are nothing less than 'ultimate symbols of their vital consciousness'.[49]

There were many other scholars of this period who perceived language as a sophisticated development of elemental emotional expressions, including Malinowski,[50] Sapir,[51] Jesperson[52] and Davis, who in 1938 published a hypothetical postulation that all languages originate in vocal sounds of 'emotional tension, conditioned by the physiology of all peoples', of which onomatopoeia and echoism are the only surviving vestiges.[53] Jung too asserted that 'language was originally a system of emotive and imitative sounds' which served to express primal affects such as 'terror, fear, anger' and 'love' and which imitated sounds heard in nature like 'the rushing and gurgling of water' and 'the roll of thunder' as well as 'the cries of the animal world'.[54]

Since the early days of such postulations and Kurth's explorations into what he called 'music psychology', the study of indigenous songs in a voluminous variety of cultures has grown to grand proportion within a field most commonly labelled 'ethnomusicology'. From such research it has been possible to discover that all cultures, no matter how diverse in other respects, create, retain and disseminate songs which express subjects fundamental to the human condition – such as love and hate, birth and dying, need and longing.

Bowra, one of the early researchers of this field, has shown that, as in the development of the infant, so in the transpersonal historical development of the species, primitive songmaking served to articulate primal emotions.[55] Bowra studied primitive songs of cultures in which, he believes, earlier sensibilities are preserved – such as the Pygmies of Gabon and Ituri, the Semang of Asia, the Veddas of Ceylon, the indigenous peoples of the North American Arctic, the Yahgans from south Tierra del Fuego and the aboriginal Australians[56] – and discovered that in many cultures song 'is often found without words or with sounds that have no meaning' and yet are still 'perfectly effective'.[57] Bowra's discovery invites a link to be forged between the culturally primitive indigenous song and the primal vocal expression of each infant throughout the ages who spends the first period of life singing without words, effectively communicating through the sounds of the sung voice alone.

A connection between the 'babble songs' of infants and primitive music is revealed by Sachs, who notices how both are extremely repetitive. The peoples of the Dim tribe in central New Guinea, for example, constantly repeat two notes with an interval of a fourth apart.[58] Sachs further points to the appearance of very simple melodies and rhythms which are repeated successively in many forms of primitive music.[59] Schneider has said that 'primitive melody' is 'scarcely more than a continually repeated and varied motive'.[60] Sachs has pointed out that the repetitive songs sung by children also have this property of repetition.[61] Furthermore, in both infant composition and primitive vocal song, the timbre and emotionality of the vocal style is more suggestive of its meaning than the compositional structure of the melody.[62]

Bowra's second observation of early songs is that 'they are essentially dramatic', revealing 'the first, faint beginnings of the theatre'. In such songs 'parts are acted, whether of men or animals or things or spirits, and the actors of these parts feel that they somehow embody them and partake of their personalities'.[63]

This also relates to the early months of each infant's life, during which the baby is completely identified with the mother, cradle and blanket, the smells, noises and visual field and all the components of the environment and does not yet possess a sense of separateness and individual entity. Furthermore, as

Erich Neumann has described, in early infant life we observe the most likely process by which human consciousness was born in the ungraspable preverbal and pre-thoughtful distant past, when men and women did not feel themselves to be separate from nature.[64]

Voice, Song and Nature

In our reconstructed preverbal civilisation, vocal sounds which were first uttered as the spontaneous exclamation of feeling states were, perhaps, latterly employed to paint in sound all physical properties of the environment, such as water, earth, heat, cold, night, day, sun and moon. Information about the environment and its contents could have been communicated through an expressive and apprehensible embodiment of the essence of their being. The act of early singing could, thereby, have preserved a close sympathetic relationship between humankind and nature in the same way that the early songs of the infant preserve an exclusive intimacy with the mother. In such a context the sensible qualities of the environs would have been understood experientially, for it would not have been possible to communicate 'about' things without, first, experiencing and, second, embodying their rudimentary nature through sound and movement.

In many early cultures where the notion of animism prevailed, every object and being was believed to be endowed with a soul or spirit and the fundamental essence of something, which was transcribed into sound and movement for the purpose of communication, was probably believed to contain this spirit. Therefore, when people sang of the bear, they became one with the animal's soul and so too they partook of the sun and the moon, the earth and the river so that to all things and all phenomena there was beholden a sound, an acoustic symbol, a vital cry.

These acoustic symbols of 'vital consciousness', which, we may speculate, were once expressed through the spontaneous vocal sounds of early peoples and later formed the core of primitive song, compare to the preverbal musical babblings of the infant, as though each new born child in a matter of months traces the development of human beings played out over thousands of years. The sounds which we place in the mouths of preverbal peoples would, perhaps, have had in common with preverbal infantile music a generic universality, giving voice to a level of human experience which constitutes a collective consciousness, a trans-cultural level of feeling. Such preverbal or non-verbal sound does not 'describe' or 'represent' phenomena but 'exposes' an immediate response to experience. Unlike the subsequent development of culture-specific languages which have generated a communication barrier between different peoples, these trans-cultural and paralinguistic expressions of affect continue to infiltrate the oral code of humankind, revealing a common experiential root to all humanity. A cry or laugh or shout is the same the world over.

With regard to this primary level of vocal expression which reveals a common depth of experience, Roche has pointed out how important it is to remember not only that it 'is perfectly comprehensible and coherent from one ethnic group to another, from one country to another' but that it 'exists in animals as well as in humans' whilst the 'secondary level' of acoustic emission which 'involves learning a verbal language' and which is 'variable and incoherent from one country to another', however, is 'specifically human'. Roche, like Kristeva, also points out that the 'primary level is never eradicated and it persists through a person's lifetime even though it often has the tendency to minimise itself, taking second place behind a verbal vocal expression'.[65] We may lose contact with feeling as we contact explanation, but feeling never leaves us.

In a study of the different kinds of these non-verbal symbols which take second place but which people use to enhance spoken language, the psychologists Ruesch and Kees remind us that 'emotional expression appears most spectacularly when verbal communication fails altogether' and that 'the inability to use words occurs when people are overwhelmed by anger, anxiety, fear, shame'. Despite the incoherency of what people say on such occasions, or 'the inability to speak at all', 'others can still understand the implications of their actions' for sounds such as 'human cries of fear' are 'correctly interpreted anywhere in the world'. The voice, in such circumstances, therefore, acts as the carrier 'of a universal and international emergency language'.[66] In 'highly charged situations' when the voice exclaims this emergency language, 'two sides of feeling often appear together' revealing an 'archetypal level' of experience; 'grief and laughter, desire and disgust, love and aggression, often combine with the same intense relationship at the very same moment'.[67] Indeed, 'often the noises made by children at play leave the parent in doubt whether pleasure or pain is the cause'.[68]

Many of these non-verbal acoustic signals communicated by adults and children in extreme states compare to the sounds made by animals, such as hunting calls, warning cries, sounds of fright and aggression or the vocal excitations of mating, for indeed 'man may also growl, howl, whimper, grunt, roar and scream.'[69]

The expression of such sounds by a modern man or woman can create the appearance of a savage and primitive revisitation to an earlier time when, in Jung's words, there was little separation between men and beasts.[70] Yet the use of such non-verbal utterances also reminds us of the use of voice by the infant who, without recourse to the sophistication of verbal discourse, cries and screams and wails as she kicks and writhes in a rhythmical song and dance.

The innovator of analytical psychology, Carl Jung, was convinced that each seemingly civilised human being has in common a deeply buried and well disguised layer of experience and behaviour which is extremely primitive. This untamed and uncultivated potential of the human condition led Jung to conceive of a time when there was no separation between human and animal, a time when we were simply another species in the panoply of beasts. Jung named this savage and uncultivated aspect of the human condition the 'shadow' and it is through the release of primal non-verbal sounds that Jung's notion of the primitive human shadow becomes audible through the animality of vocalisation.

The rehearsal for this spectrum of acoustic emissions takes place in the early days of the infant's life, during which sound making is an elementary means by which primitive ideas and endemic affects are expressed. The experience of the neonate is one of primal sensations such as hunger and cold and the non-verbal nature of its song suits the content of its communication, which is no more articulate than the voiced sounds of the animal kingdom. The imitation of animal sounds is also subtly evident in the latterly-acquired childlike word-sounds for certain species. A dog bow-wows, a cat purrs, a sheep goes baa-baa and a cockerel goes cock-a-doodle-doo. However, such sounds are not universal. In French a cat goes ron-ron and a dog goes gnaf-gnaf; in Vietnamese a dog goes won-won; in German a cockerel goes kikeriki and a cat goes schnurr-schnurr.[71] The moment inarticulate vocal compositions are made phonological, they become culturally specific and disconnected from the universality or collectivity of human experience.

The research of Iona and Peter Opie has shown how songs have formed a vital part of children's playing, often being an aspect of games which reflect primal elements such as chasing, catching, duelling and pretending and often containing their ideas on a variety of subjects from murder to mating. Unlike the cognitive use of language which, through dialect, accent, vocabulary and articulation tends to reveal the social status of children, songs seem to act as an equaliser and, according to the Opies, 'children with homes and backgrounds as different from each other as mining community and garden suburb share jokes, rhymes, and songs, which are basically identical'.[72] Furthermore, this commonality within the song-making capacity of children reaches beyond the Western hemisphere. John Blacking, for example, has bequeathed a remarkable study of children's songs amongst the Venda people in South Africa, where infantile songmaking is constituted around many of the same archetypal themes of which English and American children sing.[73]

Language and Separation

With the development of language the acoustic composition of words becomes abstracted from the essence of that which they seek to express, so that eventually it is not necessary to experience and embody something in order to make it the subject of communication. With the increasing abstraction of words it becomes possible to communicate the danger of an approaching bear with simply the phonological production of the sound 'bear', the meaning of which remains unaltered even when uttered with an emotional detachment, a vocal monotone and a physical stasis. With the word 'storm', the leaping and twisting of the body with hands sweeping from above the head to the floor, accompanied by great roaring breaths and guttural belches, becomes condensed into a single syllable.

If there was a period of human history which was vocal but preverbal, then, perhaps in the course of language development and acquisition, it became unnecessary for people to experience the essence of a subject in order to expressively identify it. It may have been that people did not need to experience and embody the essence of fear or triumph, a bear or a horse or the river or the night in order to communicate about them, for the words which had come to stand in their place were understood abstractly. Consequently, humankind may have ceased to express through sound and begun instead to describe with words. If this is so, then something was truly lost.

The effect of this abstract nature of words may well have been threefold. First, it could have put an end to the sympathetic relationship with the essence of natural elements which had hitherto been enjoyed. On a grand scale this separation between human and nature mirrors Kristeva's assertion that language separates the child from the mother. Second, it could well have distanced men and women from the experience of their own emotions.

Third, it may have replaced the tonal range of acoustic qualities and rhythms which have been described as the earliest form of singing with the comparatively monotonal system of words. This predicated development from the phono-physical vocal dance to verbal linguistics underpins a cultural move from a spontaneous and experiential process of communication based on expression of fundamental essences and affects to a system of comminication based on a fixed code of abstract significication, from emotive expression to cognitive communication, from the semiotic to the symbolic.

It is one of the aims of my approach to Therapeutic Voicework to reclaim a little of what is lost as a result of this process.

Therapeutic Voicework Methodology: The Instinctual Developmental Postural Cycle

The Instinctual Developmental Postural Cycle is a variation on the kinetic cycle of postures and movements which I named as the Personal Developmental Postural Cycle in Chapter 3. Its purpose is to provide a system of physical, respiratory and vocal exercises which enables the client to achieve maximum malleability of vocal expression by learning to control the lengthening and shortening, dilation and constriction of the vocal tract. The method also assists the client in finding the three distinct elementary vocal timbres of flute, clarinet and saxophone by grounding these deeply in the body and its movement.

During this work attention is drawn to the lengthening of the vocal tract whereby the drop of the larynx vertically in the neck is used as the basis for an ideokinetic image of the tube of vocal resonance extending further down the body. By this method the natural movement of the larynx in the neck is amplified to create the imaginary picture of the vocal tract actually lengthening down the entire torso. In addition, the client is enabled to dilate the vocal tract, orally and sub-orally.

The first stage by which clients enter this process involves closing the vocal tract to its flute configuration and vocalising on different vowels within a comfortable pitch range. The physical position during this is similar to that which in personal developmental work I have called 'Walking Position'. The client stands erect with straight legs and arms hanging by the sides, with a concentrated expression of the physiognomy and the eyes focused on a particular object in space. The client imagines the length of the tube to run from the lips down to the concave indent between the clavicle at the base of

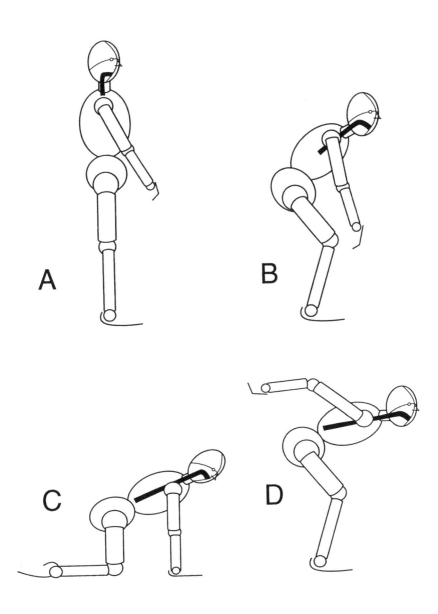

Figure 4.1

the neck (Figure 4.1a). In addition, the tube is conceived to be of minimal diameter, as it would be if whistling or blowing a kiss. This posture and its accompanying flute configuration is called 'Homo Erectus'.

The concentrated facial expression is a highly important part of Homo Erectus for a number of reasons. First, the narrowing and shortening of the vocal tract during the articulation of language demands tensile activity of the physiognomical muscles which form facial expression. Speaking, therefore, influences facial appearance by physiologic necessity. Second, speaking serves to articulate thought by sculpturing cognitive conceptual information into acoustic segments. The concentrated expression of the face in the Homo Erectus posture helps to compound and amplify the experience of such a relationship between thoughtful activity and narrow vocal tract dimensions.

From Homo Erectus the client is enabled to enter into the second posture, which in personal developmental work I have called 'Squatting Position' and which in instinctual work is further developed into what I have called 'Primate Position'. Here the legs bend slightly at the knees, the pelvis tilts forwards, the space under the arms increases, the physiognomy relaxes, the eyes lose specific focus and readjust to peripheral vision where the entire optical span is given equal attention, the jaw drops passively, as in the excessive salivation during drooling, the tongue falls forwards onto the bottom lip, the oropharynx and pharyngeal space falls open into passive dilation, the larynx descends in the neck and the vocal tract moves from flute to clarinet configuration with an accompanying shift in acoustic quality. As clients drop down into Primate they are encouraged to imagine the tube lengthening so that it now extends down to the bottom of the sternum (Figure 4.1 b). In addition, clients allow the vocal tract to dilate, increasing its diameter along its entire length, as they might if steaming a pair of glasses.

Central to the effective use of this posture to facilitate vocal tract expansion is the willingness of clients to give up conscious cognitive concentration as they drop down into the Primate Position. Because the predominance of thought in the mind tends to prepare the mouth for the articulation of that thought through language by causing a narrowing of the vocal tract, it is difficult to let go of the necessity of such preparation whilst thought predominates. Clients are, therefore, required to allow an expression of bland, vacant emptiness cover the face as the muscles around the forehead, jaw and cheeks relax. To mirror the relaxation of the thought process further, the eyes stare out into infinite space, letting go of directed vision as the mind releases itself from directed thought.

As the client physically drops down into Primate they notice the sensation of a deeper, fuller stream of breath. They also hear a radical change of vocal timbre, which sounds resonant with more harmonic content. To assist in the achievement of a discernment between the flute and clarinet timbres, clients are enabled to return to Homo Erectus, experiencing the gradual contraction and shortening of the vocal tract as the legs straighten, the armpit space closes, the eyes re-focus on a specific object, the face resumes its expression of cognitive concentration and predominance of thought returns. The client then moves back and forth between the two positions of Homo Erectus and Primate, experiencing a regression to a preverbal mode of functioning expressed physically through the ape-like postural position and acoustically through a semi-articulate, but resonant, vocal expression. When clients have successfully managed to allow a genuine dilation and lengthening of the vocal tract into the clarinet configuration, the next stage is to attempt to allow the vocal tract to dilate and lengthen to its maximum potential during vocalisation, producing the timbre referred to as saxophone. To assist with this, the client moves into a third animal position known as 'Feline-canine', which is similar to that which I have named 'Crawling Position' in relation to personal developmental work.

Whilst the animal image for the Primate position is the great ape, here the client imagines a combination of lion and wolf. From Primate Position, the pelvis tips completely, the arms fall towards the floor, the legs bend from the knees, the body moves into being supported on all fours, the head raises, the vocal tract actively dilates to its maximum diameter, the larynx descends further in the neck and the voice expressed is fully resonant. As clients drop down into the Feline-canine position, they imagine that the tube extends from the lips all the way down into the abdomen, as though the lungs have dropped into the belly (Figure 4.1c). In addition, clients aim to dilate and expand the diameter of the vocal tract to its maximum potential, as they might if yawning. The quality of the consequent saxophone voice is imaginatively comparable to the baying and howling of a wolf and the stretched soporific sounds of the great cat. It is also similar to the sound produced when one sings and yawns simultaneously and that produced during deep and prolonged sobbing.

The drop from Primate into Feline-canine represents a further regression from the semi-articulate acoustics of the great ape to the completely inarticulate expressions of the wild cat and dog. Indeed, because in saxophone the vocal tract is so expanded, the articulation of consonants as well as the production of distinctive vowels is barely possible.

To further enable the discernment between the three distinctive timbres, the client can now pass back from the Feline-canine position through Primate and return to Homo Erectus before journeying again regressively down through Primate into Feline-canine. The client repeats this descent and ascent whilst the practitioner meanwhile assists and supports, guides and instructs until the client is able to expand and contract, lengthen and shorten the vocal tract by their own volition, producing an ever more distinctive vocalisation of three elementary timbres.

In moving from Homo Erectus to Primate there is an initial feeling of a drop in the centre of experience from the head to the chest, as though in Homo Erectus one is focused on the articulation of the thoughts which abound in the mind whilst in Primate there is a letting go of this sensation and an awareness of the moods and sentiments of the heart. Then, finally, as the client drops into Feline-canine, the entire gravitational relationship of the body to the world shifts and the belly which has hitherto been held vertical to the ground now falls horizontal to the earth with the organs hanging down off the spine. The belly is now the under-belly. In Feline-canine there is, therefore, a sense of the centre of experience dropping down into the gut emotions of the lower regions.

The client now has three distinct bodily positions correlating with three animal images which utilise three distinct vocal tract dimensions. It is important to remember that the configurations of flute, clarinet and saxophone are arbitrary and extreme positions of the vocal tract which, obviously, can form an infinite variation of combined lengths and diameters. The aim of the three timbres is not to imply a limitation but to offer distinct sensate positions and articulations against which the infinite possibilities of vocal timbral expression can be measured, experienced and adapted.

Having introduced the three animal positions which constitute the Instinctual Developmental Postural Cycle, a further vocal liberation can be provided by training the client to control the passage of breath through the nasal cavities. The technique used to facilitate this is to introduce a fourth animal image: the Bird.

From the Feline-canine position clients gently ease back onto two legs, raising the squat half-way towards Primate, lift the spine approximately forty-five degrees to the floor, raise the arms up and out to the side of the body, lean forward onto the toes and imagine the kinetic choreography of the great bird. Whilst the vocal tract remains lengthened and dilated as in the saxophone configuration, the velum moves to increase nasal resonance and the saxophone timbre is produced with the new added ingredient of violin whilst the body suspends as in flight (Figure 4.1d).

When clients have achieved the production of the violin quality in saxophone, they are encouraged to repeat the process of passing through the other animal positions, going from Homo Erectus through Primate into Feline-canine, infusing the timbres of flute, clarinet and saxophone with the acoustic quality I have called violin. Clients then soon discover that through careful control of nasal resonance, each of the three elementary timbres of flute, clarinet and saxophone can be vocalised with a greater or lesser degree of violin, bringing spectral variation to them.

With the introduction of the bird image as a stimulator for the spectral quality of violin, the pedagogical system of movements and postures which constitute the Instinctual Developmental Postural Cycle is complete.

Therapeutic Voicework Methodology: Primal Archetypal Regression

On one level, the Instinctual Developmental Postural Cycle is simply a pedagogic technique to enable clients to expand vocal tract dimensions. However, needless to say, the work presents the client with challenges which invariably provoke highly affective responses. Therefore, it is necessary to understand that beneath the pedagogic layer of the methodology is another dimension which instigates a therapeutic process.

In an attempt to rescue the regressive tendencies of non-verbal Therapeutic Voicework from the confines of personalised autobiography and provide a means to excavate a collective strata of the psyche, I have developed a body of investigatory processes within a systematic modality of Therapeutic Voicework which I call 'Primary Archetypal Regression'. This body of work consists of using the system of physical and imaginative movement exercises which I have called the Instinctual Developmental Postural Cycle as a springboard from which clients can explore a menagerie of animal movements and sounds, shifting the tendency for regressive activity which non-verbal Therapeutic Voicework inevitably inspires into a collective and archetypal framework. In Primary Archetypal Regression the tendency towards personal regression to infantile vocalisation is located in an archetypal regression to an animalistic form of vocalisation. In other words, rather than expressive regression to personal infancy, there is an archetypal regression to a human primitivity and instinctuality.

Clients begin by standing quietly in the Homo Erectus position, vocalising with little effort. The practitioner then verbally guides the clients through the Primate, Feline-canine and Bird movements, encouraging them to vocalise with the distinctive qualities of flute, clarinet and saxophone with and without the spectral dimension of violin. As clients move and vocalise, they are asked to experience having animal qualities and sensations which are synonymous with the three key animal positions. Aside from assisting the expandability of the vocal tract, the animal positions somatise the journey from the superficial transactions of thought to the depthful quagmire of affect. These animal positions and images are of further importance because each of them represents a core archetypal fantasy within the collective unconscious; the ape, the lion, the wolf and the bird represent human potentialities in a network of legends, myths and parables world-wide. The werewolf, for example, is an image which has occupied a dominant place in the collective psyche from Paleolithic animal cults to the myths of ancient Egypt, from European societies to Hindu cultures.[74] The primitive and underdeveloped human self is mirrored in stories of human beings, particularly men, turning into wolves and, more frequently, women turning into cats; no less proliferate are the myths of the human that can transform into a flying bird. Moreover, one of the most frequently recurring motifs in the dreams of all peoples is the animal and there is not an adult alive who has not at some time dreamt of wild creatures, both real and imaginary. These animal constructs, therefore, go to the heart of the imaginative collective unconscious and assist the client in paving the way for an exploration of the deeper strata of the psyche through sound and movement.

As clients move through the animal positions, they develop a kinetic choreography which emulates the great bird, the great cat, the great dog and the great ape. Through careful guided instruction, clients are enabled to personalise their own mythic creature and develop an acoustic pattern and physical choreography through which they personify animal essences. As clients enter into this process, the sounds become wild, unformed, savage and primal and the vocal tract instinctively lengthens and dilates.

Throughout the guided journey the practitioner continually intervenes with containing instructions and eventually brings the session to an end, creating a period of silence in which clients can return to a sense of conscious cognition. In utilising this work I am attempting an acoustic and somatic realisation of Jung's concept of an archetypal human shadow, that part of the human which is still primitive, savage and little separated from the animal.

Jung believed that the 'lowest levels of the shadow are indistinguishable from the instinctuality of the animal', reminding us of a time when the distinction between humanity and animality was not so great.[75] All of the dark, chthonic and downward-pointing aspects of ourselves converge in the collective unconscious as the archetypal shadow. The more society demands humanity to be ordered, tamed, controlled, passive and civilised, the more the shadow tends to become chaotic, savage, wild, ferocious and primitive. Primal Archetypal Regression asks the client not only to shed language and enter into the primality of non-verbal vocalisation but, by implication, to shed the developed and matured social and psychological graces, mannerisms and constructs which language is adept at describing.

A minor acknowledgement of the psyche's animality is perceivable in common English usage where animal metaphors provide a vivid representation of qualities integral to our human nature: sly as a fox, cunning as a shrew, stubborn as a mule, slow as a snail, dog tired, strong as an ox, beavering away, slippery fish, dirty rat, filthy pup, lion-hearted, lone wolf, dark horse, stupid ass, fly like an eagle, feeling sluggish, frightened as a rabbit. Many of these metaphoric usages, however, are not employed to openly express one's own animality but to berate, belittle or degrade the person to whom such a metaphor is applied. Such use is made of animal metaphors to degrade women who are variously described as bitches, cows, dragons and pussies and nowhere was an animal image more heinously employed than in Nazi propaganda where Jews were portrayed as rats to further disseminate the anti-Semitic comparison between the Jewish race and vermin to be exterminated. Such demeaning projections remind us that consciousness actively seeks to avoid identifying with the shadow and, therefore, the beasts. Primal Archetypal Regression provides an opportunity to overcome this conscious resistance by appealing to what one Jungian analyst has called our propensity for 'animal empathy',[76] which is, perhaps, exemplified most vividly in the myth of Tarzan, who could communicate with animals.[77] The idea that humans share the same language as animals is also epitomised in the story of Dr Doolittle[78] and brought somewhat closer to reality in the testimony of Diane Fossey, who liaised with the Gorillas in the mist.[79] Since Freud's study of the so-called 'wolf man', animal aspects of human nature have always been lurking in the background of psychotherapy and Douglas Candland has compiled the stories of many similar cases of humans being found living as animals,[80] including the infamous Kasper Hauser, who was confined to a dungeon from his birth to adolescence before being released into the world.[81] Candland proposes that by understanding the way that animals and non-speaking humans think, we hold up a mirror to an aspect of our own functioning.

Primal Archetypal Regression is not only a doorway into the shadow lands of savagery but also provides access to some of the most glorious and beauteous aspects of life. For in contacting the dark side one often discovers the glittering diamonds which have been lost as a result of one's fear of the dark: the instinct to protect and to nurture, the combination of grace and strength which we recognise in the elephant, the powers of peaceful observation and wisdom which we project onto the owl, the sense of the expansiveness of time which facilitates restful sleep, the absence of the need to act which provides slumber as seen in the hippopotamus and the quality of peace represented by the dove. Working with a sense of animality provides an opportunity to recapture the fundamental essences of life which have become overlaid with centuries of cognition, by which the immense differentiated spectrum of our emotions become entrapped.

Amongst the various speculations upon the elements which distinguish humans from the animals is the proposal that only human beings have cultivated a complex acoustic communicative code of language which is culturally specific and trans-culturally decodable. This code is distinct from the sounds made by other animals by the advanced ability to vary the acoustic signal made by the larynx with subtle articulations of the mouth, lips and jaw with incredible precision and dexterity. Consequently, language and the capacity to articulate is a predominant psychological symbol for conscious development. Conversely, therefore, inarticulate sound making – the grunts, groans, screeches and calls of the voice unshaped by the speech apparatus – provide an acoustic reflection of psychological primitivism and Primal Archetypal Regression provides a container and an expressive framework for such a process. To enter into a matrix of non-verbal vocalisation is, therefore, not only to reverse the developmental process on a personal level but also to entice the shadow-laden aspects and instinctual propensities of the collective unconscious forward into the arena of therapeutic and artistic investigation. This, naturally, leads to resistance. The more primitive vocal sounds heard in daily life, such as yawning and belching, lead us to literally place our hands over our mouth. This may, in part, be because these preverbal utterances remind us of the primal and untamed aspects of ourselves which, deep down, still growl like the bear, roar like the lion and screech like the hawk. If so, relocating the capacity for such vocal utterances provides a container for the exploration of the instincts and nothing could be more therapeutically pertinent.

Therapeutic Voicework Case Study: To Be Wild and to Be a Mother

Mary was 52 when she first came to work on her voice. She was a woman of petite proportion and slim dimension who spoke gently and quietly and whose reason for attending was a tiresome irritation with frequently feeling 'small', 'quiet' and somewhat 'taken advantage of', describing her image of how people perceived her as 'a soft touch'. In addition, she suffered from an overwhelming shyness, a feeling of inferiority and what she described as a 'paralysing lack of confidence'. She had, in the past, suffered two periods of debilitating depression for which she had been prescribed anti-depressant medication.

Mary had not had the opportunity for formal education beyond her late teens, despite a deep interest in, and aptitude for, the sciences. When she was fifteen her mother died and she was forced to look after her younger sister and brother. Shortly after her siblings had left home, her father had fallen ill with Parkinson's Disease and she had nursed him until he died.

During the period of nursing her father she had met a man eight years her senior whom, after her father's death, she had married and with whom she had three children. During my taking of her case history she said that she had enjoyed motherhood and that she maintained a close relationship with her children. Shortly after her last child had left home, her husband became very ill with cancer and she nursed him for two years before he died. Since her husband's death, one year prior to our meeting, she had felt 'completely at a loss'.

Mary had always wanted to sing but had been discouraged by her husband and her children due to her sounding 'out of tune' and had, in addition, felt it imprudent to spend money on singing lessons when the children already needed more than the family's financial resources could bear. Now, however, she had taken a job and had decided to explore her voice. She had chosen to investigate her issues through Therapeutic Voicework because she felt that it was primarily through her voice, which she described as 'shaky', 'trembly' and 'thin', that her unassured personality was expressed; epitomising this, she said that during her depressive periods she had remained 'almost dumb'. She also said that she had been told that she was 'too quiet', 'too slow' and that her voice was 'monotonous' and 'difficult to listen to' by a number of people close to her.

As we began working with simple exercises involving Mary in the intoning of single notes ascending and descending the pitch scale, I noticed that there was no violin in any of the sounds. Thus I asked Mary to try to imbue her voice with a quality of childlikeness, which I knew, from experience, usually stimulates the component parameter of violin in the voice. However, this was to no avail.

When we discussed her difficulty in finding the child's voice it became apparent that Mary felt that her childhood had been taken from her and that she had been untimely and prematurely propelled into adulthood by the death of her mother, upon which she was forced to assume adult duties before her time. She had raised her younger sister and brother almost single-handedly and buried deep beneath Mary's brave face of 'having come to terms with this' there was an 'anger and a resentment' which she felt she had put out of sight.

In a later session, after considerable analysis of the effect of her lost youth, I asked her to sing the highest note of her comfortable pitch range, imbuing it with an attitude of 'spiteful resentment'. When she did this the sound became drenched in violin and there emerged a voice more intense and emotive than I had heard her sing before 𝆔 ♩.

Taking Mary through the Instinctual Developmental Postural Cycle, I encouraged her to linger in the Bird Position and helped her individualise her experience. Over the next 20 minutes Mary composed an extravagant dance of her voice, rushing like a tornado up and down the pitch scale, singing and moving and creating a panoply of winged creatures. She became a hot-blooded prehistoric 'ravenasaurus', soaring at top-speed across valley and plain, brandishing her beak and bellowing out the cries of hunger. She became a great winged compound, part heron and part stalk, perched and poised. She became a screeching pink flamingo, a squawking magpie, a wild black crow and a parrot with the full prism of plumage (Figure 4.2). As Mary journeyed through the matrix of bird imagery, her voice became very loud and extremely powerful and she became particularly engaged in the transformation back and forth between the stalk and the crow. The former, she felt, symbolised the role of nurse and midwife she had played all her life whilst the crow somehow stood for the 'blackness' and 'anger' which she felt. During our analysis of the work Mary spoke about her memories of the role of surrogate mother which she had played to her sister and brother and began to reveal her unexpressed resentment, not only towards her mother for dying but also towards her brother and sister for requiring care, her own

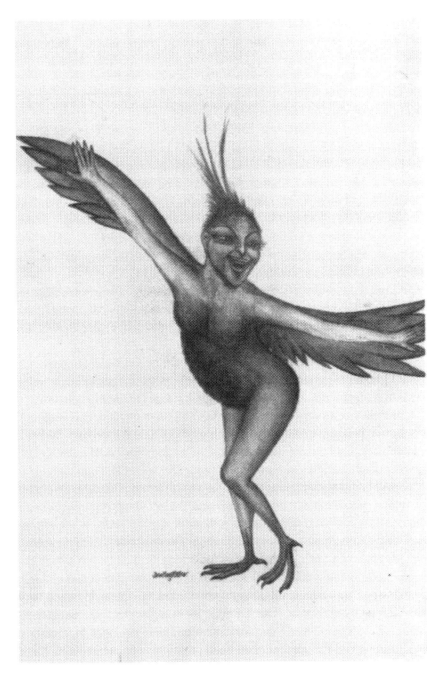

Figure 4.2

During our analysis of the work Mary spoke about her memories of the role of surrogate mother which she had played to her sister and brother and began to reveal her unexpressed resentment, not only towards her mother for dying but also towards her brother and sister for requiring care, her own children for 'taking every ounce of energy she had' and towards her husband for falling ill and leaving her 'unprovided for'.

During her reportage Mary happened to say that her sister had always accused her of being spiteful and she had, in fact, been quite malicious during her own childhood. Furthermore, after the death of her mother, she had recurring dreams in which her sister died, releasing Mary from the burden of care-giving. In addition, during the mothering of her own children she often had sporadic 'spiteful' feelings towards them and she often felt that they kept her from 'living her own life'. However, Mary had repressed all this because it was 'negative and destructive' and, anyway, she said that she loved her children dearly.

As we continued working I guided Mary through a process of Primary Archetypal Regression, encouraging her to embody animal images and essences which gave a framework within which to release and explore her sense of repressed spite and resentment.

As she passed down into Feline-canine position, her head dropped, her hands gripped tight and she held her posture with her sight line passing down her torso, as though looking through her legs. Then she began to cry.

The Feline-canine position had caused Mary to experience the weight of her breasts hanging from her chest and this physical sensation had somehow encapsulated and crystallised her feeling of having been 'sucked dry' by her brother, sister, children and husband leaving her 'shrivelled' and 'empty'.

I gave Mary the image of a drought-weary lioness, fatigued with heat, worn and exhausted with well-suckled nipples, prowling through the bush (Figure 4.3). She sang soporifically, with wide gaping yawns in saxophone and a very slow vibrato ⋀⋀⋀ ⟨⟩. Then, as she explored the Feline-canine movements, she seemed to discover a fresh energetic quality with which she began to move and vocalise with complete engagement. She hissed and spat and clawed, her voice manifesting extremely fast vibrato as it passed back and forth across the modal-falsetto bridge ⋀⋀ M ⫶ ⋀⋀ F. She concocted a liquid voice made of arsenic and strychnine and there emerged the character of a creature half cat and half crow, with an acidic voice which burned and bleached with every note. Then, as she rolled over onto her back, she sang like a viper, like a boa constrictor. I asked her to decrease the loudness and

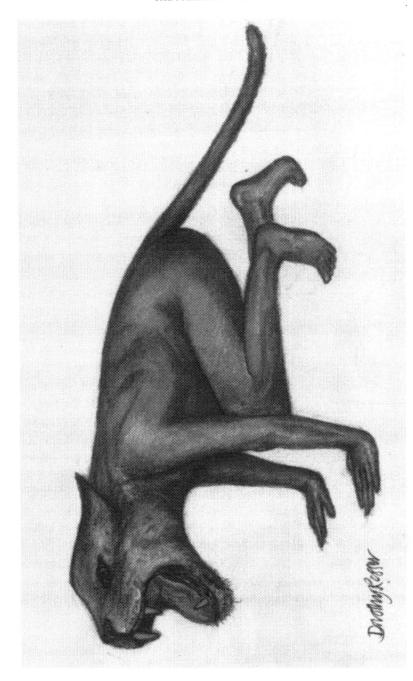

Figure 4.3

make the spite more conniving and ensnaring, like a spider slowly and cautiously spinning a web of death and then as a scorpion quickly and impulsively injecting the poison. The images of insects increased both the quality of spite and the intensity and strength of the voice. Now, as we worked, a fresh network of images unfolded in the voice which built up an emotional field composed of a premeditative revenge against an oppressor and she became a character, half insect and half crow, with a fatal sting that aimed to kill, slowly.

Gradually, these emotions and images birthed a voice nearly one and a half octaves higher than when we had started and which sounded calm, strong and self-possessed.

The next time we worked together she manifested the violin component of the voice with comparative ease and explored sounds associated with childhood. Her voice gurgled and effervesced with innocence and naïveté, she sang with the freshness and purity of a kitten untouched by trauma and, as she sang, Mary's face took on an open and inquisitive smile which I had not seen before.

The discovery and liberation of the vocal component parameter of violin had been, in Mary's case, connected to the release of spite, resentment and anger, which also acted as a discharge of, and an absolution from, the bottled-up energy which its repression had caused. Meanwhile, the animal work had provided a framework within which Mary could explore the shadow side of the good nurse and the good mother, an entirely necessary process for someone who had been prematurely denied her own mother and forced into assuming the role of a good mother herself. For Mary, to explore such issues could have been a terrifying process and the animal work provides a means of distancing it from the personal, thereby offering a degree of safety. Furthermore, it helps the client to sense that, despite the magnitude of personal trauma, there is often a universal structure lodged beneath the personal narrative which reflects broader issues.

In Mary's case, such issues were not composed of elements of her own neuroses but were, in many respects, political factors arising from the way circumstances had made functional use of her at the expense of so much of her soul.

Conclusion: Back to the Roots

Utilising non-verbal vocal expression to investigate and reclaim aspects of a person which have been deeply effected by historical circumstances and personal trauma, as in the case of Mary, naturally demands of the Therapeutic Voiceworker an exceptionally diligent, sensitive, compassionate and analytic point of departure.

One can utilise the Instinctual Developmental Postural Cycle as an aid to pedagogic and technical procedures, helping a client to develop vocal expressivity. But, as with many vocal techniques, the work can often move into an area where training the voice to express the self meets with an exploration of the self itself. In all forms of Voicework we are, by facilitating increased vocal expression, naturally facilitating increased self-awareness. This can be extremely uplifting but can also be challenging and at times frightening or overwhelming for the client as well as for the practitioner. There is a need to recognise, therefore, that at a certain level and under certain circumstances, creative Voicework and technical Voicework can become Therapeutic Voicework and the lines between them can be very difficult to see. Recognising this can place Therapeutic Voicework in a psychotherapeutic framework and begs us to consider the way in which vocal work might connect to psychological work.

One domain of psychological investigation of the self is psychotherapy, a field of enquiry which originates from principles which were first articulated by Sigmund Freud and which birthed an entire professional arena. To understand more the connection between Therapeutic Voicework and the field of enquiry initiated by Freud, I shall now turn my attention to his early work and look at the role of vocal expression in psychoanalysis, hoping to throw light on the psychological dimension to Therapeutic Voicework – a theme which I will be deepening as this book progresses.

Notes

1   Harris, J. (1990) *Early Language Development: Implications for Clinical and Educational Practice.* London: Routledge, p.8.

2   Marleau-Ponty, (1970) cited in P. Lewis, 'Marleau-Ponty and the phenomenology of language.' In J. Ehrmann (ed) *Structuralism.* New York: Anchor Books, pp.9–31, (p.19).

3   Hymes, D. (1971) 'Competence and performance in linguistic theory.' In R. Huxley and E. Ingram (eds) *Language Acquisition: Models and Methods.* London: Academic Press.

4   Skinner, B. (1957) *Verbal Behaviour.* New York: Appleton-Century-Crofts.

5   Pinker, S. (1994) *The Language Instinct.* London: Penguin.

6   Smith, W. (1996) 'Voice, psychotherapy and feminism.' Paper presented to the International Association Therapeutic Voicework. London, October 1996.

7   Smith, (1996) 'Voice, psychotherapy and feminism.' Paper presented to the International Association for Voice Movement Therapy. London, October 1996.

8   Kristeva, J. (1987) *Tales of Love* (Trans. by L. Roudiez). New York: Columbia University Press, p.27.

9   Moi, T. (1985) *Sexual–Textual Politics: Feminist Literary Theory.* London: Routledge.

10   Silverman, K. (1988) *The Acoustic Mirror: The Female Voice in Psychoanalysis and Cinema.* Bloomington and Indianapolis: Indiana University Press, p.105.

11   Eagleton, T. (1983) *Literary Theory: An Introduction.* Oxford: Blackwell, p.188.

12   Smith, W. (1996) 'Voice, psychotherapy and feminism.' Paper presented to the International Association for Voice Movement Therapy. London, October 1996.

13   Eagleton, T. (1983) *Literary Theory: An Introduction.* Oxford: Blackwell, p.188.

14   Grunwell, P. (1982) *Clinical Phonology.* London: Croom Helm.

15   Schneider, M. (1957) 'Oriental and primitive music.' In E. Wellwsz (ed) *The New Oxford History of Music,* vol. 1. Ancient and Oriental Music. London: Oxford University Press, pp.1–82.

16   Picken, L. (1957) 'The music of Far Eastern Asia 1: China.' In E. Wellwsz (ed) *The New Oxford History of Music,* vol. 1. Ancient and Oriental Music. London: Oxford University Press, pp.83–134.

17   Aitchison, J. (1996) 'A web of deceit: the origin of language.' The 1996 Reith Lectures: Lecture 2. Broadcast on BBC Radio 4, (Tuesday 13 February 1996).

18   Gardner, H. (1979) 'Developmental psychology after piaget: an approach in terms of symbolisation.' *Human Development,* 22, pp.73–88, (p.76).

19   Gardner, H. (1994) *The Arts and Human Development.* New York: Basic Books, p.45.

20   Winner, E. (1982) *Invented Worlds: The Psychology of the Arts.* Cambridge, Massachusetts: Harvard University Press.

21   Bamberger, J. (1982) 'Revisiting children's drawings of simple rhythms: a function for reflection-in-action.' In S. Strauss and R. Stavy (eds) *U-Shaped Behavioural Growth.* New York: Academic Press.

22   Moog, H. (1976) *The Musical Experience of the Preschool Child.* London: Schott.

23   Dowling, W.J. (1982) 'Development of Musical Schemata in Children's Spontaneous Singing.' In W. R. Crozier and A. J. Chapman (eds) *Cognitive Processes in the Perception of Art.* Amsterdam: Elsevier.

24   Davidson, L. (1985) 'Tonal structures of children's early songs.' *Music Perception,* 2, pp.361–74.

25   Berryman, J.C. with Hargreaves, D., Herbert M. and Taylor, A. (1991) *Developmental Psychology and You.* London: British Psychological Society/Routledge, pp.157–58.

26   The Voices Foundation (1996) 'Developing children through singing.' Publicity Brochure.

27   Law, M. (1996) 'The practice of voice: an investigation into the diversity of approaches to vocal work as exemplified by current practitioners.' Unpublished research project prepared for the International Association for Voice Movement Therapy.

28   Armstrong, F. (1995) Unpublished information leaflet on current voice teachers.

29   Programme notes to *Folkworks' Vocal Chords Festival.* Newcastle-upon-Tyne 3–5 May, 1996 and London 4–6 May 1996.

30   Programme notes to *Folkworks' Vocal Chords Festival.* Newcastle-upon-Tyne 3–5 May, 1996 and London 4–6 May 1996.

31   Law, M. (1996) 'The practice of voice: an investigation into the diversity of approaches to vocal work as exemplified by current practitioners.' Unpublished research project prepared for the International Association for Voice Movement Therapy.

32   Law, M. (1996) 'The practice of voice: an investigation into the diversity of approaches to vocal work as exemplified by current practitioners.' Unpublished research project prepared for the International Association for Voice Movement Therapy.

33   Law, M. (1996) 'The practice of voice: an investigation into the diversity of approaches to vocal work as exemplified by current practitioners.' Unpublished research project prepared for the International Association for Voice Movement Therapy.

34   Mothersole, A. (1920) 'La Rythmique est-elle une lubie?' *La Rythme* 5, p.23 (p.23).

35   Choksy, L. (1988) *The Kodály Method.* New Jersey: Prentice Hall.

36   Lissau, R. (1987) *Rudolf Steiner: Life, Work, Inner Path and Social Initiatives.* Stroud: Hawthorn Press.

37   Gardner, H. (1994) *The Arts and Human Development.* New York: Basic Books.

38   Gardner, H. (1993) *Multiple Intelligences: A Theory in Practice.* New York: Basic Books.

39   Cassirer, E. (1953–59) *The Philosophy of Symbolic Forms,* 3 vols. New Haven: Yale University Press.

40   Goodman, N. (1976) *Languages of Art.* Indianapolis: Hackett. (1978) *Ways of Worldmaking.* Indianapolis: Hackett.

41   Langer, S. (1963) *Philosophy in a New Key,* 3rd Edn. Cambridge, Massachusetts: Harvard University Press, p.88.

42   Langer, S. (1963) *Philosophy in a New Key,* 3rd Edn. Cambridge, Massachusetts: Harvard University Press, pp.260–261.

43   Langer, S. (1953) *Feeling and Form.* London: Routledge & Kegan Paul, p.27.

44   Langer, S. (1953) *Feeling and Form.* London: Routledge & Kegan Paul, p.27.

45   Langer, S. (1963) *Philosophy in a New Key,* 3rd Edn. Cambridge, Massachusetts: Harvard University Press, pp.246–247.

46   Lonsdale, S. (1981) *Animals and the Origin of Dance.* London: Thames and Hudson.

47   Jesperson, O. (1922) *Language: Its Nature, Development and Origin.* London: Allen & Unwin, pp.436–437.

48   Spencer, H. (1922) *Essay on the Origin of Music,* cited in O. Jesperson, *Language: Its Nature, Development and Origin.* London: Allen & Unwin, p.434.

49   Kurth, E. (1931) *Musikpsychologie.* Berlin: M. Hesse, p.291.

50   Malinowski, B. (1927) 'Supplement 1.' In C. K. Ogden and I. A. Richards (eds) *The Meaning of Meaning.* New York: Harcourt and Brace.

51   Sapir, E. (1921) *Language: An Introduction in the Study of Speech.* New York: Harcourt and Brace.

52   Jesperson, O. (1922) *Language: Its Nature, Development and Origin.* New York: Holt.

53   K. Davis, (1938) 'Sounds in language.' *Journal of Nervous and Mental Diseases,* 4, pp.491–99, (p.499).

54   Jung, C.G. (1953) *The Collected Works of C G Jung,* vol. 5, pp.12–13.

55   Bowra, C. (1962) *Primitive Song.* New York: World Publishing.

56   Bowra, C. (1962) *Primitive Song.* New York: World Publishing, pp.4–5.

57   Bowra, C. (1962) *Primitive Song.* New York: World Publishing, p.29.

58   Sachs, C. (1943) *The Rise and Fall of Music in the Ancient World: East and West.* New York: Norton.

59   Sachs, C. (1962) *The Wellsprings of Music.* The Hague: Martinus Nijhoff.

60   Schneider, M. (1957) 'Oriental and primitive music.' In E. Wellwsz (ed) *The New Oxford History of Music,* vol. 1. Ancient and Oriental Music. London: Oxford University Press, pp.1–82 (p.3).

61   Sachs, C. (1958) *Our Musical Heritage.* New York: Prentice Hall.

62   Sachs, C. (1962) *The Wellsprings of Music.* The Hague: Martinus Nijhoff.

63   Bowra, C. (1962) *Primitive Song.* New York: World Publishing, p.29.

64   Neumann, E. (1970) *The Origins and History of Consciousness.* Princeton: Princeton University Press, Bollingen Series XLII.

65   Roche, J. (1980) 'La Voix de 'enfant', *Le Journal d'Audiophonologie,* p23, (p.23).

66   Ruesch, J. and Kees, W. (1971) *Nonverbal Communication: Notes on the Visual Perception of Human Relations.* Berkeley and Los Angeles: University of California Press, p.64.

67   Hillman, J. (1980) *Jung's Typology – The Feeling Function.* Dallas: Spring Publications, p.101.

68   Plutchik, R. (1955) 'The emotions: facts, theories, and a new model.' *Psychosomatic Medicine,* pp.15–42, (p.27).

69   Schafer, R. (1994) *The Soundscape: Our Sonic Environment and the Tuning of the World.* Vermont: Destiny, p.40.

70   Jung, C.G. *The Collected Works ,of C G Jung* vol.9 pt. 2. (Bollingen series XX). H. Read, M. Fordham, G. Adler and Wm McGuire (eds). Princeton, New Jersey: Princeton University Press and LondonL Routledge and Kegan Paul, pp233–34.

71   Schafer, R. (1994) *The Soundscape: Our Sonic Environment and the Tuning of the World.* Vermont: Destiny, p.41.

72   Opie, I. & Opie, P. (1959) *The Lore and Language of Schoolchildren.* Oxford: Oxford University Press, p.3.

73   Blacking, J. (1995) *Venda Children's Songs: A Study in Ethnomusicological Analysis.* Chicago: University of Chicago Press.

74   Douglas, A. (1993) *The Beast Within: Man, Myths and Werewolves.* London: Orion.

75   Jung, C.G. *The Collected Works ,of C G Jung* vol.9 pt. 2. (Bollingen series XX). H. Read, M. Fordham, G. Adler and Wm McGuire (eds). Princeton, New Jersey: Princeton University Press and LondonL Routledge and Kegan Paul, pp233–34.

76   Whitcher, D. (1978) 'Animal empathy.' Unpublished graduating thesis for the Jung Institute, Zurich.

77   Farmer, P. (1972) *Tarzan Alive: A Definitive Biography of Lord Greystoke.* New York: Doubleday.

78   Lofting, H. (1950) *The Voyages of Dr. Doolittle.* Philadelphia: Lippincott.

79   Fossey, D. (1983) *Gorillas in the Mist.* Boston: Houghton Mifflin.

80   Candland, D. (1993) *Feral Children and Clever Animals.* Oxford: Oxford University Press.

81   Pies, H. (1833) *Kasper Hauser.* London: Simpkin and Marshall.

CHAPTER 5

The Talking Cure
Therapeutic Voicework and Psychoanalysis

Introduction: Sigmund Freud

Sigmund Freud is probably one of the most loathed, revered, despised, studied, respected and scrutinised men of the twentieth century. Certainly, he has escaped being ignored. He is responsible for completely reshaping the way novels are read, the way seemingly innocent remarks are echoed, the way sexuality is perceived to be implicitly present in everyday affairs and the way we talk about ourselves and others. He introduced terms which are now part of the vernacular vocabulary amongst educated privileged westerners: terms such as ego, libido and id. He made an entire nation, then an entire continent and now almost an entire world conscious that there were many things unconscious. But, most significantly, he initiated the practice of psychoanalysis, which, in turn, augmented the profession of psychotherapy, a form of medicine in which the cure is contained by the words which the patient speaks. Freud discovered the Talking Cure. Indeed, early psychoanalysis is as much a study of language as it is of the psyche.[1]

In recent years widespread criticism of Freud – particularly his perception of women, originating from educated, respected and discerning theorists – has instigated a re-examination of psychoanalytic and, therefore, psychotherapeutic practice, its clinical viability, political integrity and its theoretical substance. Despite this wave of interrogation, psychoanalysis and its various descendent therapeutic strategies – which invite one person to pay another to listen – is still a widely disseminated form of curative activity practised all over the world. And, central to the modality of this psychotherapy is the process by which the client or patient gives voice to thought, feeling, fantasy and fact. It is an act of vocalisation and audition.

Some would say that mistakes or misdeeds weaken a person's successes. Others would say that we should be judged by our achievements rather than our faults. For the purposes of this study, the most apposite point from which I shall depart is that it was the words which women voiced that provided the materials from which Freud proclaimed to have found a cure; a talking cure. Therefore, I am suggesting that we should not allow the evident and alleged inconsistencies and misbehaviours of the man to veil the unwitting insight which his patients have bequeathed. It was their voices, their tales and their phrases and secrets, uttered in a consulting room of Vienna, which hold a key to understanding the voice of present day women and men. Moreover, in order to mentally comprehend and historically locate the multitudinous dimensions of Therapeutic Voicework, it is vital that Freud's attention to the human voice as a medium for the talk which cured, be acknowledged and explained. I shall, therefore, without ignoring the issues pertaining to a contemporary political analysis of Freud's stance, outline the aspects of his early work, before the detailed and complex unfolding of psychoanalytic principles, during which his focus was upon the nature of voice, word and emotion. Further to this, I will locate the act of psychoanalytic vocalisation in the context of contemporary feminist analysis in order to intimate the future for Therapeutic Voicework within a politicised psychotherapeutic framework.

Hysterically Talking the Cure

The most common complaint amongst Freud's early patients in the late-nineteenth century consisted of bodily pains for which there appeared to be no physiological explanation. These included headaches, paralysed limbs, stomach upsets, respiratory problems and disturbances of speech, sight and hearing. Freud proposed to have discovered that the cause of these 'phantom diseases' usually consisted of a psychological trauma which the patient had experienced in the past, in some cases many years prior to the occurrence of the physical problem which had brought her to the doctor. Indeed, quite frequently it was a distressing childhood event, the emotional effects of which continued to disturb the patient long after it had apparently been forgotten.

Freud referred to these patients as hysterics: those in whom the emotional reaction or affect provoked by a specific psychological trauma had been converted into a physical symptom which persisted for many years afterwards. The hysteric seemed genuinely unable to recollect the precipitating event and had no idea of the causal connection between it and the bodily dysfunction.

Freud's discovery of the connection between apparent physical dysfunction and predisposing psychological trauma originated from his studies and research first with Jean Martin Charcot and later with Josef Breuer, which culminated in an analysis of the women whom they named hysterics. Freud and Breuer published the results of these analyses under the title *Studies in Hysteria* in 1895 and their case studies marked an important departure in psychological analysis, from the pictorial emphasis in the work of Freud's predecessor and teacher Charcot to the auditory skills of listening and attending to women's stories and voices.

Jean Martin Charcot worked in the Salpêtrière Clinic in Paris, where his studies in hysteria began in 1870 and where he was the first theorist to see hysteria as psychological rather than physiological in origin. He also showed that hysteria was suffered by men and was, therefore, not limited solely to women. Nonetheless, although this proved hysteria was not related to the female biological disposition, the etymological significance of the word hysteria – which literally means 'wandering womb' – continued to influence the perception of the condition and hysteria remained predominantly and symbolically a 'female malady'.[2] Charcot frequently presented his female hysterics to audiences in public lecture theatres, encouraging them to perform *attitudes passionelles* – the physical mime and replay of their lives and emotions – with the result that several patients became stars or celebrities of his 'hysteria shows', later becoming immortalised in the collection of photographed gestures and hysterical expressions called *Iconographique de la Salpêtrière*.

The importance of the female hysterics to the development of psychoanalysis has been described by Elaine Showalter in *The Female Malady*, where she points out that 'while we have a full pictorial record of Charcot's hysterical patients' only a 'few fragments of their words' remain recorded. However, 'with the case studies of Josef Breuer and Sigmund Freud, women's voices, stories, memories, dreams, and fantasies enter the medical record'. Thus psychoanalysis begins with intimate conversations between hysterical women and male psychiatrists, that is verbal dialogues rather than exhibitions or voice rather than picture.[3]

In many ways, Freud gave women a voice, or rather he listened to their voices, which only makes the process by which he allegedly distorted and misrepresented them more tragic.

The Body of the Word

Freud identified two distinct processes by which psychological trauma became converted into physical symptoms. The first process occurred when a person experienced a particular mental trauma whilst suffering from a genuine physiological disease. Although the person recovered from the disease, the physical symptoms recurred whenever he or she was reminded of the traumatic event which originally accompanied it. Let us take, for example, someone suffering from the severe abdominal pains caused by appendicitis during which time the person suffers the mental trauma of being bereft of a close relative, which naturally arouses a strong affect of grief. If this person has a 'hysterical disposition', he or she may continue to experience the abdominal pains whenever grief is aroused by new situations involving a bereavement, even long after the appendix has been removed. In such an example a physical symptom originally generated by organic causes is later revived as an expression of a psychological affect, simply because, by chance, they originally occurred simultaneously.

The second process involved the patient's unwitting translation of a verbal phrase from its metaphorical into its literal meaning. For example, a traumatic event which morally disgusts and revolts the patient may precipitate sporadic fits of vomiting because the linguistic term 'to be sick' is translated from its metaphorical description of psychological disgust into its literal designation of vomiting. A man who is being continually pressurised by his colleague to agree to a transaction that he feels is conspicuous may begin to suffer from numbness in his arm because his work partner is metaphorically 'twisting his arm' over the deal. A 'slap in the face' describes both a severe facial neuralgia and the affect of a swiping insult and 'feeling choked' describes both respiratory constriction about the larynx and the affect of deep sadness. By converting such linguistic metaphors into a literal somatic experience, the hysteric could genuinely feel severe spinal pain when people 'got his back up', experience agonising shooting pains in the fore limbs when colleagues 'twisted his arm' over an issue at work or be caused to vomit when morally disgusted. Hysterical patients, therefore, possessed a particular susceptibility to the power of suggestion or imagination. Through careful aural observation of the patient's speech, Freud noticed that many linguistic phrases which patients used to describe physical symptoms at the same time denoted emotional responses. This provided the key to the precipitating trauma.

Freud believed that in both processes the persistence of the bodily symptom was caused by the patient's insufficient active emotional reaction to the original event or scene, which had consequently become 'strangulated' or 'bottled up'. Freud compared the psyche to an electrical system which becomes charged with a certain amount of energy when it is effected by an event. For example, a patient who is insulted becomes excited in such a way as to increase the amount of energy in the nervous system. In healthy situations this increase in energy is immediately expended by the individual's responsive reactions, which can be verbal or physical – such as a bout of abusive swearing or a histrionic waving of fists. Freud described such active responses as 'motor activity' because they were stimulated by the neurological impulses of the motor neurons which stem from the central nervous system; the function of such activity was to bring the energy level of the psyche back to a state of balance or neutrality. If, however, for reasons of social prohibition or personal inhibition, the individual represses the response, refrains from responsive motor activity and retains the increased energetic excitation, it becomes bottled up and seeks expression by converging upon a weak spot localised in a part of the body. Freud described the ideal expenditure of increased energy through motor activity in response to the original event as 'abreaction' and proposed that the physical symptoms of hysteria were the result of the emotional affect having been insufficiently abreacted.

Freud proposed to have discovered a method of curing the somatic disease by assisting the patient to remember the original upsetting experience which had accompanied the genesis of the physical symptom. This involved a thorough psycho-archaeological excavation of the patient's past in search of a single precipitating trauma which, when remembered and articulated, allegedly caused the symptom to vanish for ever.

However, the somatic cure was not achieved through recollection without affect. The patient had to revive and re-enact the same intensity of emotional response to the memory of the event as was evoked by its original occurrence. Freud thus claimed to have discovered that 'each individual hysterical symptom immediately and permanently disappeared' when he succeeded in 'bringing clearly to light the memory of the event by which it was provoked', in 'arousing its accompanying affect', in enabling the patient to describe 'that event in the greatest possible detail' and in successfully facilitating the client to put the 'affect into words'. But, most significantly, Freud asserted that recollection of the event 'without affect almost invariably produces no result' and that the event 'which originally took place must be repeated as vividly as possible'.[4]

In encouraging the patients to not only verbally remember, that is to put back together the original event, but also to imbue the text of this memory with expression of the full emotional excitation which had been denied at the time of its first occurrence, Freud gave the patient a second chance to 'complete his reaction'[5] and, in so doing, release both the stored affect and, along with it, the somatic symptom which had hitherto served to contain it. Freud described this process of giving vent to stored-up feelings as 'catharsis', a word which he took from the effect upon the audience which Aristotle said was achieved by ancient Greek theatre. Thus Freud proposed that the hysterical phenomenon 'comes to an end as soon as the patient has spoken about it'.[6] Even if the original abreaction would have normally involved a muscular or physical reaction, such as, for example, a punch or other kinetic display of aggression, the full abreaction could be achieved the second time around through words alone. Thus, according to Freud, 'words are substitutes for deeds'.[7] However, because the verbal memory of the precipitating trauma had to be experienced in full emotional depth, the patient was encouraged not to remember in a cool detached and reflective way but to speak as though he or she were experiencing it all over again. If the patient simply spoke the words which described the remembered event with no emotional recollection, the cure was ineffectual. It was, therefore, not the words alone that performed the cure but the voice which expressed all the emotions associated with the memory through its acoustic tonal and timbral quality, ranging from sobbing to rage, from bitter grief to intimidated fear. Freud's medicine was not, in fact, a talking cure but a vocal cure.

We experience this fundamental tenet of catharsis every time we repeat to ourselves the things we wished we had said in an argument. Whilst involved in a quarrel with someone, we often remain calm and objective, asserting only a fraction of the aggression we feel. Then, later, when we are alone, we rant and rave to ourselves as though we were back again at the scene and afterwards we feel relieved. In such a situation, just as in Freud's consulting room, it is not the words themselves that become a substitute for deeds but the voice which utters them with an acoustic vocal tone equivalent to the emotional tone of the affect. In many cases of abreaction the tone of the voice is actually more important than the words, as, for example, when bottled-up pressure and frustration are released through yelling, screaming, laughing or crying. Freud referred to such non-verbal processes as providing an important opportunity for 'letting off steam' but, for him, non-verbal sound making was not sufficient to facilitate genuine and complete cathartic abreaction because words were essential to remembering and describing the specific historical event which had caused the physical problem. It was here that Freud may be said to have ignored a fascinating line of enquiry for he did not consider the relationship between the act of vocalisation and that of verbalisation, neither did he relate abreaction to the discharge of phonated breath divorced from articulation. Though his reasons for this originated from his desire to detect precipitating trauma, such a desire was predicated on the assumption that psychosomatic symptoms originate from such traumatic specificity rather than from an accumulation of affect from continuing life experience.

Therapeutic Voicework Methodology: From Story Through Affect to Song

At times when we we break into tears, or indeed into laughter, during the telling of a story, the natural tendency is to stop, to 'compose' oneself and begin again when the affect underlying the expressive volatility has passed. However, if one listens to a client through the ears of a composer, these times of highly charged affect which disturb the controlled continuity of the voice are the most musical and the most expressive.

In Therapeutic Voicework a client who discharges affect during the telling of a story – such as in the report of a tragedy or during the disclosure of a delicate piece of personal history – is encouraged to continue speaking in such a way as to amplify and heighten the vocal expression of the affect. This amounts to talking whilst crying or laughing, shouting or yelling, gasping or sobbing and it enables the speech to be turned into song.

In some cultures there is no separation between emotionalised vocalisation such as crying and the process of singing – as, for example, amongst the Kaluli peoples of Papua New Guinea, where weeping forms the basis for song structure and singing style.[8] In Therapeutic Voicework this interface between crying and other forms of emotional vocalisation and the process of singing provides both a container for intense affect and, at the same time, inspiration for the composition of artistic form. The process of wroughting song from trauma develops Freud's observation that vocalised affect facilitates therapeutic process. In Therapeutic Voicework, however, the affective component of vocal utterance is magnified so that, metaphorically speaking, the talking cure becomes a singing cure.

The Language of Dreams

Freud's preoccupation with language and the significance of words, which had originated in his analysis of psychosomatic disorders, continued to colour his beliefs during his subsequent work regarding the nature of dreams. In 1900 he published a book entitled *The Interpretation Of Dreams*, which rescued the nocturnal opticality from the clutches of superstitious and amateur dabbling and brought to it a new respectability; for Freud realised that the dream presented a rare opportunity to perceive the elements of a person's unconscious unrestrained by the censoring devices of consciousness. In fact, Freud applied the same framework of linguistic analysis to dreams as he had done to the hysterical symptoms which resulted from converting semantic phrases from their metaphorical to their literal meaning. Freud said that after his work on hysterical symptoms 'it was then only a short step to treating the dream itself as a symptom and to applying to dreams the method of interpretation that had been worked out for symptoms'.[9]

According to Freud, thought is a linguistic activity reliant upon words, whilst the dream is primarily concerned with 'representability in visual images'.[10] Thus he proposed that the process of dreaming consists of the 'transformation of thoughts into pictures'.[11] This process of transformation from thoughts, which operate through language, to dream images, which operate through pictures, was described by Freud as a form of 'displacement' and he proposed that 'the direction taken by the displacement usually results in a colourless and abstract expression in the dream-thought, being exchanged for a pictorial and concrete one'.[12]

The interpretation of dreams in the psychoanalytic consultation, therefore, involved a process of translation, which sought to decode the visual dream image by converting it back into the linguistic thought which had allegedly originally created it. Consequently, the analysis of the pictorial dream image divulged by the patient was much less important than the analysis of the words with which the patient voiced it. For example, within Freud's framework of analysis the dream image of a tennis racket may imply a patient's preoccupation with a 'shady deal', an important financial transaction about which the patient feels uneasy and suspicious regarding its legality. The analysis of the dream involves translating the pictorial image of a racket into a linguistic code, which, in turn, points to its meaning. In the psychoanalytic consultation, the focus of the interpretation centres on the word 'racket' as a signifier for immoral transactions which the dream has transformed into a pictorial image of 'an object for sport' in order to give it visual presentation.

This interpretative decoding and unravelling of linguistic transformations, or displacements, consequently demanded a scrutinising attention to the multiplicity of simultaneous potential meanings contained within a single linguistic phrase, for many single words signify a number of different things. A racket, for example, may also signify 'a terrible noise' and could, therefore, lead the psychoanalytic process to an entirely different conclusion regarding the patient's mental preoccupations. Faced with this multiplicity, Freud proposed that the 'correct interpretation can only be arrived at on each occasion from the context'[13] and he turned his attention to the patient's own specific personal history and its determination of the particular associations evoked by certain words.

In the same way that Freud had sought the genesis of hysterical symptoms in the autobiographical history of the individual patient, so too the contents of dreams were perceived as an expression of the patient's unique and idiosyncratic experience of the world. Thus Freud proposed that the significance of dream images depended upon the varying personal circumstances which have informed each patient's psychological disposition. In other words, two patients may have exactly the same dream but the significance of the images contained therein will be entirely different as a result of specific and distinct life experiences. For Freud, therefore, dreams were ultimately composed of the residue of life's events and he further proposed that they presented to the dreamer the fulfilment of wishes which had not been achieved during waking hours. So, for example, the appearance of a tennis racket in another person's dream may signify that the patient is preoccupied with the unbearable noise or racket generated by a local night-club which has recently opened near his home and his wish that it would close.

However, Freud's theory regarding the individual determination of dreams was called into question when he discovered that the meaning of some dreams involved the use of linguistic metaphors of which the patient could not possibly have had knowledge in waking life. Of course, most people knew the various meanings for 'racket' but often Freud believed he had discovered images which originated in word meanings which could not possibly be known to the patient. On occasions this involved a translation from a foreign language which the patient could not speak. For example, Freud pointed out that 'the commonest expression in German for male sexual activity is 'to bird' and that 'the male organ is actually called "the bird" in Italian'. Freud thus proposed that when people dream of being able to fly it is 'only a disguise for another wish' which is 'nothing else than a longing to be capable of sexual performance'.[14] Freud further added the fact that small children are told that babies are delivered by a stork and that the ancients portrayed the phallus with wings as further evidence to connect the dream image of a bird with sex. Freud believed that it was irrelevant whether or not the dreamer was aware of these word meanings or ideas in waking life and that the significance of the bird was trans-cultural, independent of language or tradition.

Sex with Everything

Despite his strong adherence to the belief in the dominating efficacy of personal circumstance in shaping mental outlook, Freud could not avoid postulating that each individual inherits a certain body of psychological information, a process known as phylogenesis. Freud was led to propose that humankind possesses what he called an 'archaic heritage'. He believed that 'dreams bring to light material which cannot have originated either from the dreamer's adult life or from his forgotten childhood' but which 'a child brings with him into the world, before any experience of his own, influenced by the experiences of his ancestors'. He further suggested that 'we find the counterpart of this phylogenetic material in the earliest human legends and in surviving customs' and 'thus dreams constitute a source of human pre-history'.[15]

However, Freud remained uncomfortable with the concept of an archaic heritage. It threatened his stringent individualistic stance and it encouraged psychoanalysts to entertain immeasurable hypotheses regarding inherited patterns, which Freud was keen to avoid. Therefore, in order to compromise his position and find a sympathetic relationship between an undeniable inherited psychological predisposition on the one hand and a belief in the primary importance of personal context on the other, Freud proposed that a universality of dream images occurred only within the field of sexuality. In seeking to validate this hypothesis, Freud traced the significance of transpersonal dream images to a strictly sexual origin, even to the point of considering that all words may have their genesis in a sexual signification. Indeed, in a footnote which he added to his essay *The Dream Work* in 1925, Freud refers supportively to the theory of Dr Hans Sperber, who was of the opinion that, originally, all words 'referred to sexual things but afterwards lost their sexual meaning through being applied to other things and activities which were compared with the sexual ones'.[16] Consequently, Freud went to great lengths to argue that just about every image you can imagine has a sexual origin and that, more often than not, the words used to describe it have a sexual connotation also.[17]

Central to Freud's strictly sexual vision of phylogenesis was his belief in the inheritance of an innate identical disposition in every child, which, for boys, consisted of an unacknowledged desire to kill the father and consummate his love for the mother. Freud took the ancient Greek myth of Oedipus, preserved by Sophocles' tragic play, who, in ignorance, killed his father and married his mother, as a literary allegory for this internal psychological disposition which no man can escape and which every man must overcome. Freud termed this innate disposition the 'Oedipus Complex' and maintained that it was central to the phylogenetic inheritance of information from previous generations. Freud proposed that young boys become so deeply stimulated by the nourishing and affectionate attentions of their mother that they preserve a deeply-buried desire to consummate their motherly love through sexual activity. They are, however, at the same time, prevented from expressing or realising this by an established and externally enforced moral code which marks incestuous desires as taboo. Simultaneously, boys have equally ambiguous relationships with their fathers, who, whilst being the object of love and respect, are nonetheless loathed and despised for their unfettered sexual intimacy with the mother. Furthermore, they fear that the father will castrate them as punishment for their intentions. The deeply-buried wish for consummation with the mother is, therefore, accompanied by an equally buried wish to murder the father, and thereby remove the preventative competition and the source of threat, held in check only by the fear of being castrated. For little girls, meanwhile, Freud prescribed a variation on the same theme, according to which they harbour deep sensual feelings towards the father but repress their desires for intimacy in response to social taboo. Such repressions allegedly lead to unconscious fantasies of sexual relations with the father, which cause some guilt, distress and abhorrence and so become inverted and transformed into a fantasy of the father himself initiating sexual contact in the form of affection, inappropriate advances or sexual abuse. Thus it was that Freud laid the seeds which would grow into the bitter grapes which posthumously taint his reputation.

According to Freud, these alleged incestual desires of the child, buried though they may be, nonetheless provoke in the child much anxiety, confusion and energetic disturbance and, in order to escape the subsequent discomfort, the desires are buried even deeper so that they are apparently forgotten. However, refraining from the motor action of incest and patricide causes an accumulation of psychic energy and, just as Freud's early patients had suffered physical and psychological impairment as a result of retaining the affective energy associated with certain events, so too the affective energy associated with the Oedipus Complex tends to manifest itself in a host of mental and physical disturbances. In this next stage of Freud's work he therefore became less interested in reviving the now seemingly minor idiosyncratic traumas suffered by individual patients. Rather, he was now intent on tracing psychological suffering to certain universal sexual traumas suffered by everyone. However, it was not the real trauma of sexual abuse by fathers, uncles, brothers and friends of the family, of which so many of his female patients complained, that interested Freud. For, despite giving women a voice and despite listening to their words, Freud did not hear the stories of abuse which they told him. Rather, he heard what he considered to be fantasy stories which revealed the inverted desire of the patient for sexual intimacy with the man whom she, in her helpless delusion, mistakenly and hysterically believed had forced sexual intimacy upon her. In recent years what was once thought to be Freud's ingenious scrutiny has been labelled blind, dishonest and, in itself, abusive for, according to some research – particularly that amassed by Masson – Freud had access to proliferate and incontrovertible evidence which substantiated the claims of his patients.[18] Indeed, it seems that sexual abuse of children by family members and associates was alarmingly widespread during his era, as it seems to be in our own time. Yet Freud proceeded with the publication of theories which effectively rendered women's voices silent in the same moment that he encouraged them to speak. In addition, Freud seemed to completely ignore the Oedipus myth in its entirety, choosing to select only the small portion which verified his hypothesis that sons wish to kill the father and sexually possess the mother and that daughters seek to sexualise their relationship with the father; for in the myth the baby Oedipus is cruelly staked to a mountain and left to die by his own father, who has already enraged the gods by sexually assaulting a young boy named Chrysipuss. Oedipus, having been saved from his fate, then later leaves his adopted parents to avoid fulfilling the oracle's prediction that he will kill his father and marry his mother. Oedipus is, therefore, in the context of the myth as a whole, entirely innocent. Nonetheless, Freud proceeded to analyse women on the basis of his vision, assuming the inheritance of specific psychosexual constructs which for the boy involved the fantasy of sex with the mother and for the girl sex with the father. For Freud, the child carries the crimes of the parent.

In limiting the concept of a transpersonal aspect of psychological functioning to innate patterns of psycho-sexual development, Freud retained his belief in the primary importance of personal history. The key to decoding the patient's psyche lay in discovering the unique way in which the fundamental inherited material had been manipulated by personal circumstances and the way in which the accumulated energy expressed itself. However, in addition to ensuring the grief of his patients and the angry animosity of those who would later investigate his work, Freud created for himself an ensnaring dichotomy between the undeniable occurrence of inherited and transpersonal elements in the psyche on the one hand and his firm belief in the primary importance of individual experience on the other. This dichotomy was never fully resolved and it formed the single most important principle which separated the intellectual foundations of Freud's thinking from those of Jung.

Therapeutic Voicework Methodology: The Family Song

In the process of working through voice and song there are many compositional genres which provide specific therapeutic containers. These include the prayer, the lullaby, the ballad and the dirge, for example, which provide containers for need or thanks, self-soothing personal narrative and extreme sorrow or mourning respectively.

One particular song structure which I have found useful is what I have called 'The Family Song'. Here, the client, usually during a period of working through personal developmental material, spontaneously writes a simple, often childlike, song about the primary family members: mother, father and siblings.

When faced with this process, clients find that they crystallise specific images associated with the primary family members in the form of a song lyric. It also offers a regressive structure comparable to the process of painting the classic picture of mummy, daddy, siblings, house and trees when we are children, only in acoustic form.

The Family Song may serve to express and contain one isolated aspect of the client's feelings towards the family or member thereof, such as love, loathing, rage or remorse, and the artistic structure serves to shape, wrought and specify hitherto unformed affects. The writing process is kept very simple and clients are encouraged to begin lines with phrases such as 'My Mummy was...' or 'My Daddy used to say...'. In the singing of the song the voice usually takes on a childlike quality, infused with free air and violin, and the feelings towards the parents as experienced during the time of childhood are often vividly recapitulated.

Words Without Voice

It would be easy to continue in the tradition of blindness by turning a blind eye to Freud's work entirely. But during this early period of investigation he identified nothing less than the power of the voice to heal, a process which has sustained dissemination as a therapeutic modality for nearly one hundred years. It is, therefore, of significance both historically and theoretically. For though Freud soon departed from a cathartic model of treatment, and though the dissemination of psychoanalytic practice does not revolve around abreactive procedures, the process of catharsis still sits at the heart of many psychotherapeutic modalities by which the act of talking provides a certain energetic discharge.

Psychotherapeutic procedures which descend in form from Freud's vision of curative verbal discourse have focused particularly on the verbal aspect of voice, despite the fact that the vocal form of utterance was so crucial to the psychosomatic therapy which Freud developed with so-called hysterical patients. However, there have been a small number of psychoanalysts who have recognised the significance of the voice within the treatment process and who, therefore, have made psychoanalysis more relevant to the practice of Therapeutic Voicework by drawing attention to the specific role of vocal quality as opposed to speech content in the psychoanalytic strategy.

The Voice in Psychoanalysis

Attention to the voice from within the circle of Freud's psychoanalytic empire was first paid in 1927 when Ferenczi[19] published notes on two cases from his consulting room. Both concerned men who displayed the ability to speak in two voices, one which was high in pitch and had a quality like the falsetto register in classical song and one deeper in pitch, like the bass or baritone in singing. Ferenczi equated the appearance of the falsetto in one patient as a manifestation of his desire to receive the affection of his mother by retaining a girlish and childlike voice which he felt pleased her. In both cases Ferenczi proposed that the voice was revealed to be related to homosexuality and the image of femininity. Despite Ferenczi's publication and its obvious significance in focusing specifically upon the vocal aspect of verbal communication, nobody from the institution of psychoanalysis responded and little more was uttered about the voice by those who specialised in the analysis of words.

Then, in 1943, another psychoanalyst of the Freudian school by the name of Morris Brody noted that 'disturbances of the voice and of voice production occur not infrequently as an outward manifestation of emotional conflict, in short, as a symptom of neurosis'[20] and he recorded a number of case studies of patients who were neurologically normal, free from the physiologic voice changes of puberty and yet manifested vocal disturbance. One of these was a 24-year-old male with a self-admitted strong dependence on his mother, who had always 'babied' him. Brody detected in the tone of this patient's voice a 'break which sounded almost like a sob' which, according to Brody, 'attested to his yearning to remain a child'. The analyst concluded that the 'bass voice was repressed in an effort to retain his mother's love.'[21]

In this case of Brody's the man allegedly used his voice as an expression of his wish to identify with a child, whilst a further case recorded by Brody sought to reveal how an adult male expressed identification with his father directly through his voice. This second patient was a man in his late thirties who had been raised a catholic by a cruel and violent father. The patient, who was very weak and timid physically, though allegedly he very much wanted to be strong like his father, had subsequently renounced his religion. According to Brody, this patient, unable to compete with the father physically, strove to become intellectually superior to him. In addition, he did what many boys do in order to disguise their competitive relationship with their father, he displaced his competition onto something and someone else – in this case the church or, more specifically, the priest. The patient was thus consumed with what Brody describes as 'ideas of a grandiose ecclesiastical nature' and, in the process, became completely celibate. However, bubbling away under this attempt to outdo his father, the patient became preoccupied with sexual ideas about women and Brody notes that 'when expressing sexual ideas the patient's voice assumed a low chanting tone as if he were praying' whilst 'at other times his voice seemed to carry all the incantations and inflections of the clergy, as if he were not really expressing his sexual ideas but were 'delivering a sermon on sexuality'. Brody believed that the low chanting voice acted as a means of avoiding punishment and that the incantations were a way of attempting to neutralise the feeling of wickedness about his sexual ideas for 'when the patient's attention was drawn to his change of voice and he felt that he was expected to speak normally, he was then unable to bring himself to talk about sexual matters'.[22] Based on cases such as this drawn from his own consulting practice, Brody concluded that 'to hear the voice solely for what it has to say and to overlook the voice itself, deprives the analyst of an important avenue leading to emotional conflict'.[23]

Further to Brody's comments, Harry Stack Sullivan, an influential Freudian analyst, said that the psychoanalytic interview 'is a situation of primarily vocal communication – not verbal communication alone'.[24] Also, in 1959 Mahl[25] noticed that extraneous vowels accompanied verbal language in psychiatric illness and since then a number of psychotherapists and psychiatrists have paid special attention to the voice as well as the speech of a patient. For example, in 1960 a group of researchers made a tape recording of the first five minutes of an interview between a psychiatrist and a patient and then made a written transcription of absolutely all the vocal sounds which the patient expressed. This included the actual words spoken, the way they were uttered and all other emissions – such as a quick gasp of breath or a contemplative 'mmm'. Words were denoted with standard phonetic and linguistic signs while paralinguistic activities, such as shifts of rhythm, tempo, inflection and other noises, were given specially-created symbols.[26] There were, consequently, major differences in the interpretations and conclusions reached by psychiatrists about the patient's predicament between those based only on the usual written case notes and those ascertained when all the paralinguistic information was available. Thus the experiment highlighted how vital it is to take into consideration an assessment of all audible noises made by the patient in order to come to a satisfactory analysis of his or her conscious and unconscious ideas. The experiment shows that an analysis of what a patient has said – based on what is written down in a transcription, such as in a patient's notes – can lead to an inaccurate diagnosis and, consequently, inappropriate treatment. Given that the psychiatric treatment of patients has always been augmented within a classic allopathic medical model composed of a multi-disciplinary team of specialists whose assessment is based upon the circulation of written notes, the results of this experiment are potentially terrifying.

Wilhelm Reich and the Mind Within the Muscle

Whilst Ferenczi, Brody and Sullivan listened to the voice, they did not work towards a cathartic utterance, as Freud had done in his very early work. It was a pupil of Sigmund Freud by the name of Wilhelm Reich who revisited the significance of catharsis and became particularly interested in the conversion of so-called psychic energy into physical ailment and psychological state.

Reich proposed that bottled-up psychic energy is expressed not only in specific physical malfunctions and extreme psychological states, such as muscular paralysis, depression or anxiety, but also in the general psychological attitude and outlook which a person holds towards the world. Reich saw a person's character as comprising certain identifiable attitudes, such as cynicism, bitterness and envy. He believed that the process of repressing the demands of the instincts in the face of moral requirements led to the erection of strong emotional guards which served to keep the two apart and which subsequently become a regular feature of the person's character. These guards were, for Reich, the mainstay of what Freud called 'resistance'. The stronger and more firmly established a certain emotional attitude, the more adequately was the person able to resist giving in to the demands of the underlying instincts which it had been erected to suppress. They also served to protect the individual from threatening attacks and demands from the outside world. Reich said that it is as if the personality has 'put on an armour, a rigid shell on which the knocks from the outer world as well as the inner demands rebound'.[27] Thus for Reich, the first aim of therapy was to break through the resilient habitual attitudes which seemed to form the nucleus of a person's character. However, the innovation of Reich's insight lies not here but in the next stage of his thinking.

Reich proposed that the elaborate armour of strongly defended emotional attitudes which the patient erects manifests in the general muscular state of posture and physical carriage, what he described as 'chronically fixed muscular attitudes'.[28] In order to bind and stem the flow of suppressed psychic energy, a person tended to develop a high degree of tensile rigidity in his muscle tone, which Reich called 'muscular armour'. This served to preserve the 'pent-up' and intransigent psychological outlook by which it was generated. So for Reich, muscular armour and character armour are 'functionally identical'[29] and reveal themselves through a host of psycho-physical expressions such as 'the manner of talking, of the gait, facial expression and typical attitudes such as smiling, deriding, haughtiness, over-correctness'.[30]

The character armour develops 'as the chronic result of the conflict between instinctual demands and the frustrating outer world' and 'the continuing actual conflicts between instinct and outer world give it its strength and continued reason for existence'.[31] The character armour therefore becomes fixed and preserved by the muscular armour of the body. Thus one of the primary functions of character armour and muscular armour is that of 'absorbing dammed up energy'.[32]

Reich, like Freud, saw the quality of these instinctual demands and their constituting energy as essentially sexual in nature and he named it 'orgone energy', a word which he derived from 'organism', 'organic' and 'orgasm'. Reich also shared with Freud the belief that the resistances which a patient concocts as a means of preventing admission to the existence of the instincts must be dissembled. However, there marks the end of Reich's synonymity with Freud.

Because Reich believed that the manifestations of this dynamic were psycho-physical, he also believed that a successful therapeutic process would have to be psycho-physical too. For this reason, Reich attacked the purely verbal strategy of Freud's work. For Reich, the nature of a patient's repressions, problems and resistances could not be ascertained or dissolved by the words which he or she spoke. Rather, the therapist had to physically investigate the movements of the body and, by manipulation of, and direct contact with, the muscles, ventilate pent-up energy. Reich said that his approach 'is distinguished from all other modes of influencing the organism by the fact that the patient is asked to express himself biologically while word language is eliminated to a far-reaching degree.'[33] But what did Reich mean by expressing oneself biologically?

Respiration and Repression

Reich believed that one of the methods employed by a neurotic individual to keep his character armour and muscular armour in place was a restricted pattern of breathing. By maintaining a shallow intake of breath or an overly quick rate of respiratory cycles, the patient was able to keep affective constructs retained and restrained. Reich therefore abandoned the couch and the static verbal dialogue and worked directly on the patient's body. Applying pressure to abdomen, chest and other areas which housed important organs, he encouraged his patients not to talk but to focus on 'letting go' of their feelings through breathing.

By releasing restricted patterns of inspiration and expiration and encouraging long, deep, free breaths, Reich caused emotions to be released in the form of sobs, tears, screams and sighs, which left the patient feeling purged, cleansed and disengaged from the previously unpliant condition to which they had become accustomed.

But it was not the process of breathing enhancement itself, but the resulting movements of the body which Reich attended to in his analysis. He believed the human body had an in-built tendency to express itself through free-flowing, unbounded, undulating physical movements, the ultimate expression of which occurred during orgasm. However, Reich believed that what most people experience as orgasm is but a tiny vestige, a minuscule moment of climactic release completely divorced from a total body experience. He observed that when a free and unbounded respiratory cycle was achieved, it was always accompanied by undulating movements of the body, which he called the 'orgasm reflex'.[34] This orgasm reflex was not equivalent to the genital climax of copulation or masturbation but was the total bodily experience of climactic release of which genital orgasm should ideally be only a part. Despite the eccentricity which characterised and, according to some, depleted the integrity of Reich's later work, one thing remains undeniably certain: it was Wilhelm Reich who initiated the breakthrough in Western psychotherapy from a purely verbal analysis to direct work with the body and central to this body work was the attendance to the process of respiration by which, it was recognised, a patient kept instincts repressed.

Furthermore, because the releasing of the restricted process of breathing caused many of Reich's patients to let out vocal sounds as an expression of feelings which had been pent-up for a long time, Reich may also be credited as having made a significant, if minor and unwitting, contribution to the significance of the voice in psychotherapeutic practice.

Alexander Lowen and Bioenergetics

It was one of Reich's pupils who developed the principles of body work into a more systematised and communicable process and, in so doing, highlighted further the importance of the human voice in psychotherapeutic methods. This was Alexander Lowen.

Lowen was Reich's pupil from 1940 to 1952 and inherited from him a dissatisfaction with the underachievement of the verbal therapy initiated by Freud. He believed that though 'much valuable information was gained through these inquiries' they nonetheless 'left untouched the most important domain of personality – namely, its base in bodily processes.'[35] Lowen alleged that 'the weakness of psychoanalytic technique is that it ignores the body in its attempt to help the patient work through his emotional conflicts'. Consequently, he claimed that 'the ideas that emerge in the course of treatment remain impotent to produce any major changes in personality'.[36]

Lowen was deeply influenced by Reich's discovery of the unity of psychological and bodily experience and went on to further extend the principles by which a person's emotional preoccupations may be read from his somatic condition. He believed that 'the functional identity of psychic character and body structure, or muscular attitude, is the key to understanding personality' for, he proposed, it enables us to 'read the character from the body and to explain a body attitude by its psychic representations and vice versa.'[37]

Lowen saw the damming-up and impediment of the body's innate physical malleability and capacity for expression not as a problem unique to neurotics or those suffering from severe trauma but as the social curse of Western humanity. He proposed that the inhabitants of the modern world have betrayed the body, that 'all our personal difficulties stem from this betrayal' and that 'most of our social problems have a similar origin'.[38] Gathering impetus from Reich's research, Lowen developed further the principles and practices by which people could be released from these psycho-physical restraints and hindrances and be enabled to rediscover an unbounded and unencumbered capacity for emotional and physical expression. Lowen called these principles 'Bioenergetics', the aim of which was 'to remove the barriers or blocks to self-expression' and thereby 'to help a person become more spontaneous and more self-expressive'.[39]

Also inherited from Reich was Lowen's understanding that the respiratory act is one of the elemental barriers to self-expression, the primary means by which instincts and feelings are repressed and therefore also the means by which the blocks and instincts can be released. As a result, central to the therapeutic method of Bioenergetics was direct work on enhancing the patient's freedom of respiratory movement. But Lowen took things one stage further than Reich.

From Breath to Voice

Lowen believed that the quality of vocal sounds which patients released as an involuntary response to the therapeutic process contained important information about their character and psychological predicament. Lowen listened, therefore, not only to the gasps, cries and sighs which were emitted during the physical manipulation of his patient's bodies but also to the timbres inherent in the patient's speaking voice, the patterns of 'inflection, tone, rhythm and gesture, which in large part are spontaneous and unique to the speaker'[40] and which often have 'greater impact than the words he utters'.[41]

Lowen therefore introduced into the psychotherapeutic process the idea that the quality of a voice mirrors the nature of underlying emotional dynamics. It was simply a logical extension of his belief that freeing the body resulted in a freeing of the psyche to propose that a loosening of the voice resulted in the same psychological liberation.

Lowen proclaimed 'that a rich voice is a rich manner of self expression and denotes a rich inner life'.[42] He identified a rich voice as one with 'the presence of undertones and overtones that give it a fullness of sound'[43] and a broad range of tonal expression. He said that 'a voice can be flat, without depth or resonance, it can be low as if lacking energy, and it can be thin and bodiless' and that 'each of these qualities bears some relationship to the personality of the individual'.[44] Lowen believed that 'the blockage of any feeling will affect its expression vocally'[45] and, consequently, 'if a person is to recover his full potential for self-expression, it is important he gain the full use of his voice in all its registers and in all its nuances of feeling'.[46]

Therefore, Lowen's techniques of physically manoeuvering the patient's body and enhancing the breathing process through methodical exercises geared itself not only to releasing the undulating movements which Reich had called the orgasm reflex but also encouraged the often inevitable vocalisation of pent-up emotions which occured as the natural outcome of muscular release, giving them acoustic form, which contributed to the overall process of catharsis.

Scream and Leave It at That

Of all the various involuntary sounds which Lowen's patients emitted, the most powerful and emotionally impacted was the scream – which he described as 'an explosion within the personality that momentarily shatters the rigidity created by chronic muscular tension'[47] and which has a 'powerful cathartic effect on the personality.'[48] Lowen also claimed that other vocal emissions like 'crying and deep sobs produce a similar effect by softening and melting body rigidities'.[49]

Lowen believed that 'because the voice is so closely tied to feeling' the process of 'freeing it involves the mobilization of suppressed feelings and their expression in sound'. He alleged that there are identifiable qualities of voice which express specific feelings: 'fear and terror are expressed in a scream, anger in a loud, sharp tone, sadness in a deep, sobbing voice, pleasure and love in soft, cooing sounds'. Furthermore, he said that 'a high-pitched voice indicates a blocking of the deep notes that express sadness' whilst 'a low-pitched, chesty voice indicates a denial of the feeling of fear and inhibition against its expression in a scream'.[50]

As with his body work, Lowen was here in the realm of catharsis, providing a release of generalised emotional accumulations. He did not attempt to shape the sounds or manipulate them as he did the body, as one might in Therapeutic Voicework. However, Lowen did record his own experience of the positive psychological benefits of singing. Working with 'a singing teacher who was familiar with bioenergetic concepts' and who 'understood the role of the voice in self-expression' Lowen was reminded of his feeling that his mother had cut his throat, which had 'created some difficulty' in speaking and crying 'but especially in singing' and, at the start of the lesson, he felt afraid that his 'voice would crack' and that he 'would start to cry'. To his surprise, Lowen found that he could open his throat 'and vocalize fully' as his 'voice became freer' and his body entered a 'constant state of vibration'. Furthermore, he 'didn't feel like crying once' and left the session with 'a sense of joyfulness' felt only on a few previous occasions.[51] Though Lowen continued his singing lessons, he, like many before him, did not further investigate the means by which the act of singing could contribute to the animation of psychotherapy.

Therapeutic Voicework Methodology: Breath, Voice and Catharsis

During Therapeutic Voicework clients will often experience heightened emotion whilst pursuing respiratory, physical and vocal exercises. Indeed, there is probably no other medium of human expression which can communicate and embody affect so intensely.

The verbal articulation of affect, which Freud believed was indispensable to the cathartic process, serves, nonetheless, to distance the emotional experience from its expression, for Freud himself admitted that words are a substitute; language signifies a lack.

In Therapeutic Voicework, by removing the necessity for verbal articulation, the gap between the expression and the instigating experience is closed and the emotion is thus intensified.

In the approach to Therapeutic Voicework which I have developed, the practitioner is sometimes required to contain the client's expression of intense affect through a number of strategies, which include physical contact with the body, instruction in ways of breathing and the facilitation of physical and vocal methodologies which help the client locate the catharsis in a structure. One of these structures is the act of singing, which gives a musical voice to neurosis.

Taking the work of Reich and Lowen a stage further, I have found it extremely beneficial to intervene whilst a client is physically undulating and vocalising intense emotion, encouraging them to shift register, change pitch, infuse the voice with free air and add or remove violin or vibrato. Additionally, it can be extremely therapeutic to assist the client in placing the cries, sobs and screams in a melodic framework whilst they are being experienced. This closes the gap between musical and songful composition and performance on the one hand and intense personal experience on the other. The client, in addition to experiencing catharsis, undergoes a creative transformation of a neurosis into a work of art. That which is originally conceived as something to be exorcised becomes the raw material from which expressively valuable form is wrought.

Paul Moses and the Voice of Neurosis

Lowen's fundamental belief that emotional disturbance is audible in the non-discursive quality of the human voice was inherited from the work of a man, whom Lowen publicly acknowledged, called Paul Moses, who was a clinical professor in charge of the Speech and Voice Section, Division of Otolaryngology, at the Stanford University School of Medicine, San Francisco. It was here in 1940 that he conducted an experiment under the auspices of the University of California Institute of Child Welfare[52] in which he analysed the personality of an adolescent boy, whom he had never met, from a phonograph record of the boy's voice without face-to-face contact.

The boy had previously been analysed by a psychiatrist and had been subjected to a psychological examination known as the Rorschach test. Based on what he perceived in the patterns of rhythm, pitch, timbre and prosody of the boy's voice, Moses gave an analysis of the character and psychological constitution of the boy which was found to agree on many points with the Rorschach findings and the psychiatrist's own report.[53] Moses believed, like many before him, that oral communication is composed of both speech and voice and was convinced that it was possible to detect in the voice alone any underlying emotional or psychological disturbance. He proposed that 'vocal dynamics truthfully reflect psychodynamics' and that 'each emotion has its vocal expression.'[54]

Moses was deeply influenced by Freud, from whom he learnt that traumatic events which occur during childhood can come back to haunt the adult in the form of physical sufferings, and disturbances in the quality of the human voice were, for Moses, manifestations of such traumas. In addition, Moses was intrigued by Freud's notion of an archaic heritage, a deeply buried layer of images in the human psyche which belong to a collective unconscious, which for him were also evident in the sound of a person's voice. For Moses, 'voice is an indicator of different phases in a person's life' because 'vocal changes accompany the development of the individual' but, additionally, 'voice contains archaic properties originating in the cradle of mankind' and thus 'one can go as far as to say that vocal expression is a record of the history of mankind as well as a record of the individual'.[55] Moses proposed that 'the child's vocal development, from its first cry' to the acquisition of speech, 'retraces the development of the species', that emotional disturbance in adult life can cause him to 'return symbolically to a phase that gave greater security' and that the regression will be expressed through the vocal characteristics which accompanied that stage.[56] Because of the synonymity between the developmental dynamics of individual infancy and preverbal humankind, Moses believed that in the paralinguistic utterances of schizophrenics one could perceive the acoustic remains of an earlier time – just as Jung had perceived such primitivity in the paintings of psychotics, which he believed mirrored those contained in ancient myths.

Moses was a laryngologist and, as such, was involved in the treatment of the voice problems of which his patients complained. However, just as Freud had discovered no organic or physiological cause for the broad range of somatic sufferings of which his early patients complained, so too Moses discovered that the larynx of many of his patients was completely healthy. Moses therefore assumed Freud's role of searching for the underlying psychological cause of physical disorder, in this case disorders which affected the voice.

Moses thus sought to encourage an inter-disciplinary approach to treating voice disorders in which psychodynamics played a central role. He believed that the 'ideal speech and voice specialist should be a combination of otolaryngologist, psychiatrist, psychologist, speech trainer, singing master, and experimental phonetician.'[57] He felt that it was important to recognise that it is often 'emotional disturbance' which causes misuse of the vocal instrument and, in turn, causes the symptoms with which the patient comes to the laryngologist. These ideas are recorded in his only book, *The Voice of Neurosis,*[58] published in 1954.

Moses' argument was that a certain amount of psychotherapeutic knowledge was necessary in order to deal with the high number of cases of vocal dysfunctions for which there appeared to be no physiological cause. Moses said that 'it is in such cases that the laryngologist must step into the realm of psychiatry and psychotherapy because it would be a technical impossibility to consult the psychiatrist for each of this group of patients.'[59] Moses believed that treatment of the voice had to run in tandem with treatment of the psyche and his prime aim was, therefore, to introduce the precepts of psychotherapy into vocal analysis.

Amongst the case studies which Moses recorded, he gives an example of a man with a persistently high voice which, he points out , 'in our culture' is associated with 'young' and 'female' whilst low voices are identified with 'old' and 'male'. Because, for a male, the 'adult range and register are acquired during adolescence', Moses interpreted the patient to be experiencing the results of an 'unsuccessful identification' with the father and an over-identification with the mother, expressed in a high voice equivalent with that of a pre-adolescent boy or of a woman. With such cases, Moses claimed that 'psychotherapy alone will not lower the voice, just as voice therapy alone will not reveal and cure the causing factors'.[60] Consequently, Moses urged all clinical professionals to seek a multi-disciplinary model for voice therapy which would combine attention to psyche and soma.

It was Paul Moses who really grounded the notion of a vocal psychology in the theoretical principles established by psychoanalysis. In particular, Moses recognised that analysts of the Freudian school believed that one of the most significant traumas suffered universally by children is being weaned off the breast and that many psychological difficulties suffered in adult life can be put down to the fact that the patient has never fully recovered from having been separated from the once reliable source of nourishment and comfort. But Moses proposed that there was another more shattering trauma which could have equally severe repercussions in later life.

Moses believed that the action of phonation at birth and the subsequent preverbal noises of a child are extremely pleasurable and releasing. The child draws sensual oral pleasure from the process of suckling at the breast which becomes associated with the vegetative sounds of sucking to such a degree that the process of vocal sound making becomes an important source of pleasure whether accompanied by feeding or not. This pleasure is unhampered by any external restriction and the sounds are composed according only to the baby's own whims, feelings and responses and as a result of involuntary physiological operations.

However, Moses also proposed that the acquisition of speech is, by comparison, a traumatic experience which interferes with this free-functioning of vocal expressivity. To learn language, the child is required to bring his feelings and instincts, moods and affects – which have hitherto been sung in a fashion reminiscent of preverbal peoples – under the jurisdiction of words.[61] This involves the child in a game of punishment and reward, which he or she finds terribly traumatic.

According to Moses, therefore, patients who have found this trans-formation from non-verbal to verbal communication particularly traumatic are subconsciously yearning for an opportunity to once again give free rein to their feelings and instincts via the spontaneous emission of inarticulate vocal sounds. The success of any vocal and psychological therapy depended on giving the patient an opportunity to once more give voice to the psychological dimensions for which no words are appropriate.

As a result of his search for a means to give patients such an opportunity, Moses believed to have discovered that the process of singing was the only adult activity which answered to these needs. It was in this connection that Moses proposed the idea of transposing Freud's cathartic method of verbal therapy onto the act of singing for he believed that just as the infant 'lets his vocal powers range to their fullest extent', so 'in archaic days, when sounds, and not abstract constructions of grammar, were the interpreter of human thoughts and emotions, the complete range of voice was used more freely' for 'primitive peoples at the dawn of society used their voices to their heart's content to express their feelings and reactions'. However, 'as we ceased to communicate in gestures, imitative sounds, cries of sorrow and jubilation, and acquired, instead, words, our vocal range began to shrink to the point where speech melody' or prosody 'is now merely a weazened emotional scale on which articulation plays its piece'. Only at times when 'our controls get out of hand, when we become excited or intoxicated, do we become savages again' and 'the primeval cry can be heard again'. For Moses, 'singing is something of a compromise, a willed recall of an echo of the pure satisfaction of primitive vocalisation' serving also to release 'the tensions built up by our repressions'.[62]

Unfortunately, it was not until towards the end of his life that Moses discovered, in theory, that singing was an aid to psychotherapeutic development and he did not, therefore, have the opportunity to practically investigate the use of singing with patients. Nonetheless, Moses is an important figure in the development of a model for Therapeutic Voicework and his book, though no longer in print, remains a classic text.

In the approach to Therapeutic Voicework which I have developed, the vocal expressions which occur during intense cathartic experience are perceived as the elements of artistic composition. This means that crying, deep breathing, shouting, wailing, laughing, chuckling, screaming and all manner of extreme vocal expressions which occur when a client is sequestered by an intense emotional sensation are repeated, rehearsed and transformed. A client is asked to scream again, cry again and gasp again, only higher, softer, with more free air and in saxophone or in clarinet. This destigmatises the process, which, for many, is perceived as 'hysterical', and heals the split between exaggerated emotional expression and artistic composition.

Semiotics and the Limits of the Word

The work of Reich, Lowen and Moses, combined with those other analysts who cast their ear upon the vocal channel of oral communication, represents a body of work which attempted to put the words of the talking cure to one side in order to hear more clearly the voice beneath. However, parallel to this field of enquiry, an equally important development has taken place within the study of the words by those interested not in voice but in language, but which ironically also ultimately points to the significance of voice by revealing the limitation of words. This field, which I will now attempt to describe, is complex and confusing because it seeks to explain in words that which is both unique to and beyond words. It is, though, an absolutely crucial component to the model of Therapeutic Voicework which I have developed.

Despite Freud's concern with the importance of language in revealing the unconscious, he was not aware of important linguistic research that was being conducted in his own time for, whilst Freud was developing the ideas presented in *The Interpretation of Dreams* which laid foundations for the new discipline of psychoanalysis, the Swiss linguist Ferdinand de Saussure was formulating the principles for a new field of enquiry which he called 'Semiology' and which were posthumously transcribed from his manuscripts in 1916.

Saussure's semiology, defined as the study of any system of signs which express ideas, is primarily concerned with the sign-system of language and the means by which this linguistic activity creates meaning. The semiotic process first necessitates that an individual formulates or conceives of a mental 'sound image', 'sense-image' or 'psychological picture' of a word, 'not phonic but incorporeal'[63] which remains unspoken and is called the *signifier*. This serves, in turn, to evoke the psychological image or idea of the phenomenon which it denotes, which is called the *signified*. The relationship between the sense-image of the word, called the signifier, and the idea of the phenomenon which it signifies, called the signified, is what constitutes the *sign* for the actual phenomenon itself. The actual phenomenon, the identification of which is the aim of the semiotic process, is the *referent*.

Thus the phenomenon of truth is a referent, which is identified by the process of conceiving first of a signifier or a mental sound-image of the word 'truth', which, in turn, creates the mental idea of truth – which is the signified – and the relationship between them activates a sign for truth itself. It is important to reiterate that this process can be silent. For Saussure, the audible process of speech is the primary, but not essential, expression of the linguistic signifier whilst writing constitutes a secondary process which exists 'for the sole purpose of representing the first'.[64]

Saussure recognised that the 'bond between signifier and signified is arbitrary' – that a certain word denotes a specific phenomenon only by way of convention – thus, with the support of the social consensus, any word could be exchanged for another without altering the signified phenomenon or referent. If we had been raised to refer to truth as 'dog', then the phenomenon of truth or of dog would remain unchanged. Thus, for Saussure, language 'is the social side of speech, outside the individual who can never create or modify it by himself; it exists only by virtue of a sort of contract signed by the members of the community.'[65] However, although the relationship between the signifier and signified was considered to be arbitrary, the relationship between the sign and referent was proposed to be direct and rudimentary, assuming the pre-linguistic reality and existence of the phenomena for which the signifier and signified are a sign. Truth is, therefore, assumed to exist in order to be signified and to which to be referred. By way of this assumption, Saussure's semiotics emanate from the same epistemological foundation as the tradition of Western metaphysical philosophy, which employs language to identify and define phenomena which it proposes exist independently of it. But this metaphysical assumption of the a priori existence of phenomena, which has provided language with a stable centre around which to operate, has been challenged by the cultural movement known as Post-modernism.

This challenge proposes that the sign created by the relationship between signifier and signified leads not to the evidence of a phenomenal referent but simply to another signifier, at which point the process of signification begins again. Language leads only to language. The word 'truth' signifies the word 'fact', which signifies the word 'actuality', which signifies the word 'truth'. Post-modernism holds that in fact there is no actual referent divorced from the signifier or word used to define it. Truth is but a word. This philosophy, which confines reality to the experience or illusion created by language, is proliferated particularly by the work of Jacques Derrida.

Derrida argues that Western metaphysical philosophy has always assumed not only, like Saussure, that the relationship between the signified and the referent is direct and rudimentary but that there is some transcendental signified which exists outside the system of language, even though it cannot be touched or experienced sensately. This signified changes according to the philosopher or period and has been at different times Will, Faith, Reason and God. In order for there to be a maintainable difference between the signifier and the signified, there has to be one term which describes and signifies itself. The assumption that there is such a term reflects the metaphysical search for a referent which is final and absolute, a unifying principle that marks the end of the chain of signifiers in search of meaning. Derrida proposes that this transcendental signifier is a fiction and that there is no real difference between signifier and signified because the only way we can come to know the signified is through another signifier. Consequently, the system of language is in a state of constant free play within a closed system. The dictionary itself is an example of such a system in which one word can only be explained in terms of another word which, in turn, can only be explained in terms of another word. According to Derrida there is nothing that one can call real beyond this finite set of words. No longer can language be seen as a system operating around a centralising notion which exists outside the system, such as truth. Rather, the system is open ended and infinite.

This state of perpetual lack of meaning in the absence of all signifieds is what Derrida called *'Dissemination'*. The application of this theorem to philosophy and linguistics, indeed to all writing, is known as *'Deconstruction'* and the effect of Derrida's deconstruction is to completely decentralise language. He says that the function of giving language and thought a centre which is assumed to exist beyond the sign which designates it is not an essential component of thought or language itself but a quality with which we invest it 'to orient, balance, and organise' a structure and provide a 'point at which the substitution of contents, elements, or terms is no longer possible'.[66] The idea of language being structured not around the relationship between signifier and signified but only between signifiers is central to the deconstructionism of Derrida and the decentralisation which it installs is, in turn, central to Post-modernism.

Jacques Lacan

Though Saussure's work was not known to Freud, a later analyst, Jacques Lacan, a student and colleague of Freud, applied Saussure's semiology to his linguistic view of the psyche. Lacan takes Freud's preoccupation with language to its limits, proposing that it is through language and language alone that the psyche is constituted and by which it reflects upon itself. In Lacan's theory of human progress there is a crucial phase of infant development, synonymous with the child first seeing himself in a mirror, called the 'mirror stage', which occurs between six months and eighteen months and during which the child begins first to be able to reflect upon himself mentally and thoughtfully as an entity. It is through the acquisition of this ability to reflect back upon himself as an individual whole being that the linguistic concept of 'I' is born. Up to this point the child is unable to distinguish between himself and his environment, his own needs and his mother's response, but, with the acquisition of language, comes personal identity central to which is the individual as a subject of his own discourse. Lacan argues that it is this acquisition of language that constitutes the unconscious, which is not only structured like a language but is born from language, constituted of language and, in fact, *is* language. Furthermore, there is no subject, no sense of what one is and no sense that one exists, independent of language. We come into being only through linguistics.

In addition to extending Freud's linguistic obsessions through the translation of Freud's psycho-sexual hypothesis into Saussure's semiotic terms, Lacan also shares with Derrida the belief that words or signifiers do not denote a definitive set of underlying signifieds with a singular meaning or truth relating to a single narrative which merely awaits excavation. In applying a decentralised view of language, synonymous with Derrida's, to an extension of Freud's linguistic description of psychological functioning, Lacan destabilises the psyche, abandoning all search for any centralising concept or definitive meaning to the patient's text. Lacan proposes that there is no centre to the self but that it is structured as a continuous process of mobility in which one signifier points to another, each one possessing a multiplicity of meanings which constantly shift in time, upsetting any notion of a fixed meaning.

One of the main structures employed instinctively by human beings to make sense of the world and of themselves is narrative. In fitting the fleeting images of our perceptive faculties, memories and ideas into a chronological series we generate a story within which we can place ourselves. There is a past, present and future which secures us in time, place and causality. Freud employed narrative as an essential framework within which to locate the patient's verbal utterance for he was concerned with mapping out the individual's own story as it appeared in verbal dialogue during the analytic session. Furthermore, he was also determined to contextualise these small stories within the grand narrative of the Oedipus myth, which meant forging an equation between the individual tales of sexual repression and the great tale of a Greek figure. Freud's reading of the individual's psychological disposition was thus based on pre-existing structures around which he sought to centre the personality.

The tendency of Freud to centralise the psyche around pre-existing structures places his work within an entirely modern aesthetic, for modernism may be defined as that which seeks to unify through the attachment of a single meaning to a given phenomenon around which it may cohere and by which it may be defined. One of the primary structures which serves to centre a subject or phenomenon is narrative, which is thus a central feature of modern aesthetics. This modern aesthetic has, however, subsided and we are presently suffering or experiencing a 'post-modern condition'.[67]

The cultural period or movement defined as Post-modernism, which departs from modernism in its opposition to centralising structures, has effected psychotherapy by challenging the fundamental tendency to nurture the idea of a single personality with a stable narrative around which to cohere and within which to be placed.

Post-Modernism

The analysis of cultural aesthetics proceeds by placing a subject under the scrutiny of an interpretative process. The substance of the subjects to which interpretative process may be applied ranges from the inanimate objects of fine art and sculpture to the psychology of the human subject in psychoanalysis, whilst the systematic methodology which has governed the interpretative process in the development of cultural history include such '*isms*' as Marxism and Feminism. Post-modernism may be defined as a cultural aesthetic which defies and denies both the subject and the interpretative process any centralising idiom, aesthetic or idea around which to cohere.[68]

As we have seen, in linguistics this process of decentralisation is manifested through the deconstruction of the illusion of phenomenal existence independent of language, whilst in psychology it consists in destabilising the idea of a single self or personality structure through deploying the efficacy of narrative or stable linguistic meaning and instead nurturing a model of the psyche based on simultaneous multiplicity of meaning within a closed system of signifiers. In architecture it entails the abandonment of any unifying principle such as symmetry, stylistic anachronism or consistency in the choice of constituting materials. In painting it means the absence of thematic links between the elemental subjects of the content and the lack of any single formal style around which the painting could be said to be structured. This shift from the Modern to the Post-modern can also be seen in theatre as reflected in the development of performance from the first to the second half of this century and which has entailed the rejection of presenting identifiable characters in the context of a comprehendible narrative.[69] In seeking to abandon any secure and stable centralising principle around which the subject or interpretation of the subject may operate, Post-modernism necessarily deploys and dissolves the efficacy of identity, which has been, historically, the primary point of reference by which the subject is defined and named in relation to a single centre.

The subject of identification involves eliciting from the subject its point, that which is at the centre of it. This process of identification, which Post-modernism seeks to obstruct, necessitates the simultaneous induction of two points of reference: first, the subject to be identified and second, the principle or principles extraneous to it within which the appropriate identification is sought. That is to say that the subject is given meaning by being identified as something else. In negating and disabling the application of identity to the subject, Post-modernism prevents analytical recourse to a conceptual field extraneous to the subject itself. It faces the interpretative process with the ontological pure presence of the subject, which, consequently, can be identified only as itself. A word is a word without necessarily denoting anything else; a sound is, likewise, just a sound. The theatre performance is not about anything nor does the dance performance describe anything outside of itself. This is post-modern art which reflects the Post-modern condition.[70]

This Post-modern condition is of major theoretical significance to the principles and practice of Therapeutic Voicework for the sounds uttered by the vocalist during non-verbal work do not partake of a schematic codified matrix of language within which one unit can be exchanged for, or translated into, another. As Barthes[71] has so eloquently described, the act of vocalisation presents exactly itself, expressing that which is woven so intricately into the grain of the voice that it is identical with it. The sound of the voice does not describe something else in the way that the word 'truth' stands for the notion of 'actuality' or the way that the word 'dog' stands for the animal. The voice is both the content and the form. It is the the 'urgh' or 'ah', the tonal and timbral expression which cannot be written here and which, if it were, could not be read. It is expression before representation.

When an audient listens to a vocalist, therefore, the listener's own linguistic reactions are of limited use in dialoguing with the sounds, just as the words of the dictionary are meaningless to the infant during the pre-Oedipal, semiotic stage. At the most elemental level, voice is untranslatable and sonorises its own language. Yet meaningful, expressive and communicative dialogue clearly takes place in the acoustic space between mother and babe. Voice is, therefore, communicative within its own compositional nature, just as post-modern dance communicates without referring to another language beyond the kinetic motion of the body in space. Therapeutic Voicework may, therefore, be understood as a particularly post-modern practice. Furthermore, it is the Post-modern precept that connects, at the deepest level, the psychological and the artistic dimensions of Therapeutic Voicework.

Feminism and the Freedom of the Word

In disposing with the process of identification, which has historically been the means by which the interpretative process has defined what the subject seeks to mean, Post-modernism presents its subject as having no need for meaning. Post-modernism turns identity in on itself, forces interpretation to give way to experience and claims no need for meaning in order to sustain its proliferation. The multiplicity of meanings inherent in language, which has been such a central focus to the Post-modern movement, has shed suspicion on the validity of any single interpretation or 'reading' of a text. Furthermore, it has highlighted the extent to which any reading or interpretation of a text tends to reveal more about the framework employed to perceive it than the inherent nature of the text itself. A Marxist critique of a novel will tend to discover a political paradigm at the heart of it, whilst a psychoanalytic analysis of the same text will be found to discover evidence of the Oedipus Complex. Because the subject of scrutiny in the traditional psycho-therapeutic relationship is the fabric of verbal discourse, this too may be viewed as a text – the analysts appropriation and interpretation of which is rendered suspect by a Post-modern view. Thus various models of psychotherapeutic interpretation reflect mainly the perceptive structures utilised by those who create them.

It is this revelation that the text which is uttered does not necessarily reveal stable structures that was so welcomed by the key psycho-analytically-orientated feminists. For, in the light of Lacan, the theorems of psychoanalysis initiated by Freud and sustained by his followers, which were so degrading to women, could be seen as self-referring linguistic structures with no a priori or definitive claim on adequately signifying, speaking for or referring to reality. Contemporary feminism thus offers a reinterpretation, a re-writing and re-working of major psychoanalytic principles. The diverse thinking of French Post-modern feminists Julia Kristeva, Luce Irigaray and Hélène Cixous endeavours to unsettle and undermine patriarchal thought, bringing together psychoanalytical theories with philosophy, politics and literary theory and feminists have, therefore, been able to reassess Freudian psychoanalysis as a self-reflecting image of patriarchal society rather than a recommendation of one.

Feminism and the Voice

In the patriarchal paradigm of Freud's talking cure, words and their utterance are proposed to be the key to psychic functioning. Feminism, however, has pointed to the preverbal voice, particularly that of the mother, as being of paramount significance in understanding the human condition as it is through this dimension that each of us first expresses and communicates. Because the compositional development of vocalisation is so often guided and conducted by the maternal voice, many feminist writers see the semiotic and pre-Oedipal rapport as an exclusively female language. However, because the mother and baby duet takes place during the phase of development before the infant recognises its own gender, other theorists see it not as exclusively female but as a 'bisexual' form of experience which 'throws into confusion all tight divisions between masculine and feminine'.[72]

In 1982 the feminist Carol Gilligan published her study of women's voices and human development in a book entitled *In a Different Voice* and in 1993 she reframed her classic work with new-found experience and understanding of vocal expression gained through her work with the renowned voice teacher Kristen Linklater. In it she says that 'to have a voice is to be human' but it 'depends upon listening and being heard' for 'it is an intensely relational act'. For Gilligan, voice is both natural and cultural and is 'composed of breath and sound, words, rhythm, and language' providing 'a powerful psychological instrument and channel, connecting inner and outer worlds'. Vocalisation is 'a form of psychic breathing' and 'provides a new key for understanding the psychological, social, and cultural order' and 'is a measure of psychological health'.[73]

Psychoanalysis is more than a form of psychotherapy. The use of a psychoanalytic model of interpretation is now employed to understand literature, to assist film criticism, to comprehend social relationships within institutions and to increase awareness of the intimate dynamics within the singing lesson. This is evidenced not only by the widespread application of the model outside the psychoanalytic institution but by the diversification of application within it. With regard to voice, for example, the Tavistock Institute in London has run a series of courses for singing teachers aiming to offer insight into the intense feelings and projections which a student is likely to have towards the teacher and the effect this can have on both parties.

The professional training in Therapeutic Voicework which I direct does not train psychoanalysts. However, students are encouraged to locate their work in a number of interpretive models, including a psychoanalytic one. Furthermore, the feminist perspective on any form of 'analysis' should, in my view, be integral to any contemporary training.

One graduate of the professional Therapeutic Voicework training who is investigating in depth the feminist psychoanalytic model of interaction is Wendy Smith, who runs a private Therapeutic Voicework practice in the north of England. Smith works almost exclusively with women who have suffered some kind of silencing due to social, political, sexual or emotional abuse or repression. Working within the contractual model of one-hour consultations and supported by psychotherapeutic supervision, Smith is discovering the particular 'semiotic dimension of women's experience which somehow speaks through voice but is distorted and corrupted by language'.[74]

Towards Post-Modern Therapeutics

Despite Freud's regrettable and, perhaps, inexcusable behaviour, from his early work we have learned to what degree psychological health is dependent upon an ability to give expressive articulation to affect through motor activity. We have come to understand that the repression of our affective reaction to individual traumas suffered in childhood or in adult life cause mental suffering which can, in turn, produce physical symptoms. We have learnt that there are certain universal instincts, of a sexual nature, which society requires us to repress and which also lead to impairment. Repression leads to bottled-up energy which, in turn, leads to pain.

Freud's legacy to those suffering from such syndromes was his discovery of the power of verbal discourse to bring to light causative trauma and his further realisation of the ability for the motor activity of emotionalised dialogue to instigate a cathartic abreaction of repressed affect. Freud's insistence on the undisposable and essential role of verbal language in this curative process remains a visible inheritance of the classic schools of psychoanalysis, where the method of communication between patient and therapist remains purely verbal. Although Freud was clearly aware that the non-verbal acts of sound making, such as screaming, shouting and yelling, were also cathartic, he did not pursue in any detail the means by which the therapeutic method might employ non-verbal communication and thus he left a major stone unturned.

Furthermore, although there were those men, such as Brody, Lowen and Reich, who did explore working through a non-verbal medium of exchange with their patients, the interpretative framework which they applied to the sounds which they heard was very closely aligned with Freud's own paradigm. And it must be remembered that such a paradigm was founded upon, extracted from and evidenced by verbal dialogue. Consequently, to change the medium of therapeutic exchange from speech to voice also necessitates an entirely new paradigm and method of listening. We cannot and should not expect to hear evidence of the Oedipus complex in the pre-Oedipal sounds of the infant as they are reactivated through the adult sounds of Therapeutic Voicework. By the same token, we cannot expect to re-enter the semiotic realm of the psyche, first unfolded in the intimate years of mother-infant sonority, through a verbal discourse which, by its nature, departs from and dispatches that realm for ever more.

My proposition is that to accept the challenge of contemporary feminist psychotherapeutics means to search for a preverbal mode of discourse, beyond the written page and beyond the spoken words, and to allow the semiotic voice to find its own contours, structures, patterns and modes of expression. It is to this challenge, perhaps, that Therapeutic Voicework can in some small measure respond.

Furthermore, because both men and women begin life as infants who sing and vocalise in a preverbal semiotic register, perhaps Therapeutic Voicework can not only assist women in reclaiming and celebrating the sonority of their identity but also help men share in that language, as they once did as babes, and, in so doing, develop a compassion and comprehension for gender difference and gender convergence.

Psychoanalytically-orientated feminists such as Gilligan invite inquiry into how the non-verbal sounds of the human voice can be reinstated and acknowledged as a language of the psyche. However, as yet, no practical work on a non-verbal acoustic therapeutic modality has been initiated from within feminist psychoanalysis. In fact, those feminists who practice as clinical psychoanalysts still do so through the medium of verbal dialogue. The work of trained Therapeutic Voicework practitioners such as Smith, though, perhaps at least set the scene for a new departure in psycho-therapeutics by which women as well as men may re-experience and re-communicate through the semiotic realm of the voice.

Therapeutic Voicework Case Study: A Journey Through Song and Sperm

During the morning of a one-day Therapeutic Voicework group, I had been facilitating the participants in the process of exploring the dramatic notion of slapstick as a metaphor for the tragedy of repetitious human mistakes. This process had particular reverberations for this group as many members presented issues connected to feelings of being caught by the same footfall over and over again.

The work took place in summer and during the lunch break the group had found a spout of celebrational energy resulting from the transformation of their personal trauma into a theatre of collective slapstick. In consequence, one of the members had, in jest, pushed an ice cream into the face of a woman participant. All of this was jokingly reported to me on their return for the afternoon session.

At the beginning of the afternoon the participants pursued and explored the Personal Developmental Postural Cycle. As the group worked, I noticed that the woman who had been smothered in ice cream was making very deliberate masticatory movements of her jaw, which went round and round as though chewing cud. These were followed by wiping movements of the fingers across the face. She then began to alternate between laying on her back with legs and arms in the air and crawling on all fours, gyrating and salivating as though about to vomit. Eventually, she began to vocalise extremely loud sounds, high in pitch with lots of violin and with quite a fast vibrato ⑪ ⑦| ∧∧∧. I was very surprised as she had found it difficult to produce anything but the faintest free air sob up until now in the work.

As the wiping movements and rolls from back to front got faster, so her face took on an attitude which I associated with angry retaliation and her voice, to me, became like a war cry. The repetition of the movements continued as the voice developed into a short melody which reminded me of a simple childlike nursery rhyme which I must have heard at some time. This seemed to me so incongruent with the extremely matured and aggressive adulthood which her body and vocal timbre displayed. In time, she came onto her two feet where she began to laugh in wild abandonment before coming to rest.

Later in the process I asked the participants to write the experience of the Personal Developmental Postural Cycle in the form of a Family Song and when the young woman in question came to present her piece, she sang: 'Sperm and cream it makes me scream cos daddy made me sucky at his big Jimmy Dean' to the childlike melody she had spontaneously invented.

Later, during the process of the group's verbal sharing, she explained that she had been repeatedly abused as a child by a father who made her engage in oral sex. The harmless prank of shoving an ice cream into her face had brought her feelings surrounding this to culmination as it reminded her of the orally-abusive experiences so palpably. During the Therapeutic

Voicework she had explored expelling the sperm, wiping it away and refusing to take it in. It was during this time that she found herself singing a childlike melody and remembering how she used to sing to herself as a means of comfort after her father had left the room following an abusive episode. However, she had also, ironically, experienced a loss of vocal expression as an adult. Indeed, when she explained why she had admitted herself to the work, she had described the sensation of something being 'glued to her voice', preventing it from 'coming out'.

During the verbal sharing the woman began to cry and sob as her body undulated and quivered in spasm. I thus began to work with her, facilitating her development of the masticatory jaw movements combined with singing her song. This gave the impression of someone trying to sing whilst chewing. I directed her body back and forth from a concave implosion to a convex protrusion at the front and this instigated her to spit out saliva, as though expelling sperm. As we worked, her body became extremely hot and she sweated profusely.

Then, at a point of quite vigorous expulsive movement, her voice jumped out of flute falsetto with free air into a modal register in clarinet on a sound that was very disrupted >K F⫯<> M 〰〰. I asked her to amplify this disrupted sound and allow the song to develop, in response to which she sang the words: 'Its not sweet, even though its white' over and over again.

In time, the song developed into a whole verse which attacked the father with contempt and rage. The song finished with lines which accused him of 'spoiling her ice cream' with the sperm from 'his big Jimmy Dean.'

For this client, the process of working simultaneously through catharsis, bodily movement and sung words was extremely beneficial for she had reached a point in her psychoanalytic treatment where the repetitious verbal analysis of the problem had most definitely served the purpose of enabling her to withdraw negative projections and displaced anger towards men, originating from her father's abuse. Yet it had not solved the problem of her voice, which still felt like something was glued to it.

By putting the affect associated with her trauma into song and working through the developmental psychomotor process, she was able to intensify her affect, undergo a catharsis and, at the same time, liberate her voice from the muscular manifestation of sexual abuse.

Conclusion: Making a Song of It

In this chapter I have attempted to locate Therapeutic Voicework in both a psychoanalytic and post-modern context and have intimated that words can be as effectively utilised to a therapeutic end in singing and free vocalisation as they can in talking. Singing clearly reanimates a primary infantile experience rooted in the relationship with the mother where the self is experienced prior to language. Singing thus offers an opportunity to access the world of feeling and sensation which exists beyond the linguistic boundary. Furthermore, the human voice is, perhaps, more than any other dimension of human expression, pure presence. It can be nothing but what it is. It reveals and exposes itself, it need not describe something else.

In order to investigate this implication in more depth, I shall now turn my attention to the nature of singing, its history, function and practice.

Notes

1   Forrester, J. (1980) *Language and the Origins of Psychoanalysis.* London: Macmillan.

2   Showalter, E. (1987)*The Female Malady: Women, Madness and Culture, 1830-1980.* London: Virago Press.

3   Showalter, E. (1987)*The Female Malady: Women, Madness and Culture, 1830-1980.* London: Virago Press.

4   Freud, S. (1953–74) *Standard Edition of the Complete Psychological Works of Sigmund Freud*, vol. 2, ed. by James Strachey in collaboration with Anna Freud, assisted by Alix Strachey and Alan Tyson. London: Hogarth Press and the Institute of Psychoanalysis, pp.6–7.

5   Freud, S. *Standard Edition of the Complete Psychological Works of Sigmund Freud,* vol. 3, p.39.

6   Freud, S. *Standard Edition of the Complete Psychological Works of Sigmund Freud,* vol. 3, p.35.

7   Freud, S. *Standard Edition of the Complete Psychological Works of Sigmund Freud,* vol. 3, p.36.

8   Feld, S. (1990) *Sound and Sentiment: Birds, Weeping, Poetics and Song in Kaluli Expression.* Philadelphia: University of Pennsylvania Press.

9   Freud, S. *Standard Edition of the Complete Psychological Works of Sigmund Freud,* vol. 4. p.101.

10   Freud, S. *Standard Edition of the Complete Psychological Works of Sigmund Freud,* vol. 5, p.344.

11   Freud, S. *Standard Edition of the Complete Psychological Works of Sigmund Freud,* vol. 5, p.344.

12   Freud, S. *Standard Edition of the Complete Psychological Works of Sigmund Freud,* vol. 5, p.339.

13   Freud, S. *Standard Edition of the Complete Psychological Works of Sigmund Freud,* vol. 5, p.353.

14   Freud, S. *Standard Edition of the Complete Psychological Works of Sigmund Freud*, vol. 11, pp.125–126.

15   Freud, S. *Standard Edition of the Complete Psychological Works of Sigmund Freud*, vol. 23, pp.166–167.

16   Freud, S. *Standard Edition of the Complete Psychological Works of Sigmund Freud*, vol. 5, p.352 (footnote).

17   Freud, S. *Standard Edition of the Complete Psychological Works of Sigmund Freud*, vol. 11, p.143.

18   Masson, (1992) *The Assault on Truth: Freud and Child Sexual Abuse.* London: Harper Collins.

19 Ferenczi, S. (1926) 'Psychogenic anomalies of voice production.' In *Further Contributions to the Theory and Technique of Psychoanalysis*. London: Hogarth Press, pp.105–109.

20 Brody, M.W. (1943) 'Neurotic manifestations of the voice.' *Psychoanalytical Quarterly*, 12, pp.371–80 (p.371).

21 Brody, M.W. (1943) 'Neurotic manifestations of the voice.' *Psychoanalytical Quarterly*, 12 (1943), pp.371–80 (p.374).

22 Brody, M.W. (1943) 'Neurotic manifestations of the voice.' *Psychoanalytical Quarterly*, 12, pp.371–80 (pp.375–76).

23 Brody, M.W. (1943) 'Neurotic manifestations of the voice.' *Psychoanalytical Quarterly*, 12, pp.371–80 (p.379).

24 Sullivan, H.S. (1955) *The Psychiatric Interview*. London: Tavistock, p.5.

25 Mahl, G.F. (1956) 'Disturbances and silences in the patient's speech in psychotherapy.' *Journal of Abnormal Social Psychology*, 53, pp.1–15.

26 Pittenger, R.E., Hockett, C.F. and Danehy, J.J. (1960) *The First Five Minutes*. Ithaca, New York: Paul Martineau.

27 Reich, W. (1948) *Character Analysis*, 3rd Edn. London: Vision Press, p.342.

28 Reich, W. (1948) *Character Analysis*, 3rd Edn. London: Vision Press, p.341.

29 Reich, W. (1948) *Character Analysis*, 3rd Edn. London: Vision Press, p.353.

30 Reich, W. (1948) *Character Analysis*, 3rd Edn. London: Vision Press, p.47.

31 Reich, W. (1948) *Character Analysis*, 3rd Edn. London: Vision Press, p.146.

32 Reich, W. (1948) *Character Analysis*, 3rd Edn. London: Vision Press, p.48.

33 Reich, W. (1948) *Character Analysis*, 3rd Edn. London: Vision Press, p.362.

34 Reich, W. (1961) *The Function of the Orgasm*. London: Panther.

35 Lowen, A. (1976) *Bioenergetics*. London: Penguin, p.44.

36 Lowen, A. (1976) *Bioenergetics*. London: Penguin, p.62.

37 Lowen, A. (1976) *Bioenergetics*. London: Penguin, p.137.

38 Lowen, A. (1976) *Bioenergetics*. London: Penguin, p.43.

39 Lowen, A. (1976) *Bioenergetics*. London: Penguin, p.263.

40 Lowen, A. (1976) *Bioenergetics* London: Penguin, p.263.

41 Lowen, A. (1976) *Bioenergetics*. London: Penguin, p.99.

42 Lowen, A. (1976) *Bioenergetics*. London: Penguin, p.270.

43 Lowen, A. (1976) *Bioenergetics*. London: Penguin, p.270.

44 Lowen, A. (1976) *Bioenergetics*. London: Penguin, p.270.

45 Lowen, A. (1976) *Bioenergetics*. London: Penguin, p.271.

46 Lowen, A. (1976) *Bioenergetics*. London: Penguin, p.271.

47 Lowen, A. (1976) *Bioenergetics*. London: Penguin, p.121.

48 Lowen, A. (1976) *Bioenergetics*. London: Penguin, p.121.

49 Lowen, A. (1976) *Bioenergetics*. London: Penguin, p.121.

50 Lowen, A. (1976) *Bioenergetics*. London: Penguin, p.274.

51 Lowen, A. (1976) *Bioenergetics*. London: Penguin, p.113.

52   Wilma, L. and others, (1942) *Analysis and Interpretation of the Creative Work of John Sanders*, Institute of Child Welfare, Study of Adolescence: University of California.

53   Jones, H.E. (1942) 'The analysis of voice records.' *Journal of Consulting Psychology*, 6, pp.254–256.
      Jones, H.E. (1943) *Development in Adolescence*. New York: Appleton-Century, pp.122–123.
      Moses, P.J. (1942) 'The study of voice records.' *Journal of Consulting Psychology*, 6, pp.257–61.
      Moses, P.J. (1954) *The Voice of Neurosis*. New York: Grune & Stratton, pp.1–3.

54   Moses, P.J. (1953) 'Speech and voice therapy in otolaryngology.' *Eye, Ear, Nose and Throat Monthly*, 32, no.7 (July 1953), pp.367–375 (pp.369–370).

55   Moses, P.J. (1954) *The Voice of Neurosis*. New York: Grune & Stratton, p.15.

56   Moses, P.J. (1958) 'Reorientation of concepts and facts in phonetics.' *Logos*, pp.45–51, (p.45).

57   Moses, (1953) 'Speech and voice therapy in otolaryngology.' *Eye, Ear, Nose and Throat Monthly*, 32, no.7 (July 1953), pp.367–375.

58   Moses, P.J. (1954) *The Voice of Neurosis*. New York: Grune & Stratton.

59   Moses, P.J. (1954) *The Voice of Neurosis*. New York: Grune & Stratton, p.6.

60   Moses, P.J. (1953) 'Speech and voice therapy in otolaryngology.' *Eye, Ear, Nose and Throat Monthly*, 32, no.7 (July 1953), pp.367–375 (pp.370–71)

61   Moses, P.J. (1954) *The Voice of Neurosis*. New York: Grune & Stratton, pp.15–20.

62   Moses, P.J. (1954) *The Voice of Neurosis*. New York: Grune & Stratton, p.41.

63   Saussure, F. (1916) *A Course In General Linguistics*. New York: McGraw-Hill, p.119.

64   Saussure, F. (1916) *A Course In General Linguistics*. New York: McGraw-Hill, pp.23–24.

65   Saussure, F. (1916) *A Course in General Linguistics*. New York: McGraw-Hill, p24.

66   Derrida, J. (1967) *L'Ecriture et la Différance*. Paris: Seuil, pp.409–10.

67   Lyotard, J.F. (1984) *The Postmodern Condition: A Report on Knowledge, Theory and History of Literature*, Volume 10. Manchester: Manchester University Press.

68   Hassan, I. (1987) *The Post-Modern Turn: Essays in Post-modern Theory and Culture*. Ohio: Ohio State University Press.

69   Silverman, H. (ed) (1990) *Post-Modernism – Philosophy and the Arts*. London: Routledge.

70   Connor, S. (1990) *Post-Modernist Culture: An Introduction to the Theories of the Contemporary*. Oxford: Blackwell.

71   Barthes, R. (1990) 'The grain of the voice' in S. Frith and A. Goodwin (eds) *Rock, Pop and the Spoken Word*. London: Pantheon.

72   Eagleton, T. (1983) *Literary Theory: An Introduction*. Oxford: Blackwell, p.189.

73   Gilligan, C. (1993) *In a Different Voice: Psychological Theory and Women's Development*. Cambridge: Harvard University Press, p.xvi.

74   Smith, W. (1996) 'Voice, psychotherapy and feminism.' Paper presented to the International Association for Voice Movement Therapy. London, October 1996.

CHAPTER 6

The Singing Cure
Song as Psychotherapy

Introduction: The Singing Psychotherapist

Psychotherapy, psychoanalysis and counselling are, in essence, verbal processes in which two people talk and listen. Within these modalities, the professional practitioner pays a great deal of attention to what is said by the patient and deduces the nature of his or her unconscious operations from the inferences and implications inherent in the words uttered. In response to the fact that such words are communicated through the musical intonation of the human voice, a number of psychotherapists have recently made a tentative move towards an investigation of the singing voice and its potential as a medium of psychological change. For example, Mary Lynn Kittelson, a Zurich-trained Jungian analyst, has eloquently and vividly described the psychotherapeutic relationship as one which takes place inside an 'acoustic vessel' where the unconscious resounds and is echoed through crescendos and tempos to which the analyst must be aurally sensitive.[1] Exploring the psychotherapeutic process in the language of music and acoustic phenomenon, Kittelson, in many ways, redresses the imbalanced emphasis on opticality and seeing deriving from Jung – an approach which a number of recent Zurich graduates have explored.[2] In sympathy with this approach, a number of other Jungian analysts have investigated the acoustic field: Barbara Bliss has documented the way a client's psychological process during analysis is reflected in the transformative relationship with the singing voice[3] and Patricia Moroney has observed the analytic process as a metaphor for the interface between silence and song.[4] The influential Ivan Fónagy, a psychoanalytically-orientated linguist, has also shown the importance of vocal prosody in communicating meaning, which has invited psychotherapists to review the manner in which they hear a client and the dimensions to which they actively listen.[5] None of this, however, has changed the technical practice of psychotherapy, which remains predicated on verbal discourse. Indeed, it has been said that in the field of psychotherapy, the importance of non-verbal aspects has been clearly realised, yet little has been done.[6]

In an attempt to alter this fixation with dialogue, the psychotherapist Lane Arye has urged all psychotherapists to take inspiration from primitive singing, its simplicity and lack of literate compositional form. She says that when a psychotherapist hears a patient wailing or gasping with tears, it is useful to perceive this as an ancient pattern of music making. The psychotherapist should, therefore, 'sing' with the patient instead of simply listening compassionately. For Arye, the broad canvas of world singing styles should remind us that only in the West do we have such a narrow idea of how the singing voice should sound. Therefore, by opening our ears to the world's songs we can come to hear the emotional sound making of all clients in distress as music and singing. Ayre believes that one of the roles which a psychotherapist should assume for their clients is 'a singing partner who can sing with them, sharing their load and harmonising, reverberating and echoing their sufferings'.[7] This proposed move away from a talking cure towards a singing cure is, perhaps, made urgent by the recognition that 'some people feel that they will never be able to find words to express their innermost feelings because no such words exist' which 'gives rise to a sense of complete isolation'.[8]

In my view an integrated methodological and analytic approach to Therapeutic Voicework is concerned with facilitating a process which compares to psychotherapy in many respects but which operates through the medium of the singing voice and the structure of the singing lesson.

The Voice of Ancient Greece

In the West the most consistently revered form of singing has, for centuries, been that displayed by the opera singer, whose virtuosity and skill exemplifies for many the most highly developed form of vocal expression.

This operatic vocalisation originates in ancient Greece, where lone players told the tales of the great myths whilst accompanying themselves with a small stringed instrument called a lyre and where they played all of the characters, giving each one a distinctive vocal quality and set of characteristics whilst retaining a neutral voice to speak as the narrator. In time, these solo renditions developed into small ensemble performances;

later, playwrights wrote the mythical stories in dialogue form and small groups of players came together and played one or two characters each. In the process of transition from solo recitals in story and music to actual musical and dramatic productions, the use of the mask was added and the vocal dance of word and song emerged from the actor through a hole cut into the mask at the mouth. The etymology of our term 'personality' is inextricably linked to this use of the human voice and originates in these masked performances. The term 'personality' comes from the Latin *per sona* which means 'the sound passes through' and was first used to describe the mouthpiece of the mask worn by actors. It then came to denote the character or person which the actor portrayed. Eventually, the word came to mean any person and, finally, 'personality' as we now understand it.

In ancient Greek theatre the mask placed over the face was fixed whilst the actor's voice was free to weave and dance an acoustic tapestry. In time, of course, masks were abandoned and the actor was able to utilise the mobility of facial expression to support and reinforce the vocal message.

Therapeutic Voicework Methodology: Voice and Mask

In singing the term 'mask' is also used to denote the vocalist's facial muscles and expression and in vocal work, as in everyday expression, the face itself can be like a mask, either fixed as the original dramatic masks of Greece or mobile as in the expressive use of the face by later actors. The term 'mask' is also used to denote a shield behind which the true Self is hidden.

The face is a primary means by which we express attitude, feeling, response and intent and can be a mobile and malleable picture of the diversity of inner experience. However, the face often becomes a rigid mask which expresses only one aspect of our Self and serves to ensure that exposure of that which lies behind it does not occur.

The degree of facial expression depends upon the mobility of the same physiognomical muscles which determine the configuration of the oral cavity, which, in turn, affects vocal timbre. Facial stasis thus often accompanies vocal rigidity whilst increased malleability of the facial muscles encourages vocal flexibility.

The holistic interconnectedness of face and voice can be used in Therapeutic Voicework to mobilise and animate self-expression when a client suffers from immobility, depression, lack of vitality and expressive reticence. The practitioner encourages the client to arbitrarily 'make faces', forming a series of masks with the facial muscles which express specific characteristics and emotions which the client experiences but has difficulty expressing, perhaps for fear of exposure. The vocal timbre consequently changes in response to the varying facial expressions, particularly the shape of the mouth, and the client thus hears voices emerge which emanate from previously dormant parts of the personality.

The Mythical Voice

The fixed masked theatre productions were one of the most significant contributions which the Greeks made to Europe's future cultural and artistic development. Moreover, it was from one of these masked dramas that Freud drew his theory of the Oedipus Complex and it was these performances that inspired the infamous Aristotle and Plato to speculate their philosophy of art and the nature of human emotions and it was from these philosophies that Freud drew the concept of 'catharsis'.

Aristotle proposed the theory that the audience who bear witness to these tragedies experience the fate of the central character intensely, as though it were their own. In particular, he hypothesised that the onlookers feel immense pity for the character's predicament and extreme fear in imagining that such a fate might befall them. According to Aristotle, such active investment of belief in the theatre of tragedy gave rise to a means by which the audience could purge themselves of the affects of pity and fear and thereby experience a genuine psychological relief which he called 'catharsis'. It was from these ideas, concocted to describe the psychological effect of theatre, that Freud drew the term 'cathartic method' which he originally used to describe his 'talking cure'.

The plays of this cathartic theatre were performed by three or four actors who played the main characters and a group of performers known as the chorus who sang, yelled, spoke and chanted in a powerful and exuberant mixture of prayer and narration, serving to work the actors and the audience into a climactic state. Many of the texts from these plays still exist, as do many vivid descriptions of the productions by the ancient philosophers, historians and politicians who attended them. From these extant writings we know that the actors and chorus recited their dialogue not in a fashion analogous with daily speech but with special intonations which were accentuated by the music of a lyre or aulos, a flute-like instrument. The bodily movements used by the performers were also stylised, forming a choreographed gestural dance which contributed to the overall arousing effect which the spectacle is known to have had on the audience. To the modern ear, this acoustic aspect of Greek theatre would probably sound chaotic and lacking in all melody. There was no concept of musical harmony and the utterances of the voice, pipes and strings served the purpose not of articulating the formal discursive logic of a musical composition but of enhancing the text with exhilarating emotive sounds. As the Greek scholar Stanford says, every play in Greek drama 'has its nexus of inarticulate sounds' which express 'grief or fear or joy or triumph and other emotions' through vocal 'sobs, groans, screams, gasps, laughs and ululations'. Among 'the most frequent and most expressive noises of Greek tragedy' were those which were 'articulate though not quite verbal' and were 'the most primitive of all human sounds, more like animal cries than speech'. These sounds 'are of supreme importance for the emotional effects of Greek tragedy, setting up physical and emotional vibrations that no articulate words could', though, of course, 'editors often ignore them and translators are commonly satisfied' with recording them as a perfunctory 'oh', 'ah', or 'alas'.[9] The use of the voice in Greek theatre was clearly acrobatic and extensive, serving to communicate emotions of extreme magnitude, the effect of which was to arouse the passions of the audience to a high degree of excitation in order that they may experience a catharsis. Indeed, the term 'audience' comes from '*audio*', meaning 'hear'.

In ancient Greece then, theatre was closely related to therapy by way of its cathartic effect; to the Greeks, the art of theatre was by its very nature medicinal and they held music in the same regard. In Greek mythology music and medicine were literally sister and brother. The Muses were divine characters who invented music and reigned over its human use and Aesculapius was the inventor of medicine capable even of raising people from the dead. Both the Muses and Aesculapius were fathered by Apollo and their charms were equally revered as being capable of affecting the health of mortals. Apollo was thus regarded as the father of medicine and of music and it was Apollo's son Orpheus who came to be regarded as the keeper of the mysteries of song and its healing powers. In the myth of Orpheus, when the hero descends into the underworld to rescue his beloved, he discovers that the power of his singing voice can pacify any aggressor, including Hades himself.

Cacophony and Oratory

We know that the Greeks did not create combinations of voice and instruments which a modern ear would describe as concordant. Although such combinations as we might call harmonious may have occurred spontaneously in the course of playing, it would not have been possible to plan it or fix it from one performance to the next because their system of writing music down was not sophisticated enough. The Greeks simply used the letters of their own alphabet to indicate notes on their scale, with some letters turned around to denote changes in the quality of a sound. When the Romans infiltrated and overpowered Greek culture, they simply exchanged the signs of Greek notation for their own alphabet, but did not significantly elaborate its complexity.

The period of classical antiquity was also characterised by the proliferate concern with oratory as a social and political art. The philosophical dialogues and problematics of ancient Greek civilisation are inseparable from their oral articulation through the effective use of the voice. Consequently, most philosophers wrote upon the subject of oratory and disseminated opinions as to how the voice should be used and its components of rhythm, prosody, stress and intensity combined to effectively present an argument. The assertion of rules and suggestions for the appropriate use of voice gave rise to schools of oratory which sprang up throughout Greece and which trained novices to specialise in the oral presentation of speeches on a variety of subjects. However, the singing voice did not attract such attention and therefore the development of singing training does not possess such a long history as does that of speech training, which originates in the classical Greek appetite for the articulation of ideas.

Roman Voices

The Romans inherited from the Greeks the use of music and drama as a form of mass public entertainment which formed an important part of pre-Christian Roman life. However, with the coming of Christianity, these great pagan tales of raging gods and supreme heroes, whose deeds were emulated in action with mask and song to the awe and wonder of the adoring masses, disappeared. Worship and admiration for the ways of the deity took on a more solemn form.

An important part of the solemnity which is associated with early Christian worship is the way in which holy scripture was uttered in such sorrowful and non-elaborate tones by the church leaders and worshippers alike. This was, indeed, a far cry from the spectacular vocal renditions which the Greeks gave of their religious stories and which inspired the theatre of Greek and Roman culture.

It was the pre-Christian Romans who invented the organ, originally a contraption about ten feet high and four and a half feet wide, blown by means of a weight of water; the later ones were air blown by hand. Although those of the Christian church did not choose to inherit the revelries and masked dramas from their pre-Christian antecedents, they did retain the organ and, by about 350 BC, the first singing schools were established in Europe to train singers to give voice to the words of God in timely synonymity with the authoritative solemnity of the organ. By this time, the organs had become gigantic affairs and required two or three players, called 'organ beaters', to thump the huge keys with gloved hands whilst a group of 'blowers' pumped the bellows. But the simultaneous combination of organ and choral singers was still a far cry from what later became known as harmony.

As a result of these musical experiments with voice and organ, which had no system of notation capable of restraining the impromptu expression of feeling on any pitch, the once solemn chants became more elaborate and often quite vigorous and the church authorities believed this to be incompatible with the reverence due to God. As a result, the church made strict rules dictating the kinds of vocal sounds and combinations thereof which could and could not be used.

It was from this desire on the part of the clergy to control the nature of the singing voice that the first singing schools of Europe sprang. Among the most renowned was that implemented by Pope Sylvester in the early part of the fourth century, who established a musical conservatory, the *Schola Cantorum*, where the principles of tone production and musical theory were taught to ordained singers. With the passage of time, the specific demands and taboos of the church with regard to the singing voice became more conservative and stipulations demanding what could and could not be sung culminated in the infamous rulings of Pope Gregory the Great during the second half of the sixth century, whose strict stipulations led to the Gregorian chant which is still in use.

Systematic instruction in the art of singing, therefore, originally served the process of ordaining those who could perform the musical services of the church according to its taste. The presence of a trained élite at the service naturally put the spontaneous vocalisations of the congregation to shame and, in 350 AD, the Laodicean Council and, later, the fourth Council of Carthage decreed that congregational singing interfered with the beauty of

the musical service as held up by the trained singers and rules were drawn up
to limit the participation in the service by the congregation.

Therapeutic Voicework Methodology: The Hymn

The hymn is another example of an artistic genre which serves to express and
contain specific affects – in this case usually praise, exaltation, exuberant
celebration and devotion.

The hymn is particularly useful because many clients raised in the West
who feel frustration because they cannot recall a song from memory to work
on in a session, seem to know a hymn. Moreover, because hymns are
associated with singing in church, where the tunefulness and virtuosity of the
rendition is not scrutinised, many clients feel that they have nothing 'to live
up to' in singing it.

The use of The Hymn in Therapeutic Voicework, like the use of Voice and
Mask, also serves to animate the spirit of those clients who are searching for
relief from depressive feelings and lack of vitality because the singing of a
hymn can stimulate exuberance, regardless of the religious or
denominational orientation of the client.

The Bards Outside the Church

During the the so-called dark ages, which followed the collapse of the
Roman Empire in western Europe during the sixth century, lone players
continued to roam the lands singing and telling their own stories with the aid
of music. These singing tale-tellers, who owed their birth to the ancient
Greeks and who remained untouched by the demands of the church, were to
become a significant part of European song culture. The most well known of
these are, perhaps, the Troubadours, singing poets who flourished in
southern France throughout the 12th, 13th and 14th centuries and whose
wandering lives, full of passion and adventure, made them the typical
romantic figures of their age. But the Troubadours are only one example of
the many kinds of singers and poets who wandered alone and in groups
throughout Europe, combining story, text and music to entertain in the
courts, in the taverns and on the streets.

Many cultures have, at various times in history, hosted travelling or local
artists whose function was to keep myth, mystery and indigenous religious
tradition alive through the oral expression of tale, narrative, parable and song
and, in many cases, their function was also a healing one. The general term

for such persons is 'Bard', who in more recent history have been seen as mere entertainers but who stem from a Shamanic tradition where mystical knowledge of the myths and insight into rituals of healing combined with the artistic skill of the singer and reciter were contained in a single person. In many ways, the Bard is the precedent for the healing artists of today. In French they were the Troubadours, in Africa they were griots, in Norse they were skalds, in Anglo-Saxon they were gleemen, in Russian they were the kaleki, in India the magahda and in Japanese the zenza. In many cultures the bardic tradition eventually became one of entertainment, losing its original connection to the priestly virtue of imparting mystical truths to the listeners through the palatable and accessible form of musical song.

Albert Lord, the renowned scholar of the oral arts, tells us that 'the poet was sorcerer and seer' before he became an artist and the roots of oral traditional narrative are not artistic but religious in the broadest sense.[10] Indeed, it was the Bard, or the 'singer of tales', who preserved not only a shamanic healing tradition in many indigenous cultures but who, in the European tradition, also preserved the great mythical epics such as Beowulf, the Iliad and the Odyssey. In the classic study of this essential and archetypal figure of the singer, Lord reminds us that the singer of tales, or Bard, preserved the tradition of a narrative whilst at the same time reinventing it anew with his own particular vocal, dramatic and interpretive features. Lord says that when we speak of an oral tradition of poetry, we refer not just to the fact that poems were performed orally but that poems and songs which told of the great narratives were composed during oral performance.[11] Despite familiar narratives, in an oral culture, 'every performance is unique, and every performance bears the signature of its poet singer'. He may have learned his song and the technique of its construction from others, but, good or bad, the song produced in performance was his own. The singer of tales is, therefore, 'at once the tradition and the individual creator'.[12] This gave the singer enormous freedom to break, ridicule and challenge the mores and ideas contained within an established narrative as well as providing an opportunity for reverence towards its essence; the Baul singers of India continue to utilise singing as a means to ridicule even today.

In ancient Greece the celebrational social life of the populace was intimately connected to the artistic and spiritual adoration of the gods. For example, wine, dancing, hymn, prayer, theatre and song were all part of the worship of Dionysus. However, during the 'dark ages' a split between the secular and the religious occurred and many singers or Bards indulged in rambling songs of love, lust and wild adventure whilst the church continued to develop its solemn and structured chants which told of Christ and the Apostles.

Therapeutic Voicework Methodology: Known Song Symbolism

Many clients will remember a song that is, for a finite period of time, 'on the tip of their tongue'. This is often because the song reflects and represents a particular mood, preoccupation or mental fixation which may, however, be unconscious. In addition, titles of songs are a predominant part of popular vernacular culture and it is surprising how many clients can reel off titles of songs with seeming infinity.

In Therapeutic Voicework the client can be asked to draw on his or her memory of songs or song titles to symbolise particular experiences, choosing songs for the way in which they represent feelings and ideas prompted by the therapeutic process. This also stimulates clients to listen to music and deepen their relationship with song outside of the consultative Therapeutic Voicework process, making the work their own and facilitating independence. For example, a client can often gain much insight by seeking a handful of songs which deal in a subject currently relevant to their journey. Bringing these songs to the Therapeutic Voiceworker, the client can work on them not to achieve formal virtuosity but to animate the Self through the process of singing songs which reflect the inner experience.

Therapeutic Voicework Methodology: The Free Ballad

One of the most moving elements of the methodological approach to Therapeutic Voicework which I have developed is what I have called the 'Free Ballad'. Here, usually in the first session or at the beginning of a group process, the client begins by telling her story, including the most potent childhood memories, major relationships, medical history and current predicament. This process is, of course, comparable to the way in which a client may introduce herself into any therapeutic process.

In the interim between this and the next session the client is required to write this story in the form of an autobiography which she then reads, either in its entirety or from which she selects passages, at the next session. The next stage, to be pursued in the interim before the third meeting, requires the client to rewrite her autobiography as a fairy-tale, which, again, she reads from at the next session. Then, finally, in the third interim, the fairy-tale is used as the basis from which to extract the lines of a ballad.

In writing the lyrics of the ballad the client is not required to consider any musical form but simply to create words upon the page which, in some dream-like fashion, depict imaginally the rudiments of her story. At the next meeting the client reads the ballad lyrics whilst the Therapeutic Voiceworker listens to the subtle prosody and timbral changes in the voice. By the Therapeutic Voiceworker's careful choosing to use either an instrument, his own voice or the vocal sounds of other members of the group, the client's rendition is then supported by a sonorous envelope of sound and she is encouraged to characterise the figures, images, moods and emotions within the story with different vocal timbres.

This work can be particularly inspiring when the person's story is composed of a major trauma or tragedy for the presenting of the ballad often stimulates intense affect, often manifested vocally through tears, sobs, gasps and groans. Yet the process of working vocally provides an artistic context within which such vocal expressions of emotion can be experienced and perceived as integral to the creative telling of the story. Furthermore, even those who consider themselves unable to write or to sing find that through focusing on the authenticity of their own story and its transposition from autobiography, through fairy-tale to ballad, it is impossible not to discover an expressive voice which has nothing to do with formal literacy or musical structure. Through this process some of the originality of the bardic singing process is recaptured, along with some of the original artistic instinct to tell a tale through vocalisation.

The connection between personal experience, particularly that of a traumatic kind, and the act of composing and writing original material which emanates from that experience has been investigated consistently by Melanie Harrold, a practising Therapeutic Voiceworker and co-teacher on the professional training in Voice Movement Therapy.

Harrold was a singer and song-writer for many years and later became a singing teacher, working with novices and non-musicians. She now runs a Therapeutic Voicework practice in London where clients with inhibitions, residual trauma, physical debilitation and other obstacles to vocal expression can explore the interface between improvised and spontaneous release of sound and the process of composing formed song. Within this process, Harrold uses a number of instruments to accompany and support the client's vocalisations.

From the Oral Song to Written Music

Around the sixth century AD the crude system of alphabetical notation which had been originated by the Greeks was superseded by a system of points, hooks, curves and lines placed above the words to be sung. These signs, called 'neumes', became formalised so that to a trained singer each had its own meaning. By this means it was possible to recall melodies already committed to memory, but it still did not enable previously unheard songs to be learnt as the notation did not indicate pitch. It was not until around the end of ninth and beginning of the tenth century that the pitch of musical notes began to be fixed by notation.

The first step towards this was attained when a person who remains unidentified drew a red line horizontally across the page. Any sign placed on this line indicated the note F while a sign placed immediately above or below it indicated G and E respectively. Soon, another line was added, in yellow, and any note placed on this line indicated C while D and B were notated by signs above and below it respectively. However, there was still a long way to go before the God-fearing men of the cloth were satisfied that the resulting sound was in tune with their master's wishes and, in the year 1020, a learned Benedictine Monk called Guido of Arezzo wrote that 'in the church service it often sounds not as if we were praising God but rather as if we were engaging in quarrelling amongst ourselves.'[13]

Guido set out to remedy this lack of harmonious concord amongst worshipping vocalists. First, he added two black lines to the existing yellow and black ones and these indicated the exact notes which the performers were to sing in more than one octave. Second, to help his pupil's memory, he taught them to remember certain syllables from a Latin hymn, each line of which began on an ascending degree of the scale C, D, E, F, A.

> UT queant laxis
> REsonare fibris
> MIra gestorum
> FAmuli tuorum
> SOLve polluti
> LAbi reatum

Ut has since been changed to doh and this gives rise to the well-known Tonic scale still in use: doh–ray–me–fah–soh–la–te–doh. Guido's success in creating the four-line stave and fixing a named scale of notes has led him to be known as the father of literate music as we now know it.

The founding of this scale had, and continues to have, an insidious, yet dominating, effect on the art of singing training and on the accessibility to song for many people for it made singing training irreversibly synonymous with musical training, an equation still visible today in the fact that singing teachers almost invariably work through the medium of set literately-notated music. Moreover, it is impossible for a student to enter any of the major Western training schools or conservatoires to study singing without the ability to read music. The fact that musical literacy has become an unquestioned prerequisite for singing training in Western culture is a testimony to our cultural arrogance and sense of supremacy for, in the vast majority of the remaining world, singing is not related to any kind of literacy at all. In the West, however, singing lessons and the act of singing is a terrifying and often inaccessible notion and vast numbers of people feel alienated from training their singing voice because they do not have a so-called aptitude for, or ability to read, music. Musical instinct has been sequestered and subsumed by musical literacy. Yet, in its origin, singing in Europe was a dramatic use of the voice to articulate story without regard for scale or fixed melody. For these reasons, musical literacy is not an entry requirement for the RSA Diploma in Voice Movement Therapy training.

Zoltán Kodály

There have been a small number of pioneering contributions from figures who have sought to find an alternative to the classic pedagogical music notation system and thereby make vocal and musical activity more accessible to a wider range of mental and creative dispositions. For example, in Germany Carl Orff pioneered his own approach to music education whilst in Switzerland Émile Jaques-Dalcroze researched the relationship of bodily movement to the conception and performance of music. However, the Hungarian Zoltán Kodály is, perhaps, the most renowned of those who have revisioned musical education and whose method of vocal literacy now forms the basis of all musical education in Hungarian schools and has also proven successful with school children in Europe and the USA.[14] The educational work of Kodály was characterised by his 'all-embracing and principal slogan' which proclaimed that 'music belongs to everybody' and his mission was to return music to the entire population by bringing it central to the curriculum of the schoolchild from the very first stages of education. Kodály believed that 'the part played by music in education should be given an equally important position' as it had 'once enjoyed in classical Greece'. However, he felt that the pedantic, systematic and complex 'musical literacy' which had come to dominate musical training, symbolised by a highly abstracted notation system, actually 'impedes musical culture'.[15] His response to this situation was to restructure musical education where it would have the most influence: at training colleges for prospective primary school teachers. It was at such centres that Kodály implemented his beliefs that 'musical culture must be introduced as early as the nursery school'[16] so that when children reach primary schools they have an enjoyment of music and an appetite to learn its structure and expression. But central to his propositions was that the 'best approach to musical genius is through the instrument most accessible to everyone: the human voice' and that 'this way is open not only to the privileged but to the great masses'.[17] For Kodály, singing was, therefore, the supreme act and he claimed that 'daily singing, side-by-side with daily physical exercise, equally develop a child's body and mind'.[18] Seeking the most accessible form of singing, one which would immediately appeal to the child's natural instinct for musical expression, Kodály founded his educational practice on the singing of traditional Hungarian folk-songs and nursery rhymes, which were introduced to the classroom through the singing voice without recourse to musical accompaniment. This meant that children learned music by developing the sensitivity of the ear to their own voice and its harmonic relationship to other voices. In the absence of a fixed note on an instrument, therefore, children learned the scale Doh, Ray, Me, Fah, Soh, Lah Te Doh but without the first sound, Doh, being permanently rooted to any specific pitch. The scale Doh, Ray, Me, Fah, Soh, Lah Te Doh in Kodály's system does not represent particular notes such as C, D or E on the tempered scale played upon a piano. Rather, it designates particular intervals. One can, therefore, begin singing the scale at any pitch with an intuitively-acquired ability to sing the following intervals.

Kodály applied this 'movable Doh' idea to the singing and analysis of folk-songs, which he combined with the rhythmic bodily movements utilised by Émile Jaques-Dalcroze and, in so doing, grounded musical education, appreciation and expression in a sensory and instinctive process.

Therapeutic Voicework Methodology: Free Interval Vocalisation

Many people are prevented from gaining access to the expressivity of their voice by a fear that vocal emissions will not conform to a particular set of notes and intervals as represented by the piano. Many people have a voice which displays slow pitch fluctuation and which, therefore, when aligned to a set musical piece, can appear 'out of tune'. However, the problem here is with the attempt to align, not with the voice itself.

In the original conception of singing as a story told to music, the voice was allowed to roam freely through all possible frequencies and with a great deal of fluctuation – as, indeed, it is in many non-Western forms of singing. In Therapeutic Voicework a client with fears regarding musicality can be enabled to take possession of a full vocal expressivity by refraining from aligning the voice to a set of intervals and allowing it to journey spontaneously.

In cases where the surrounding silence proves as intimidating as the dominance of a piano, the Therapeutic Voiceworker can provide a constant tone or drone on an accordian, open-tuned guitar, harmonium or other instrument, which provides a platform from which the client can meander.

This process allows the voice the same freedom as it takes in speech, where there is no concern for being in tune. When the method of Free Interval Vocalisation is combined with rehearsing the Free Ballad, beautiful turns of musical phrases often arise from this freedom, which can create the atmosphere of a multi-cultural melody, as though all the intervals possible in every conceivable culture have been combined in a kind or archetypal music of the world. A number of contemporary rock groups and singers are beginning to utilise a conglomeration of non-Western intervals in combination with Western musical instruments and melodic patterns. These include the band *Enigma*[19] and the singer Lisa Gerrard, lead singer with *Dead Can Dance*.[20]

The technical approach to this is introduced on the set of audio cassettes *The Singing Cure: Liberating Self Expression Through Voice Movement Therapy*[21] and I have shown its use in musical expression and composition on the CD *Prayers and Prophecies*[22].

The Genesis of Opera

Around the ninth century the Christian church began to introduce music and drama into its services where Easter Passions and Christmas Nativities which contained spoken text and sung choruses became a part of Christian ceremony throughout Europe. The origin of the idea of a religious story told in music, speech and song, which constituted the fundamental concept of these Christian performances, is rooted in the ancient history of Greece but the formal structuring of music, which was developed primarily in the hands of the church, completely altered the way that the voice was used. In Greek tragedy it was unbound by fixed musicality and served instead to encapsulate the emotional tones, rhythms and atmospheres of the myth being played. In Christian service, however, the voice now served to articulate the written score, which was attached to the words arbitrarily and in a manner completely dislocated from the emotive impulse generated by the utterance of the word.

However, in Italy, towards the end of the 16th century, there lived an influential man of music, Giovanni de' Bardi the Count of Vernio, who invited to his house the most celebrated and learned men of music and letters where they gathered to form a society of fellows whose shared aim was to rediscover the way in which the ancient Greeks had used voice, movement, music and drama in their theatre. It was from the meetings of this exclusive musical society, called the *'Camerata'*, which took place over a period of thirty years in seventeenth century Florence, that opera, as people know it today, was born. When Count Bardi moved to Rome in 1592, the meeting place of the *Camerata* changed to the house of the younger Jacopo Corsi, who kept his house open like a public academy for all those interested in the liberal arts. It was here in 1598 that what is considered to be the first true opera was performed.

The opera was called *'Dafne'* with music composed by Peri and the text or libretto by the poet Ottavio Rinuccini. We know that it told the story of a Greek myth in which the god Apollo slays the great Pythian monster but, unfortunately, only a few segments of this score remain. The manuscript of Peri's second opera, *Eurydice*, however, has survived in full and tells the Greek Myth of Orpheus who descended into the underworld to rescue his beloved Eurydice, after whom the opera is named.

Peri was convinced that the ancient Greeks had used a form of vocal expression, more musical than that of ordinary speech but less melodious than song as the church had conceived of it, to produce an 'intermediate form'. Peri said that he too wanted to 'imitate speech in song' and use 'elegances and graces that cannot be notated' and in his preface to *Eurydice* he said that he was aiming for something between 'the slow and suspended movements of song and the swift and rapid movements of speech'.[23]

Therapeutic Voicework Methodology: From Prosody and Speech Rhythm to Music

Prosody, or the pitch contours of intonation which give colour and stress to the speaking voice, is a musical phenomenon. Imagine all the possible ways of saying 'Hello, my name is Paul' by varying the prosody alone. For clients who believe that they do not possess any musicality and are thus unable to bring themselves to sing, pointing out and exaggerating the prosody in the speaking voice is, therefore, an enlightening way of opening the doorway to song.

The Therapeutic Voiceworker asks the client to speak the text at hand, imbuing it with different expressions by varying the prosody. Over time, the Therapeutic Voiceworker helps the client extend the phonation times so that each unit of sound is extended. Gradually, therefore, the speaking turns unnoticeably into singing. This also inspires the client compositionally because the melody which arises from the methodology is a genuine extension of the prosodic intonation which, in turn, emanates from the authenticity of the client's communication of the text.

A similar process can be pursued with rhythm. The client begins by speaking the text at hand, exaggerating the intensity and distinctness of the articulate rhythm of the speech. The Therapeutic Voiceworker then assists the client in amplifying the musicality of the text by creating a rhythmic rendition.

Bel Canto

Those members of the *Camerata* who sought to achieve a renaissance of the primal vocal expression which they believed to have been at the heart of ancient Greek performance had, by their own admission, failed. The forthcoming composers of Italy sought to make music itself the carrier of emotion and not merely an accompaniment to heighten the emotive vocal power of the text. The new opera makers were seeking to combine musical instruments and voices in a total harmony and therefore a fresh demand was placed upon the performer, one that would make him a singer first and a vehicle for the expression of emotion and experience second.

These new demands required a new kind of teaching that would nurture singers to retain some of the ability to communicate a primacy of emotional experience whilst at the same time remaining formally responsive to the specifically-notated music which brought instrumentalists and vocalists together into a harmonious whole.

Amongst the members of the *Camerata* was the great vocal soloist Giulio Caccini, who became the academy's authority on solo singing technique. Caccini was also inspired by his belief that the ancient Greeks had possessed a natural ability to express human emotions through the voice and he combined this with his development of fixed notated musical composition. The aim of his teaching was to nurture singers to bring full expression to the portrayal of human emotions whilst retaining musical harmony with the supporting instruments. It was from this objective of Caccini and others that the school of composers and singers known as Bel Canto arose.

Bel Canto is an Italian term which literally means 'beautiful song' and was the particular art of singing and vocal training which flourished in Italy throughout the seventeenth and eighteenth centuries in response to the need for emotional genuineness and authenticity combined with musical precision and virtuosity. Bel Canto singing was passed on through the classic singing schools of Florence, Rome, Naples, Bologna and Milan, though the term 'Bel Canto' was not used until towards the end of the 19th century.[24]

The techniques used to teach singing in this period are known to us through the writings of three teachers and singers: Caccini's *Nuove Musiche*, dated 1601; Pietro Francesco Tosi's *Observations on the Florid Song*, dated Bologna, 1723; and Giovanni Battista Mancini's *Practical Reflections on the Figurative Art of Singing*, dated Milan, 1776.

The special art of the Bel Canto singers consisted in their ability to communicate a genuine expression of human emotion by singing precisely notated musical phrases with a wide range of qualities or timbres, spanning a vocal range of three octaves, without losing refinement and eloquence of verbal diction. Unlike more recent classical singing for the opera, where the singer is trained to specialise in or is restricted to a single timbral quality, the Bel Canto singer could sing a vast array of qualities, covering tenor, baritone, soprano and mezzo-soprano, for example. Bel Canto, according to one historian, meant to have 'not three, four or five sonorities but in fact, ten, twenty, or thirty. The voice had to be moulded in an infinite degree, passing through all the colours of the sound prism'.[25]

Lucie Manen makes the crucial point that the extensive range of timbres possessed by the Bel Canto singers was not a cosmetic trick of virtuosity to make the range of emotions depicted in opera more interesting. Rather, the range of timbres or qualities was born out of the spectrum of human emotions 'for it is only from the primeval sounds and exclamations' such as 'joy, surprise, grief, passion, annoyance, anger' and 'hatred' which people use to 'express their inner feelings and reactions to impressions from the world around them' 'that the colourful timbres of Bel Canto can emanate.'[26]

The tuition and teaching methods of the Bel Canto singing teachers 'was not based on any explicit theoretical method'.[27] Rather, the teachers, who were all expert singers themselves, 'relied heavily' on a process of 'trial and correction' in which the student and teacher had to listen acutely with an attentive ear.[28] However, some of the exercises invented by these Bel Canto teachers are preserved in books such as Alessandro Busti's *Studio di canto: Metodi classica del Conservatorio Reale di Napoli*, first published in 1865 and the manual of exercises with explanations, *Metodo pratico di vocalizzazione*, by Gaetano Nava of Milan, published in 1876. There are also a number of teachers in the modern era who claim lineage from this tradition and offer techniques which allegedly correlate with the method of voice production used by the Bel Canto singers.[29]

The core principle of the Bel Canto technique rests in the malleability and articulation of the resonating spaces above the vocal folds, particularly the pharynx. The shape of the vocal tract, which acts like an elastic tube, influences the timbre of the sound made by vibrating vocal folds. By nurturing the maximum malleability of this tube, acquiring the ability to lengthen and shorten it as well as controlling its diameter, the Bel Canto singers produced a panoply of timbres which could represent the full canvas of human emotion. It is this articulation of the vocal tract that gives rise to the set of vocal timbres which form the system of voice training, profile and analysis which I have developed, which sits at the heart of the Voice Movement Therapy system and which I have described in Chapter 1.

Therapeutic Voicework Methodology: The Practice of Timbre and Tone

Within this system is a methodology which I have called 'The Practice of Timbre and Tone', which is quite a rigorous process suitable only for those seriously committed to training their voice to a level of maximum malleability. The process consists of taking one note at a time, usually sustained by an instrument such as the piano for the purposes of practice, and vocalising each note with all possible component parameter combinations. Each note is therefore sung with different degrees of pitch fluctuation in flute, clarinet and saxophone, each time with and without free air, with and without violin, with varying degrees of loudness and glottal attack in different registers, on different vowels, with and without disruption.

The effect of this training process is the opposite to that of a contemporary classical training in that it despecialises the vocal quality and gives it access to heightened timbral flexibility. It is, in part, this training process which enables graduates of the Voice Movement Therapy training to achieve their vocal malleability and I have demonstrated some of the consequent timbral styles on the CD *Prayers and Prophecies*[30] and the set of audio cassettes *The Singing Cure: Liberating Self Expression Through Voice Movement Therapy.*[31] In addition, the behaviour of the vocal tract during the making of this range of sounds can be seen on the video *Shouting for Jericho: The Work of Paul Newham on the Human Voice*[32] through a fibre optic recording of my larynx during extended vocalisation.

The Discovery of the Vocal Folds

The emphasis on the malleability of the vocal tract which underpinned Bel Canto teaching was countermanded by an alternative focus on the significance of the vocal folds. Leonardo da Vinci was one of the first to attempt to analyse the larynx, which he did by extracting respiratory tracts from cadavers.[33] But it was the French anatomist, Antoine Ferrein, who discovered, while dissecting corpses in 1741, two 'shelves' in the larynx and who assumed that the human voice was caused by their vibration induced by air being blown forward from the lungs like bellows. He named these shelves the *cordes vocales* and his discovery of the production of vocal sound received widespread recognition.[34] This attention drawn to the vocal folds as the most significant aspect in the production of vocal tone contributed to the erosion of Bel Canto techniques, which had been concerned with the elasticity of the resonating spaces.

Manuel Vicente del Popolo Garcia was a great singer and singing teacher who trained his son in the Bel Canto style but treated him harshly, beating him and degrading him regularly. While his sisters became famous for their singing, Manuel Garcia junior was a failure. Seeking to find the answers to his own lack of success, he took up the vocal fold theory of Ferrein and conducted some experiments on the larynxes of poultry in which he produced sounds with bellows. Inspired by the sight of a dentist using a mirror, he then constructed a contraption by which he could observe his own vocal folds. Although he had not received recognition as a singer, he now became famous as the inventor of the laryngoscope – a small metal instrument which is placed in the mouth and enables the larynx and vocal folds to be observed. It was the development of the laryngoscope that instigated the diagnostic techniques developed by Tuerck and Czermak and which provided the foundation for contemporary laryngology.[35]

When his father died in 1832, Manuel Garcia junior took on the role of director of his father's singing school, assuming, without justification, a reputation for being a great singing teacher. In his teaching techniques and through his manual, *Traité complet de l'art du chant*, Garcia altered the Bel Canto techniques which focused on the malleability of the vocal tract, claiming to proliferate a method based on the true physiology of the vocal instrument. By 1856 he was so famous that his methods, by now articulated in his new book, *Nouveau traité sommaire de l'art du chant* became acknowledged as the finest in Europe.

The decline of Bel Canto may be attributed, in part, to Ferrain and Garcia who, with a dangerously small and historically premature knowledge of laryngeal function, abandoned the intuitive and emotional insight of the anatomically blind singers. But another reason why the emphasis on flexibility of vocal characteristics or timbres was not to last long in the development of opera was because composers began to demand voices specialised in one particular quality of sound. Operas were written which contained the demand for one voice high as a nightingale and another low as a bear, both with precise musical phrases, and from this development came the operatic specialisations of soprano, mezzo, contralto, tenor, baritone and bass.

Whilst the Bel Canto singers were intent on mastering the arts of extending the different possible emotive qualities and imagistic characteristics on each note, later singers have sought to specialise in the perfection of a single operatic quality of voice and have been loath to try and extend the range associated with it. Furthermore, the increasingly elaborate complexity of musical composition has led to a process of training operatic singers which has become more influenced by the technical demands of the music and less connected to the primal and fundamental role of the voice as the expression of emotion, narrative and experience.

There are, of course, some exceptions to the composer's demand for the primacy of beauty and logically encoded symbols of meaning, such as Verdi's instruction that during the famous madness scene in his opera *Macbeth*, the singer playing Lady Macbeth should not sing but 'gasp, whisper and sob'. A number of these diversions from beauty in the history of twentieth century classical music have been discussed by Anhalt and they remain exceptions buried amidst an array of rules.[36]

With the decline of Bel Canto another significant aspect of performance was lost: that of trans-sexualism in character playing. In the classic Bel Canto operas, parts were not allotted according to gender as they are in the later genre of operatic realism. During the Baroque period, in both ballet, theatre and opera, men would play women's characters and vice versa and a male castrati, that is a castrated male singer with a high pitched voice in a falsetto register, would dress as a woman to play a female part.[37] Now, however, the voice was allotted according to gender and this very quickly began to infiltrate the way that singing was taught.

The Classical Vocal Compartments

The classical European operatic voice has a number of distinct voice qualities or specialisations allotted according to gender and which sing within specific pitch ranges. For women, the three most significant are the Soprano, which is the highest female voice and usually ranges upwards for two octaves from Middle C on the piano, the Mezzo-soprano, from the Italian *mezzo* meaning 'middle' which is the middle female voice ranging two octaves upwards from the A just below middle C on the piano and the Contralto, which is the lowest female voice ranging two octaves from the F below middle C to F an octave and a half above it. For men, meanwhile, the three most significant are the Tenor, which ranges from the C below middle C to the C above it, the Baritone, which is the middle male voice and ranges from G an octave and a half below middle C to the F above it and the Bass, which is the lowest male voice ranging from middle C down to E almost two octaves below.

It will be apparent that there is some overlap of notes between these classifications. For example, while one person may sing middle D as a tenor, another may sing it as a baritone. Though both sing the same note, however, they will both possess very different qualities, colours or timbres. The same may be said of a group of notes between the female mezzo and contralto. Therefore, the operatic specialisations cannot be described only as being defined by pitch ranges, they also constitute particular timbres. Furthermore, a note can also be sung in timbres which do not correspond to any of the operatic registers; both Elton John and Phil Collins have the same range as a tenor but their voices would not be described as tenors in the operatic sense. Moreover, those contemporary rock singers who have had a classical training can sing with two completely different acoustic qualities, both in the same pitch range. Michael Bolton, for example, has sung classical tenor duets with Pavoroti followed by his own contemporary songs during the same concert; both were sung in the same pitch range but the first was in the classical timbre of the tenor and the latter in a timbre more suitable to rock songs. The operatic voice is, therefore, one which operates within certain given pitch ranges and, at the same time, has a particular timbre. The registers of modal and falsetto may be defined as particular types of timbre. In opera the tenor, baritone and bass are all sung in modal. In this operatic tradition of singing, male modal voices are only permitted to rise in pitch to a certain level. Taking this to extremes, some teachers say that exclusive use of the modal register above middle C is potentially damaging to the vocal folds,[38] for which there is in fact no evidence whatsoever.

Above the male modal tenor is the counter-tenor, which is sung entirely in the falsetto register and for which there are a few parts written. The male falsetto register is also a major component of the voice quality produced by a young boy prior to the pubertal voice changes characterised by a descent of the larynx and a slackening of the vocal folds, and it was this quality that the castrati, male singers who were castrated to prevent such pubertal changes, sought to preserve. In the Baroque and Renaissance culture of seventeenth and eighteenth century Europe such a voice was greatly admired and the castration of pre-pubescent boys was common practice, producing the so-called castrati singers. Due to the prevention of hormonal release by removing the testicles, these singers conserved the quality of a child's voice in an adult body. They had both the larynx of a boy and the resonators of a man, which, according to musicians of the period, gave the castrati's voice a unique quality neither male nor female but angel-like and androgynous. The most well-renowned castrati is Farinelli, who was employed by the queen of Spain to cure her husband, Philip V, of madness. There are obviously no recordings of what this voice sounded like, though Gluck's opera *Orfeo* has a role written for a castrati and thus gives an idea of its range. As well as singing in concerts and at the courts, the castrati were also employed by the Vatican, who needed high voices but did not allow women to sing. However, Pope Leo XIII banned the castrati from the church towards the end of the 18th century. The adoration for the voice of the castrati is eloquently expressed in Balzac's story of *Sarasine* and though the castrati no longer exist, we come close to it in the male falsetto counter tenor. Among the most known of these counter tenors is Aris Christofellis, who has recorded pieces from the repertoire which the castrati are known to have sung.[39]

For women, meanwhile, the falsetto is the register in which soprano and mezzo-soprano are sung whilst the contralto is usually blended with some modal quality. Again, for women, there is an overlap area where the same range of notes can be sung in both falsetto and modal. The aim of singing training in western Europe has always been to reduce or even eliminate the changes in timbre between one register and another which characterise so many non-European song traditions. This has led to the production of voices which can sing the widest possible pitch range without any audible change in timbre. This is achieved by a process known as blending, which eliminates the dramatic opposition between modal and falsetto and blends the qualities along the whole length of the pitch range. This blending is particularly utilised in training women singers.

One of the primary factors which distinguishes female singers in the operatic tradition from those in the popular tradition is that in the latter the predominant sung register is modal, with falsetto used as an embellishment on certain notes or phrases, particularly in the higher pitch ranges. For singers wishing to traverse both traditions, this presents confusion and technical difficulty which few classical singing teachers are prepared to take on.

For most untrained singers, male and female, the modal register is the most natural, for it should be remembered that for both men and the majority of women, the speaking voice is predominantly modal, with occasional peaks of falsetto during moments of excitement. Despite this, male performers often assume a falsetto quality when impersonating women, such as that used by the Australian comedian, Barry Humphries, in his characterisation of Dame Edna Everage, the characterisation of Mrs Doubtfire by Robin Williams and of Tootsie by Dustin Hoffman. It is also frequently used in the classic pantomime dame caricature.

Because the speaking voice is rooted primarily in modal, the training of a falsetto voice is, therefore, one which demands an aesthetic adaptation of the natural speaking voice to meet a particular set of demands. Many of the great mid-century film actresses who also sang, such as Rita Hayworth, Gloria Swanson and Judy Garland, can be heard moving from their modal speaking voice into a falsetto singing voice.

Those trained in the operatic tradition are thus taught, if not indoctrinated, to perceive vocal acoustics within a register spectrum running from vocal fry to chest, or modal, through mixed to head, or falsetto, up to the loft or whistle register. However, there are some key opponents to such a framework of perception from within the operatic tradition itself. For example, the renowned German soprano Lilli Lehmann, who sang throughout the late nineteenth and early twentieth century and who was coached by Wagner and achieved international fame for her performances which included 600 lieder and 170 operatic roles, bequeathed her opinions and her advice in a short manuscript entitled *How to Sing*, in which she admits that registers are not found in nature but are acquired through use of the voice.[40] Indeed, in my experience, the training which classical singers have received, particularly in the field of register, is often, later in life, retrospectively perceived as an imprisonment.

Therapeutic Voicework Methodology: Register Malleability

Included in the Practice of Timbre and Tone is the search for Register Malleability, which involves training the voice to sing both modal and falsetto registers on as wide a pitch range as possible. Starting with a note in the middle of the range, the trainee sings in modal and then, half-way through singing the note, changes the register into falsetto without ceasing to sing. Then the vocalist inspires, sings the same note in falsetto and this time changes it to modal half-way through. The trainee repeats this process on each note ascending and descending up and down the pitch range. The higher the voice ascends in pitch, the more difficult the modal register is to master. Conversely, the falsetto register becomes more difficult to achieve the lower in pitch the voice descends. Part of the training process, therefore, involves the Therapeutic Voiceworker in helping the trainee to achieve both registers at the extremes of the scale. In addition, the trainee then attempts to blend both registers together, singing the broadest pitch range without any perceivable register break.

Finally, at the very top of the pitch scale, the trainee attempts to close the glottis and vocalise the whistle register whilst, at the bottom end, allowing the voice to crumble into the vocal fry register.

I have demonstrated this process on the set of audio cassettes *The Singing Cure: Liberating Self Expression Through Voice Movement Therapy*[41] and I have shown their musical application in singing on the CD *Prayers and Prophecies*[42].

The Singing Lesson

From the late eighteenth century through to the present day, techniques for singing teaching have been developed and recorded primarily by successful singers who have committed their methodology to writing in the form of hints and exercises.[43] In addition, other singers have dedicated their life to teaching pedagogical methodologies which assist the sustaining of a classical voice, such as the renowned British teacher Esther Salaman.[44] Of course, no classical singer has been more consistently admired and analysed than Enrico Caruso, who, when he died in 1921, left behind his own hints on singing[45] and whose methods are recorded by the laryngologist Dr P Marafioti, Caruso's medical adviser and friend who learned from Caruso the techniques upon which his natural art of singing were built. Marafioti passed on these techniques in his advice to other singers and students who were referred to Marafioti in times of difficulty in a book completed just before Caruso's deat.[46]

Despite the intimate nature of the singing lesson and the deeply emotional nature of the material therein expressed, few singing teachers from the classical tradition have articulated or spoken of the relationship between training the voice and the therapeutic development of the person. One of the first exceptions to break from this pretence that the singing lesson has nothing to do with the psyche is Cornelius Reid, who, during the second half of this century, taught and wrote about techniques for training the singing voice based on his modernising of the Bel Canto principles. Reid believed that the aim of the training process was to provoke 'organic movement', causing 'fundamental changes within the coordinative process' which give rise to vocalisation. But he pointed out that 'any programme designed to promote organic movement when such movement has been held in check will constitute a threat and arouse anxiety'. For Reid, 'the training process necessarily and unavoidably upsets both the physical and emotional equilibrium to which the student has become accustomed', forcing the student to ask 'Is the "I" I think myself to be truly me ?' Consequently, the training process touches 'upon a very sensitive area, as correction of a vocal problem is equivalent to an attack on the student's emotional core'. Yet by viewing the voice as an extension of the person, it becomes apparent that working on the voice can be a remarkably inspiring way of working on one's self and that 'vocal growth' inevitably facilitates 'emotional growth'.[47]

For Reid, 'inner tensions are the single greatest obstacle to vocal development' and the effect 'of one's emotional constitution on phonation cannot be overestimated'.[48] However, Reid remains an exception to the approach of most singing teachers in the classical tradition whose focus is on the pedagogical imparting of technical virtuosity. This usually occurs in a one-to-one consultation of between thirty minutes and one hour, during which little acknowledgement or investigation of emotional issues, or psychological concerns, including those pertaining to the relationship between teacher and student, takes place. But the format of singing teaching and its contract of a paid-time period in which the experienced singing teacher instructs the student is by no means any more universal than the singing style which this contract perpetuates. Neither the style nor the method of imparting it is appropriate to the songs of the Alaskan Eskimos, the north American native song culture, the secular song culture of Iran and the Arabic Near East, the folk music and its dissemination in Ethiopia, the drum accompanied songs and their teaching in Ghana, the narrative story songs and their passing on in the South Sahara, the ancestral dream time songs and their preservation amongst the Australian Aborigines or the dance songs and their imparting in Polynesia. The way that the songs of another culture can challenge the sensibility and move the heart of a Westerner is told in the poignant tale of Louis Sarno, who lived amongst the Ba-Benjellé Pygmies in Africa. This story reminds us how narrowly many Westerners perceive the meaning of singing.[49]

Women's Voices

The development of a literary music, like many cognitive systems which replaced intuitive ones, was primarily a male-directed project and the subjugation of non-formal, non-discursive oral traditions of musical presentation and dissemination in favour of literary music inevitably involved the subjugation of the women who were the keepers of oral song.

Just has said that, for the Greek patriarchy, the lamentations of women caused disruptions, posing a threat to the order and survival of society by introducing the unrestrained, the emotional and the illogical.[50] Indeed, in the first century BC, Plutarch tells us that the Athenian lawgiver, Solon, forbade women to perform their 'composed dirges'.[51] Plato, meanwhile, stated that lamentation is 'weak and feminine', stood against the vocal expression of grief[52] and said that 'ideal lawgivers' would prohibit public outcries at funeral processions.[53]

In classical mythology the feminine realm of song is symbolised in the figure of the bird-bodied Siren, who personifies the use of voice to both seduce and to impart knowledge. In Homer's *The Odyssey* the Sirens lure Odysseus toward their 'rocky shores' with their knowledge of 'all things', tempting him with the words: 'Come hither Odysseus' and 'listen to our song', for 'never has any man passed this way in his dark vessel and left unheard the honey sweet music from our lips'.[54] The Sirens reveal the power of the voice to enter or penetrate and wound, as well as to move or impart knowledge for we can be 'damaged by what comes in through sight and hearing', yet 'what comes in' also 'stimulates' and sows the seeds for 'skill and power'.[55] The fact that the Sirens offer knowledge is the essence of their 'sensuous magnetism'[56] and, like the Muses, they are images of illumination and inspiration.[57] In time, the Sirens shed their wings and claws, lost connection with wisdom and knowledge and were transformed by popular culture into *femmes fatales* and mermaids. The power of a woman's voice to impart wisdom is also evidenced by the oral tradition of fairy-tales, which represent a form of knowledgeable wisdom passed down to a young audience by older women who, in giving voice to the tales, are breaking a silence and refusing subjection.[58]

In Greek mythology the Muses and the Sirens, both emblems of song, were women, yet the female tradition of song has been obscured by the political oppression of the supposed illogical emotionality that vocal expression contains when compared to the articulate verbality of patriarchal linguistics. The roots of patriarchal repression which can be found in ancient Greece have continued to the present day in Greek society where women do not have the same freedom to enter folk dance and song as men. To this day, women are prohibited from playing instruments in rural Greece and are 'the designated guardians of vocal forms' where 'they preserve folk songs as the keepers of traditional lore and perform laments in their capacity as chief mourners'. The process of growth from girlhood to womanhood involves an education by which they are 'socialised to respond to changing family circumstances with shifts in vocal expression, from songs of carefree youth to the musical restraint and laments of middle and old age'. The village men, meanwhile, by contrast, are forever free to 'sing, dance, and play certain instruments throughout their lives, but never lament'. In other words, 'the free exercise of musical joy is essentially a male privilege, while lamenting, the antithesis of music-as-joy, is seen as women's expressive hallmark.'[59] Simultaneously, women are also, in many cultures, excluded from other singing acts, such as the exclusion of women from Hasidic ceremony in synagogues among orthodox Jews.

In Western Christian culture women's voices have also been considered dangerous and seductive. In the Biblical Garden of Eden, Eve 'sinned through speech by tempting Adam to eat with her words'.[60] She is then tempted by speaking to the serpent and she, in turn, seduces Adam. Eve thus 'sinned by mouth', reminding 'us of the misogyny that loquacity is a woman's vice, silence a woman's virtue.'[61] Although silence can be a stratagem for women and the powerless can use speechlessness as a strong line of defence, this is no substitute for the right of women to reclaim the full resonance of their vocal power and, through the emergence of a feminist musicology, womens' musical traditions are being acknowledged and their role as preservers of the oral arts remembered.[62]

In many regions 'most aspects of daily life that are accompanied by songs are the domain of women.'[63] For example, 'women are the principal transmitters of the song tradition'[64] throughout the Balkans which, because the womens' hands are constantly occupied with 'weaving, knitting, carrying, and cooking tasks', are vocally composed and embellished rather than instrumentalised.[65] Women are also the exclusive singers and preservers of traditional Hispanic wedding songs amongst the Moroccan Jews in Canada,[66] they are the exclusive singers and preservers of the rich array of lullabies amongst the Hazaras in Afghanistan,[67] they are the leading vocalists accompanying Gamalan music in Java[68] and they are traditionally the keepers of songs which relay wisdom and foreboding, parable and education to children throughout Europe and the USA.

The Contemporary Challenge and the World Perspective

There are a number of contemporary practitioners who implicitly challenge the traditional nature of singing and the singing lesson, and the political injustice within which so much singing activity has been couched, by offering group workshops where all people, regardless of age, race, mental and physical disposition, economic or social status and musical ability, literacy and experience, can discover an authentic voice and learn songs through oral memory without recourse to any kind of notation.

One such practitioner is the Czechoslovakian singer and actress Ida Kelerova, who was a member of the legendary Czechoslovakian experimental theatre company, Theatre on a String. The eastern European performance style, as exemplified in the work of Bertolt Brecht and Kurt Weil, is one that uses song to highlight emotional and political constructs and Kelerova's work is grounded in this tradition. However, her workshops are directed towards non-singers as much as performers and enable participants to find an authentic voice regardless of musical ability. Kelerova, who worked in the UK for some years but has now established the International School for the Human Voice in the Czech Republic, works to 'precipitate the personal process' which will 'free body and voice towards openness of fullest expression'. She says that in her work she encourages participants to form an understanding 'that not only are our feelings not negative, but also, once we know them, they are a vital and dynamic part of our life and our performance.'[69]

Another contemporary practitioner who extends the boundaries of singing and songmaking is Ysayé Barnwell, one of the singers with the popular American Gospel group *Sweet Honey in the Rock*, and who is, by training, a speech and language therapist. Working with large groups of people, particularly young adults who cannot read music, she exercises her belief that the history of a person, of a community and of a culture is evident in songs, exemplified most poignantly in the way that the politics of the black slave movement is documented through ballads and choral melodic verses. Thus teaching a group of workshop participants or schoolchildren to sing co-operatively and in harmony is, for Barnwell, a political act.[70] In their own concerts the essence of their intentions is 'to convey social, political and emotional passion through the fundamental medium of the human voice', singing songs which 'are an uncompromising campaign for justice, equality and peace.'[71]

In workshops for children run by Barnwell and other members of the performing group, songs are taught in such a way as to educate the students not only musically but politically. For example, one song called 'Juba' illustrates for children the importance of rhythm in the body but, in addition, provides a context for historical teaching. The singer first explains how, historically, the drums were taken from the slaves to disempower them, make them less defiant and make it harder for them to communicate their musical messages over distances. Juba is, says the singer, 'the drum rhythm in the body'. 'Juba cannot be taken away'. 'Juba can remind you at any time of your own stand, the right to your own voice'.[72] The children then learn the song, the rhythm and the words and experience Juba first-hand. A further illustration of defiance and sense of justice from *Sweet Honey in the Rock* is Ysayé Barnwell's commitment to performing *The Halleluljah Chorus* from Handel's *Messiah* with a mass choir of individuals who do not read music but who are enabled to learn and perform it through oral abilities alone.[73]

The commitment to a sense of community and its right to enjoy and communicate through sung music is also central to the work of London-based Maggie Nichols, who leads regular groups for anyone who wants to experience singing through group improvisation. The groups are usually held at the London Musicians Collective, which continues a movement instigated by, among others, John Stevens in the 1960s. The loose relaxed organisation and democratic structure of her workshops offer an empowering framework for musical expression.[74]

Nichols is a singer and her own performance background is rooted in a jazz tradition which makes use of scats improvisation, where the voice works rhythmically through a spontaneous collage of staccato and sustained sounds. It is this tradition that Nichols has extended in her workshop teaching where she facilitates the ability for all people to create free improvisation using all vocal sounds, including coughs, burps and sneezes. Her work is politically motivated by an allegiance with socialism and feminism and her belief is that political and social consciousness can be mobilised through the act of singing.

The community-orientated work of Maggie Nichols compares to that of Richard Roberts, who has been leading workshops in London for sixteen years. Initially inspired by his participation in a Roy Hart Theatre workshop, Roberts began to lead singing groups for those who could not read music – out of which he formed the Bath Choir, which enables all those who sing in the bath but rarely venture beyond it to join with others in a community celebration of the singing voice. Roberts, unlike Nichols, however, also offers one-to-one work which he describes as 'voice and healing work'.[75] The interface between singing for pleasure, singing for social empowerment and singing for therapy or healing is complex and each practitioner has a different set of boundaries within which they seek to work.

The Community Singing Revival

The wave of interest in vocal expression and singing for pleaure and social activity is exemplified in the increasing number of choirs which are being formed all over the UK.

A choir tradition which has been consistently popular in the USA, and which has recently found a revival in the UK, is shape note singing, where sounds are recognised and sung literally in response to the shapes of the written notes. The style originates in the country parish churches of the 18th and 19th century and most of the songs sung by this means are still based on the scriptures, though this is said to be no barrier to the participation of the non-believer.[76] Another increasingly popular choir style is that of gospel choirs, which have spawned many high-profile popular singers, such as Aretha Franklin.[77] In complete contrast, many choirs are beginning to recapture the Gregorian Chant.

Law says that there is 'a new freedom within group singing' born 'from enthusiasm for natural vocal expression' and 'the general feeling of well-being reported by most regular singers during and following energetic vocal activity' and perpetuated by those choir leaders committed to a non-judgmental approach to the provision of singing workshops, choirs and lessons.[78] In addition, there is an increasingly widespread network of those who facilitate Voicework in groups and in individual sessions throughout the UK which extend the notion of the singing lesson and the act of singing to incorporate political, educational and social processes. In Britain the major preceding pioneering contributor to the revisioning of singing teaching is Frankie Armstrong.

Frankie Armstrong

No one has done more to reframe the singing lesson, lifting it from the one-to-one contractual encounter and relocating it as a community celebration and simultaneously fashioning the process in a multi-cultural and multi-ethnic aesthetic, than Frankie Armstrong.

As a teenager, Armstrong lost her sight. Despite training as a social worker, her present career began as a singer in a skiffle band, with whom she sang about 'the black and poor white peoples of the United States' and 'the peasantry: land workers of the British Isles and Eire'. These songs 'spoke of the happenings of everyday life – loving, feuding, working, suffering, dreaming and hoping' and though when she first sang them she 'knew little or nothing of their history and background', something inside her was 'stirred by these stories, by the cries for freedom and affection'.[79]

It was the process of singing these songs which opened her 'small-town eyes' to 'universal issues such as Civil Rights, the appalling conditions in mines and factories, the brutality and dangers of life at sea over the past centuries and women's outrage and sorrow as their husbands and sons were sent to war'.[80] Later, after travels through Europe, a formal social work training and encounters with European folk culture, she sang with Ewan McColl and Peggy Seeger as well as developing a solo career singing political and social issue songs in various community settings, including drug rehabilitation centres, prisons and hospitals, where she adjusted her repertoire to respond to the audience at hand.

While in the USA, Frankie met Ethel Raim, who gave workshops for groups of artists and others who wanted to experiment with singing. This meeting launched Frankie into a long career of providing workshops for all those who want to discover their indigenous voice.

Central to the style which Frankie has developed involves using the human body to simulate industrial working actions that would have accompanied many folk songs, such as hoeing, planting, weaving and hurling. She points out that 'the idea that singing involves standing or sitting still' is probably 'of very recent origin'. In fact, 'throughout most of human history, it's probably true that some kind of movement went with giving voice'.[81] Frankie's workshops 'encourage the open-throated style of singing found in cultures that sing in the open air, singing as naturally and spontaneously as they speak.'[82] Frankie realises that she is 'also drawing on those years of social work and group work' and that part of what she offers 'is a sort of fearlessness about what people may bring to the groups'. In her workshops 'participants have wept, screamed, found themselves totally silent and literally climbed up the walls as they found themselves in touch with old, repressed events' that bring with them deep emotions. She perceives her job to be to 'contain and allow this to happen and then get the person and the group back to voicing and singing'. 'After all', she says, 'I have deliberately chosen to call them 'Voice Workshops', not voice therapy'.[83]

Whilst Frankie distinctly defines her work as 'not therapy', there are other practitioners of Voicework who do not make such stipulation but who promote the healing nature to their work and which I will explore later.

Singing in the Field

The rich history of singing, in its broadest possible aesthetic and cultural sense, is being reclaimed and celebrated through the current proliferation of workshops, courses and events facilitated by an increasing number of practitioners who work with groups through various strategies drawing in some way upon the act of singing.

Mary Law points out that the idea that everyone has a right to sing together in a choir and that the addition of any voice, 'even an untutored voice or one that has difficulty in keeping pitch', is not a hindrance but 'an asset' is a relatively new approach to singing activities for a major part of the present-day Western world. Few 'choirs in the classical tradition accept new members without first submitting them to an audition' and 'potential members frequently are rejected because of lack of musical skill' or 'more often because the voice offered will not blend appropriately with the whole choir'. Even today, in what Law describes as 'these relatively vocally enlightened times', choir leaders are seeking voices which fit within a very narrow corridor of the human vocal capacity'. Today's 'community choirs', however, are 'unlikely to turn away new members other than for reasons of over-subscription'. Moreover, the reported experience of such choirs is 'that peoples' diverse voices merge and blend extremely well for a whole range of songs of many different styles and origins whilst retaining what is individual within the overall group sound'.[84]

Among leaders who direct community-based choirs in the UK are Andrew Scott, who directs the youth choir *The Swing Bridge Singers* in Tyneside,[85] Katherine Zeserson, who directs the *Newcastle College Choir*,[86] Sian Croose, who works as a workshop leader and directs the choir called *Big Sky* in Norwich,[87] Dorota Kotz, who runs the *Queer Choir* in London,[88] Jenny Goodman in Scotland, who runs of *The Voice House Choir* and offers workshops,[89] Alison Burns in Edinburgh, who is a singer, songwriter and voice teacher who also runs choirs, Sammy Hurden, based in Dorset, who rewrites classic soul and jazz songs for choral groups,[90] Sandra Kerr, who formed a 35-piece choir consisting of Northumberland women which performs a wide range of material both traditional and newly written[91] and Liz Hodgson, who runs voice workshops and directs a choir in Oxford.[92]

In addition, there are many facilitators who work with transient groups for a finite period of time, using song as a means to revive and celebrate. These include Douglas Coombs, who teaches a broad catalogue of vocal music to people of all ages from infants to adults,[93] Barbara Swetina and Kate Holly O'Connell, who teach secular and religious but non-denominational songs at the Findhorn community in Scotland,[94] Mick Sands, a song writer, teacher, community worker and voice coach who sings with people who have learning difficulties,[95] Venice Manley, who teaches a wide repertoire of songs from many parts of the world to workshop participants,[96] Harriet Buchan, who runs voice workshops in Glasgow,[97] Helen Chadwick, who works with theatre groups as a voice and singing teacher and teaches a mixture of her own compositions and songs from many parts of the world to workshop participants[98] and Joan Mills, a voice coach offering workshops who organises regular conferences.[99] In France, meanwhile, Brigitte Cirla and Kozanna Lucca lead voice workshops with similar aims and intentions.[100]

Within the ever-growing field of voice and singing activities is a body of work where the practitioner passes on and teaches songs from the villages and towns of the world, an increasingly popular component of many voice workshops – some of which are led by those whom Armstrong has influenced. For example, one workshop leader in the Armstrong tradition is Rowena Whitehead, who, together with her colleague Sue Parlby, runs workshops called 'Talking in Tune' for singers at all levels of experience in the Cambridge area of the UK and leads a choir called *Women of Note* which

sings a repertoire drawn from many parts of the globe,[101] Vivien Ellis, who
sings black African songs and other world music and runs workshops,[102] Tran
Quan Hai, an ethnomusicologist based in Paris but originally from Vietnam,
who teaches Tibetan-originated overtone chanting,[103] Erin McDonnell, who
regularly visits Zimbabwe to refresh and extend her repertoire and runs
workshops which teach African songs through oral exercises,[103] Eugene
Skeef, who specialises in disseminating South African songs and rhythms,
often working with very large groups,[105] Pinise Saul, who is a professional
singer and dancer who leads groups of performers in Zulu and other African
dances and songs and passes on indigenous songs to workshop
participants,[106] Bosco de Olivera, who is an instrumentalist and singer of
South American music, including bossa nova and salsa, and runs
workshops,[107] Brigitte Cloareg, who introduces Breton songs and dances
and other folk music from the British Isles to workshop participants,[108]
Christine Kidd and Janet Russell, who run workshops to teach their native
Scottish songs and singing style,[109] Sianed Jones, who is a singer and
composer who plays 'distorted funk hoe down fiddle' and runs singing
workshops with a particular slant towards voice rhythms and vocal
improvisation,[110] Eddie Upton, who specialises in singing and teaching
English folk song[111] and Brenda Rattray, former director of the Oval House
Music School and now Education Officer for the *Grand Union Orchestra*, who
sings jazz, blues and soul with the ensemble Darker than Blue and runs
singing workshops drawing from a repertoire of vocal music from all over the
world.[112]

These disseminators of ethnic music and esoteric vocal styles, who are
essentially singers working to share and pass on songs from their own
inherited musical tradition, are often committed educators but may not have
around them the structures of formal education which one finds in the
conservatoire or music college. The work of these and other practitioners is a
testimony to the current surge of interest in the human voice as a means of
expression rightfully available to all.

In addition to these artistically-orientated practitioners, there are many
workshop leaders and facilitators throughout the UK who specifically
declare that their approach to vocal work facilitates personal growth and
who imply either a psychotherapeutic or a healing dimension to the process.
These include Derek Gale, based in Essex, who works with voice as a
'medium for personal growth',[113] Susan Osborn, who runs workshops to
'help people unlock the power of their voices and open to a process of deep

healing and transformation,'[114] Jenni Treeves-Curran, who uses chants and other forms of vocalisation to 'release the inner voice',[115] Jackie Summers, a social worker based in London, who uses singing to 'support assertiveness training' and 'heighten self esteem',[116] Nina Chandler, based in Bristol, who describes her work as 'voice therapy',[117] Rosey Vallack, based in Huddersfield, who runs vocal groups for women which facilitate 'confidence and self-expression',[118] Jill Rakusen, who facilitates 'self-expression through vocalisation to mobilise each individual's response and forward the instinctual process'[119] and Rae Levy, who runs singing groups for women.[120]

In addition to these practitioners, workshops which offer 'healing with the voice' are offered by a growing number of local practitioners, some of whom have developed their abilities via spiritual and physical practices from the East and others whose musical training and research has led them to discover the healing power exerted by the vibrations of the human voice. Among them is Peter Wright in Bognor, a qualified music therapist working within the Health Service as well as from his own private practice[121] and Susan Lever in Middlesbrough, who offers workshops in healing with voice.[122] Many of these practitioners are members of The UK Sound Healers Association, of which Simon Heather is the secretary as well as being a practising member who combines massage, acupuncture and sound healing in workshops based in Powys.[123]

Within the expanding field of vocal investigation pursued by diverse practitioners there is thus a place where singing for social pleasure intersects with singing to aid self-knowledge, which intersects with singing as a form of healing, which, in turn, intersects with singing as a spiritual act. It is this latter field of enquiry and activity, which uses voice and song within the framework of spiritual healing, that I shall investigate in the next chapter.

Singing and Sickness

Singing, to another or to oneself, is an immensely soothing process which is most familiarly symbolised in the lullaby. A mother with a sick child will often sit at the infant's bed-side and hum or sing a simple refrain which, like the original sonorous envelope, creates the sensation of being held, rocked and assuaged. The healing power of song is also symbolised in the fact that to sing is often considered to be a way of discharging cares and worries.

Furthermore, songs often provide a context for the musicalisation of pathology, negative experience and bodily dysfunction. A nursery rhyme as simple as 'Ring a Ring of Roses' is based upon the bubonic plague, the jazz and blues song tradition is predicated upon tales of depression and anguish, many musical theatre productions comprise songs about death and dying and the vast majority of British and North American folk ballads tell the tale of a 'poor' or 'poorly' fellow or maiden. Somehow, the song makes darkness tolerable for the singer as the process of music making made illness tolerable for so many great composers.

Handel was plagued with paralysing rheumatism and contracted cataracts which rendered him blind. Mozart, who died at thirty-six years of age, was continually ill from infancy when he suffered from fevers, skin rashes and recurrent streptococcal tonsillitis as well as contracting smallpox in his adult years. Beethoven, aside from deafness, suffered from chest infection, asthma and bowel disease which tyrannised him with painful diarrhoea leaving him frequently exhausted and dehydrated; he died of cirrhosis of the liver. Paganini, who had all of his lower teeth removed by an incompetent dentist and lived on a diet of liquid and medication, spent the last years of his life in agony with laryngeal disease and severe abdominal pain, eventually dying of symptoms initiated by syphilis. Rossini suffered from chronic gonorrhoea, respiratory and cardiovascular diseases. Schubert suffered from syphilis and typhoid fever. The entire Mendelssohn family died of strokes. Chopin suffered from a debilitating lung disease which killed him at the age of 49. Liszt suffered from chronic bronchitis, arthritis, poor vision and heart disease. Grieg had respiratory illness and terrible rheumatism. Bizet died at 36 after a lifetime of ill health, including chronic streptococcal throat infections and chronic rheumatic fever. Brahms died of cancer of the liver. Britten died of a stroke. Debussy died of rectal carcinoma and Shostakovich died of motor neuron disease.[124]

Yet the intimate relationship between pathology and creativity provides inspiration and encouragement for clients of Therapeutic Voicework. The process of allowing clients to vocalise all aspects of themselves, rather than just the beautiful and the healthy parts, means that sickness can be perceived as part of life's journey and contributory to the creative process.

Therapeutic Voicework Methodology: The Healing Song

One of the methodologies which I have found useful when working with clients who have an identifiable illness is the composition of a Healing Song. This consists of allowing the creative imagination to write freely upon the fantasy of the illness, including descriptions of bodily organs and their condition.

The client begins by taking hold of a part of the body which is painful and proceeds to rub it, stroke it and attend to it in a soothing fashion. Simultaneously, the client makes sounds which express the sense of illness: groaning, moaning, crying and gasping in the way many people do when alone in their sick bed. In time, the client begins to verbalise these sounds, which may, to begin with, consist simply of identifying the bodily part with words such as 'my stomach', in the case of gastrointestinal problems, or 'my head', in the case of migraine, for example. With the support and encouragement of the practitioner, the client develops these initial words into vocalised descriptions of the body and its sensations, repeating lines as they emerge and building up a song which originates in the authentic vocalisation of disease or discomfort.

This song can then be rehearsed using instruments or other voices and often acts as a container and a medicine for the sensations which instigated it.

Therapeutic Voicework Case Study: I Heard the Plane Came Down

Richard was one of a few who had survived an aeroplane crash. Though he had remarkably and miraculously not sustained any serious physical injury, the event had severe consequences regarding his mental and emotional life.

His symptoms included insomnia, nightmares, periods of extreme depression, suicidal fantasies and panic attacks. Prior to the accident he had been married and held a job carrying considerable responsibility at a major financial institution. However, he had never returned to work and one year after the crash he was divorced.

Richard had received counselling twice a week for the first three months after the accident and once a week for a further two months. Since then he had not pursued any further therapy but visited his General Practitioner frequently for a variety of medications, including analgesics and tranquillisers.

Prior to the accident, Richard had been a member of a choir where he often sang solo and which was his central social and recreational pursuit. Since the accident, however, he had not sung and said that he felt as though his voice had dropped out of him.

The only optical memory which Richard had of the plane crash was seeing the head of the person he was sitting adjacent to, separate from his body. The rest was, he said, 'complete darkness' until he was placed upon a stretcher by the medical team.

What Richard did have was a complete spectrum of acoustic memories: engine noises, announcements of the pilot, the screams of the passengers and the sirens of the emergency team. Indeed, when Richard told the story, most of his sentences which described the three minutes leading up to the point of impact – at which he became buried by debris and contained by darkness – began with the words: 'I heard'. For example, he said: 'I heard the pilot announce his apologies for the difficult take-off'; he said: 'I heard the crashing of the glasses in the steward area'; he said: 'I heard the sirens of the emergency team and I knew I was alive'; and he said: 'I heard someone say: "It's all right we are going to get you out."'

Richard had come into Therapeutic Voicework because he wanted to rediscover his singing voice in order that he could rejoin a choir and 'begin to put his life back together'. Moreover, he was somewhat guarded about working directly on the experience of the crash because, he said, he had 'been through it over and over again in counselling'.

During the investigation of his voice, Richard experienced intense sensations of fear and anxiety when vocalising high in pitch with lots of violin, which, for some reason, provoked his acoustic memories of the incident.

I could not help being struck by the rhythm and tonality of the repetitious use of the motif 'I heard' which began each of his sentences. I therefore asked Richard to write them down in a long list and read them out aloud. I then reflected back to him the prosody underlying his speech, which read like a combination of a protest song and a folk ballad, so that he could hear the music inherent in what he had created. Then I asked him to sing the lines with the prosody exaggerated into melody. Whilst Richard's most familiar voice was a classical tenor, which he had used in the choir, he now sang in a strong but calm and collected folk-style voice which reminded me of Ewan McColl.

As I listened, I noticed that Richard was tapping his foot to enhance the beat of the rendition, so I asked someone in the group to play the rhythm in time with the foot tapping on a single note on a clarinet. In addition, another member beat a drum in the same time. Richard smiled and said: 'wow, this is new'.

After the clarinet and drum-accompanied version, Richard was extremely animated and reported that he remembered hearing muffled speech over some kind of loudspeaker and suggested that we add this to the musicalisation; so a group of three people sang Free Phonetic Improvisation with lots of violin resembling inaudible articulation on a fluctuating pitch, which alternated between being harmonious and being discordant with the clarinet. In addition, a woman with a beautiful soprano voice elaborated on the idea of a siren by singing up and down the pitch range very softly in the background.

The effects were, in Richards words, 'absolutely electric'. The atmosphere in the room was highly charged and the musical form was like an epic folk ballad as Richard's voice curved and turned, called and whispered through every nuance. As he did so, tears ran silently from his eyes.

Later that year I received a letter and a tape from Richard. The letter said that he had decided not to rejoin a choir but that he was now singing solo unaccompanied folk songs in folk clubs where he was discovering a new way of using his voice. He had also performed the ballad, which he called 'I Heard the Plane Came Down', at one club and it was this that was on the tape.

For Richard, the act of singing about a most serious trauma, which had changed his life and suppressed his voice, was a healing process which served to make an artistic form from a negative experience and excavate his voice from traumatic shock.

Of course, it was not the same voice; perhaps the tenor voice which he once had will never return. Sometimes, the voice is changed irreversibly by what happens to us. However, for Richard, something else was gained in its place that enabled him to move on with a newly discovered voice without pretending that the extreme circumstances which had befallen him had never happened. Indeed, he had something to sing about.

Conclusion: From Song to Vocal Healing

Although there are many workshop leaders and choir leaders using songs from a variety of cultures, they do not necessarily seek to perpetuate indigenous religious or spiritual practices for healing purposes. This is, perhaps, what distinguishes such work from that of others who, in addition to passing on a repertoire of songs, most of which are spiritual, also aim to effect healing by utilising systems of psychosomatic perception drawn from non-Western cultures.

It is this body of work to which I shall now turn the reader's attention.

Notes

1   Kittelson, M.L. (1996) *Sounding the Soul: The Art of Listening*. Einnsiedeln: Daimon.

2   Clarkson, A. (1978) 'Creative listening: an archetypal attitude to musical experience.' Paper presented to the 13th World Congress of the International Society for Music Education (Ontatrio, 12-20 August 1978).

3   Bliss, B.(1984) 'The singer and the voice.' Diploma Thesis for C G Jung Institute, Zurich.

4   Moroney, P. (1980) 'Apples on a lilac tree: silence and song in the individuation process.' Diploma Thesis for C G Jung Institute, Zurich.

5   Steiner, R. (1987) 'Some thoughts on "La Vive Voix" by Ivan Fónagy.' *International Review of Psycho-Analysis*, 14, pp. 265–272.

6   Crystal, D. (1969) *Prosodic Systems and Intonation Systems in English*. Cambridge: Cambridge University Press, p.66.

7   Arye, L. (1988) 'Music the messenger.' Unpublished Master's Thesis for Antioch University. Zurich, Switzerland.

8   Killingmo, B. (1990) 'Beyoantics: a clinical study of isolation.' *International Journal of Psychoanalysis*, 71, pp.113–126, (p.120).

9   Stanford, W.B. (1983) *Greek Tragedy and the Emotions*. London: Routledge & Kegan Paul, p.57.

10   Lord, A. (1960) *The Singer of Tales*. Cambridge: Harvard University Press, p.67.

11   Lord, A. (1960) *The Singer of Tales*. Cambridge: Harvard University Press, p.5.

12   Lord, A. (1960) *The Singer of Tales*. Cambridge: Harvard University Press, p.5.

13   Stowell, G. (ed.), *The Book of Knowledge*, vol. 5. London: Waverly, Date unspecified, p.303.

14   Choksy, L. (1988) *The Kodály Method*. New Jersey: Prentice Hall.

15   Szönyi, E. (1990) *Kodály's Principles in Practice*. Budapest: Corvina, p.11.

16   Szönyi, E. (1990) *Kodály's Principles in Practice*. Budapest: Corvina, p.14.

17   Szönyi, E. (1990) *Kodály's Principles in Practice*. Budapest: Corvina, p.12.

18   Szönyi, E. (1990) *Kodály's Principles in Practice*. Budapest: Corvina, p.12.

19   Enigma, *Enigma* CD. Virgin Records.

20   Lisa Gerrard and the Victorian Philharmonic Orchestra, *The Mirror Pool* CD. Beggars Banquet Music.

21   Newham, P. (1998) *The Singing Cure: Liberating Self Expression through Voice Movement Therapy*. Boulder: Sounds True.

22   Newham, P. (1997) *Prayers and Prophecies*. London: Tigers Eye Press.

23   Peri, J. 'Preface to Eurydice', translated by O. Strunk in *Source Readings in Music History*, p.373. London: 1952. Cited in part in C. Headington, R. Westbrook & T. Barfoot, *Opera: A History*. London: Arrow Books, 1991, p.22.

24   Manen, L. (1989) *Bel Canto: The Teaching of the Classical Italian Song-Schools, its Decline and Restoration*. Oxford: Oxford University Press, p.3.

25   Hahn, R. (1920) *Du Chant*. Paris.

26   Manen, L. (1989) *Bel Canto: The Teaching of the Classical Italian Song-Schools, its Decline and Restoration*. Oxford: Oxford University Press, p.23.

27   Manen, L. (1989) *Bel Canto: The Teaching of the Classical Italian Song-Schools, its Decline and Restoration*. Oxford: Oxford University Press, p.3.

28   Manen, L. (1989) *Bel Canto: The Teaching of the Classical Italian Song-Schools, its Decline and Restoration*. Oxford: Oxford University Press, p.3.

29   Reid, C. (1971) *Bel Canto: Principles and Practices.* New York: Joseph Patelson Music House, p.34.

30   Newham, P. (1997) *Prayers and Prophecies.* London: Tigers Eye Press.

31   Newham, P. (1998) *The Singing Cure: Liberating Self Expression through Voice Movement Therapy.* Boulder: Sounds True.

32   Newham, P. (1997) *Shouting for Jericho: The Work of Paul Newham on the Human Voice.* London: Tigers Eye Press/Class Productions.

33   Panconcelli-Calzia, G. (1943) *Leonardo als Phonetiker.* Hamburg.

34   Ferrein, A. (1741) 'De la formation de la voix de l'homme'. In *Mémoires de l'Académie Royale des Sciences.* Paris, p.422.

35   Brodnitz, S. (1954) 'One hundred years of laryngoscopy: to the memory of Garcia, Tuerck, and Czermak.' *Transactions of the American Academy of Ophthalmology and Otolaryngology,* 53, p663.

36   Anhalt, I. (1984) *Alternative Voices: Essays on Contemporary Vocal and Choral Composition.* Toronto: University of Toronto Press.

37   Celletti, R. (1991) *A History of Bel Canto.* Oxford: Clarendon Press, pp.7–8.

38   Phillips, K. *Teaching Kids to Sing.* New York: Schirmer Books, p.48.

39   Aris Christofellis, *Farinelli Et Son Temps* CD. EMI Records.

40   Lehmann, L. (1993) *How to Sing.* New York: Dover, p.54.

41   Newham, P. (1998) *The Singing Cure: Liberating Self Expression through Voice Movement Therapy.* Boulder: Sounds True.

42   Newham, P. (1997) *Prayers and Prophecies.* London: Tigers Eye Press.

43   Hines, J. (1982) *Great Singers on Great Singing.* New York: Doubleday.

44   Salaman, E. (1989) *Unlocking Your Voice: Freedom to Sing.* London: Gollancz.

45   Caruso, E. & Tetrazzini, L. (1975) *The Art of Singing.* New York: Dover.

46   Marafioti, P. (1981) *Caruso's Method of Voice Production: The Scientific Culture of the Voice.* New York: Dover.

47   Reid, C. (1975) *Voice: Psyche and Soma.* New York: Dover, p.13.

48   Reid, C. (1975) *Voice: Psyche and Soma.* New York: Dover, pp.13, 15.

49   Sarno, L. (1993) *Song from the Forest: My Life Among the Ba-Benjellé Pygmies. London: Penguin.*

50   Just, R. (1989) *Women in Athenian Law and Life.* London: Routledge, pp.198–200.

51   Plutarch, *The Life of Solon,* 21. 90. 4.

52   Plato, Republic, 3.395 d-e.

53   Plato, Laws,12.960 a.

54   Homer (1980) *The Odyssey.* Oxford: Oxford University Press, p.147.

55   Padel, R. (1992) *In and Out of Mind: Greek Images of the Tragic.* Princeton: Princeton University Press, p.65.

56   Padel, R. (1992) *In and Out of Mind: Greek Images of the Tragic.* Princeton: Princeton University Press, p.65.

57   Warner, M. (1994) *From the Beast to the Blonde: On Fairy Tales and their Tellers.* London: Chatto & Windus, p.401.

58   Warner, M. (1994) *From the Beast to the Blonde: On Fairy Tales and their Tellers.* London: Chatto & Windus, p.30.

59   Auerbach, S. (1989) 'From singing to lamenting: women's musical role in a Greek village.' In E. Koskoff (ed) *Women and Music in Cross Cultural Perspective*. Illinois: University of Illinois Press, pp.25–43, (pp.25–26).

60   Warner, M. (1994) *From the Beast to the Blonde: On Fairy Tales and their Tellers*. London: Chatto & Windus, p.30.

61   Warner, M. (1994) *From the Beast to the Blonde: On Fairy Tales and their Tellers*. London: Chatto & Windus, p.31.

62   Smith, W. (1996) 'Voice, psychotherapy and feminism.' Paper presented to the International Association for Voice Movement Therapy. London 1996.

63   K. Marshall (ed.) (1993) *Rediscovering the Muses: Women's Musical Traditions*. Boston: North-eastern University Press.

64   Shehan, P. (1989) 'Balkan women as preservers of traditional music and culture.' In E. Koskoff (ed) *Women and Music in Cross Cultural Perspective*. Illinois: University of Illinois Press, pp.45–53 (p.48).

65   Shehan, P. (1989) 'Balkan women as preservers of traditional music and culture.' In E. Koskoff (ed) *Women and Music in Cross Cultural Perspective*. Illinois: University of Illinois Press, pp.45–53 (p.46).

66   Cohen, J. (1989) 'Ya Salió de la Mar': Judeo-Spanish wedding songs among Moroccan Jews in Canada.' In E . Koskoff (ed) *Women and Music in Cross Cultural Perspective*. Illinois: University of Illinois Press, pp.55–68.

67   Sakata, H. (1989) 'Hazara women in Afghanistan: innovators and preservers of a musical tradition.' In E. Koskoff (ed) *Women and Music in Cross Cultural Perspective*. Illinois: University of Illinois Press, pp.85–96.

68   Anderson Sutton, R. (1989) 'Identity and individuality in an ensemble tradition: the female vocalist in Java.' In E. Koskoff (ed) *Women and Music in Cross Cultural Perspective*, ed. by . Illinois: University of Illinois Press, pp.111–130.

69   Kelerova, I. (1995–6) Publicity brochure for the International School of the Human Voice.

70   Programme notes to *Folkworks' Vocal Chords Festival*. Newcastle-upon-Tyne 3-5 May, 1996 and London 4–6 May 1996.

71   Barnwell, Y. Lecture given at Songs of Heaven and Earth Conference (Findhorn Foundation, Forres, 30 March–6 April 1996).

72   Sweet Honey in the Rock (1992) *All for Freedom*. Cassette. Warner Bros. Records Inc.

73   Barnwell, Y. (1996) Lecture given at Songs of Heaven and Earth Conference. Findhorn Foundation, Forres, 30 March–6 April.

74   Nichols, M. cited in Law, M, 'Interviews with contemporary voice practitioners.' Unpublished research papers prepared for the International Association for Voice Movement Therapy (1996).

75   Roberts, R. cited in Law, M, 'Interviews with contemporary voice practitioners.' Unpublished research papers prepared for the International Association for Voice Movement Therapy (1996).

76   Roberts, R. cited in Law, M, 'Interviews with contemporary voice practitioners.' unpublished research papers prepared for the International Association for Voice Movement Therapy (1996).

77   Law, M. 'The practice of voice: an investigation into the diversity of approaches to vocal work as exemplified by current practitioners.' Unpublished research project prepared for the International Association for Voice Movement Therapy (1996).

78   Law, M. 'The practice of voice: an investigation into the diversity of approaches to vocal
      work as exemplified by current practitioners.' Unpublished research project prepared for
      the International Association for Voice Movement Therapy (1996).

79   Armstrong, F. (1992) *As Far as the Eye Can Sing: An Autobiography.* London: The Women's
      Press, p.16.

80   Armstrong, F. (1992) *As Far as the Eye Can Sing: An Autobiography.* London: The Women's
      Press, p.16.

81   Armstrong, F. (1992) *As Far as the Eye Can Sing: An Autobiography.* London: The Women's
      Press, p.107.

82   Armstrong, F. (1992) *As Far as the Eye Can Sing: An Autobiography.* London: The Women's
      Press, p.107.

83   Armstrong, F. (1992) *As Far as the Eye Can Sing: An Autobiography.* London: The Women's
      Press, p.115.

84   Law, M. (1996) 'The practice of voice: an investigation into the diversity of approaches to
      vocal work as exemplified by current practitioners', Unpublished research project prepared
      for the International Association for Voice Movement Therapy.

85   Law, M. (1996) 'The practice of voice: an investigation into the diversity of approaches to
      vocal work as exemplified by current practitioners.' Unpublished research project prepared
      for the International Association for Voice Movement Therapy.

86   Law, M. (1996) 'The practice of voice: an investigation into the diversity of approaches to
      vocal work as exemplified by current practitioners.' Unpublished research project prepared
      for the International Association for Voice Movement Therapy.

87   Law, M. (1996) 'The practice of voice: an investigation into the diversity of approaches to
      vocal work as exemplified by current practitioners.' Unpublished research project prepared
      for the International Association for Voice Movement Therapy.

88   Programme notes to *Folkworks' Vocal Chords Festival.* Newcastle-upon-Tyne 3–5 May, 1996
      and London 4-6 May 1996.

89   Programme notes to *Folkworks' Vocal Chords Festival.* Newcastle-upon-Tyne 3–5 May, 1996
      and London 4-6 May 1996.

90   Programme notes to *Folkworks' Vocal Chords Festival.* Newcastle-upon-Tyne 3–5 May, 1996
      and London 4-6 May 1996.

91   Programme notes to *Folkworks' Vocal Chords Festival.* Newcastle-upon-Tyne 3–5 May, 1996
      and London 4-6 May 1996.

92   Armstrong, F. (1995)Unpublished information leaflet on current voice teachers.

93   Law, M. (1996) 'The practice of voice: an investigation into the diversity of approaches to
      vocal work as exemplified by current practitioners.' Unpublished research project prepared
      for the International Association for Voice Movement Therapy.

94   Barnwell, Y. Lecture given at Songs of Heaven and Earth Conference (Findhorn Founda-
      tion, Forres, 30 March–6 April 1996).

95   Programme notes to *Folkworks' Vocal Chords Festival.* Newcastle-upon-Tyne 3–5 May, 1996
      and London 4–6 May 1996.

96   Armstrong, F. cited in Law, M (1996) 'Interviews with contemporary voice practitioners.'
      Unpublished research papers prepared for the International Association for Voice Move-
      ment Therapy.

97   Law, M. 'The practice of voice: an investigation into the diversity of approaches to vocal
      work as exemplified by current practitioners.' Unpublished research project prepared for
      the International Association for Voice Movement Therapy (1996).

98   Barnwell, Y. (1996) Lecture given at Songs of Heaven and Earth Conference. Findhorn Foundation, Forres, 30 March-6 April.

99   Conference series notes and information leaflet to Giving Voice, four annual conferences held at Cardiff, Centre for Performance Research (1993–96).

100 Conference series notes and information leaflet to Giving Voice, four annual conferences held at Cardiff, Centre for Performance Research (1993–96).

101 Law, M. 'Interviews with contemporary voice practitioners', unpublished research papers prepared for the International Association for Voice Movement Therapy (1996).

102 Law, M. 'The practice of voice: an investigation into the diversity of approaches to vocal work as exemplified by current practitioners.' Unpublished research project prepared for the International Association for Voice Movement Therapy (1996).

103 Conference series notes and information leaflet to Giving Voice, four annual conferences held at Cardiff, Centre for Performance Research (1993–96).

104 Armstrong, F. (1995)Unpublished information leaflet on current voice teachers.

105 Programme notes to *Folkworks' Vocal Chords Festival*. Newcastle-upon-Tyne 3–5 May, 1996 and London 4–6 May 1996.

106 Programme notes to *Folkworks' Vocal Chords Festival*. Newcastle-upon-Tyne 3–5 May, 1996 and London 4–6 May 1996.

107 Programme notes to *Folkworks' Vocal Chords Festival*. Newcastle-upon-Tyne 3–5 May, 1996 and London 4–6 May 1996.

108 Conference series notes and information leaflets to Giving Voice , four annual conferences held at Cardiff, Centre for Performance Research(1993–96).

109 Law, M. 'The practice of voice: an investigation into the diversity of approaches to vocal work as exemplified by current practitioners.' Unpublished research project prepared for the_International Association for Voice Movement Therapy (1996).

110 Publicity leaflet for Talking in Tune workshops, (1996).

111 Programme notes to *Folkworks' Vocal Chords Festival*. Newcastle-upon-Tyne 3–5 May, 1996 and London 4–6 May 1996.

112 Programme notes to *Folkworks' Vocal Chords Festival*. Newcastle-upon-Tyne 3–5 May, 1996 and London 4–6 May 1996.

113 Conference notes and information leaflet to Giving Voice conference, four annual conferences held at Cardiff, Centre for Performance Research,1993–96).

114 Barnwell, Y. (1996) Lecture given at Songs of Heaven and Earth conference. Findhorn Foundation, Forres, 30 March–6 April.

115 Armstrong, F. (1995) Unpublished information leaflet on current voice teachers.

116 Armstrong, F. (1995) Unpublished information leaflet on current voice teachers.

117 Armstrong, F. (1995) Unpublished information leaflet on current voice teachers.

118 Armstrong, F. (1995) Unpublished information leaflet on current voice teachers.

119 Rakusen, J. cited in Law, M, 'Interviews with contemporary voice practitioners.' Unpublished research papers prepared for the International Association for Voice Movement Therapy, (1996).

120 Armstrong, F. (1995) Unpublished information leaflet on current voice teachers.

121 Wright, P. cited in Law, M, 'Interviews with contemporary voice practitioners.' Unpublished research papers prepared for the International Association for Voice Movement Therapy, (1996).

122 Lever, S. cited in Law, M, 'Interviews with Contemporary Voice Practitioners.' Unpublished research papers prepared for the International Association for Voice Movement Therapy, (1996).

123 Heather, S. cited in Law, M, 'Interviews with contemporary voice practitioners.' Unpublished research papers prepared for the International Association for Voice Movement Therapy, (1996).

124 O'Shea, J. (1993) *Music and Medicine: Medical Profiles of Great Composers*. London: Dent.

CHAPTER 7

The Healing Voice
Voicework in Ancient and Contemporary Healing Practices

Introduction

Song making and singing has, for thousands of years, formed part of healing ceremonies performed by cultures all over the world.

In recent years some of these practices, including the use of vocal expression, have been appropriated and disseminated by contemporary practioners. This has given rise to a proliferate and influential movement which may be called the 'New Age Sound Healing Movement'.

In this chapter I will describe its development, background and origin as well as identifying its major proponents and their work.

Songs of the Shaman

In many indigenous cultures that have been relatively untouched by the ways of Western medicine, the use of vocal sounds to heal the sick is, or was, often the guarded practice of a select member of the community - a medicine woman, a magician, a sorcerer, a witch-doctor or a shaman. There are two seminal texts on shamanic practice, Mircea Eliade's research into Shamanism as a religious phenomenon[1] and the collection of interviews and writings with and about Shamans by Joan Halifax.[2]

Shamanism is still practised in different parts of the world, including Siberia and Central Asia,[3] the Malay peninsula,[4] Alaska[5] and Central America.[6] This is, however, a small vestige of what was once a world-wide phenomenon covering many other regions. One of the significant similarities between the rituals of all cultures with a shamanic content is the role played by the human voice in the process of healing.

In cultures where the medicinal services of Shamans or other chosen individuals have been or still are employed, the process of healing is intimately connected with belief in a spiritual cause for physical illness and the treatment issued by the healer is aimed not at allaying the physical symptom but at ridding the body and soul of the spirits which are thought to be its cause. Central to the act of spiritual exorcism, by which the Shaman flushes causative evil from the sick patient, is the process of catharsis, by which the patient discharges pestilent and violating spirits and emotions and is thereby purified. These bottled up fragments of emotion and spirit often emerge in the form of terrifying vocal noises which the patient emits whilst in a state of semi-consciousness. In cultures where trance and spirit possession play a role in the religious, ritual and healing activities, song and non-verbal utterance are often central to the curative process. Sometimes the utterance is expressed using a vocal emission totally different from the ordinary singing voice representative of a particular culture;[7] such vocal sounds often have no articulate words but are a string of syllables, cries, screeches and improvised sonic forms which sustain the trance experience.

In shamanism this spiritual aspect to disease brings a religious dimension to the healing process, in which the healer is not the objective and detached representative of science but an active participant in the liaison between the earthly life of the patient and the spiritual world. This means that the Shaman must sometimes take the evil spirits from the patient into his own body and later coax them out through a self-exorcism. Kalweit points out that 'in tribal society, the healer experiences the illness that he cures, often initially in his own body' and 'if they are holy, then their wounds heal by themselves' and thus they 'provide proof of their healing ability', an approach 'that has completely fallen into disuse in modern medicine'.[8]

Eliade reminds us that one of the most crucial gifts of the spirit world to the shaman is the song which is believed to be the lost language of the animals that everyone could speak long ago.[9] Such Shamanic songs, which have a 'therapeutic role', are believed to be 'charged with a magical power'[10] and Shamans from a variety of cultures give form to vocal utterance through words and melody.

In their original indigenous context, such shamanic songs may accompany the summoning of a guardian spirit or may express the search for union with a particular animal considered to possess a special quality of power.[11] During healing ceremonies the Shaman usually dances deliriously, singing the healing songs and uttering piercing cries or chanting a maniacal and indecipherable spirit language. Often such rituals are aided by an onlooking audience, who enforce the atmosphere of climactic purgation by chanting, yelling, sobbing and screaming. All of this contributes to a cathartic experience which is often central to Shamanic ritual.

The anthropological explorer and researcher Rasmussen provides a report of a case which occurred amongst the Eskimos and which consisted of a process of cathartic verbal confession very similar to Freud's talking cure. A woman had become physically ill but told the Shaman that she believed her sickness was due to a failure to 'fulfil her duties' and a continual participation in 'bad deeds'. The Shaman asked her to reveal these deeds and after her confession was considered complete, she allegedly recovered.[12] Another case of the curative power of Shamanic confession is reported in an anthropologist's observations made amongst the Guatemalan Indians in 1946. The patient was a 63-year-old woman who had become consumed, first by anxiety, then by depression and, as a result, had withdrawn from all social contact. She also suffered from diarrhoea, stomach pains and loss of appetite. The Shaman began his healing process by confirming local suspicion that she was suffering from 'magical fright', after which he urged the woman to confess. The woman subsequently gave vent to a flood of emotion. The Shaman then drank some curative liquid and then spewed it all over her naked body and face. He then massaged her body with eggs and sent her to bed where she was told to rest underneath blankets. By the next day the woman had allegedly recovered.[13]

Here, as in the previous case, one of the key elements is the opportunity for cathartic confession, which plays a part in many magical healing processes in indigenous cultures. For example, amongst several different American Indian tribal healing ceremonies there is a common therapeutic strategy of talking about guilts and worries to a willing listener.[14]

The culture of the American Indians also has a long history of using voice and song as an integral part of their healing rituals. In many of the northern tribes, for example, part of the cure for illness involves finding the person who knows the correct song appropriate to a particular illness. These medicine songs come to certain 'chosen ones' in special prophetic dreams which warn of the havoc that will be wreaked by the coming of a particular disease. Often, the singing of these songs is accompanied by the ritual chanting of the whole family to the rhythmic beat of a rattle held by the medicine man.[15] Only by remembering and guarding the life-long existence of the song can the dreamer protect the tribe from impending destruction and these songs are, therefore, preserved by being passed down orally through the generations.

But it is not only amongst the American Indians that singing forms, or has once formed, part of the curative rituals for disease. Anthropologists report the medicinal use of music, song and voice in many indigenous peoples, including the tribes of Papua New Guinea, the nomadic peoples of the Sahara and the Sudan as well as the Aborigines of Australia,[16] where, among the Wurajeri peoples, the process by which a novice becomes a doctor includes having a spirit companion 'sung into' him by an elder.[17] This 'singing transmission' enables the power of the elder to duplicate itself in the novice, enhancing the latter's power without depleting that of the former. Among the medicine men of the Yamana of Tierra del Fuego, singing also plays a crucial role and is an 'indispensable activity'[18] in initiation practices where only through vocalisation can an initiate acquire the power of a healer and activate his Shamanic soul.

Workshops and Western Shaman

In recent years the role and function of the Shaman has been emulated, appropriated and sequestered by a number of practitioners within the New Age Sound Healing Movement throughout the UK, Europe and the USA. This has, however, led to confusion and it has been said that 'it is no wonder that thousands of troubled men and women' no longer seem to 'know whether they need psychological or spiritual help.'[19]

Through the provision of workshops, what was originally an indigenous socially-contextualised ritual woven into the cultural fabric of a community becomes a method of self-enlightenmnent for Westerners in search of a soul. For example, many original Shamanic songs have been collected from anthropologists' recordings and freely adapted by David Cloutier, who has disseminated them for use among modern Western people thirsty for a Shamanic experience.[20] Moreover, there are a number of texts which overtly facilitate the reader's attempt to follow in the Shaman's footsteps and discover inner powers of insight, knowledge, self-awareness and healing. Such texts have a number of literary precedents, including the works of Carlos Casteneda, which, in the form of a novel, take the reader through the journey of a pilgrim in search of Shamanic status and awareness[21] and the psycho-philosophical text by Aldous Huxley, which asserts the idea that each of us contains the potential to enter through the 'doors of perception' into an alternative state of consciousness.[22] However, many texts have appeared more recently which actually instruct the reader in exercises which are allegedly drawn from a study of indigenous Shamanic practice. For example, Michael Harner in *The Way of the Shaman* offers readers exercises by which they can allegedly reach a 'Shamanic State of Consciousness'.[23] The aim of Harner's writing and his training workshops is to introduce the reader and participant 'to some of the basic shamanic methods of restoring and maintaining personal power' and to show people how to use these methods 'to help others who are weak, ill or injured'.[24] Included in these methods is the use of a 'Power Song'.[25] To discover a power song, Harner advises that the reader fasts for a day before wandering through the countryside discovering what animal he or she 'feels like' and allowing a 'song, melody, words or both' to arise and then to 'repeat it'.[26]

Another practitioner who runs workshops based on a notion of shamanism is Gabrielle Roth, who aims to 'awaken the Shamanic dimension' in people.'[27] Unlike Harner, and many like him, Roth does not claim association with the actuality of indigenous shamanic practice but draws her experience from life in the city, describing herself as an 'urban Shaman'. In her teachings Roth uses movements which accord with what she names 'sacred rhythms' and which allegedly enable people to discover the 'singer within'.[28] She says that 'if we could full-throatedly wail our grief as mourning Spanish peasant women do, or shout our joy like celebrating Zulus, we'd begin to feel the pulse of emotion once more.'[29] To Roth, the aim of her workshops and the modality which she has developed is the peak experience, what she describes as 'ecstasy', which is central to the experience of the indigenous Shaman.[30]

Roth's teaching work is offered as 'a journey to an ecstatic level of consciousness' because she believes that ecstasy is 'what we need to heal our psychic dismemberment'.[31] Roth describes her work as a 'kind of Zen/Tantra/Shamanism'.[32] By observing and facilitating the dance of archetypal patterns of movement, Roth claims to 'articulate maps which are designed to find how the psyche was wounded, and how it can be healed'.[33] Roth expands the meaning of 'shaman' to include pop stars, such as Patti Smith, or playwrights like Sam Sheppard, both of whom, she says, lead people through a map to ecstasy.[34] But, with regard to how she perceives her own therapeutic responsibility, she says that she calls her work shamanistic 'so people will be prepared for what we do here, because it isn't easy', its what she calls 'a warrior path' and she asserts that 'nobody's going to sit and hold your hand' or 'go through hours of process to get you ready to go for the ecstasy', that's why she says she 'can't' call her workshops 'dance therapy or anything but shamanic'.[35]

The problem with Roth's propositions is that the work of Patti Smith is that of a singer who works in the context of performance, at which the audience are implicitly offered a different quality of invitation to those accepted into a workshop. Whilst the contemporary rock concert models itself upon the healing ecstasy of the performance event, the modern workshop is often perceived as comparable to group psychotherapy. Consequently, many of those coming to a workshop bring with them an expectation that they will receive the quality of attention more comparable to the way a group psychotherapist would treat clients than to the way a rock performer would treat her fans.

Musician, Priest and Psychotherapist

The ambivalent and often confusing relationship between the workshop leader as therapist and workshop leader as performer perhaps stems from the potential healing function of performance in some cultures where therapy and theatre blend in a single ritual event. It is significant that Freud drew his notion of catharsis from the effect which Greek theatre allegedly had on the audience. This aspect of healing is also rooted in non-Western indigenous Shamanic practice where, in many instances, songs form both a medicinal and an artistic role where singing rituals are observed and witnessed by an audience who hear them for their artistic content whilst simultaneously witnessing them perform a healing function.[36] This notion has been approriated by modern performers. For example, Mickey Hart, the drummer with rock and roll band *The Grateful Dead* for over twenty-five years, has explored the Shamanic and spiritual underpinnings of percussion in the context of his own autobiographical discovery of music as a means to inner work on his Self. Drawing inspiration from Eliade, Hart draws attention to the public performability of the Shaman's transformations. He says that 'far from being a private, solitary act, this ecstatic transformation is undertaken in full view of members of the community' the presence of whom 'is as necessary to the successful completion of the Shamanic journey as is the Shaman's ability to enter trance'.[37]

Many of the New Age healers and writers who draw upon vocal work are, in training and practice, musicians and composers, such as Patrick Bernhardt[38] and Steven Halpern,[39] who generate live and recorded works which aim to have healing effects on the listeners. The aim of many of these musicians is, perhaps, more equatable with a priest than it is with a psychotherapist in that they seek to contact the spirit and soul of the listener and to facilitate a kind of pilgrimage which, as Kopp has pointed out, mirrors the psychotherapeutic process to some degree.[40] Such practitioners reach their clients via the dissemination of recordings or through the medium of live performance within what has been called the 'New Age Music Movement'.

This movement can be traced to the music produced during the 1960s by British rock bands such as *Yes, King Crimson, Hawkwind* and *Pink Floyd* and individual composers such as Mike Oldfield whose album *Tubular Bells* is very much an iconographic precedent for contemporary New Age electronic music. The 1960s British groups and artists had their parallels in European work, such as that of the band *Tangerine Dream* and the composer Jean Michel Jarre as well as in the work of Americans such as Philip Glass. Much of this music aimed to take the listeners on a journey comparable with both a drug-induced psychedelic experience and a spiritual awakening. Later, Brian Eno investigated and analysed the electronic and synthesised melodic pattern which arose from 1960s psychedelic music and reduced it to its elemental nature, producing minimalism within a popular form. This later developed into his 'ambient music', which aimed to create atmospheres and moods which would effect the listener subliminally rather than consciously. In fact, the ambient, mystical and atmospheric notions which underpinned this music had been preceded by the explorations of more classical composers, particularly Stockhausen.[41]

The recordings of the genre of current New Age music descendant from the work of 1960s rock bands originally entered into therapeutic modalities by serving to accompany movement and meditation workshops offered by leaders of various kinds. As leaders began to invite musicians to perform original compositions live, replacing the cassette tape recorder, so the composers began to realise their own contribution to the healing process facilitated by the workshop. As a result, there are now leaders such as Nevill Drury,[42] whose workshops focus primarily on facilitating an intensified and concentrated mode of listening to music. Another such leader is Helen Bonny, who originated something she named 'Guided Imagery and Music'. This aims to lead people into an 'altered state of consciousness' from which 'deep spiritual wholeness' may arise,[43] a method which has been further developed by Carol Bush.[44] Such approaches draw on what the eminent British psychiatrist Anthony Storr has called the profound and universal effect of music upon the mind.[45]

The Shaman: Drug User, Psychotic and Psychotherapist

The state of consciousness which anthropologists believe Shamans to experience has been compared to that state which can be induced by hallucinogenic drugs. Indeed, in many Shamanic practices hallucinogens, such as certain mushrooms, mescaline and opium, are used to assist the Shaman in entering into another level of consciousness[46] and in many ancient and indigenous cultures drug-induced trances were, and are, experienced by the entire community partaking in the ritual at hand.[47] From this Shamanic State of Consciousness many communities utter spontaneous songs and melodies which serve to provide an acoustic container for the ritual process. Again, the use of such drugs in cultures which have revered the Shaman are usually very precisely controlled and sanctioned by ceremonies and processess which remind the entire community of the sacred and awesome power of the drug and the importance of giving it the respect due to a god.

This aspect of Shamanism too has been explored in modern times and the relationship between drug-induced states and spontaneous songmaking was ignited and investigated by many Western rock musicians during the 1960s. Rock bands such as *Pink Floyd, Tangerine Dream, Camel* and even the *Beatles* produced albums which, rather than a series of individual songs, presented a conceptual acoustic journey through heightened moods, dream-like themes and ideas, much of which was rooted in the musicians' own exploration of drug-induced states, though without the spiritual sanctions and boundaries to the use of drugs present in indigenous ritual.

Often, the hallucinated visions seen by the Shaman are experienced both as an outward manifestation of his inner soul and, at the same time, a genuine appearance from the outer world of the spirits. Because of this hallucinogenic experience of there being no boundary between inner and outer, the practice of Shamanism and the so-called Shamanic State of Consciousness have often been compared to what an allopathic diagnosis would define as an extreme psychotic state,[48] a schizophrenic condition[49] or other mental disorder requiring psychiatric treatment.[50] In contradistinction, the Shaman has also been described as an 'indigenous therapist'[51] and Shamanic practices, compared to that of psychotherapy by a number of serious academic researchers, including Peters,[52] Murphy[53] and Gatheru.[54] The Shaman, it seems, could be both a psychotic patient, a drug user and a psychotherapist.

In addition to academic research into indigenous Shamanic use of drugs, the practical use of LSD to assist psychotherapeutic work has been consistently advocated by Stanislav Grof, who was at one time married to the scholar of Shamanism, Joan Halifax, with whom he co-wrote a book on the encounter with death.[55] For Grof, LSD induces states which, only in certain superficial respects, are comparable to psychosis but which otherwise, he claims, can provide a means to health and well being.[56] In recent years he has continued to research therapeutic work substituting the client's ingestion of LSD with the guided facilitation of a breathing technique which he calls Holotropic Breathwork. This allegedly puts the client into a state of heightened awareness in which regression to an intrauterine experience is possible.[57] The common thread which connects Grof's early and more recent work to that of contemporary workshop leaders such as Roth and which, in turn, connects this contemporary body of work to the ancient practices of the Shaman is a focus on the ecstatic peak experience as a means to therapeutic development. In contradistinction to the prolonged and protracted work of psychotherapy which methodically analyses life-patterns through a series of weekly consultations or group processes, the peak experience is often a once-only opportunity or is, perhaps, repeated only a half a dozen times, aiming to purge, exorcise or cathartically vent emotions associated with specific trauma. Of course, such a dimension of therapy perfectly suits the format of a workshop as well as the life of a workshop leader and participants who meet only rarely. This is very different to the role of a Shaman, who remains domestically and socially embedded in the fabric of the village community.

In the methodological approach to Therapeutic Voicework which I have developed, I do not draw directly or explicitly on the so-called Shamanic tradition. I have a great respect and interest in anthropological research into all cultures but retain some skepticism and concern for contemporary dissemination of ritual, religious and medicinal processes which have been separated from their context.

A New Age Insult to Indigenous Culture?

There have been courageous and entirely necessary attacks on the New Age repackaging of ancient indigenous wisdom for commercial gain. Particularly enlightening retaliation comes from a member of a team working with the elders of the American Indian Hopi people, who points out that 'the past twenty years have seen the birth of a new growth industry' in the USA known as 'American Indian Spiritualism' which 'began with a number of literary hoaxes undertaken by non-Indians', including Carlos Castenada. According to the author, this era has given birth to a new generation of healers, workshop leaders and persons whom she describes as 'Plastic Medicine Men and Medicine Women' who, she says, 'do not teach traditional Indian spirituality and ceremonies which are in close connection to the land and the community' but, in most cases, 'teach a mixture of a New Age Mother Earth philosophy and elements of European occult traditions' serving only to 'lead their followers – mostly young, idealistic people – away from the political struggle of traditional American Indians'.[58] Some of these defendants have been accused of proclaiming themselves to be 'official spiritual representatives' of various Indian peoples'[59] and, in 1993, the National Congress of American Indians issued a declaration of war against such workshop leaders, whom they described as 'self-styled new age shamans'.[60]

Despite articulate protests from those living communities whose archaic heritage has been appropriated by contemporary practitioners, a Western appropriation of indigenous shamanic practices constitutes a significant segment of the current alternative culture of New Age Sound Healing and all students of Therapeutic Voicework should, in my opionion, be encouraged to know of this field and form their own opinion regarding its efficacy.

Music, Number and Vibration

The shamanic dimension to contemporary practice is complimented by another strand, which also draws influence from other cultures but with less focus on vivid, active ecstatic activities and with more concentration on the European Pythagorean tradition and the contemplative and meditative disciplines of the eastern hemisphere.

To the ancient Greeks, who were inspired particularly by Pythagoras, the fundamental principles of music, such as rhythm, melody and proportion of high and low, soft and loud, all had their equivalent in the human soul or psyche. The right music could, therefore, bring the soul into order and integration whilst the wrong sounds could throw the whole person into confusion, madness and disarray.

During Roman times, Cicero, in the tradition of Pythagoras, proclaimed that every emotion had a corresponding vocal sound and he compared the tones of the voice to the strings of the lyre, both of which he believed could be tuned to represent perfectly changes in human mood and temperament. Later still, during the Renaissance, the notion of a soul-map for the voice was further developed into principles for the composition of vocal music. Renaissance composers took the four elements of earth, water, air and fire, originally depicted by the Greek philosopher Hippocrates, and equated them with different classical vocal ranges: earth was bass, water was tenor, alto was air and soprano was fire. Each of the Hippocratic elements was thought to correspond respectively to four humours in the body: blood, phlegm, yellow bile and black bile, the balance between which was thought to be crucial for the healthy functioning of the body. Vocal music was thus composed in such a way as to create a harmonious and proportionate combination of the four vocal timbres and thus induce an analogous equilibrium in the corresponding humours of the body.

For Pythagoras, the laws of music were also laws of both the universal movement of the planets and the inner motion of the soul. By studying the physics and musicality of the monochord – a single string stretched across a piece of wood – Pythagoras observed some fundamental principles which continue to underpin many musical traditions to this day.

Imagine Pythagoras' string vibrating at 440 times per second or c.p.s. when plucked and giving off a certain note, call it A. When Pythagoras' string is cut in half, it now vibrates twice as fast – at 880 c.p.s. – and the consequent note produced is perceived as having the same identity as A, only higher by what we would measure as an octave. If that string is then halved again, it will vibrate at 1760 c.p.s. – that is exactly twice as fast as 880 – and will again produce the note A an octave higher still. The Pythagorean law teaches us that halving the string on the monochord doubles the speed of its vibration and produces a note of equal identity but an octave higher. The problem for our monochord player, of course, is that he is only ever able to produce the note A and his only opportunity for variation is a jump through the octaves.

In the absence of measuring equipment, and with only a feel for simple proportion, the next most obvious way of dividing a string is not into two but into three. Simple, yet with profound results. If our Pythagorean musician's monochord string vibrates at 440 times per second, then, when cut down to two-thirds of its length, it will vibrate one and half times as fast at 660 c.p.s., producing a note with a very different identity to A. If this string is then cut to two-thirds of its length, it will vibrate again at one and a half times as fast at 990 c.p.s. In musical terms, the relationship or interval between the notes produced by the two-thirds string length is no longer an octave but what is known as a musical fifth. This notion of a fifth, however, has nothing to do with string length, which is, in fact, two thirds.

Our monochord player is now in a problematic situation, the reverse of that created by halving the strings, which only ever produces the same note an octave higher for now the two-third string lengths simply continue to produce ever higher notes, each with completely unique identities and never returning to a higher octave pitch equivalent to the A produced by the original string length vibrating at 440 c.p.s.

If we were to lay a series of monochords on the ground adjacent to one another, each one with half the string length of the one before it, in an attempt to create a crude multi-stringed instrument, we could only play tunes made up of A in different octaves. On the other hand, if we were to lay out our series of monochords, the string of each one two-third of the length of the one before it, then we would have no octaves, only a spiral of ever higher notes – in musical terms, a spiral of fifths. Yet this non-repetitive spiral of notes which never repeats a sound of equal identity to any other is the natural outcome of the simple ratio 3:1 or 'one and a half times as fast'.

There is a further problem with our arrangement of monochords, each one with a string two-thirds of the length of its preceding one. The jump or interval between notes is too great for us to sing with our limited vocal range. In moving from our first note of A, produced by a string vibrating at 440 c.p.s., to our third note, produced by a string vibrating at 990 c.p.s., we have already jumped more than an octave. If we added two more notes we would be beyond the range of the average singing voice, yet with only five notes to compose with. To overcome this problem, we have to use the natural ratios of two-third string lengths vibrating one and a half times as fast as the previous one but somehow make them all slow down in equal proportion to produce a set of notes within a singing range. We know that continually halving the string length just makes the note higher by an octave without changing its identity and that doubling the length of the string makes the note lower by one octave with a similar lack of change. So, in order to bring the series of two-thirds length monochords into a singing range, maintaining the identity of each note, we simply halve the length of the strings originally produced by cutting a string to two-thirds of its length.

The length of string vibrating at 660 c.p.s. is halved to vibrate at 330 c.p.s. and the string vibrating at 990 c.p.s. can be halved so as to vibrate at 495 c.p.s. Combined with the original string vibrating at 440 c.p.s., we then have three notes, each sounding very different but close enough together to be able to sing with plenty of vocal range left. This is how we arrive at our crude stringed instrument which becomes the piano.

However, we have only solved half of the problem: that of range. We still have an instrument that goes on forever producing new notes but never repeating a sound an octave higher because no string will be vibrating exactly twice as fast as any other. Indeed, it has been said by one of the most perceptive musical scientists of the twentieth century that the history of music is also the history of varying attempts to resolve the discrepancy between the natural vibrations and proportions in nature's mathematics and the need for simplicity and repetition in music.[61]

In order to overcome this problem and make an instrument that was capable of repeating a cyclical octave whilst, at the same time, retaining the rich variation produced by the spiral of musical fifths or line of string thirds, tempered tuning was introduced, whereby the string lengths were adjusted a little and the natural vibrational frequencies altered slightly. Consequently, the current Western musical scale, as represented by the keys on the piano, is a bastardisation of a scale formed by nature and a false system of tuning. In this scale the A above middle C vibrates at 440 c.p.s. and its equivalent an octave higher at 880 c.p.s. But the E which in our ancient array of monochords was naturally vibrating at 660 c.p.s. is adjusted to vibrate 659.26 c.p.s., with its equivalent E an octave higher vibrating twice as fast at 1318.5 c.p.s. With this tempered tuning, or adjustment, a certain natural order is lost. In addition, it should be noted that to equate the note A with a vibrational frequency of 440 c.p.s., which was agreed at the Standard Pitch Conference in London in 1939, is itself arbitrary. Mozart's A tuning fork vibrated at 421.6 c.p.s., Handel's at 422.5 and Bach's at 415.5.[62] We could equally denote A as 450 c.p.s. and move all other notes and their frequencies up by ten c.p.s. Indeed, this is the premise of classical Indian music where the musician or singer can begin on any note and the players adjust themselves in relation to it according to precise intervals indigenous to that culture.

The Indians, instead of the twelve tones and semi-tones constituting a Western octave, have 22 notes called 'shrutis' which provide tone intervals of various sizes. As Hamel says, the notes of this scale arose not mathematically but out of their psychic awareness and an ear more subtly attuned.[63] Indian music is passed on orally and there is no set external measure against which to check the correctness of the fundamental, that is the note against which singers and musicians are measuring their atunement. There is, therefore, no fixed pitch in India and the unchanging drone is individually decided with the instrumentalists and singers adapting accordingly. Furthermore, the singers are not under the Western pressure of 'hitting the note' exactly but may slide into the note from a little above or a little below.

The work of the French singer, musician and teacher Gilles Petit is grounded in a study of this Indian music.[64] Petit reminds us that 'the western larynx has had the structure of tones and semi-tones imposed upon it' whilst 'the physical voice' is capable of 'moving between pitched notes in any intervals including seamless slides'.[65] Another practitioner utilising the singing of Indian intervals for healing effect is the native Indian Vemu Mukunda, a nuclear physicist and classical musician in the Indian tradition who runs a one-to-one client practice in London, taking on people with emotional and physical problems, where his focus is 'on clearing blockages of emotionally charged energy, utilising specific notes for different organs'.[66]

The musicalisation of vibrating strings in India has produced a very different scale and genre of music to that of classical western Europe and the different cultural styles of music which we immediately recognise as, for example, Arabic, Egyptian or Persian, are actually responses to different ways of dividing up mathematical frequencies. Moreover, the different methods of so doing, and their resulting scales, are responses to a universal problematic of making ordered repetitive scales of music from the natural infinite and non-repetitive spiral of physical vibration inherent in nature.[67]

Therapeutic Voicework Methodology: Infinite Intervals

In speech the voice is permitted to slip and slide through any intervals, landing on any note. However, in the West the intervals used during singing in alignment with the tempered scale are dictated by specific rules that prohibit certain notes and certain intervals, prohibitions which do not apply to talking. This is one of the reasons why so many people find the process of learning to sing intimidating and bemusing.

Voicework can provide an opportunity to release the voice from the constrictions of the Western tempered scale by musicalising the full range of notes and intervals which the phonation of the vocal folds are able to produce and do produce during speaking.

Taking a single note and sustaining it over a period of time, the client attempts, first of all, to keep the note consistent so that the vocal folds vibrate at one frequency only. Because this is a physical impossibility, the client will notice tiny slides up and down – in response to which the natural tendency is to return to the original constant tone again. However, with the support of the practitioner, the client is asked to continue the fresh note which arises out of the impossibility to sustain the first until this new note slides again. Then this note is subjected to the same process, by which the space between what the West recognises as two adjacent notes, for instance C and C sharp, is broken down into many notes which have no keys on the piano.

Through this process, the musicality of the voice is returned to its biological reality and the client gains a sense of authenticity without imposed structure. As a result of this process, clients can begin to redeem the process of singing and rescue it from the framework of right and wrong, which is often the primary cause of insecurity.

All That Moves is Sound

For Pythagoras, anything which moved or vibrated gave out a sound, including the planetary bodies such as the moon, sun and earth – which all hummed on notes equivalent to their frequency of orbital movement and moved in harmony with every other. This is the harmony of the spheres. For Pythagoras and his school of followers, 'music was number, and the cosmos *was* music'.[68]

Pythagoras distinguished three sorts of music in his philosophy, which were (to use the nomenclature of a later era): *musica instrumentalis*, the ordinary music made by plucking the lyre, blowing the pipe and so forth; *musica humana*, the continuous but unheard music made by each human organism, especially the harmonious or inharmonious resonance between the soul and the body; and *musica mundana*, the music made by the cosmos itself, which would come to be known as the music of the spheres. There was no more of a difference among his three classes of music than there was among a triangle traced in the palm of the hand, a triangle formed by the walls of a building and a triangle described by three stars. For Pythagoreans, 'triangleness' is an eternal idea and all expressions of it are essentially the same.[69] The classic account of Pythagoras's vision of the harmony of the spheres comes to us from Aristotle's treatise, *On the Heavens*, where he tells us that the Pythagoreans believed that the planets, like any moving or vibrating object, produce sound and that the sound given forth by the circular movement of the planets is a harmony.

The mathematical nature of Pythagoras' cosmic philosophy and its relationship to sound has, in recent years, been ingeniously explored by the maverick Swiss scientist Hans Cousto.[70] Using the fundamental law of octave equivalence, Cousto brings the dimensions of light, sound and planetary movement into convergence. Cousto equates planetary orbiting times with vibrating frequencies. For example, take the earthly rotational frequency of 23 hours, 56 minutes and 4 seconds, which has been conveniently made into our 24-hour day in the same way that our piano is an adjustment of nature's eternally specific numbers. This period is equivalent to 86, 164 seconds. Because frequency equals one divided by time, 1/86164 gives us the frequency of the earth's orbit as 0.000116 c.p.s. The frequency of the earth may, therefore, be set at 0.000116 c.p.s. whilst the frequency of an object giving off the note middle A is 440 c.p.s. Obviously, whilst the note produced by something vibrating at 440 c.p.s. is within the range of hearing, the note produced by 0.00016 c.p.s, if there is one, is certainly not audible. To bring this within the range of hearing we would have to double it 21 times, or transpose it upwards by 21 octaves, giving 24.33 c.p.s., which is close to the G just below the bottom of the piano keyboard, but which is still too low to sing. However, if we double this frequency again we get 48.67 c.p.s., which is very close to the lowest G on the piano; if we double it again we get 97.35 c.p.s., which is the G an octave higher and if we double it once more we arrive at 194.71 c.p.s., which is close to the G just below middle C and which is within most people's singing range. The earth therefore sings G and when we sing G we are, allegedly, in tune with our planet. By working out the frequencies of other planets through the same method, it is accordingly possible to tune into Mars, Pluto, Venus and the rest.

Cousto and his mathematical musings, which connect the orbiting times of planets with the frequencies of sound vibrations, belongs to a tradition which stretches from Ancient Greece through the Middle Ages, the Renaissance, Baroque, Enlightenment and Romanticism for Pythagoras has inspired, and permeates the philosophy of, numerous speculators from each of these periods, including Ptolemy, Aristeides Quintilianus, Marsilio Ficino, Johannes Keppler, Robert Fudd, Isaac Newton and Arthur Schopenhauer.[71] Moreover, the relationship between music, mysticism and magic is not unique to the European tradition inspired by Pythagoras but has been proclaimed by many masters from other world traditions, including those of ancient Judaism and Islam as well those of the twentieth century such as Isaac Ben Solomon Ibn Sahula, Majd Al-Din Al-Ghazali, Rudolf Steiner,[72] Marius Schneider, Rudolf Haase and Hans Erhard Lauer.[73] The work of many of these people has been collected and annotated by the scholar Jocelyn Godwin, who has also elucidated the universal principles of the spiritual dimension of music in his seminal text *Harmonies of Heaven and Earth*.[74]

Cousto's renaissance of Pythagoras' cosmic music of the spheres provides a bedrock upon which the contemporary interest in holistic thinking, disseminated and perpetuated by texts and teachers within the current New Age workshop movement, are erected. Within this field of thought there is a belief in a fundamental level of connection between microcosm and macrocosm, between the nature of the planets and the nature of being human. By using the voice to reflect the Pythagorean frequencies of the planetary cosmos, we can, it is proposed, encourage harmony in a world victimised by so much discord.

The Colour of Sound

The human being perceives only a certain range of vibrations as heard sounds which is approximately between 20 and 20,000 c.p.s. and we are thus able to hear a range of sound spanning in excess of ten octaves. The eye, meanwhile, perceives as light frequencies between around 375 trillion c.p.s. and 750 trillion c.p.s. (375,000,000,000,000 −750,000,000,000,000), covering a range of only one octave. The frequency of light occupies the 49th octave of vibration and when we see light we are perceiving the entire spectrum of the octave, comparable to hearing all possible frequencies of sound within the ear's range of receptivity at once. But when light passes through a prism it is split into frequency bands producing colour similar to the frequency bands which produce different notes in sound.

Using Cousto's methodology, various practitioners of the current New Age Sound Healing Movement have taken the frequency of a particular colour, continually halving it until it reaches the range of heard sound, and equating the colour with the consequent note. For example, the colour with the lowest frequency in the light spectrum is a very dark red with a frequency of 430×10^{12} c.p.s. If we halve this forty times, or transpose it downwards by forty octaves, we arrive at 391.3 c.p.s. Using the standard tempered tuning, the closest note to 391.3 is close to the G with a frequency of 392 c.p.s. Thus, dark red is analogous with G both of which correspond to the frequency of the earth. Within the tempered tuning system, few of the colour/tone relationships are this precise and many of the practitioners seeking to use such a correlation advocate abandoning the tempered system and working with the infinite spiral of tones and intervals which are naturally occurring.[75]

The combination of colour and sound using paint, cloth, objects and light combined with music, sound and vocalisation for healing effects has been named 'chromatherapy'. Again, like many contemporary alternative healing modalities, it has its history in ancient practices of China, Egypt, Greece, Tibet and India and some practitioners have combined eclectically the mystical beliefs of various cultures in an idiosyncratic way to provide what one practitioner has called a 'system for Self-Awareness and Soul Evolution'.[76]

The Shape of Sound

One project which has, in some ways, seemed to verify a connection between the behaviour of sound vibration and the movement of matter and which has provided motivation and verification for the New Age Sound Healing Movement is the body of work developed by Hans Jenny in the field of Cymatics. In the eighteenth century a German Physicist, Ernst Chladni, mounted a thin metal plate on a violin and placed a small amount of fine sand on it. When he drew the bow across the strings of the violin, sustaining the note for a prolonged period, he discovered that the sand formed geometric patterns; and changing the note caused the patterns to alter formation, therefore making audible structures visible.[77] Chladni's experiments were further pursued many years later in the twentieth century by the Swiss scientist, Hans Jenny.

Jenny subjected a variety of different substances, such as water, iron filings, mercury and other liquids, to sound vibration, including those produced by the human voice intoning on single vowels. His discovery was that randomly scattered particles of various substances are called to tune to form geometric patterns in response to sound. Mandalas, spirals, circles and elaborate webs and mazes form and change in response to fluctuating frequency of sound vibration.[78] Jenny's work culminated in his plea for further investigation into the effect of sound on genes, cells and other structures of the body.[79]

The effect of sound vibration on matter is in keeping with the discoveries of physics which have shown that at the subatomic level there is no reliable distinction between matter and energy. Consequently, Jenny's discoveries have been utilised as inspiration within the New Age Sound Healing Movement. Because Jenny caused particles to form structure in response to sung tones, so it has been speculated that singing directly at a person can cause a chemical restructuring at the physical level and an energetic restructuring at a more subtle or 'etheric' level. Such a use of 'intoning' is prevalent amongst contemporary voice workshop leaders and is claimed to offer a healing effect.

Taking this field of enquiry to extremes, the equatability between all vibrational frequencies and their synonymous musical tones when multiplied or divided has been used by Sharry Edwards to suggest synchronicity between certain notes and brain wave frequencies.

In 1929 the German neurologist Hans Berger discovered that the field of neuro-electrical waves generated by the brain clustered and peaked within a number of spectral parameters. Using the same principle of transposing downwards through the octaves, Edwards finds the equivalent brain wave frequency for a particular note. From this starting point, she has created a body of work known as Bio-acoustics or 'life sounds'. Her premise is that all human beings radiate a unique tone measurable as a precise frequency of vibration which is a combination of 'genetic coding, geographical locale, brain and neural functions, biochemistry, emotions, physical structure and environmental influences'.[80] This sound is named their 'signature sound'. Edwards has claimed that illness, negative social influences, diet and a host of other factors can cause disturbance in the signature sound. By bathing the client in a reproduction of their signature sound, either by electronic musical instrumentation or through a practitioner's own voice, a wide spectrum of diseases and dysfunctions can allegedly be healed. However, many of the claims made by Edwards regarding the therapeutic efficacy of her methods are considerably more advanced than the available substantiating evidence.

Through Sound to the Self

Both the European mystical tradition underpinned by Pythagorean speculation, particularly as interpreted by Cousto, and the broad multi-cultural canvas of musical mysticism and spirituality are present in the current New Age Sound Healing Movement, which is predicated on the proposal that vocalisation can serve 'as bearer and vehicle of a spiritual message' from an inner and outer place which is 'totally other', thus guiding a person through the perilous passage from one phase of life to another. This function of sound is, according to Peter Michael Hamel, immanent in all musical form if we are open to hear it. Therefore, music can assist 'the way to individual self-discovery' helping us pass 'through suffering' and 'the dark night of the soul' and into a realised spirituality that facilitates the dawning of true selfhood.[81]

The human voice is used to such a spiritual end in traditions where singing or chanting sits at the centre of a religious or esoteric discipline, such as that practised within Tibetan Buddhism and that originating in Mongolia. In both of these traditions, the singer is able to sound two notes at once by humming or singing a single pitch whilst altering the shape and size of the oral cavity, thus varying the harmonic spectrum of a single note. Among these harmonics is often a very high overtone which is as piercing and shrill as the fundamental is basal and dark. Such focused vocalisation is also widely pursued in Indian Hindu contexts where the chanting articulates a mantra, that is a Sanskrit prayer, and the repetition of the mantra, often on a single tone, awakens the spirit and its ability to facilitate contemplation.

Body Map, Body Score

The Sanskrit chanting is connected to a perception of the human body quite different from the Western allopathic body map where the body is perceived as containing centres or wheels of energy spaced vertically parallel to the spinal column. These wheels, known in Sanskrit as 'chakras', each have a specific quality of energetic fabric and each effect the functioning of specific bodily parts and organs. These chakras underpin the system of breath and movement work known as yoga.

The chakras are connected to each other by fine threads or routes of energetic matter called 'nadis' and each main chakra is associated with a major nerve plexus and an endocrine gland. Consequently, according to this discipline, blockage or impedance in the flow of energy through the nadis or problems with the receptivity and energetic permeability of the chakras can result in general spiritual and emotional disturbance as well as physiological pathology in a specific endocrine gland, nerve plexus or organ directly associated with it.

In Hindu and yogic literature the unique source which activates the energy of the chakras and assists in the awakening of higher consciousness is called the 'Kundalini', which, in Sanskrit, means 'coiled serpent'. This snake lies at the bottom of the chakra system in the region of the first chakra, in many people sleeping and dormant. However, when the snake is awakened, the energy rises up through the chakras, passing through each one in turn facilitating enlightenment and higher consciousness.

The most widely practised means to achieve this awaking and rising of energy is that of meditation, which, when practised regularly over a long period of time causes the chakras to open and clear from the root upwards to the crown. One of the means to achieve this meditation is through vocalisation and, in the Hindu chanting, certain sounds stimulate and purify the chakras, serving not only to awaken the soul to the spirit but to awaken the body to its aspiration to health. In the most probing study of non-allopathic medicinal systems, Gerber states that repetition of mantras 'helps to clear the mind of conscious thoughts' and 'are actually special higher vibrational sonic energy signals which have unique effects in lifting consciousness to higher spiritual levels of being' as well as perhaps having the capacity 'when repeated over time' to 'cause subtle changes within the nervous system'.[82]

Many renowned North American Sound Healing practitioners draw on the chakras and relate them to chanting in such a way as to suggest that specific vowel sounds awaken the energy of particular chakras. Whilst this idea is widespread within the movement, there is little, if any, agreement between practitioners with regard to which vowels relate to which chakras. For example, Randall McClellan, Jonathan Goldman, Peter Hamel and Kay Gardner, some of the more renowned figures who begin from the premise that 'just as music affects us physically, emotionally and mentally, so it also influences us on a spiritual level'[83] all use vowel chanting and a body map composed of the chakras, but each draws on a different vowel-chakra relationship. For example, Gardner relates the vowel 'OH'[84] to the second chakra located about two inches above the naval, whilst for McClellan[85] it is stimulated by 'OOO' and for Hamel[86] it is 'UH'. Furthermore, the acoustic description of the vowels which such practitioners provide is very non-specific and bares little relationship to the phonetic transcription of speech sounds from the linguistic cultures in which the chanting modalities originate.

Despite differences in eclectic combinations of techniques and tools, another aspect shared by nearly all New Age Sound Healing practitioners is the concept of energy, a vital life force which can be activated through song, voice and chant and which is an importation from non-Western cultures where it is common to find a system of medicine based on a fundamental energy source. In Sanskrit this is known as prana, in Chinese it is chi, in Japanese it is ki and in Tibetan it is thig-le or rlung. Another body map which relies upon a flow of energy through certain key points is the ancient Chinese system which perceives a flow of an energy known as chi through pathways known as meridians which have nexus points around the body and which are utilised in acupuncture and acupressure. The chi energy, which is perceived as physically and spiritually nutrient, enters the body at the acupuncture points and seeps deeper into the organs of the body. There are twelve pairs of meridians linked to specific organ systems. When the flow of the chi becomes blocked at or near a particular acupuncture point, the relevant organ system to that point becomes dysfunctional or diseased. This body map, like that which is predicated upon the chakras, is also used in New Age Sound Healing modalities.

The repetition of words, syllables or spontaneous free vowels on a tone or tones in a meditative and repetitive fashion is not unique to the Sanskrit language or the Indian, Chinese, Tibetan and Mongolian traditions but is found in many other religious cultures, including those of Turkey, Israel and Central Africa. Many sacred traditions from various countries include belief in the sacred potential of certain sounds and words to invoke deities or provoke spiritual states. These too have been repackaged for the modern workshop attendee or avid book reader and made available to the novice who wants to experience the power of such invocation through repetitious utterance of the words. For example, Brian and Esther Crowley have collected what they call 'words of power' from Egyptian, Hebrew, Sanskrit, Tibetan, Arabic, Greek, Latin and other languages with advice on correct pronunciation and instruction as to useful meditative techniques. The authors say that their 'own personal conviction is that participation in sacred sound, by its very action, results in stimulation of individual intuitive insight'.[87]

Among the chants most recognisable to contemporary ears is that which accompanies a Buddhist meditation and which consists of repetitious utterance of the sound 'OM'. Moreover, whilst the Sanskrit use of chakras has permeated the New Age workshop movement, Buddhism has, in the UK, found its place closer to the mainstream of psychotherapy, with one institution offering a full psychotherapy training based on the principles of Buddhism which is accredited by the United Kingdom Council for Psychotherapy. This is part of a more general movement towards exploring the interface between Eastern spirituality, particularly Buddhism, and Western psychotherapy – which has been investigated through a number of essays by Welwood.[88] In another exploratory work, Brazier asserts that Buddha himself described Buddhism as anything which led to the true cessation of suffering. Consequently, he wonders whether Buddhism is 'perhaps primarily, a therapy'.[89]

Jenni Roditi, the first practitioner to graduate from the professional training in Voice Movement Therapy and to found a one-to-one practice upon the methods which I have developed, has been studying Tibetan Buddhism for many years under her mentor, an exiled Tibetan Lama. Roditi's approach to Therapeutic Voicework is quite deeply influenced by the principles of Tibetan Buddhism yet, in addition, she supports her work with a classical psychoanalytic process of supervision. Roditi's journey, therefore, involves seeking a careful balance between the psychotherapeutic model of therapist and client and the spiritual model of guide and pilgrim. In addition, Roditi is an accomplished composer in the contemporary classical tradition and her approach to Therapeutic Voicework also incorporates facilitating the client's ability to locate vocalisation in a structured melodic framework. Roditi's model of work is thus complex and multifaceted yet reflects the position of many practitioners who are serious about developing an integrated approach to facilitative work.

Voice and Spirit

In the Persian and Arabic region from Turkey to Afghanistan it was within the secret schools of Sufism, which formed the mystical roots of Islam, where music and singing was used as a path to enlightenment. Indeed, singing is central to the Islamic prayer in which the muezzin intones the holy Koran from the minaret, with both hands on his temples as he implores the great Allah. Sufi mysticism has also influenced contemporary practice in the field of voice and music workshops, primarily through the Sufi musician and master Hazrat Inayat Khan's book *The Music of Life*, which draws attention to the subtle vibrations which, though outside of the threshold of sight and hearing, may, allegedly, still effect the human spirit. Sufi principles have also provided the foundation for a formal psychotherapy training institution in Britain. For Khan, to be enlightened means, among other things, to be receptive to such vibrations through a special sensitivity of the spirit or soul. The voice holds a special place in Khan's vision, being for him 'not only indicative of man's character' but also the 'expression of his spirit'.[90]

A further key author in the field of spiritual vocalisation is Joachim-Ernst Berendt whose texts, *The Third Ear*[91] and *Nada Brama – The World is Sound*,[92] have provided intellectual underpinnings for contemporary experimentation with chant, song and breathing as a means to enlightenment and personal growth. For Berendt, like his contemporaries, the world is literally sound and the path to consciousness involves discovering the receptivity to the sound of the world, which may be beyond the threshold of hearing but which is capable of being received through the subtle channels of our 'third ear'. Another spiritual teacher who has placed great store on the use of voice and song is Edgar Cayce, for whom the voice is the 'highest vibration in the whole nerve system' and who also advocates breathing and singing as a means to enlightenment.[93]

Toning and Healing

A common tool within voice and music healing workshops is 'toning', a term coined by a minister in Colorado, Laurel Elizabeth Keyes. Experimenting with the members of her congregation, Keyes felt she had discovered the power of the human voice to effect spiritual healing. One day, whilst standing alone in a room, Keyes 'noticed a sensation' in her 'chest and throat as though a force were rising, wanting to be released in sound'. She found her lips parting and her 'mouth opened very slightly in an easy relaxed manner', then, unexpectedly, 'a sound bubbled up, like something tossed upon a fountain spray', which became the sung syllable 'Ra'. As she sang continuously, she did not 'take a deep breath, as a singer, but the note was sustained as though supplied by a limitless source and it went into heights' that she 'couldn't have reached normally' since her voice was naturally rather low.[94]

Wittingly or not, Keyes initiated what is now the widespread use of toning in voice workshops led by an array of teachers who claim the healing effects of vocalisation. A key figure in this movement is Kay Gardner, who runs workshops and gives performances of her New Age Healing music. Applying an eclectic combination of chant, toning, rhythm, melody and meditation, Gardner seeks to facilitate healing.[95]

One of the most renowned and long-established practitioners of an approach to vocalisation which is predicated on the alleged healing benefit of toning is Don Campbell, who runs workshops using voice and music throughout the USA and who has become known through the books which he has edited, drawing together articles by theorists and practitioners in the field of healing music.[96] One of Campbell's premises is that 'we in the west have lost the art of contemplation and meditation because of the rapid rate at which we assimilate facts and information.'[97] Campbell draws eclectically from the world-wide mystery schools of music which 'used patterns of tone, movement, and breath to open the inner gates where awakened energy could flow between the subconscious and conscious worlds'.[98] Campbell's workshops attempt to rediscover the mystery through music and vocalisation which he believes can 'directly and efficiently affect the limbic system', creating a positive 'response within the hypothalamus, which, in turn, affects the immune system'. Thus, by 'prolonging tone in the body for two or three minutes, there is a tremendous change in both psychological and physiological response', and 'perhaps even in the T-cells and endomorphins within the blood.'[99]

Campbell was a founder of the now defunct Institute for Music, Health and Education in Colorado where a number of experiments have been pursued to investigate the healing effect of sound and where he initially collaborated with Jonathan Goldman, author of the popular text *Healing Sounds*[100] and who claims to have 'witnessed amazing healings with sound therapies, particularly using vocal harmonics'.[101]

In the USA there are many other practitioners who utilise voice as an aid to healing within an eclectic multi-cultural framework who have written books to accompany their workshops. Among them are Ted Andrews, whose premise is that 'the voice has a tremendous ability to be an instrument for healing'[102] and who, like many of his contemporaries, offers techniques for healing which includes a repackaging and renaming of ancient spiritual practices. For example, drawing on the chanting of mantras in yoga, he disseminates what he calls 'Directed Esoteric Toning',[103] which involves chanting 'the appropriate vowel', which can restore balance and health to those parts of the body which may be pained or in need of revitalisation.[104]

In similar vein, but with more grandiose claims, the work of Laeh Maggie Garfield is also predicated on a belief in the healing powers of voice. She cites one case where 'a long-time quadriplegic had the use of one arm and her hand partially restored by toning and crystal healing.'[105]

Such use of crystals, particularly quartz, is wide-spread in the New Age Healing Movement, which draws its inspiration both from the technological discoveries regarding the conductive properties of quartz and mythological accounts of their healing powers. Another exemplifying practitioner who uses toning combined with crystals is Joy Gardner-Gordon, who instructs a reader on how to become a healing practitioner by following her guidance recorded in her short book. She tells the novice to hold a single-terminated smoky quartz over the painful part of a patient's body and vocalise a tone that feels appropriate to break up the pain or make the corresponding sound for the chakra that is closest to the painful area.[106] However, the book through which Gardner-Gordon offers a basic training in healing, which utilises various combinations of colour, sound, chant, crystals and body work, is preceded by a foreword from the publisher which states that 'the exercises described' are provided for information 'and not as a a prescription' because 'they have not been tested on a broad sample of individuals, nor scientifically established'. Therefore, 'neither the author nor the publisher can take responsibility for any positive or negative results which may be produced by using these exercises'.[107]

Despite such warnings, many of the publications within the New Age Healing Movement act as a substitute for therapeutic procedure. A typical example of this is exemplified in the Sound Therapy Manual by Dewhurst-Maddock, which gives advice on de-armouring, a term taken from the tradition of body work initiated by Wilhelm Reich. She suggests that the reader begins by vocalising during daily life 'while walking, bending, stretching and turning.' By noticing 'how your voice responds when a certain part of your body is involved in the motions', she says you can locate areas of 'armouring', that is 'parts of your body that seem to be stiff, tense and tough', which is often 'the residue of painful (usually forgotten) experiences, frozen into muscular resistance'. She instructs the reader to 'give voice to these frozen feelings' in order to dissolve them and 'free yourself'.[108] There are also a number of books, such as those by Lingerman[109] and Watson and Drury, [110] which have been published and which select certain recordings from a classical and contemporary repertoire and which come with suggestions as to which particular ailments or conditions they might be suited to relieve, leaving the reader to choose the music and effect their own healing.

Many practitioners in this field not only combine body-maps, frameworks of perception, exercises and disciplines from various international sources but also construct their own particular voice profile and analysis. Andrews, for example, listens for voice qualities which he equates with the elements. He associates water with a voice which is soothing, healing and intoxicating, air with a voice which is uplifting, calming and detached and fire with a voice which is arousing, exciting and frightening.[111] This use of the primal elements is made by many contemporary voice practitioners as a diagnostic tool for working with the voice and has been elaborated by John Beaulieu, who asserts, for example, that 'water has the timbre of being connected and flowing' and a watery voice 'lacks substance' and 'will absorb anything.' Beaulieu says that yelling, which requires fire with air, is therefore difficult for a water voice because it 'causes the voice to become steamy'. If fire is continually applied to water, it will, he says, 'eventually boil or erupt'.[112] In his case studies, Beaulieu typifies the approach of practitioners who use an elemental framework. By applying a subjective interpretation of acoustic properties based in an astrological framework, he teaches his clients to vocalise missing qualities and, therefore, bring their soul into balance.[113] Such approaches are, in many ways, like a reappropriation of renaissance equations between Hippocratic elements and vocal sounds.

In Australia the most renowned exponent of Voicework as a healing modality is the 'ex-monk, rock singer, martial arts expert, breath therapist and body worker and musician' Chris James, who runs workshops at home and in the UK which he succinctly describes as 'oral acupuncture'.[114] James, like many contemporary workshop leaders, draws his inspiration from non-Western religious practices which involve toning and chanting' and says his work is motivated by 'the desire to know God'.[115] The name he uses to describe the vocal expression which he facilitates in his workshop participants is 'sacred sound',[116] which he traces back to 'the ancient mystery schools in Greece, Rome, Ancient Egypt and Tibet' and the aboriginal culture of his home, Australia.[117] Inspired by the work of a Steiner music therapist, James began teaching singing to individuals and small groups, which led him to work as a choirmaster. He found that when singing a single note to students, they would often 'start catharting, having visions or crying' and when he touched people they would have 'electric shocks'. From this, James deduced that he 'had very strong healing powers'.[118] James, like Campbell, asserts that particular tones can reach specific organs of the body and claims a somatic as well as a psychological therapeutic effect for his work.[119]

In the UK, meanwhile, probably the longest standing practitioner in the field of healing through voice is Jill Purce, who claims to have taught many of those who now lead workshops and teach overtone singing themselves.[120] Purce originally trained as a classical singer and was subsequently a close collaborator with Stockhausen. Describing herself as part of a shamanic tradition, Purce's work is informed by an interest in the mystical history and nature of music and, like many in the field, she does not describe herself as a therapist but as a 'facilitator of healing'.[121] She says that her 'aim is not modest', that 'nothing short of the transformation of humanity is what is necessary' and that 'since the voice is an instrument of transformation that we carry about with us all the time, it is one of the most powerful and also readily available means for this'. Her intention is to 'open people's ears , so that they can hear their own voice'. This then, according to Purce, 'can become a means of transformation'.[122]

Among those who acquired this use of voice from Purce is James D'angelo, an American workshop leader, musician, composer and educator, who moved to Europe in 1990, where he now conducts workshops which he describes not as therapeutic but as healing. He is also lecturer in music at Goldsmiths College, London. In his workshops D'angelo combines a number of practices, including overtone chanting, body movements, which originate from Sufi spiritual disciplines, and the use of crystals. His approach to workshop facilitation also involves teaching a repertoire of chants which he has collected from from Indian, Islamic and Christian traditions. He also uses the now widespread process of 'toning the chakras' and believes that 'sound is one of the most powerful forces that can heal not only the physical body, but can change perceptions and link individuals to spiritual evolution'.[123]

Also in the UK, Chloe Goodchild has developed a body of teaching work known as 'The Naked Voice',[124] which facilitates the combination of free vocalisation, sung chants from Eastern traditions, the use of physical movement and a focus on the body which is rooted in the Chinese body map of chakras and channels of energy. She describes her workshops as 'a force for healing through sound, performance and recording art form, a doorway for meditation and a metaphor for living.'[125]

Further UK practitioners of 'vocal healing' include Tim Ward-Jones, a craniosacral therapist based in Somerset who has studied vocal music in South India with Sivasankara Pannikar, who has worked extensively in Europe with Gilles Petit and teaches overtone chanting and singing as a spiritual and creative expression in workshops which 'provide a safe space and time'[126] to 'explore a sense of self through voice and sound';[127] Amanda Relph, an actor and singer based in Bradford-on-Avon who, for the past ten years, has been running workshops combining her early training in voice production with the use of toning, overtone chanting and colour therapy both independently and under the aegis of The College of Psychic Studies in London;[128] and Rollin Rachel, originally from Amsterdam, who is a performer and teaches the classic vocal music which originates in Northern India combined with the overtone singing, or throat singing, which has its roots in the Mongolian Altai mountains. His stated objective in the workshop is 'to slow everything down and observe closely where the sound originates in the body', thereby gaining 'new insights' into the 'power and beauty of sound.'[129]

There are also many singers who have turned away from professional, élite singing to find greater reward in leading workshops and offering therapeutic services in institutions caring for disabled and mentally ill patients. A story which exemplifies such a journey is that of Deforia Lane, once an opera singer, who turned to using her singing voice to rejuvenate the spirits of people suffering from cancer.[130]

The first generation of initiators in the field of spiritually-orientated vocal healing are now being followed by a second generation of workshop leaders, singers and performers who have been influenced by them, such as Susan Hale, who gives a digestible overview of song as a means to healing oneself in her 'Song and Silence'.[131] Another musician who, in more light-hearted fashion, facilitates personal growth is Mathieu, who draws on the presence of the music inherent in everyday life – toothbrushes on teeth, fence posts, empty jars and garbage cans – and advises on utilising them as the foundation for one's own composed music.[132] Thus the contemporary New Age Sound Healing Movement contains a vast cacophony of activities ranging from the grandiose, through unwavering optimism regarding the healing power of sound, through commited attempts to comprehend the relationship between the behaviour of matter and the nature of spirit, to the work of those creating music to lift the spirits with the objects of mundane and everyday life.

Sung in the Name of Jesus

In 1994 the Benedictine monks of Santo Domingo de Silos in Spain released a recording of a Gregorian chant called 'Canto Gregoriano' which sold a quarter of a million copies in Spain and over two million copies in total world-wide. In many ways the stage was set for this, given the receptivity to the healing power of chant,[133] and Katherine Le Mee has revisited the phenomenon of Gregorian chant, its development and healing uses in her book 'Chant' which was inspired by the 1994 recording.[134]

Indeed, the Old Testament contains many references to the power of music and singing. Genesis connects the farewell of loved ones with 'joy and singing to the music of tambourines and harps':[135] Moses and his sister, the prophetess Miriam, worshipped and praised God in triumphant song during the miracle of the parting of the Red Sea as God brought the Israelites into the promised land.[136] To celebrate the victory of David over Goliath, women and children joined in a procession of singing and dancing accompanied by tambourines and lutes.[137] In the New Testament, the tradition is continued: Jesus sang the Hallel with his disciples at the close of the first communion service just before his death,[138] the apostle Paul urged his converts in their new faith to admonish each other with 'psalms and hymns and spiritual songs, singing with grace' to the Lord[139] and ecstatic songs in unknown languages were sung 'in the spirit'.[140] In the Apocalypse an oratorio of redemption is sung by the throng of believers, or bride of Christ, to the accompaniment of angels.[141] Finally, the power of the human voice is nowhere more perfectly illustrated than in the story of Joshua, who, after marching around the city a total of thirteen times, commanded the people to shout and, with that, the walls of Jericho 'fell down flat'.[142] This story exemplifies a widespread idea behind a lot of primitive and oriental music: that sound governs matter.[143]

The human voice comes to the fore most poignantly in Christian activity through the phenomenon of Glossolalia, or speaking in tongues. Several days after the death of Christ and his ascension to heaven, the disciples were gathered to wait for the fulfilment of Christ's promise to return. Suddenly 'there came from heaven a sound as of the rushing of a mighty wind' and 'there appeared unto them tongues parting asunder, like as of fire and it sat on each one of them, and they were all filled with the Holy Ghost'. So it was that all the disciples of Christ 'began to speak in other tongues as the Spirit gave them utterance'.[144]

The notion of Christian vocalisation has been investigated in modern times by Iégor Reznikoff, professor of the Art and Music of Antiquity at the University of Paris and a specialist in early Christian song. He says that 'the sounds of natural resonance are found in music that has preserved the spirit and tradition of Antiquity, now still living in oral traditions' such as those of Eastern church music and the music of India, Iran and Turkey.[145] Reznikoff considers that the restructuring of musical intervals to produce the equally-tempered scale in the 19th century has resulted in the loss of human ability to hear natural intervals. By returning a sense of such intervals through teaching workshop participants to sing ancient chants, Reznikoff believes that a healing effect can be achieved.[146] He is keen to emphasis that what he does is not 'music therapy 'in the way it is practised as an adjunct by psychotherapists and psychoanalysts'. However, he has worked with those who have severe physical handicaps, in whom he has facilitated articulate vocalisation. His journey into the discovery of early forms of Christian song has revealed to him, his students and, subsequently, patients and staff at hospitals in Paris that pure, gentle sounds can penetrate coma and bring about physiological changes in a patient's medical condition.[147]

A Practitioner's Struggle

It seems to me that a study of and respect for other cultures and their mores are essential in understanding the breadth and depth of the human condition. Yet, in the development of my own work, I have remained sceptical towards an esoteric approach to Voicework. First, I have had consistent suspicions that Western therapeutic practitioners such as myself run the danger of becoming commercial tourists, taking a small part from a cultural whole and selling it on without regard for the complexities of an originating context. Second, Voicework is an extremely powerful mode of expression and I have never felt comfortable combining the components of varying spiritual practices because such a powerful act, in my opinion, requires grounding not elevating.

In my own life I am struggling to be a Christian, and this naturally affects me at a deep level. However, it is not something which I incorporate directly into my teaching. I teach many people from diverse spiritual backgrounds and respect their individual commitment to the depth of their beliefs. For me, I believe that Christ is the way but, unlike the good pilgrim, I do not believe that he is the only way. I am also fully aware of the shadow of Christianity, its inexcusable political history and the residue of its intolerance. Such contentions remain my personal struggle.

I have, however, developed a physical and vocal exercise which seems to respond to a fundamental dimension in people regardless of their religious and spiritual persuasion which was inspired by own journey.

Therapeutic Voicework Methodology: The Spiritual Developmental Postural Cycle

The notion of prayer is, in part, predicated on two primary elements – to ask and to give thanks – and these two conditions permeate the nature of everyone's psychic disposition.

This prayerful construct is frequently evident in therapy, in relationships between friends and between lovers and is woven into the fabric of our being and our need to heard and answered. One person asks another for something and, where such requests are answered, gives thanks and expresses gratitude. Of course, our requests are often not granted and in such cases we all experience frustration, rage and despair, as Job experienced these feelings towards God upon the mountain.

The prayer is also a vocal form, like the lullaby and the ballad, and in Therapeutic Voicework this artistic structure can provide a context for the expression of asking, the utterance of thanks at receiving and the release of negative feelings in response to sensing that one's needs or prayers have not been answered.

The use of the prayer in my approach to Therapeutic Voicework is grounded in the matrix of positions and movements which I have called the

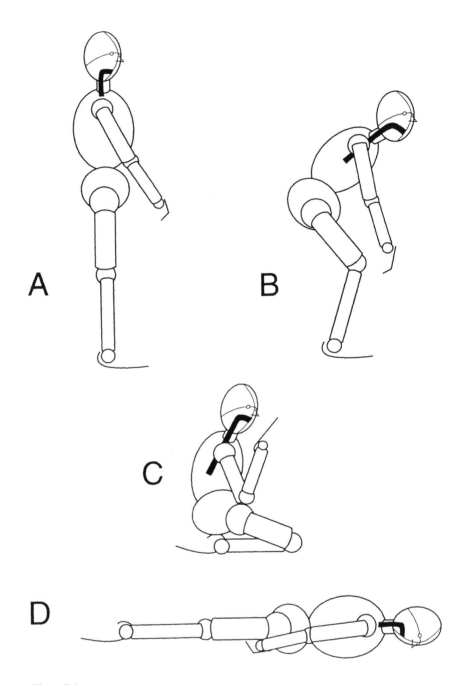

Figure 7.1

'Developmental Postural Cycle' and which I have explained in relation to developmental work in Chapter 3 and in relation to instinctual exploration in Chapter 4. In the prayer a variation of these positions is explored in relation to the process of praying, where I have called it the 'Spiritual Developmental Postural Cycle'.

First, the client stands upright in what I have called the 'Walking Position' in relation to developmental work and 'Homo Erectus Position' in relation to instinctual work. In this position the client explores choreographed movements of arms and hands which express the act of asking and receiving. This position is called the 'Standing Prayer'. (Figure 7.1a). Second, the client allows the knees to bend and the torso to descend into the position which I have called 'Squatting' in developmental work and 'Primate' in instinctual work. Here the client drops the head, tilts the pelvis forwards and allows the torso to implode into a concave configuration as though praying in a sitting position. This is called the 'Sitting Prayer' (Figure 7.1b). Third, the client drops down into what I have called the 'Crawling Position' in developmental work and the 'Feline-canine Position' in instinctual work (Figure 7.1c). Here the client bends down, placing the hands and knees on the floor, and explores the notion of praying on the knees. This is called the 'Kneeling Prayer' position. Fourth, the client slides down onto the floor so that the entire body is stretched out facing downwards, as though praying prostrate. This position is called the 'Prostrate Prayer' (Figure 7.1d). The client then comes back up through the Kneeling Prayer and Sitting Prayer position, arriving at the Standing Prayer position, before beginning the wheel again.

As the client proceeds through this choreography he allows the voice to journey through Free Phonetic Improvisation and Infinite Intervals, covering as wide a pitch range as possible and allowing all vocal component parameters to embellish the vocalisation, discovering an original language without recourse to specific linguistic signification.

Through this work, clients are enabled to contact the universal nature of need, want, receipt, thanks and frustration independent of specific transient contents, subjects or issues. Moreover, one of the inspiring aspects of this work is that, in the instinctual work of Primal Archetypal Regression, the process of moving from Homo Erectus down to the floor serves to bring the client closer to the animality of the psyche and its tendency for primitive descent. The same downward movement in the prayer work, however, serves to bring the psyche closer to the core of its most spiritual aspiration. The work can, therefore, provide an opportunity to heal some of the split between the animal and spiritual within us.

Voicework Case Study: A Prayer for Jonathan

Jonathan was mentally handicapped, a term which, as Valerie Sinason has pointed out, descends from a terminological lineage which has included 'imbecile' 'stupid', 'retarded' and 'backward'.[148] Jonathan had been in a residential home for thirty years and, in that time, only the name used to describe his condition had changed. He was thirty-eight years old, had deep green piercing eyes, gigantic teeth and hands like plates and the first time I saw him he was sitting in a circle in the common room of his home with thirty-seven men and women ranging in age from twenty-two to sixty-one, who had gathered obediently to take part in a voice workshop.

Jonathan had been classified 'non-verbal'; he had spent some time with a speech therapist in his early twenties but to no avail. Though he was non-verbal, he was certainly highly vocal; his voice sporadically emitted a stream of guttural sounds accompanied by an undulating and wave-like dance of his arms, as though he was saying goodbye to a departing loved one knowing he or she will never be seen again. Jonathan had been abandoned at the age of six; his parents were still alive but had not visited him for twenty-three years. The staff at the centre thought his sporadic vocal emissions to be harmless but meaningless.

As I said in the foreword to this book, I was once travelling in Turkey during the festival of Ramadan. It was a hot and dusty evening and the town was deserted. As I turned a corner to buy some water, I heard a sound which grabbed my attention: a moaning, pleading, yearning sound which had a pump-like pulse to it. I could not understand the words uttered and I do not know even if they were words. The sound was neither despairing nor euphoric, it was neither melodic nor was it lacking in musical form. It was, in essence, spiritual.

I retraced my steps a little way and took upon myself the audacity to peer in through a hole in the blinds of a small house, where I saw a man kneeling with tears in his eyes and beads in his hands. I looked only for a moment then I turned and listened once more. At this point my entire interpretative faculties went into overdrive in an attempt to classify and comprehend this sound. Was he crying? Was he singing? Was he praying? And the movements I saw him make with his arms? Were they the spontaneous expression of uncontrollable grief? Or were they the orderly gestural accompaniment to worship? I could not answer any of these questions but could only imagine that the ambiguity and unclassifiable nature of his vocal dance was somehow an important part of why it moved me so much.

In the centre for mentally handicapped adults we went around the circle one by one, each member calling out a sound which the group called back. When it came to Jonathan's turn, something happened that caused me to experience a deep sense of awe. He called out a sound which I had not heard since the time I had stood on that hot dusty street corner in Turkey and I thought only one thing: if we had taken Jonathan to Turkey and placed him in a room with blinded windows and asked him to call out his sound, passers by may have asked all kinds of questions– is he praying? Is he chanting? Is he singing? – but they would not for a moment have thought to ask: is he handicapped?

Jonathan's sound was not handicapped. It was full of religiosity, yearning, needing, pleading and worship. It was also full of music. However, because the linguistic content of Jonathan's day-to-day acoustic emissions were not understandable, 'the baby had been thrown out with the bath water' and his entire vocal faculty had been disqualified and rendered insignificant.

In most parts of Europe singing teachers teach with what they consider to be the indispensable aid of the piano; any vocal sounds made by the student which do not correspond to the black or the white notes are considered unmusical. Western classical music is, to a certain extent, black and white. It only takes fifteen minutes in Turkey, Egypt, Argentina, India or Bali to discover how limited this view of music is. In those countries whose musical traditions have been unaffected by the black and white philosophy they bend notes in continual defiance of a single pitch.

This is one of the qualities which Jonathan's voice had in common with the man I had heard in Turkey. Jonathan's sounds were not black and white, neither were they meaningless.

I asked Jonathan to wheel himself into the centre of the circle and asked him to sing with me. As he did so, I choreographed the perseverative and involuntary movements of his arms which always accompanied his vocalisation into a dance of praying. I had been studying and practically experimenting with various non-Western forms of singing for some time and I began to employ some of what I had learned with Jonathan. I began by singing very quietly in such a way as to create the mood and image of a Turkish prayer. I asked Jonathan to sing with me and to develop the movements of his arms into a dance of praying, bending down from the waist in his wheelchair as though kneeling. The group looked on amazed as he composed a voicedance of exquisite authenticity.

It was clear that the wheelchair was restricting him and preventing fluid and liberated physical expression of the imagistic patterns which Jonathan spontaneously yielded so we helped him out of the chair and into a comfortable kneeling position on the floor. I knelt behind him and held him around the waist with my cheek resting in the small of his back. Together we arose and descended as though in prayer and chanted together in an improvisation of wavering and undulating notes which turned the common room into a sacred space, a temple, a mosque, a synagogue, a church.

After some time, Jonathan became quite excited and enthused by the process, and this was expressed vocally in little spasmodic peeping noises in a falsetto register. I began to mirror these sounds until our musical improvisation gradually transformed into a rhythmical and semi-operatic melody with a xylophone-type quality. In order to ease out the falsetto sounds, I massaged and patted his back. Eventually I was playing his body like a drum. Each time I struck a part of his back, a clear note would emerge.

These notes became stronger, clearer and longer as time went on and it finally became apparent that not only did Jonathan have an awe-inspiring capacity to work in lower pitches but he also had a wonderful upper range akin to a choir boy's.

Over the next eight weeks Jonathan and his fellows rehearsed with me for a performance based on the story of *Sidhartha* by Herman Hesse. There were no words and no music that was not vocal other than the sounds of electric wheelchairs, which we incorporated into the composition.

When the stage was set, the lights adjusted, the audience settled and the atmosphere formed, Jonathan wheeled himself out, raised his arms as he did every day, opened his mouth and drooled saliva, as he did every day, and then vocalised continuously as in prayer whilst ten of his peers walked into the performing arena quietly humming. It was so simple, yet it was so moving. And it was not so much that they were doing anything very different to what they did every day, it was more that we had managed to shift the perspective of the audience – as mine had been shifted in Turkey. Sometimes, I feel, that to educate the ears of the beholder is a more effective Therapeutic Voicework than effecting radical changes in the sounds of the vocalist.

Conclusion: From the Globe to the Self

One of the most renowned figures who struggled to understand the fundamental roots of the human soul, the dimensions of experience which we all share, regardless of cultural and religious context, was Carl Jung, who spent his life seeking to comprehend the nature of the relationship between the psychological and the spiritual. It seems to me that Jung found a way of seeing all cultural frameworks as various expressions of something universally human. In fact, he wondered if this was not indeed the spirit, but preferred to call it the Self. It is to Jung's work that I shall now turn my attention.

Notes

1 Eliade, M. (1989) *Shamanism: Archaic Technique of Ecstasy*. London: Penguin.

2 Halifax, J. (1991) *Shamanic Voices: A Survey of Visionary Narratives*. London: Penguin.

3 Eliade, M. (1989) *Shamanism: Archaic Technique of Ecstasy*. London: Penguin.

4 Winstadt, R. (1951) *The Malay Magician*. London: Routledge & Kegan Paul.

5 Rasmussen, K. (1958) 'An Eskimo Shaman purifies a sick person.' In Lessa and Vogt (ed) *Reader in Comparative Religion*. Evanston, Illinois: Row, Peterson, pp.362–67.

6 Frank, J.D. (1961) *Persuasion and Healing*. Baltimore: Johns Hopkins Press.

7 Frank, J.D. (1961) *Persuasion and Healing*. Baltimore: Johns Hopkins Press.

8 Kalweit, H. (1992) *Shamans, Healers and Medicine Men*. Boston: Shambhala, p.36.

9 Eliade, M. (1989) *Shamanism: Archaic Techniques of Ecstasy*. London: Penguin.

10 Rouget, G. (1985) *Music and Trance: A Theory of the Relations Between Music and Possession*. Chicago: University of Chicago Press, p.142.

11 Cloutier, D. (1973) *Spirit, Spirit: Shaman Songs, Incantations*. Rhode island: Copper Beech Press.

12 Rasmussen, K. (1958) 'An Eskimo Shaman purifies a sick person.' In Lessa and Vogt (ed) *Reader in Comparative Religion*. Evanston, Illinois: Row, Peterson, pp.362–67.

13 Gillin, J. (1958) 'Magical fright' in Lessa and Vogt (eds) *Reader in Comparative Religion*. Evanston, Illinois: Row, Peterson, pp.353-62.

14 LaBarre, W. (1964) 'Confession as cathartic therapy in American Indian tribes.' In A . Kiev (ed) *Magic Faith and Healing*. New York: Free Press of Glencoe, pp.36–49.

15 Densmore, F. (1948) 'The use of music in the Treatment of the sick by American Indians.' In D. M. Schullian and M. Schoen (ed) *Music and Medicine*. New York: Henry Schuman, pp.25–46.

16 Schullian, D.M. and Schoen, M. (1948) *Music and Medicine*. New York: Henry Schuman.

17 Berndt, R.M. 'Wuradjeri Magic and "Clever Men".' *Oceania*, 17 (1946–47) pp.327–65 and 18 (1947–48) pp.60–86.

18 Gusinde, M. (1992) *Die Feurland Indianer*, 3 vols. (Vienna: 1931–74) cited in H. Kalweit, *Shamans, Healers and Medicine Men*. Boston: Shambhala, p.32–33.

19 Needleman, J. (1983) 'Psychiatry and the sacred.' In J. Welwood (ed) *Awakening the Heart: East/West Approaches to Psychotherapy and the Healing Relationship*. Boston: Shambhala, p.7.

20   Cloutier, D. (1973) *Spirit, Spirit: Shaman Songs, Incantations.* Rhode Island: Copper Beech Press.

21   Casteneda, C. (1968) *The Teachings of Don Juan: A Yaqui Way of Knowledge.* Berkeley: University of California Press.
      (1971) *Separate Reality: Further Conversations with Don Juan.* New York: Simon and Schuster.
      (1972) *Journey to Ixtlan: The Lessons of Don Juan.* New York: Simon and Schuster.
      (1974) *Tales of Power.* New York: Simon and Schuster.

22   Huxley, A. (1963) *The Doors of Perception and Heaven and Hell.* New York: Harper and Row.

23   Harner, M. (1990) *The Way of the Shaman.* New York: Harper Collins, p.65–66.

24   Harner, M. (1990) *The Way of the Shaman.* New York: Harper Collins, p.xviii–xix.

25   Harner, M. (1990) *The Way of the Shaman.* New York: Harper Collins, p.72.

26   Harner, M. (1990) *The Way of the Shaman.* New York: Harper Collins, p.73.

27   Roth, G. (1990) *Maps to Ecstasy: Teachings of an Urban Shaman.* London: Harper Collins, p.3.

28   Roth, G. (1990) *Maps to Ecstasy: Teachings of an Urban Shaman.* London: Harper Collins, p.81.

29   Roth, G. (1990) *Maps to Ecstasy: Teachings of an Urban Shaman.* London: Harper Collins, p.82.

30   Lewis, I.M. (1989)*Ecstatic Religion: A Study of Shamanism and Spirit Possession.* London: Routledge.

31   Roth, G. (1990) *Maps to Ecstasy: Teachings of an Urban Shaman.* London: Harper Collins, p.1.

32   Gruen, K. & Virato, S. (1992) 'An interview with Gabrielle Roth.' *New Frontier.* (February/March 1992), pp.11–47, (p.45).

33   Gruen, K. & Virato, S. (1992) 'An interview with Gabrielle Roth.' *New Frontier.* (February/March 1992), pp.11–47, (p.13) .

34   Roth, G. cited in M. Albert, 'Teachings of an urban Shaman.' *Yoga Journal.* (December 1990), pp.71–73, (p.73).

35   Roth. G. cited in M. Albert, 'Teachings of an urban Shaman.' *Yoga Journal.* (December 1990), pp.71–73, (p.73).

36   Barbeau, M. (1974) 'Tsimsyan songs.' In E. Garfield (ed) *The Tsimshian: Their Arts and Music.* (American Ethnological Society Publication 18, 1974).

37   Hart, M. (1990) *Drumming at the Edge of Magic: A Journey into the Spirit of Percussion.* San Francisco: Harper Collins, p.167.

38   Bernhardt, P. (1991) *The Secret Music of the Soul.* Québec: Imagine.

39   Halpern, S. (1985) *Sound Health.* San Francisco: Harper and Row.

40   Kopp, S. (1972) *If You Meet Budha on the Road, Kill Him: A Modern Pilgrimage Through Myth, Legend, Zen and Psychotherapy.* London: Sheldon Press.

41   Stockhausen, K. (1989) *Towards a Cosmic Music.* Trans. by T. Nevill. Dorset: Element.

42   Drury, N. (1985) *Music for Inner Space: Techniques for Meditation & Visualisation.* Dorset: Prism.

43   Bonny, H. & Savary, L. (1990) *Music and your Mind.* New York: Station Hill Press.

44   Bush, C. (1995) *Healing Imagery and Music.* Portland: Rudra Press.

45   Storr, A. (1992) *Music and the Mind.* London: Harper Collins.

46   Harner, M. (ed) (1973) *Hallucinogens and Shamanism.* Oxford: Oxford University Press.

47   Furst, P. (ed) (1972) *Flesh of the Gods: The Ritual Use of Hallucinogens.* New York: Praeger.

48   Kroeber, A. (1940) 'Psychotic factors in Shamanism.' *Character and Personality*, 8, pp.204–15.

49   Silverman, J. (1967) 'Shamanism and acute Schizophrenia.' *American Anthropologist*, 69, pp.21–31.

50   Devereux, G. (1980) *Basic Problems of Ethnopsychiatry*. Chicago: University of Chicago Press.

51   Torrey, E.F. (1969) 'The case for the indigenous therapist.' *Archive of General Psychiatry*, 20, pp.365–73.

52   Peters, L. (1978) 'Psychotherapy in Tamang Shamanism.' *Ethnos* 6, no. 2, pp.63–91.

53   Murphy, J. (1964) 'Psychotherapeutic Aspects of Shamanism on St. Lawrence Island, Alaska.' In A. Kiev (ed) *Magic, Faith and Healing*. New York: The Free Press of Glencoe.

54   Gatheru, R. (1960) 'The Medicine Man as Psychotherapist.' In W. Goldschmidt (ed) *Exploring the Ways of Mankind*. New York: Holt, Rinehart and Winston.

55   Grof, S. and Halifax, J. (1978) *The Human Encounter with Death*. New York: Dutton.

56   Grof, A. (1975) *Realms of the Human Unconscious: Observations from LSD Research*. New York: Viking Press.

57   Grof, S. *The Adventure of Self Discovery*. New York: State University of New York.

58   Schweidlenka, R. (1993) 'Spirituality for sale: plastic medicine men invade Europe.' *American Indian Community House Bulletin VIII*, No. XIII, pp.4–8, (p.4).

59   McCloud, J. (1993) in 'Spirituality for sale: plastic medicine men invade Europe.' *American Indian Community House Bulletin VIII*, No. XIII, pp.4–8, (p.4).

60   Shaw, C. (1995) 'A theft of spirit?' *Kindred Spirit*. (July/August 1995), pp.84–92, (p.86).

61   Pierce, J. (1992) *The Science of Musical Sound*. New York: Freeman.

62   Berendt, J.E. (1992) *The Third Ear: On Listening to The World*. New York: Holt, p.91.

63   Hamel, P. (1986) *Through Music to the Self: How to Experience Music Anew*. Shaftsbury: Element.

64   Goodchild, C. (1989) 'A servant of voice and sound.' *Human Potential*, October1989–May1990, pp.14–16.

65   Ibid., pp.14–16.

66   Mukunda, V. Lecture given at Songs of Heaven and Earth Conference. (Findhorn Foundation, Forres, 30 March–6 April 1996).

67   Daniélou, A. (1995) *Music and the Power of Sound: The Influence of Tuning and Interval on Consciousness*. Vermont: Inner Traditions.

68   James, J. (1995) *The Music of the Spheres: Music, Science and the Natural Order of the Universe*. London: Abacus, p.31.

69   James, J. (1995) *The Music of the Spheres: Music, Science and the Natural Order of the Universe*. London: Abacus, p.31.

70   Cousto, H. (1988) *The Cosmic Octave: Planets, Tones, Colours – The Power of Inherent Vibrations*, trans. by C. Baker. California: Life Rhythm.

71   Godwin, J. (1993) *The Harmony of the Spheres A Sourcebook of the Pythagorean Tradition in Music*. Rochester: Inner Traditions.

72   Godwin, J. (1987) *Music, Mysticism and Magic: A Sourcebook*. London: Arkana.

73   Godwin, J. (1989) *Cosmic Music: Musical Keys to the Interpretation of Reality*. Rochester: Inner Traditions.

74   Godwin, J. (1987) *Harmonies of Heaven and Earth The Spiritual Dimension of Music from Antiquity to the Avant-Garde*. London: Thames and Hudson.

75   McClellan, R. (1991) *The Healing Forces of Music: History, Theory and Practice*. Shaftsbury: Element, p.193.

76   David, W. (1980) *The Harmonics of Sound, Color and Vibration: A System for Self-Awareness and Soul Evolution*. Santa Monica: DeVorss.

77   Jenny, H. (1967/1972) *Cymatics*, vol. 1 & 2. Basel: Basilius Press.

78   Cymatics: *The Healing Nature of Sound*. (Pts. 1, 2 & 3). Video produced by Jeff Volk (Brookline, MA: Macromedia, 1986).

79   Jenny, H. (1967/1972) *Cymatics*, vol. 1 & 2. Basel: Basilius Press.

80   Edwards, S. 'Bio-acoustics: the potential to reverse disease using individual signature sounds.' In *Sharry Edwards: Signature Sound – Published Papers 1982-1993*, pp.12–17, (p.12).'

81   Hamel, P. (1986) *Through Music to the Self: How to Experience Music Anew*. Shaftsbury: Element, p.11.

82   Gerber, R. (1988) *Vibrational Medicine: New Choices for Healing Ourselves*. Santa Fe: Bear & Co., p.396.

83   McClellan, R. (1991) *The Healing Forces of Music: History, Theory and Practice*. Shaftsbury: Element, p.161.

84   Gardner, K. (1990) *Sounding the Inner Landscape*. Stonington, ME: Caduceus.

85   McClellan, R. (1991) *The Healing Forces of Music: History, Theory and Practice*. Shaftesbury: Element.

86   Hamel, P. (1986) *Through music to the Self: How to experience Music Anew*. Shaftesbury: Element.

87   Crowley, B. and Crowley, W. (1994) *Words of Power: Sacred Sounds of East and West*. St. Paul, Minnesota: Llewellyn, p.xiv.

88   Welwood, J. (ed) (1983) *Awakening the Heart: East/West Approaches to Psychotherapy and the healing Relationship*. Boston: Shambhala, p.7.

89   Brazier, D. (1995) *Zen Therapy*. London: Constable, p.19–20.

90   Inayat Khan, H. (1983) *The Music of Life*. Lebanon: Omega, p.93.

91   Berendt, J.E. (1992) *The Third Ear On Listening to the World*. New York: Holt.

92   Berendt, J.E. (1988) *Nada Brama: The World is Sound*. London: East West.

93   Cayce, E. (1972) 'Music as the bridge.' In S. R. Winston (ed) *Music as the Bridge*. Virginia: A R E Press, pp.1–7.

94   Keyes, L.E. (1973) *Toning, The Creative Power of the Voice*. Santa Monica: DeVorss.

95   Gardner, K. (1990) *Sounding the Inner Landscape*. Stonington, ME: Caduceus.

96   Campbell, D. (1991) *Music: Physician for Times to Come*. Wheaton: Quest Books.
     Campbell, D. (1992) *Music and Miracles*. Wheaton: Quest Books.

97   Campbell, D. (1990) *The Roar of Silence: Healing Powers of Breath, Tone and Music*. Wheaton: Theosophical Publishing House, p.15.

98   Campbell, D. (1990) *The Roar of Silence: Healing Powers of Breath, Tone and Music*. Wheaton: Quest Books, p.2.

99   Seagren, R. (1991) 'Overtones of health: an interview with Don Campbell.' *Open Ear*, (Fall 1991), pp.2–5, (p.3).

100 Goldman, J. (1992) *Healing Sounds :The Power of Harmonics*. Shaftsbury: Element.

101   Goldman, J. (1992) *Healing Sounds :The Power of Harmonics*. Shaftsbury: Element, p92.

102   Andrews, T. (1994) *Sacred Sounds: Transformation through Music and Word*. St. Paul, MN: Llewelyn Publications, p.74.

103   Andrews, T. (1994) *Sacred Sounds: Transformation through Music and Word*. St. Paul, MN: Llewelyn Publications, p.76.

104   Andrews, T. (1994) *Sacred Sounds: Transformation through Music and Word*. St. Paul, MN: Llewelyn Publications, p.77.

105   Garfield, L.M. (1987) *Sound Medicine: Healing with Music, Voice and Song*. Berkeley: Celestial Arts, p.60.

106   Gardner-Gordon, J. (1993) *The Healing Voice: Traditional and Contemporary Toning, Chanting and Singing*. Freedom, CA: Crossing Press, p.131–3.

107   Gardner-Gordon, J. (1993) *The Healing Voice: Traditional and Contemporary Toning, Chanting and Singing*. Freedom, CA: Crossing Press, Publishers 'Note to the reader', first leaf page.

108   Dewhurst-Maddock, O. (1993) *The Book of Sound Therapy: Heal Yourself with Music and Voice*. London: Gaia, p.47.

109   Lingerman, H.A. (1983) *The Healing Energies of Music*. Wheaton, Il.: Quest Books.

110   Watson, A. & Drury, N. (1989) *Healing Music: The Path to Inner Wholeness*. Bridport: Prism.

111   Andrew, T. *Sacred Sounds: Transformation through Music and Word*. St. Paul, MN.

112   Beaulieu, J. (1987) *Music and Sound in the Healing Arts: An Energy Approach*. New York: Station Hill Press, p.66.

113   Beaulieu, J. (1987) *Music and Sound in the Healing Arts: An Energy Approach*. New York: Station Hill Press, p.72.

114   James, C. (1993) 'I'd like to teach the world to sing: an interview with Chris James.' *Kindred Spirit, 2,* 10, pp.16–18.

115   James, C. (1993) 'I'd like to teach the world to sing : interview.' *Kindred Spirit, 2,* 10, pp.16–18.

116   James, C. (1993) 'I'd like to teach the world to sing : interview.' *Kindred Spirit, 2,* 10, pp.16–18.

117   James, C. (1993) 'I'd like to teach the world to sing : interview.' *Kindred Spirit, 2,* 10, pp.16–18.

118   James, C. (1993) 'I'd Like to teach the World to Sing.' *Kindred Spirit,* 22 (Spring 1993), pp.16–18.

119   James, C. (1993) 'I'd Like to teach the World to Sing.' *Kindred Spirit,* 22 (Spring 1993), pp.16–18.

120   Purce, J. (1996) Publicity leaflet for workshops.

121   Purce, J. (1996) cited in M. Law, 'Interviews with contemporary voice practitioners.' Unpublished research papers prepared for the International Association for Voice Movement Therapy.

122   Kumar, S. (1986) 'Sound in mind and body.' *Resurgence, 115* (March/April 1986).

123   D'angelo, J. (1994) 'Resonances of the cosmos.' *Caduceus 23,* May 1994), pp.6–9.

124   Goodchild, C. (1993) *The Naked Voice*. London: Random House.

125   Goodchild, C. (1993) *The Naked Voice*. London: Random House.

126   Ward-Jones, T. (1996) cited in M. Law, 'Interviews with contemporary voice practitioners.' Unpublished research papers prepared for the International Association for Voice Movement Therapy.

127   Ward-Jones, T. (1992) *Journal for South Asian Dance 16* (December 1992).

128   Relph, A. (1996) cited in M. Law, 'Interviews with contemporary voice practitioners.' Unpublished research papers prepared for the International Association for Voice Movement Therapy.

129   Rollin Rachel, Workshop publicity, (January 1996).

130   Lane, D. (1994) *Music as Medicine.* Michigan: Zondervan.

131   Hale, S. (1995) *Song and Silence: Voicing the Soul.* New Mexico: La Alameda Press.

132   Mathieu, W. (1991) *The Listening Book: Discovering Your own Music.* Boston: Shambhala.

133   Wright, C. (1995) 'The resurrection of Gregorian Chant.' *Open Ear,* Winter 1995, pp.6–10.

134   Le Mée, K. (1994) *Chant: The Origins, Form, Practice, and Healing Power of Gregorian Chant.* London: Random House.

135   Genesis 31:27.

136   Exodus 14: 15-22.

137   1 Samuel 18:7.

138   Matthew 26:30.

139   Colossians 3:16.

140   1 Corinthians 14:12-15.

141   Revelation 5.

142   Joshua 6.

143   Sachs, C. (1942) *The History of Musical Instruments.* London: Dent.

144   Acts 2.

145   Reznikoff, I. cited in 'Therapy of pure sound, reaching deep consciousness to heal: Iégor Reznikoff interviewed by Caduceus.' *Caduceus, 23,* May 1994, 16–18.

146   Reznikoff, I. Lecture given at Songs of Heaven and Earth Conference, (Findhorn Foundation, Forres, 30 March–6 April 1996).

147   Reznikoff, I. cited in 'Therapy of pure sound, reaching deep consciousness to heal: Iégor Reznikoff interviewed by Caduceus.' *Caduceus, 23,* May 1994, 16–18, (p.18).

148   Sinason, V. (1992) *Mental Handicap and the Human Condition: New Approaches from the Tavistock.* London: Free Association Press.

CHAPTER 8

Voice, Image and Archetype
Therapeutic Voicework and Analytical Psychology

Introduction: From Freud to Jung

In Chapter 5 I outlined the aspects of Freud's early work which are pertinent to the subject of vocal expression, traced the adaptation of psychoanalysis to meet the demands of vocal and respiratory processes by some major pioneers and described some contemporary perspectives on psychoanalytic theory and practice which are apposite to a new discipline such as Therapeutic Voicework. In this chapter I shall follow similar lines of enquiry applied to the field of Analytical Psychology, that is the framework of psychological investigation initiated by the Swiss psychiatrist Carl Jung.

At the end of his life and work, Freud discouraged psychoanalysts from further considering the process of phylogenesis as a primary determining factor in the psychological constitution of the individual. He remarked that 'it is not easy for us to carry over the concepts of individual psychology into group psychology' and he did not believe that anything was to be gained by introducing the concept of a 'collective unconscious'.[1] The negative reference to this transpersonal realm of psychic activity was, of course, a direct attack on the work of Jung, to whom psychological inheritance was the primary determining aspect of a person's psychological make up. For Jung, the Oedipus Complex was only one of many psychological structures which gain allegorical expression through the myths of ancient traditions, and few of them displayed a direct relation to sexuality as far as Jung was concerned.

The close friendship, eventual rivalry and ultimate infamous split between these two men is widely known and extensively described in numerous publications and the precise parallel developments of the two men's theoretical postulations is recorded with extreme diligence by Frey-Rohn.[2] Yet despite the abundant scholarly study, one of the lesser stated facts about the original connection between Freud's early work and the initial professional research investigations carried out by Jung was that both shared a mutual concern with verbal language. Furthermore, it was from Jung's early linguistic research that he momentarily turned his attention to the sounds of the human voice and their capacity to carry information about the psyche. As with Freud, therefore, I will commence by describing the nature of Jung's very early work as a point of departure from which to analyse the place of vocal expression and Therapeutic Voicework within the broad field of Archetypal Psychology as developed by subsequent pioneers.

Jung's Cacophony of Voices

In 1904 Jung conducted some remarkable experiments with words which led to the discovery of the 'complex'. Jung took a group of healthy adults and read to each one in turn a list of 400 words. After hearing each word, the subject was asked to respond with the first word which came into his or her head; this response and the time it took was recorded. Sometimes the responses to certain words were simple and predictable, for example to the word 'window' a volunteer would reply 'pane' and to the word 'house' the reply would be 'roof'. However, some of the responses seemed at first rather unusual, for example to the word 'window' the volunteer would say 'cat' and to the word 'house' the reply would be 'lost'. Closer examination of the person's personal circumstances revealed that certain words produced seemingly odd reactions because they were connected to a specific emotionally-charged preoccupation which the subject had, but of which he or she was unaware. For example, the person may respond to the word 'house' with 'lost' because of having narrowly escaped a fire, when a child, in which the house was lost or destroyed by the blaze. In similar connection, the reply of 'cat' to the word 'window' may originate in the memory of seeing the pet cat in the window of the blazing furnace. Because of the extreme emotions associated with such an event, words which represent aspects of the experience serve to reanimate a faint and unconscious memory of it, including the re-experiencing of the appropriate emotions in mild form. This is what Jung named the 'complex', which he defined as a network or cluster of half-forgotten single images which are held to together by an emotional tone, in this case terror, which, though a person is not aware of it, can continue to affect him or her for a long time.

In each person there are many complexes which arise and dissolve as part of the natural process of shifting preoccupations. It is from them that we draw our moods, our feelings and our reactions. However, because the complexes are unconscious, we are often at a loss to know where these forces come from. Many of the complexes, arising as they do from traumatic circumstances, are too painful to be allowed to remain in our field of attention but they sustain a certain dormant life of their own. When things or events around us stimulate the recollection of previous experiences, and thereby provoke a memory of the emotion originally attached to that experience, the complex is then activated and we experience feelings and behave in ways which seem strange. Complexes then are not a disease, they are not a sign of disorder or disturbance. On the contrary, they are the very means by which we feel. As Jung said, 'there is no one who has no complexes, just as there is no one who is without emotions'.[3]

Ego in the Middle

Though we have many complexes, there is one particular network of images which is, at least in the healthy individual, dominant and central and to which Jung referred as the 'ego'. Thus although the complexes dance a tango upon the stage of the psyche, the ego is at work like an organising centre, without which we would have no constant identity and, consequently, our changes of mood would make us feel like a completely different personality each time an emotional transition occurred.

The ego is not one thing but a complex of sense impressions and images, networks of ideas which we associate with the 'feeling-tone' of our own body. For Jung, the ego is, to a large extent, a conglomeration of the information which we receive through sight, hearing, taste, touch and smell.[5] It is by way of the ego's association with the body that 'I' feel bunged up when my body is bronchially congested or that 'I' feel aggravated when my skin is irritated. Jung said: 'one's own personality is therefore the firmest and strongest complex' and, 'good health permitting', it 'weathers all psychological storms'[5] because 'the ego-complex, by reason of its direct connection with bodily sensations, is the most stable and the richest in associations'.[6]

The ego is, however, influenced by the other complexes which constantly guide us in what we do; for even though they are unconscious they actively cause us to carry out certain modes of behaviour. This gives them the appearance of independent beings, acting of their own accord, which is why Jung described the complexes as the 'little people', 'mini-personalities' and 'splinter psyches'.[7] This autonomy is due to the affect, feeling-tone or emotion that binds the constituting images of the complex together. Emotion is such a strong influence compared to the reason of the ego that any group of images which are united by a strong affect will always have their way. The emotion of terror at our house being burnt down is much stronger than the reason which tells us that it is all in the past. It is this very strength that causes us to bury it, but it lives on with its own independence. Jung said that because emotion 'occupies in the constitution of the psyche a very independent place', the complexes are 'relatively independent of the central control of the consciousness, and at any moment liable to bend or cross the intentions of the individual'.[8]

Sometimes, if there are two or more complexes at work at the same time, the ego may become confused, feeling pulled first this way and then that. In a healthy individual the ego is so strong that it can take account of these voices and have the final say. But, if the ego becomes weakened, it gets lost, becoming only one voice among many. In such cases the psyche splits up into a multitude of voices all clamouring for domination. This is precisely what happens in some kinds of psychoses, where, Jung says, 'the psychic totality falls apart' and 'splits up into complexes' such that 'the ego-complex ceases to play the important role among these' but 'is now just one among several complexes which are all equally important, or perhaps even more important than the ego'.[9]

Because the ego is affirmed and maintained primarily through its association with the body, such a swallowing of the ego by the other complexes gives rise to a so-called 'mind-body split' where the body becomes the seat of sensations which come from the complexes and not only from the outside world. This is also what can happen in schizophrenia. If our subject who lost her house becomes schizophrenic, her body may genuinely feel burned when she touches a cat and she may refuse to touch any windows for fear of getting burnt. In these circumstances the voice of the fire-complex is stronger than that of the ego and, to the outside world, these imaginings are so illogical that we cannot hope to penetrate their meaning; the hot cat remains an absurdity to us. This resulting experience of the domination or submersion of the ego by one or more of the complexes is called a 'dissociation of personality'.

It is not irrelevant that Jung referred to the emotional binding of the complex as a 'tone', which is a musical, acoustic and, therefore, a vocal phenomenon; for Jung himself was to observe the activity and expression of the complexes through the timbral and tonal quality of the human voice.

The Voices of the Dead Speak Through

For his medical thesis, Jung studied the extraordinary case of a fifteen and a half-year-old girl who acted as a medium for the voices of the dead. Jung attended her regular seances where he witnessed these dead people express themselves through the girl's voice. Each time the girl expressed a different character, the quality or timbre of her voice would completely change. On occasions this involved major transformations of dialect and accent from German to French or Italian. Furthermore, though the girl displayed only a faint knowledge of High German in her normal life, in her trance she spoke the language faultlessly.[10] Jung later understood that these characters were different aspects of the girl's own personality, ramifications of her autonomous complexes, for she was undergoing a dissociation of her personality and it was through her voice that the complexes took on an identity which could be communicated to those observing as well as to our own consciousness.

Later, Jung noticed how those who, in his day, were diagnosed as schizophrenics often talked to themselves in voices with very different qualities and he noted that in severe cases of psychotic disturbance the words of the voices degenerated into a pure muddle with no linguistic meaning. For example, he observed a catatonic who used to sing a religious song 'for hours on end' with the refrain 'Hallelujah', which, over a period of months, 'gradually degenerated' into 'Hallo', then 'Oha', and finally simply 'ha-ha-ha' which was 'accompanied by convulsive laughter'.[11] Jung concluded that in Schizophrenia 'eventually all words can be replaced by a 'hm-hm-hm' which is 'uttered in a stereotyped manner'.[12] What remained was the tone in both senses: the emotional tone of the complex, which was expressed through the audible vocal tone of the voice for the psychotic does not hear or express a jumbled semi-verbal word salad in monotone but in pitches and timbral qualities expressive of the affect of the complex. One is aggressive, spiteful and provocative, the other luring, sly and seductive; another Italian, confident and full of bravado, the other English, polite and reserved. The voices of psychoses each have characteristics expressed vocally through an acoustic tone whether there are words present or not. Thus in vocal terms we might describe the concept of 'tone' as the affective nucleus of a complex as expressed through the acoustic quality of the voice.

The degeneration of a word salad into a purely vocal composition, which Jung observed in schizophrenia, has a parallel in bodily movements. The psychotic patient will, in the early stages of the disorder, repeat movements which have their genesis in some domestic gestural act, such as smoking a cigarette or combing the hair. Eventually, however, these movements become more and more abstracted until it is impossible for a newcomer to recognise where they originated. Jung observed such a choreographic degeneration in a patient who 'used to comb his hair a few hours every day in a stereotyped manner' claiming that he was seeking to remove the 'plaster that had been rubbed into it during the night'. Then, as the years went on, 'the comb got further and further away from his head' until, after three years of this dance, the patient 'beat and scratched his chest' with the comb.[13]

It is interesting to note that the process of gradually abstracting physical movements from a domestic act until they become a dance is an established choreographic principle by which Postmodern dance is devised. This is a very useful tool when working with clients, who can turn a gestural perseverative and semi-conscious gesture into a mode through which it can be made conscious and explored.

Therapeutic Voicework Methodology: Complex, Rhyme and Association

The process of making up rhymes emanates from a primary universal infantile act and rhyme making is, of course, central to the process of song-writing. In addition to rhyme making, the process of freely associating one word with another in a continuous stream without concern for conscious narrative structure is also the means by which many artists compose. Therapeutic Voicework can provide an opportunity to investigate the unconscious by applying this compositional technique in action.

The client starts singing something very simple, usually a word or phrase to which the Therapeutic Voiceworker has drawn attention from observing the client's expressions. This is repeated a number of times until it naturally provokes an association.

The associated word or phrase is then itself repeated in combination with the original word or phrase until another association is provoked. This is then also added to the first two units and the process continues until the client has accumulated a vocabulary of phrases which provide a text. This text can then be spoken and the prosody and rhythm enhanced to provide a song. Such a process can be extremely enjoyable and amusing, yet often simultaneously containing associations emanating from uncomfortable feelings or events.

Indeed, the nonsense rhyme is exemplified in the writing of Spike Milligan[14] as well as in the songs of Syd Barrett,[15] upon whose inspiration the rock band *Pink Floyd* was founded and who, like Milligan, has suffered extreme mental anguish. Yet, for both of them, their seemingly superficial compositions served to contain deep conflict.

Archetypes

Though the complexes are often formed as the result of personal memories, usually of a distressing nature, there are other networks of images which have not been formulated through experience but have been inherited as so-called instincts. These may be described as patterns of behaviour, ways of reacting to things that you can guarantee observing in all human beings. These instincts are readily observed in animals. For example, Joseph Campbell exemplifies inherited instincts in young hen chicks, whom we know are killed and eaten by hawks but not by gulls. If you take a group of chicks and enclose them in a cage before they have had any contact with the world and draw a stuffed gull along a wire above them, the chicks will not react. If you take a stuffed hawk and draw it backwards across the cage, they still will not react. But if you draw it forwards, the chicks begin digging and scratching, cooing and clucking in an attempt to get away. In this tiny creature there is, therefore, an inherited instinct of fear and flight that is attached to a certain image both in form and motion.[16] If such an animal can possess such complicated inherited information, imagine what the human being inherits.

These inherited instincts are like complexes in that they cause us to react in a certain way. They lie beneath the personal unconscious in a stratum of the psyche called the 'collective unconscious'. They are known as 'archetypes' and cause us to execute certain modes of behaviour at certain times. For example, in every person there lies a certain appetite or instinct for childlike mischief which may be expressed as a playful desire for frivolity or by playing devil's advocate in a conversation; it may manifest as an evil desire to mock or ridicule someone's success; it might cause us to contemplate stealing something for the sheer thrill of it or to torment someone by hiding their belongings. At such times we might say that the Trickster Archetype is dominating our behaviour. However, Jung looked not only at the way these archetypes gain expression through the way people behave but also through the images contained in dreams, fairy-tales, myths, legends, poetry and painting. In writing we see the Trickster Archetype reflected in characters such as Dickens' Artful Dodger from the novel *Oliver Twist*, who dances quick-foot between the crowds picking the pockets of the local gentry; in the fairy-tale character of Rumpelstiltskin, who plays a wicked trick of mischief in posing the riddle of his name; in Puck of Shakespeare's *A Midsummer Night's Dream*, who pours love juice into the wrong eyes and causes the havoc of infatuation; in Eros of Greek mythology, who causes people to fall into the mischief of love by infecting them with his poisonous arrows; or in Penguin from the Batman story, who incessantly devises more mean tricks to outwit the hero. All cultures have their examples of the childlike mischiever, for it is a universal and primordial instinct, it is the archetype of the Trickster.

Another important archetype is The Mother, a central figure to the art, culture and mythology of all peoples and always characterised by certain qualities. The Mother is the great nourisher, nurturing our growth with the milk of human kindness, she provides warmth and comfort reminiscent of the womb; she is the protector and life-giver. However, all archetypes have a positive and a negative side. Just as the Trickster is not only the harmless pick-pocket but also the wicked conniver, causing death in the trail of his traps, so too the Mother has a dark side. Just as we would all love a taste of that ultimate dependence upon the Mother reminiscent of the womb, so too we fear our independence being consumed by the mother's arms, for part of the Mother's dark side is her inability to let her children go. She is the suffocator who swallows her children whole, thwarting their independence and thus threatening their very life.

The representation of the archetypes often takes the form not of a character but of an object or an animal. The Trickster may appear as a magpie or a fox. The Mother, in her bright aspect, may appear as a safe haven, a cave where the evil men on our trail will not find us, or as a cool pool of water in which we swim, kept buoyant by the nourishing minerals. In her dark aspect the Mother may appear as the dragon that will swallow us up or the great hole in the earth of our dreams that we fall into just before we wake up with a jump. All these archetypes play themselves out through our behaviour at different times and thus Jung discovered two levels to the unconscious psyche: the first he called the 'personal unconscious' and the second the 'collective unconscious'. In the personal unconscious reside all the complexes of images grouped according to our personal experience, whilst the collective unconscious houses the patterns that we have inherited. Jung therefore defined the personal unconscious as 'the totality of all psychic phenomena that lack the quality of consciousness' including 'all lost memories', 'all contents that are still too weak to become conscious' and 'all more or less intentional repressions of painful thoughts and feelings'. Meanwhile, he defined the collective unconscious as a receptacle for those 'qualities that are not individually acquired but are inherited', such as the 'instincts as impulses to carry out

actions from necessity, without conscious motivation'. In addition, the collective unconscious houses the 'archetypes of perception and apprehension'
for 'just as his instincts compel man to a specifically human mode of existence, so the archetypes force his ways of perception and apprehension into
specifically human patterns'.[17]

The constant appearance and influence of both the personal complexes
and the collective archetypes led Jung to propose that each of us is not one
but many and that we all have multiple voices which need to have their say.
Jung believed that the original state of the psyche is 'one in which the psychic
processes are very loosely knit and by no means form a self-orientated
unity'.[18] Jung asserted that daily life consists of a continuous dialogue
between the many voices of the psyche and that this dialogue is absolutely
crucial to a healthy and balanced life. Only through 'hearing out' the different possibilities, needs, moods, complexes and archetypal influences that a
person has can he or she appreciate what it is to be alive.

The One and the Many

In the schizophrenia of his day, Jung observed merely an exaggerated form of
the dialogue, necessary for healthy living, between different voices in the
psyche. But whereas for most people this dialogue is chaired by the dominating strength of the ego, in schizophrenia and other forms of psychotic
experience each of the voices acquire such an increased intensity that the ego
becomes swamped and the psyche becomes saturated with a chorus of voices,
each wanting to instigate a different mode of behaviour. For the healthy person with a strongly affirmed ego, however, Jung proclaimed the importance
of maintaining a dialogue between the many voices. To this end, Jung proclaimed that 'one should nurture the art of conversing with oneself' and
openly encouraged people to develop the ability to give each of their complexes a voice.[19] Indeed, for Jung, this was one of the primary roles of
psychotherapy. Furthermore, for Jung, anything which enabled a balanced
conversance and interplay between the different voices was in itself therapeutic. Jung was therefore keen to observe many processes which gave
outward manifestation to the inner psychic voices, including painting,
poetry, drama, opera and, above all, dreaming.

A Mythical Language of Dreams

Jung believed that the psyche retains many ideas, images and linguistic symbols which originate from humankind's earliest days through a genealogical
inheritance. The Oedipus complex is, for Jung, only one of a vast spectrum of
image-matrices comprising emotions, instincts, ideas and characters to which
the human psyche or imagination plays host. For Jung, all the characters and
narratives which formulate religious mythology reflect the structure of, and
thus provide; an allegorical metaphor for internal psychological processes as
it is from them that they emanate. In replacing the Oedipus complex as an
equal amongst an extensive pantheon of other myths and figurative manifestations in legend, tale and folklore, Jung both de-sexualised psychoanalysis
and, at the same time, depersonalised it.

Freud's psychoanalysis reconstructed a specific autobiographical narrative in which he contextualised the psychological images central to the
patient's psychological constitution, tracing the origin of the symptom and
the cause of the neuroses to a specific event or events in this narrative of the
patient's past. Jung, on the other hand, rather than contextualising the
images in the patient's narrative, conducted extensive cross-references
between individual dreams and fantasies, observing how their structure was
represented in different guises in every individual in every culture. He consequently revealed how the roots and significance of symptoms and
dream-images originate not in the sociological circumstances which influence the development of individual consciousness but in unconscious
universal structures, a system of 'genetic blue prints'[20] or archetypes, which
are continually re-invented through the personages which appear in myths
and are continually re-animated through the process of dreaming. Jung
believed that in dreaming, as in psychoses, there are 'numberless interconnec-
tions to which one can find parallells only in mythological associations of
ideas' or 'poetic creations' which have often been borrowed from myths.[21]

Instead of tracing the significance of a dream to the idiosyncratic stories
of the patient's daily life, Jung traced them to the larger stories of the myths
to ascertain which archetypal pattern the dream originated in. Thus, for Jung,
there were 'not only typical dreams but typical motifs in the dreams' which
may be 'situations or figures'.[22] Further to this challenge to Freud's individu-
alist hypothesis, Jung placed less emphasis on the significance of linguistic
description than had Freud. For Jung, words were less important than the
analysis of the dream contents as a pictorial symbol. Language was but the
necessary means by which analyst and patient communicate, a transcription

of the actual material, which, for Jung, was always symbolic. For Jung, a dream of flying, for example, was not an indication of a particular sexual problem but took place in the context of universal myths where flight symbolised freedom, spirituality, heavenly ascension, escape and a host of other non-sexual significations. Jung's method of dream analysis amplified the patient's image of flight and looked at all the other motifs which often occur alongside flight in mythical stories and he was thereby able to relate the age-old wisdom contained in the relevant myths to the life predicament of the patient.

In tracing patients' dreams to myths, Jung consequently raised their attention above a preoccupation with their own problems and dilemmas and enabled them to see that they were not alone in their suffering but that they were temporarily hosting the eternal problems of humanity. For Jung, the individual suffering revealed through the psychotherapeutic process 'is archetypal and collective' and can be 'taken as a sign 'that none of us is 'suffering for himself, but rather from 'the spirit of the age', that is 'from an objective, impersonal cause' or, most succinctly, from a 'collective unconscious which' each of us has 'in common with all men'.[23] Jung therefore developed an ever-deepening respect for the ability of ancient myth to offer a timeless, figurative and allegorical reflection of a person's inner psychic life.

Therapeutic Voicework Methodology: Singing the Dream

Singing the Dream is a process by which the optical components of a client's dream are given acoustic form through vocal sounds using the full timbral range of vocal component parameters. This process is especially useful in excavating the affective component of the dream scene.

Through this process, the Therapeutic Voiceworker helps the client find timbral qualities of voice in combination with facial expressions and bodily movements which personify figures and objects from the dream.

To begin, the client usually stands in Homo Erectus and develops a neutral vocal timbre which expresses the condition of the dreamer as observer.

Standing in the centre of Spherical Space, the client ventures physically and vocally, occupying the role of the various dream contents and returning to the centre regularly to personify the observing dreamer. The Therapeutic Voiceworker, meanwhile, guides, instructs and assists the process of exploration and investigation.

Cracking rock, swaying trees, roaring sea, old women, young children, animals and insects all become vocal figures which interact through the dream opera giving acoustic and musical form as well as emotional depth to hitherto optical constructs.

The Self

Jung's vision of men's and women's psychological functioning was one which perceived the psyche as essentially multiple, a matrix of individual images, part personal, part archetypal, which 'do not form a self-orientated unity'.[24] Jung observed the most overt example of this disorientated mass of images in the behavioural manifestations of the so-called psychotic, in whom the extreme degree of autonomy in the emotion or affect which cemented the various image matrices led to the appearance of a number of separate personalities, 'autonomous complexes', 'splinter psyches' or 'little people'.[25] Jung's later work brought him to realise that the 'character' of these different personalities, far from being constituted of idiosyncratic components arising solely from the patient's experience, in fact demonstrated elemental similarities which arose from a collective depth.

It was in people suffering from psychoses that Jung witnessed these components erupting and interfering with conscious mental functioning and which Jung alleged occurred as a result of too wide an abyss between the unconscious treasure-house of images and the conscious process of assimilating and understanding the impulses which motivate our behaviour. The more the mental chasm widens, the more likely that the images from the depths will burst forth upon us in a way thoroughly arresting of all reasonable faculties. This is why Jung was adamant to encourage any process which nurtured and facilitated the methodological admission of unconscious contents into consciousness for this enabled the sequestered and insensible images of the deeps to be unearthed, observed, wrought, formulated and incorporated into conscious life, rendering neutral their tendency to burst forth pathologically. It would be a misunderstanding, however, to assume Jung believed that therapy should nurture the multiplicity and disorientation of psychological elements, producing people who could not maintain any consistent sense of identity but were this one minute and that the next. Far from this, Jung believed that despite the innate tendency for personal and archetypal characteristics to cluster into complex structures which appeared as distinct personalities, there was an equally strong, or, perhaps, stronger tendency for the psyche as a whole to hold all these elements in orbit around a single centre, the unifying presence of which is ideally experienced by the patient as overriding the identities of any of the smaller parts.

Jung called the sense of being 'one' in the face of continual disruptions and interruptions from the unconscious 'Self' and, despite diverse beliefs as to the subtle nature of the Self, this term is widely used by psychologists, psychiatrists and psychotherapists from different theoretical and practical fields to denote this 'sense of I' which remains regardless of the transient quality of internal or external circumstances.

But Jung's notion of the Self was more than 'a sense of I'. First, he proposed that as the ego is for the conscious, so the Self is for the unconscious. While the ego acts as the central point around which the feelings and actions of which we are conscious orbit, the Self provides the same centre for all those influences of which we are unaware. He described the Self as the 'most important and most central of archetypes'[26] with 'the significance of a ruler of the inner world' or of 'the collective unconscious.'[27] Whilst the ego keeps our conscious world of abstract thought and sensible impressions coherent, the Self, we hope, will organise the populace of our deepest mental canyons, it will stop us falling apart at the seams.

To complicate matters, Jung proposed that whilst the Self acts as a centre, it also represents the psyche as a whole, being both the centre and the circumference of the psychic circle and containing the conscious and, therefore, along with it the ego. As we cannot perceive anything but through the ego's faculties, it is, in fact, impossible to have a complete sense of Self because the parts cannot comprehend the whole. However, this sense of whole which accommodates but does not yield to the dominance of the parts was, for Jung, something that must nonetheless be forever strived for and is comparable to the Buddhist's search for Enlightenment or the Christian's search for God. Indeed, the search for the Self was, for Jung, as much a spiritual journey as it was a therapeutic procedure and, in recent years, Sheldon Kopp, in extending this idea, has described the psychotherapeutic process as a spiritual journey with great eloquence.[28] This journey represents our striving for wholeness and unity, the universal search for the true sense of who we are and the promise of a feeling of having found ourselves. Indeed, Jung at one point defined the Self as the 'God within us.'[29] The Self is a longed-for perspective, a place from which we will be able to see with an inner eye and perceive the order of things. Jung, in naming this centre the Self, admitted that it 'is no more than a psychological concept, a construct that serves to express an unknowable essence which we cannot grasp as such, since by definition it transcends our powers of comprehension'.[30]

Just as for Freud, his investigations led to a conflict between personal context and inherited patterns, so Jung arrived at conflict between the notion of multiplicity and that of a single cohering self. By 1959, when Jung was nearing the end of his life, he said that 'so far' he had 'found no stable or definite centre in the unconscious' and had come to believe that no such centre exists.[31] For Jung, the Self had become 'an ideal centre' representing humanity's 'dream of totality'.[32]

The Selves

In recent years this dream of totality, which remained central to Jung's psychotherapeutic practice, has been publicly questioned, challenged and dismantled by a number of renowned therapists working within the framework of Analytical Psychology, namely Joseph Redfearn, Michael Fordham and James Hillman. It would be wrong to imply that these therapists share an identical vision or even a common terminology, but underlying the linguistic complexities in which all of their work is couched there is a single fundamental revisioning of the notion of mental health. In this vision the dream of totality is substituted for a dream of multiplicity. In other words, the tendency for the constituting material of the psyche to fragment into partially autonomous units appearing as discreet personalities which impregnate the 'sense of I' is not viewed as pathological but as the natural and intended state of mental functioning. In this view the psyche is composed of many 'I's' or many selves which Fordham calls 'de-integrates', which Redfearn refers to as 'sub-personalities' and which Hillman refrains from naming in any consistent fashion. Common to all is the steering of the therapeutic process towards tolerance of multiplicity. Fordham, for example, says that 'any concept of mental health' must include acknowledgment of the fact that the psyche is 'a periodically unstable system' the growth of which 'must involve periodic experiences of disorder felt as dangerous or even chaotic'.[33] Redfearn, meanwhile, has continued the mission of establishing a polycentric vision of the psyche in which it is accepted as a factor of mental health that 'the basic feeling of unity and continuity and of being a person is subject to marked fluctuations and disruptions'[34] by which a person experiences himself or herself not as one person but as a different person at different times. Further to this, James Hillman's work not only redirects the psychotherapeutic procedure to tolerate multiplicity, he transforms such a goal into the code for a way of life, implying the futility of a search for any kind of exclusive centre. For Hillman, no individual can 'provide a norm even for himself'[35] because the psyche is deliberately structured by the grace of the gods 'to save the diversity and autonomy of the psyche from domination by any single power.'[36] Hillman, like Fordham and Redfearn stresses that the manifestation of multiplicity is not a sign of pathology, but asserts that 'because we have come to realize that each of us is normally a flux of figures, we no longer need to be menaced by the notion of multiple personality', such that 'I may see visions and hear voices' and 'I may talk with them and they with each other without at all being insane'.[37]

Hillman's reference to multiple personality, which, in many contexts, is perceived as a severe disorder, is a salient provocation which points to the actual clinical context of psychotherapy and is an issue over which the advocates of polycentricity, Hillman particularly, have been questioned and challenged.

Multiple Personality Disorder

Beyond the field of psychotherapy in the wards of psychiatric hospitals, and in the consulting rooms of psychiatrists and clinical psychologists, the notion of being composed of many selves still retains its pathological colouring and has implications of such a nature that any philosophy proposing to nurture such a model of health appears dangerous and morally irresponsible. Aldridge-Morris has published a review and study of people who have had a tendency to behave as different personalities to such a marked degree of differentiation that one does not remember what the other has done; many of these cases have involved criminal activity. In the USA, Multiple Personality Syndrome has been the source of considerably extensive investigation by lawyers and psychologists and Aldridge-Morris suggests that because of the lenient consideration with which the United States legal profession treats those diagnosed as mentally ill, intelligent criminals are potentially able to use the deliberate manifestation of multiplicity as a shield from execution or imprisonment.[38]

Hillman refrains from approaching the subjects of criminology, or extreme manifestations of multiplicity which cause pain and suffering to the withholder. Redfearn, on the other hand, has recognised that 'many destructive actions' seem to be performed as though 'the person is possessed by a violent sub-personality' or in a state of which he says afterwards 'I don't know what came over me'.[39] But even though Fordham and Redfearn have included clinical material from their own cases to support the process of tolerance towards multiplicity, there is still an epistemological fissure between the research of the various branches of Post-Jungian Psychology into a polycentric model of health and the implications of multiple personality in the field of psychiatry and the treatment of psychoses.

It should be pointed out, though, that those patients who select or who are referred for psychotherapy as their primary treatment tend not to be those whose 'little people' manifest themselves in behavioural tendencies with criminal or heavily anti-social consequences or who do not remember what one of their selves has done. In fact, one of the most common conditions which emerges in the course of psychotherapy is precisely the reverse: what we might call a monophrenia, a state in which a person becomes stifled by the dominating influence of a single aspect of his or her self. Redfearn himself says that 'if all one's sub-personalities were spread out like a map or landscape' there would be places 'which were often visited by the conscious "I" and others which would never have been visited' and many 'people are stuck in one role much of the time, especially if that role has paid dividends in the past'.[40]

It is here that Therapeutic Voicework can offer a primary contribution to psychotherapy for by facilitating a malleability of vocal timbre which can express a diversity of characteristics, we can facilitate expressively the journey through the selves of which Redfearn speaks.

However, it is also of vital importance that a Therapeutic Voiceworker appreciates that the diversity of voices, and, therefore, of self-experience, which Therapeutic Voicework can facilitate, makes it unsuitable for those with an unstable or poorly formed ego. In my view, a Therapeutic Voiceworker should, therefore, be able to recognise the signs of such a condition and should know exactly how to handle the necessary referral so that the client is treated with care and compassion.

A Post-Modern Jung

In the same way that the notion of a centralised psychic language has been undermined by Lacan, who has dismantled Freud's notion of a psyche orientated around a fixed structure as defined through linguistics, so the idea of an integrated or 'whole' self has been challenged by Hillman, Fordham and Redfearn. As Lacan moves Freud into the Post-modern arena through the application of a decentralised view of language similar to Derrida's, so a Post-modern dimension to Jung's work is introduced by Hillman, Fordham and Redfearn through the proposal of a model of the psyche which incorporates the freeplay and multiplicity of a number of identities or Selves. This progression away from a concern with centralisation through coherent narrative, transcendental signification and singular monocentric identity established by Freud and Jung, towards a polycentric view of the psyche based on the mobility of language and the multiplicity of identities constitutes a fundamental shift from a modern to a Post-modern aesthetic in contemporary psychotherapy, which reflects the epistemology of the present cultural position, for the dream of Post-modernism is a world without centre.

Active Imagination and Amplification

One of the primary clinical roles of a polycentric Analytical Psychology, such as that propounded by Hillman, Redfearn and Fordham, has been to entice the patient's sense of 'I' to embark upon a journey through which it may temporarily identify with the various free-floating images of the unconscious. This brings the patient in close relation to the actor, playing different roles, all of which manifest different aspects of the person he or she is – aspects which are so diverse that many of them appear to be incompatible or even mutually exclusive. Moreover, whilst a polycentric psychology may differ from Jung's original vision by way of its shift of emphasis from wholeness to decentralisation, each remains faithful to Jung's practical approach to encouraging the unconscious images to be admitted into consciousness.

Whilst the mainstream of Analytical Psychology in Europe and the USA remains committed to an essentially verbal strategy, there has been a complimentary development of more practical and creative applications of Jung's vision within other artistically-orientated therapeutic practices, of which dramatherapy, dance movement therapy, art therapy and music therapy remain the most significant and which I will later investigate. Despite their differences, these four major artistic therapies all have one fundamental principle and practical procedure in common: they seek to invite and admit unconscious contents into consciousness through an artistic medium. The contents may be dream images, personal memories, generalised compounds of feeling and mood, characters, caricatures, animals and symbols of different kinds. Regardless of their shape and form, these contents, which gain expression through the dramatic scene, through kinetic gesture, through melody and pitch or through colour and shape, are all emblems, icons or representative expressions of different aspects of the Self. My proposition is that Therapeutic Voicework can facilitate the same process, where the medium of expression is the acoustic emission of the human voice.

This process of expressing the Self and its contents through a variety of media is not a post-Jungian phenomenon. In fact, it was pioneered by Jung and he called it 'active imagination'. Andrew Samuels succinctly describes active imagination as 'a channel' for 'messages' from 'the unconscious by any means', such as painting, sculpturing or writing. Furthermore, 'these products are not viewed aesthetically but valued for the information they contain'[41] about the deeper strata of the psyche. This absence of aesthetic judgment in active imagination may constitute that which is the fundamental difference between the arts and the arts therapies. In therapy the client's acting, dancing, painting or musical rendition is not passively witnessed or judged according to the degree to which it entertains, inspires or demonstrates a formal virtuosity but is actively nurtured to honestly convey the deeper influences, fears, concerns and preoccupations which usually remain hidden behind the histrionics of day-to-day expressive communication. The emphasis, then, is not on the product – painting, dance, score or play – but on the process.

In Jung's practice, active imagination was intricately connected to another vitally important process which he called 'amplification'. For Jung, although the images which emerged from the patient's psyche were considered to be partly collective or archetypal, in the therapeutic session they tended to be perceived by the patient as largely personal, the ramification of a particular problem. Therefore, Jung needed a process by which to make the transition from the saturation of personal associations which an image held to the point where the patient realised that the image and problem or dynamic therein represented was, in fact, a typical or archetypical one. This process was what Jung called amplification.

For example, a patient may begin speaking about feeling insecure, fragile, lost and frightened but the therapist asks for an image which captures such a feeling. The patient describes a dream she had about being only eight years old and running through a dense dark wood in which the trees towered above her and appeared to speak with their rustling leaves. The therapist asks what she was frightened of and the patient says that she felt as though she was being pursued by a threatening animal. When the therapist asks why the girl cannot escape, the patient replies that the animal is too clever and that in the dream it felt as if the animal was everywhere but that she couldn't identify it. The therapist now amplifies this personal network of images by comparing it to the widely known fairy-tale of Little Red Riding Hood who is threatened by the wolf but does not recognise him due to his disguise. The image of the wolf echoes with significance in the patient and she elaborates on her feelings to the point of recognising that she relates to men as though they were wolves 'hot on her tail', disguising themselves in sheep's clothing and waiting to pounce. The therapist now begins to introduce motifs from other fairy-tales or myths in which a woman is pursued by an animal until what began as a personal admission becomes a journey of discovery amongst the world-wide myths and stories which provide exemplifications of the way women experience men's pursuit.

But the point of amplification is not simply to make the patient feel better in the knowledge that she is not the only one. Rather, it is to discover a means of overcoming the fear of threat by learning from the images contained in stories of a universal significance. For example, in many stories and myths where someone is threatened by an awesome creature, the victim overcomes not by violence or retreat but by cunning, as in the case of Oedipus who defeats the Sphinx by answering her riddle or the children's character Brer Rabbit who continually defeats the fox through cantankerous plots. The story of a fearful victim overcoming threat through cunning, intelligence, wit and skillful manipulation of the circumstances has been, and still remains, a universally popular archetypal idea in all cultures. Now the patient recognises that the wolf in Little Red Riding Hood is also very cunning and therefore will take some beating and she further refers to men as being cunning and difficult to ward off. But the therapist points out that the animal in her dream and the wolf in the fairy tale are also parts of her because everything we dream is not only a representation of our perception of something outside of ourselves but also a manifestation of a part of our inner life. So now the patient recognises that she too is the pursuing animal, the wolf, and is able to locate potentialities in herself that compare to the qualities of the victor, as opposed to the victim. In the course of this mythical seminar the therapist introduces the Greek goddess Artemis, 'Lady of the Wild Things', who lived in the forests forever chaste and with the power to hunt and tame the most ferocious of beasts. But Artemis was also protector of young nymphs and had a maternal sovereignty – one, however, that was needless of paternal intervention. The patient now begins to relate herself to the qualities of Artemis and considers how she has distanced herself from seeking relationships with both men and women and has become quite frightened at the prospect of intimacy. However, as a result of such recognition, over a period of time, the patient is able to visit parts of herself that have been hitherto ignored and incorporate them into her life and perception of herself.

Hillman states that to effect active imagination the practitioner needs to focus not on words as concepts but on words as images.[42] This approach pays no heed to the grammatical, syntactical or narrative context in which the patient couches the words, but instead expands them to take into consideration 'the full extension of any word, all its meanings and possibilities' and 'any context in which the word occurs'.[43] This means that the image of a girl being chased by a wolf may be seen as containing multiple notions. The morpheme 'wolf' appears also in the term 'wolfing it down', describing ravenous and frantic eating. The word 'chased' also occurs in association with the notion of ingestion, for we talk of 'a chaser', an alcoholic spirit which we 'chase' down and, perhaps, underlying the girl's fear of the wolf is the idea that it will ingest, devour and chase her down his own gullet. But the sound of the word 'chased' is also equivalent with that of 'chaste', signifying an abstinence from sex, and the image of running from the wolf may be expanded to incorporate the notion of virginity and innocence or of fear of being raped.

This process of reading the patient's words involves an imagistic perception which liberates the parts of speech 'from their narrational obligations which link them into time sequences for storytelling. The imagistic view of words frees them from having to submit to logical reason and operational definition.'[44] For Hillman, the image of the wolf may also contain the residual experiences of all those 'wolfy' people the patient has known, all those chased and chaste experiences which are not translatable into conceptual and definitive concepts or memories but which simply remain as images. It is a transformation of the discursive nature of words into a non-discursive mode of reading them. The purpose of Hillman's non-narrative and ontological perception is not to tie the image down to a single meaning but to tolerate and entertain the 'unfathomable analogical richness of the image'.[45] For him, the dream, the poem or the painting is a Post-modern phenomenon, 'which is not about anything, not even about the poet or the painter'. The painted lemons on the plate need not refer to any actual lemons but 'may analogize with and evoke all sorts of lemony experiences'. By the same token, 'the lemon in the dream' need not 'posit an objective psyche to which the lemon refers and from which it is a message' for 'the psyche is there in the lemon, located nowhere else than in the actual presented image'.[46]

The primary strategy by which Hillman and Jung facilitated active imagination and amplification was verbal discourse, though Jung did incorporate other forms of expression and encouraged patients to employ artistic media

to assist in the process. One of the aims of the arts therapies is to make participation in creative activity the cardinal means by which active imagination
and amplification can be achieved. Dance and bodily movement, painting,
dramatic role-playing and musical improvisation can and are all used to give
amplified, active and imaginative expression to inner psychic contents. In my
view, Therapeutic Voicework can also be effectively used to enable the clients
to embody and acoustically express the sub-personalities or aspects of
themselves which are pertinent to the psychotherapeutic process.

Therapeutic Voicework Methodology: Vocal Amplification and Active Imagination

From my early investigations I began to discover that the vocal channel is
capable of giving the shape of an acoustic image to all psychic contents and
that the process of amplification and active imagination could be applied
vocally.

Integral to this process was the use of what I have named 'Vocal Amplification and Active Imagination', a process by which the practitioner helps the
client take a personal image, expressed physically and vocally in their pedestrian behaviour, and amplify it to mythical proportion, but without losing its
individuality.

Hillman's paradigm departs from Jung's not only by way of its polycentricity and insistence on non-conceptual and non-referential relationships
between word and concept but by its intention to 'make specific', as opposed
to 'make typical'. In Jung's work the process of amplification sought, in a
sense, to generalise the patient's images in order to arrive at the archetypal
roots. The particular individual wolf became the archetype of the wolf, wolf-
ness. Hillman, on the other hand, uses the therapeutic dialogue to make the
wolf more distinctly idiosyncratic, more specific and more precisely emblematic of the withholder's unique conception of it. What sort of eyes? What sort
of fur? How fast is it running? How does it prowl, sit turn and look? How
does it feel, smell and sound? For Hillman, 'images that are generalised and
conventionalized' suffer from having 'had their characteristic peculiarity
erased'[47] which needs to be returned because 'the more precision, the more
actual insight'.[48]

For example, to continue with the the wolf imagery we may imagine that
the client, in the course of the Therapeutic Voicework session, makes a sound
that appears to the practitioner and to the client wolf-like, it has a howling to
it. The aim of the Therapeutic Voicework process is not to amplify towards

generalisation but to request of the client that it becomes a wolf, *her* wolf, with its particular teeth, legs, glistening eyes and gnashing jaw, expressed through a particular quality of voice that is entirely her own. The client repeats the sound over and over until it assumes a personalised precision, an imagistic eloquence. The client is on all fours, the head turns with a languid fluidity, the eyes blink slowly and catastrophically and a sound emerges, seemingly from somewhere deep in the client's body, that is undeniably rooted in a sensible and somatic embodiment of the image of wolf and all it means to her.

In the methodological approach to Therapeutic Voicework which I have developed, the practitioner enables the client to locate her vocalisation and physicalisation in an actively imagined and amplified framework by reflecting back images which appear to be present and by asking the client to further embody them. For example, the therapist asks the client to sing, without effort or tension, without demonstration or histrionics. She sings as herself. The patient utters first this note, then that, ascending and descending a scale in which the practitioner can hear or imagines she can hear distinct qualities. For the practitioner, the sound may appear genial and tender with a wispy emission of free air; the higher the pitch the more gentle, soft and unassertive it becomes. It has a girlish frivolity and fragile delicacy to it. The practitioner can see that the client is swaying slightly from side to side and has an ingenuous expression on her face that seems to enhance the innocence of the sound. The Therapeutic Voiceworker asks the client to exaggerate the swaying, as though she were on a swing, and to increase the childlike quality of the voice, as though she were only eight years old. The client begins to enter into the embodiment of this image and the Therapeutic Voiceworker leads the client's pitch up the scale into a higher octave to assist in excavating and refining a sonic and authentic neonatal and infantile image. As the notes begin to get higher, and more difficult to sing, the client contorts the face and clenches her fists, which serves to bring to the quality of the sound a degree of raucous and commotion, as though the baby were having a tantrum. The practitioner asks the client to sing as though the baby were spoilt, irritable, incensed and protesting and, as a result, the indignant spectacle becomes more animated and multiphonic. The client opens and closes her fists and stamps on the ground. Her voice increases considerably in volume and height on the pitch scale and sears through the studio like a siren.

In order to facilitate the sensible experience and personification of the instinctive, natal and primal quality which is emerging, the client moves to a position on all fours and dances the back and shoulders in an undulating ripple of waves as the Therapeutic Voiceworker asks the client to imagine that she howls as though from the abdomen and that the sound resonates inside her belly which is lined with white gold. The sound now assumes a canine quality like that of a howling wolf. The practitioner asks the client to imagine that her hackles are up and that she howls a warning and protecting shield of sound around her cubs which lay curled beneath her belly. The pitch descends and the sound becomes guttural and marauding and echoes as though in a cave. In the deeper pitches the sound is wolf-like; in the higher pitches it is feline; in the middle there is an ambiguous animalistic quality, half wolf, half cat, like a beast from a beguiling world of creatures concocted from an amalgam of animal instincts.

The practitioner, having paid passive attention to the client's tendency to open and close the fists during this vocal dance, now asks the client to develop this movement as though she were a creature extending and retracting her claws in preparation for a fight. At the same time, she is asked to decrease the volume of the sound and to sing with an alluring, tantalising and ravenous tone, part lion, part Siamese kitten, part wolf. As the client sings, the Therapeutic Voiceworker continues to suggest tonal images: feline, predatory, devouring, spiteful, provocative, protective. The creature has offspring and is prowling around her young. She spits, with venom, with foreboding and intimidation. Her voice is made of acid, it is caustic, ungracious and scathing.

The practitioner now influences the melodic direction of the sounds by singing different notes. As the vocal dance assumes a more formal structure, the sounds become humanised, without losing their arresting and compelling intensity. The client stands and the therapist suggests the image of a gigantic Parisian chain-smoking animal trainer with six children who wears furs and bellows and bawls. The client's voice becomes darkly enfolding, which the practitioner amplifies by suggesting a collage of images: mouth full of caviar, a voice like molasses or tar, an attitude of belligerent certainty. The voice is that of a prolific and world-famous Parisian lion tamer. A new character emerges and the studio now thunders with the voice of 'Madam Felineou'. The client now struts around the studio singing improvised arias on the words 'I am Madam Felineou', like a prima donna. She mimes smoking with a cigarette holder. Her whole face has altered radically from the attitude it expressed at the beginning of the session and any visible or vocal signs of innocence and vulnerability have long since receded. The voice and physicality of the client is dominant, proud and unnerving.

The Therapeutic Voiceworker watches the movements of the arm, which mime the backwards and forwards motion of putting cigarette to mouth, and asks the client to magnify and inflate it. It now becomes the whip that spurs the horses and the client is now driving a chariot away from the circus into the forest. The voice now takes on a hot-blooded, ambitious and barbarous tone. The practitioner encourages this transformation by suggesting tonal images: Boadicea, the wild woman of the forest, revengeful war cry, leading the warriors into battle, rounding up a tribal mass of agitated protesters. The client's voice and body is now involved in an opera of blood-curdling melody, as though the studio were full with an army of female revolters.

The client is becoming tired and the Therapeutic Voiceworker slows down the pace through gentle instruction. The dead lay scattered and the wild woman now feels sorrow for the victims. The voice returns to a higher pitch and whimpers. The Therapeutic Voiceworker suggests tonal images: pangs of regret, mourning and melancholy, a prayer for the dying and a contemplative chant on the futility of war. The client now stands swaying, as she was at the beginning of the session, and the Therapeutic Voiceworker asks her to blend in different aspects of the acoustic journey into a single tone. The irritable child, the vulnerable kitten, the howling wolf, the wild woman of the forest, Madam Felineou, the unbridled warrior and compassionate mourner become less separate and distinct voices and more aspects audible in a single tone. The voice sounds and feels to the practitioner and client that it belongs to her. But it is multi-faceted, embracing and containing a spectrum of images any one or combination of which could emerge as the dominant factor at any time.

The process from the child image through the wolf image to the image of Madam Felineou, through the warrior to the compassionate mourner is a slow one in which every stage of the transformation is fleshed out, filled in, satiated and made specific through precise alterations in phonational quality and kinetic gesture. For example, from wolf to wolf-dog and then to wolf-cat, from wolf-cat to cat and from cat to cat-woman and, finally, from cat-woman to the cat-like woman Madam Felineou. This has nothing to do with the generalised mimicry of putting on different voices, such as that heard in pastiche cabaret, and when the vocalist succumbs to the superficial option of mimicry, not only the attuned therapist and the client but anyone else who may be present in a group session can hear it.

The professional practitioner must help to amplify, embellish, fertilise, enrich and refine the timbral qualities which are present in the voice but must not generalise and abstract all detail. He must remain attentive to specifics, what Hillman calls 'sticking to the image'.[49] Furthermore, the practitioner must not be influenced by his own modalities or imagistic preoccupations. He must not trespass eagerly forward according to his own tastes. He must not adorn and decorate through suggestions which emanate from the prejudice of his own ears. The images supplied by the therapist must originate in the acoustic information supplied by the client and must be amplified to embody images of a genuine significance, culturally and personally, and not to reflect the widespread social stereotypes to which modern men and women have become prey. This requires of the practitioner an intimate and well-tested exploration of his own psyche.

The issue of training in this field of working with image is, therefore, as Hillman has pointed out, a contentious one. There is no training process which will guarantee the client freedom from the therapist's projection of his preoccupations. Neither is there a training that will ensure that the therapist is able to respond extensively and analytically to what he hears in the client's voice. The therapist must do nothing less than put all his effort into increasing the reservoir of images from which to draw in the process of nurturing a voice. Films, books, plays, music, songs, paintings, dreams, myth — everywhere there are images there is important food for the artistically- and therapeutically-orientated practitioner.

Alfred Wolfsohn and the Sounds of Psyche

The idea that the human voice might render psychic contents audible was first discovered and investigated by one of the most significant pioneers in the field of vocal experimentation, whose story is little told and whose work is known of only within certain circles. His name is Alfred Wolfsohn.

In 1959 Paul Moses, to whom I referred earlier, came to London as a delegate at the The London World Voice Conference, an interdisciplinary forum at which a singing teacher called Alfred Wolfsohn gave a pioneering presentation. Paul Moses, respected in many fields for his work on the psychodynamics of the voice and yet still in search of the practical representation of his ideas on singing, saw in this presentation the practical confirmation of all that he had formulated in theory. Later, Moses wrote to Wolfsohn acknowledging him as 'one of the greatest experts in problems of the human voice in the world' whose achievements he considered to 'encompass entirely new areas of expression and communication'.[50]

Alfred Wolfsohn was born in Berlin of Jewish descent in 1896 and at the outbreak of the First World War he was called to serve as a medic in the front-line trenches, during which time he became both horrified and fascinated by the incredible sounds which the adverse conditions and suffering prompted from the voices of dying and wounded soldiers. He was thus led to ask: 'how can a human voice utter such a sound, a voice in extremis'.[51] Like thousands of others, Wolfsohn returned from the war in a state of mental disturbance and was classified as suffering from 'war neurosis' or 'shell-shock' — terms which he resented as he felt that they deprecated and minimised the severe experiences which he and his comrades had suffered. During the year following the war his illness worsened and he became plagued by aural hallucinations of the extreme vocal sounds which he had heard in the trenches. His inner world became bombarded with a minefield of sounds which recalled the cacophony of the front line. At the centre of this hallucinated landscape of sound were the pleading screams and groans of the dying. Wolfsohn became convinced that his illness arose from an intense feeling of guilt at having denied help to a dying comrade and the voices continued to sound in his mind despite prolonged psychiatric treatment. He felt, therefore, that there was no choice but to search for his cure in himself.

Through constant and painful contemplation of his own mental state, Wolfsohn became convinced that if he could actually sing the sounds that haunted his mind, he would be able to bring about a cathartic release of the unabreacted emotion of terror and guilt associated with the voices and, by so doing, silence them.

In extending the range of his voice and holding in mind the extreme emotive sounds he had heard in the trenches, he realised that his voice could express an extensive collage of emotions, moods and characters which embraced not only the dark and agonising sounds of suffering but those of the utmost joy and pleasure. As a result of vocal catharsis, not only did he cure his illness but he became convinced that 'there exists a universal human voice of much broader circumference than has hitherto been imagined'.[52]

In 1933 a renowned Jewish opera singer and teacher, Paula Salomon-Lindberg, gave Wolfsohn a job teaching teaching singing to some of her younger students, which enabled Wolfsohn to embark on the process of passing on to others the results of his own investigations. One of the students who attended his classes in these early years had been a patient of Jungian psychotherapy prior to working vocally with Wolfsohn and recorded that 'the road taken' towards the development of her voice which she underwent when working with Wolfsohn 'was similar to that taken in following the psychology of Jung', where 'the singer penetrates deeper and deeper into the depths of his body and so arrives at the new, unknown sound of his voice, to which he listens as to a strange voice'.[53] Around fifteen years later Wolfsohn acknowledged the importance of his encounter with this student in contributing to his belief that his approach to working with the human voice 'ran parallel to the basic principles of psychotherapy'.[54]

In 1939 Wolfsohn escaped Germany and fled to London. When the war was over he gathered a fresh set of students and began teaching his work from a small studio in Golders Green, where he achieved the practical realisation of his vision. Through consistent and in-depth work, Wolfsohn enabled his pupils to exceed the boundaries of vocal expression as hitherto believed. Wolfsohn's intention was not to nurture the diligence and technical proficiency of the 'voice beautiful' but to utilise the potential range of the human voice as a probe and a mirror, investigating and reflecting the many aspects of the human psyche. Therefore, those who took lessons with him committed themselves not only to a thorough psycho-archeology of their psyche but to the process of acquiring the courage and the ability to express the many aspects of themselves through the voice.

Wolfsohn was particularly inspired by Jung's views on the collective nature of psychic experience, which enabled him to consider that the sounds that he had heard and the pain he had endured were not his own but those of humankind. However, whilst Jung was preoccupied with the pictorial expression of archetypal motifs in dreams, Wolfsohn felt he had discovered a way of making them audible through the sounds of the human voice. Wolfsohn proposed that the dream forms the foundation, the constituting material, for all art of every form and that 'art is the possibility to dream and to be able to fashion one's dreams'.[55] An important part of Wolfsohn's work, therefore, involved a translation of visual dream-images into sound and his pupils were asked to record and recount their dreams throughout their training for he believed that 'every human being has the capacity to sing, just as everybody is given the ability to dream in waking and in sleeping'.[56]

Wolfsohn had become particularly interested in an archetype which Jung called 'the shadow' and which represents the 'dark side' of our personality, that which we would never wish to become and which personifies everything that the subject refuses to acknowledge about himself'.[57] The shadow is present in every aspect of human life because nothing can be brought to light without casting a shadow.[58] Everyone has a personal shadow, an image of themselves which they hate to become or parts of themselves which they know stem from their dark or unsophisticated and undeveloped side. But the shadow is also an archetype, embodying the dark or primitive side of humanity as a whole. For Jung, one of the definitive and universal aspects of the shadow is its animalistic quality, being the sum total of those aspects of our psyche which preserve the residue of an earlier time in the evolutionary process, a time when the distinction between humanity and animality was not so great.[59] By shadow, Jung meant 'the inferior personality, the lowest levels of which are indistinguishable from the instinctuality of an animal.'[60] It has been said that the dangerous, disorderly, fugitive, distasteful, sensual, stupid and unspiritual nature of the shadow reflects precisely the nature of the genes.[61] Concerned only with securing the survival of the organism into the next generation of its species, the genes are a biological realisation of the ultimate shadow. If this is so, then the shadow may be perceived as something entirely integral to our being human.

The psychological concept of the shadow corresponds to the aesthetic concept of ugliness. Wolfsohn recognised that if the voice was to be employed as an expression of the true nature of the psyche in its entirety, it would have to establish a connection with the shadow. This meant that the voice had to be permitted to yell, scream and sob and give voice to the animalistic, primal, preverbal utterances which are part of the rightful expression of the shadow. Wolfsohn's psychologised approach to singing training thus led to the 'spontaneous emergence' of an 'extraordinary variety' of animal sounds 'which had a very special meaning for each pupil' as though 'a deeper strata of a past evolutionary process had been touched upon and was being relived'.[62] For his pupils, 'this was a far cry from singing beautifully. In the beginning it was a squeaking and a squeezing, a screaming and a peeping; and out of this developed a different kind of beauty'.[63] From this process 'something emerged that was not only beautiful, it was authentic, and this authenticity was nurtured, polished and repeated until the ear got accustomed to it'.[64]

Continuing in this vein, use of the voice to give expression to the shadow, particularly through the empathic utterance of animal sounds, has been further investigated by Noah Pikes – a long-standing member of the Roy Hart Theatre, which was born from Wolfsohn's research. Opposing the heavenly sounds of the church, Pikes draws attention to the hell of Dante, which the poet describes as a place full of terrible noises and, equating these noises with the inner hell of the shadow, Pikes seeks to relieve their pressure upon the psyche by allowing them to be voiced.[65] This serves the search for what he calls the 'whole voice', which 'can reveal inner dissonances, imbalances and the roots of duality and can thereby effect liberation and healing'.[66] Such a journey, which Wolfsohn initiated, 'is less a means to an end than it is the way and aim in one; namely to discover, hear and appreciate moods and vibrations, emotions and sensations, impressions and expressions. It is to bridge the mind and body, spirit and instinct, the re-animation of the tonalities and tonicity of one's own personality; the meeting with one's self'.[67]

Wolfsohn was keen to systematically oppose the tradition of specialisation upon which classical singing had been founded and which allotted certain qualities according to gender – soprano, mezzo-soprano and contralto for women and tenor, baritone and bass for men – considering it an unnecessary way of artificially restraining the voice.[68]

Wolfsohn thus challenged the popular preconceptions regarding the expressive limits implied and imposed by human gender and drew further support from Jung and the latter's belief in the existence of the archetypes anima and animus. Jung proposed that a man 'has in him a feminine side, an unconscious feminine figure' of which 'he is generally quite unaware', which he called the 'anima', and its counterpart, which is the male figure in a woman he called the 'animus'.[69] Wolfsohn further conceived of the idea that the anima and animus, in their contra-sexual aspects, were potentially audible through the human voice and believed that by giving a voice to the anima or animus they could be projected into sound, confronted audibly and aurally and, finally, accepted and integrated into consciousness. Thus he nurtured a bass voice in women and a soprano voice in men.

Many people became suspicious, not only that Wolfsohn's approach was 'unnatural' but that he was causing damage to his pupils' vocal apparatus. In order to assuage these fears, some of the pupils had their voices subjected to scientific measurement whilst producing their extended range. Among these students was a young woman called Jenny Johnson, who, in 1955, had her voice examined by Professor Luchsinger of the Zurich Otolaryngological Clinic using X-ray, high-speed film and a stroboscope. This examination confirmed a range of six octaves and discovered no abnormality in the anatomical structure or physiological functioning of the larynx.[70] Luchsinger's discoveries corroborated Wolfsohn's deepest belief that the range of the voice depended not on any exceptional physical virtuosity or on an unnatural or maladjusted anatomy but on psychological investigation of the deepest regions of the psyche. He declared: 'physical training only plays a secondary role in my work with students, the main task is a psychological one' for he believed that 'the range, strength and timbre of the voice' are determined 'solely by emotional factors.' For 'nobody will dispute the fact that the human voice can lose in range, power and tone-colour as a result of particular emotional events'. 'Why,' Wolfsohn asked, 'are there then doubts about the voice being capable in exactly the same way of taking advantage of another set of emotional circumstances?'[71]

In order to demonstrate his achievements to a wider audience, Wolfsohn and Jenny Johnson gave a demonstration in Paris to the psychotherapist Dr Eric Weiser, which was then reported in the Swiss Newspaper *Die Weltwoche* in an article entitled 'The Unchained Voice'. At this demonstration, Weiser claimed to have heard Jenny Johnson display a range in excess of eight octaves, from the 'impossibly high notes of a colouratura soprano' to 'a full, deep male voice', a range which incorporated 'both the male and the female ranges', enabling her to 'sing all the parts of the *Magic Flute*, from the colouratura soprano role of the Queen of the Night right the way down to Sarastro's bass'. Weiser described 'the psychic relationship between Wolfsohn and his students' as not easily definable 'using the normal psychological terms' but alleged that 'suggestion and psychoanalysis undoubtedly play an important role'. However, Weiser felt that 'Alfred Wolfsohn's profound knowledge of the connections between body and soul' were 'the hard-worn harvest of a long and painful journey: the trenches of two world wars, wounding and years of illness, persecution in Berlin, escape to London, and later – a new beginning'.[72]

Wolfsohn claimed to have found that 'each individual is variously prey to a whole host of psychic inhibitions and conflicts, anxieties and complexes, the elimination of which leads to the opening out of the personality and the voice'. By helping his students to 'overcome their inner tensions and difficulties', Wolfsohn was able to 'loosen the inhibitions' which held their 'personalities as well as their voices in chains'.[73]

Wolfsohn wrote to Jung early in 1955 enclosing manuscripts which described his work, but on 3 May 1955 Aniela Jaffe wrote back to say that Jung himself would not be able to take note of his investigations. This was a great blow to Wolfsohn, who felt that he may never get his work formally appreciated in more established circles. However, the psychotherapeutic benefits of singing and sound making under Wolfsohn's direction are preserved in the testimony of many of his students who are still living, some of whom are themselves still teaching the work which he pioneered.[74]

When Wolfsohn died, the direction of his work, and the leadership of the group which had grown up under him, was taken over by an actor called Roy Hart, who had worked with Wolfsohn for over fifteen years. What had begun as a therapeutic investigation with performance dimensions now became a theatrical investigation with therapeutic implications as Roy Hart began to steer the work towards presentations of experimental vocal performances. It was from this transition that the Roy Hart Theatre was born. Among those who trained with Roy Hart, and who has brought the work initiated by Wolfsohn into a Post-modern Archetypal Framework, is Enrique Pardo.

The Hillman and Pardo Collaboration

Since the mid-1980s, Enrique Pardo, James Hillman and Paul Kugler have taken part in a number of projects which have sought to look at the use of theatre to sensibly generate image. Pardo's specific contribution, both to the theatrical application of voice and to the psychological understanding of image, lies in his experiments to show in action how images of audible integrity and emotive density can convey meaning to an audience through the non-verbal channel of vocal sound and the non-demonstrative movements of the body. Applying Hillman's view of a polycentric psyche to an extensive malleability of the human voice which he achieved through his training with Roy Hart, Pardo utilises a dance of vocal sound to paint images in space which, to an audience, resound with an uncanny recognisability and yet defy reduction to a linguistic or otherwise codified schema. In one of Pardo's performances, entitled *Hymn to Pan*, one reviewer said that he had shown how one can use an extended vocal range to create 'a mythological and poetic language'[75] which consisted of using the singing voice, taken in its broadest sense to include the ugly and the beautiful, to 'embody' the images of the psyche. For Pardo, 'image at this level means personified archetypes, creatures, characters, elements'. For Pardo, they are not visual images but 'vocal images' which conjure ideas such as 'the screeching witch, the fat dirty baritone, a laser-beam tenor, a broken-motor sound, a multiphonic ghost, a high-alto laughing hysteric, a feeble hermaphroditic soprano, an inhuman robot, a cracking rock.'[76]

This embodiment of psychic contents through the voice often involves a direct parallel to the process of amplification and active imagination as conceived by Jung, except where the medium of expression is vocal rather than verbal. Moreover, the work of Pardo and Hillman reminds us that there is a distinctly theatrical and artistic dimension to such a process.

Therapeutic Voicework Case Study: Blind Bats and Tantrums

Up to the age of ten, Sally had led a so-called normal childhood, then, shortly after her tenth birthday, she walked into a stone pillar at her local church, where she had attended service with her mother.

Over the next few years Sally bumped into objects with increasing frequency and found that when indoors, particularly in poorly-lit places, her vision was somewhat impaired and at school she had to strain to see to read and write. The doctors whom Sally visited were unable to provide any definitive diagnosis for this slow deterioration of her eye sight but told her that she should be prepared for an eventual total loss of vision. Sally later discovered that she had a form of retinitus pigmentosa.

When Sally became adolescent, she noticed that, unlike the other girls with whom she mixed, she was not developing breasts, neither was she menstruating. Sally needed to talk to someone about this but was isolated by the fact that neither her mother nor her father were particularly liberal speakers but, instead, tended to keep things 'brushed under the carpet' and 'in the dark'. The subject of Sally's blindness was hardly ever mentioned and the parents attempted to pretend that everything was 'normal'.

When Sally finally approached her mother on the subject of her hormonal development, her mother briefly said that she should not worry and that many girls were 'late developers'. However, when Sally reached sixteen years of age, she still had not developed any breasts, neither was she menstruating, so she went to the doctor with a fresh problem.

Sally's mother had accompanied her to all her doctor's appointments and Sally had often 'sat dumb' during the consultations. The doctor now said that the visual impairment and the hormonal problem were probably related and there followed several months of hospital tests. In addition to these problems, Sally had stopped growing in height after the age of fourteen and she remained a slight four foot eight inches. Eventually, Sally was given drugs to encourage the growth of her breasts and to increase her height by several inches, but nothing was done to enable her menstruation.

After leaving school, Sally's father persuaded a friend to give Sally a job in a supermarket, he also opened for Sally a bank account in his name and took charge of all her finances. He was very protective towards her and both he and Sally's mother discouraged her from pursuing any social life for fear she would be ridiculed or shamed.

By the time Sally was nineteen she was completely blind. One evening her boss at the supermarket went 'behind her back' to see her parents and to establish the fact that Sally would have to leave her job. She has not worked since.

Sally was thirty-four when she came to work on her voice. In singing or extended vocalisation, Sally's voice was confined to an exceedingly high pitch range and easily produced an extremely loud high-powered piercing scream in the whistle register Π̂ W. Her speaking voice, meanwhile, was very quiet with lots of free air and hardly any force of glottal attack and her vocal tract was narrowed into flute configuration >|< Π̲̂ |ɜ.

On asking Sally for associations for the two distinct voices, she described her speaking voice as that of 'a wispy little girl', which she hated, and her singing as 'horrible whiny screaming'. Indeed, for me, I associated her speaking voice with frail childlikeness and her singing with infantile rage.

A voice which to the client sounds childlike often acts as a manifestation of a psychological regression or return to childhood. In cases where childhood has been a happy time in which the parents nurtured and encouraged the child's expressive faculties, this regression could be based on a deep-set desire to return to this glorious infancy when a parental figure or figures were there to listen and respond to every need. In such cases this regression is often precipitated by a feeling of not being heard as an adult and is a retreat from the competitive nature of adult vocalisation or from the situation in which one's voice is not valued. In cases where expression has not been nurtured in youth but has rather been thwarted and stifled, the childlike voice may derive from the process of being psychologically propelled back to childhood by the recurrence of an event or series of events which revive the memory of this insensitivity – as though childhood has been thrust upon the person once again.

In Sally's case there was a combination of both of these reasons for regression at work. On the one hand her childhood had been a temptingly protective and satisfying time, where her every need had been taken care of by the parents who were scared to let Sally assume responsibility for the tasks befitting her age in case she should get hurt. But, on the other hand, she now recalled her childhood with a frustrated sense of irritation, recognising the fact that her parents had further contributed to the 'stunting of her growth' by their mollycoddling.

Unable to enjoy a visual appreciation of the way she looked based upon the feeding of her self-image with the aspects open to a sighted person, such as choice of clothes and hair-style, Sally relied upon the sound of her own voice to create an impression of who she was. But, because her voice was, for her, so steeped in childlike elements, her image of herself as a child had proven to be impossible to eliminate.

Furthermore, she had, it seemed, located the two aspects of her inner child in two distinct vocal timbres: the frail and over-protected soft speaking voice and the raging, screaming voice of the child that is not allowed the freedom she needs which came alive through her singing.

The aim of our work together was to assist in the overcoming of her regressive condition and bring vocal components to both her singing and her speaking which enabled her to hear herself and thus experience herself as an adult.

As she entered into Primate Position and opened the vocal tract into the clarinet configuration, her childlikeness took on a certain wild vagrancy and she said she felt like a 'mischievous monkey'. Having created a safe Spherical Space, she turned and twisted and became what she called the 'monkey thief' and then the 'conniving hairy ape boy' (Figure 8.1).

The image of herself as 'hairy' and a 'boy' was interesting and I asked her to develop both notions. In fact, she said that her hormonal difficulties had not hindered the growth of body hair and, with a bitter chuckle, she said she would 'rather have had the breasts and not the hair'.

Having enabled the vocal tract to open and lengthen into clarinet configuration, <>, I guided Sally down into Feline-canine position and her vocal tract formed saxophone configuration with a consequent change of timbre, (). In addition, the register of her voice now changed from falsetto to modal, F⫶M (Figure 8.2).

Guiding her back up through Primate and into the Homo Erectus, I asked her to allow the tube to return to flute configuration but to try and sustain the modal register. In addition, I suggested that she allow the hair to become the feathers or fur of a lady's expensive attire.

Sally now produced a vocal quality in flute, which, she said, sounded 'the opposite to childish', like 'a kind of very sophisticate old English aunt' (Figure 8.3). In order to bring some sense of solidity into the voice, which still seemed to be a little frail, I encouraged Sally to introduce the quality of violin entering into the Bird Position and I asked her to allow the image of the feathers to develop into a magnificent plumage (Figure 8.4). It was at this

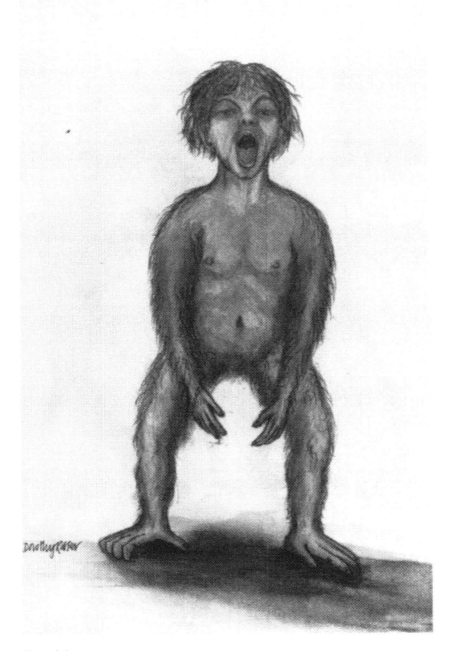

Figure 8.1

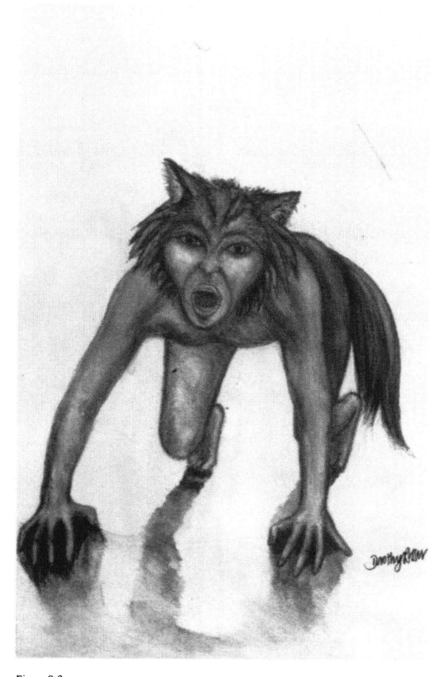

Figure 8.2

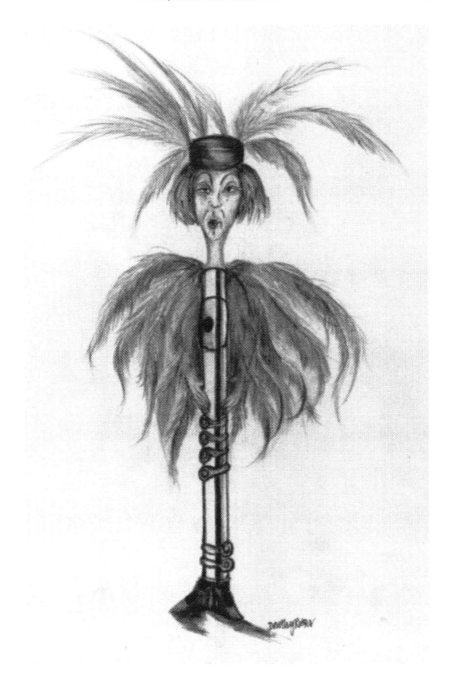

Figure 8.3

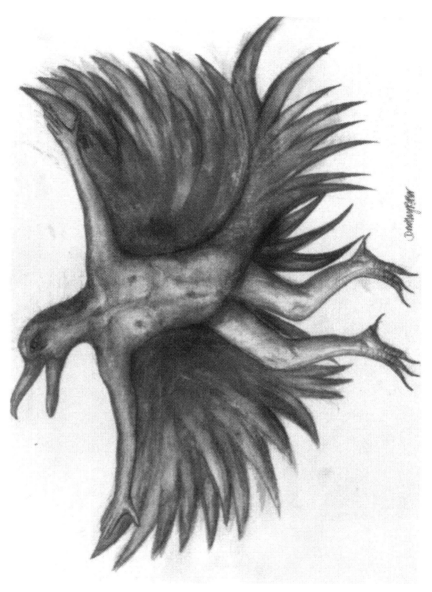

Figure 8.4

point that the most incredible alchemical transformation seemed to occur. The original raging irritability which we had both heard in the screaming whistle register, the frail free air sound which we had heard in her speaking voice, the modal saxophone quality which she had discovered in Feline-canine and the new quality of violin seemed to blend into a single sound, which, if someone had entered the room, they could easily have been mistaken for the sounds of an experienced contralto in rehearsal.

At the next session Sally reported a dream, which she had dreamed in the interim, in which a famous singer had fallen ill and was unable to give a scheduled performance and Sally was asked to replace her. However, when she appeared on stage the audience was composed entirely of children and Sally worried that they would not understand the language she was singing in. After we had done some preparatory work, I asked Sally to sing in this language of the dream singer and she began articulating a strange exotic tongue in an operatic-style voice with lots of vibrato. I then asked her to sing as the sick singer who had been unable to give the performance and she produced a timbre which was disrupted, low-pitched and quiet, 〰〰 ⨅. Then she stopped and realised that this was what her mother sounded like. Enlightened by this discovery, Sally played with going back and forth between the disrupted mother's voice and her newly-discovered singing voice, working with Free Phonetic Improvisation. I then asked Sally to sing as though performing for the children of the audience in the dream and she proceeded to sing a simple melody in the high-pitched, free air voice that I had originally heard her vocalise in.

Sally felt that she had never really grown up and that she had been expected to remain a child by a mother who really let her down when it came to engaging with her on issues of womanhood. Stranded upon a stage without being properly prepared, containing experience and speaking in a language too sophisticated for children, yet without adult friends or an adult audience to hear her, her childlike voice remained until she discovered that she could sing as a diva. Then, having discovered this new language of vocal strength and maturity, she felt somehow an adult in a children's world, for which she blamed her mother. Over the period of our work together we thus cultivated her strong singing voice, working on set pieces from opera as well as on pieces of her own writing. During this period much in Sally's environment changed and she eventually started a relationship with a partner. As her voice matured, so did her ability to express her adult needs and, more importantly, her ability to ensure that they were met.

Conclusion: Therapeutic Voicework as a Performing Art

The analytic and practical tenets introduced by Jung and developed by the post-Jungians provide an invaluable framework of analysis with which to understand what is happening during the expression of a broad canvas of vocal sound. Indeed, throughout the professional training in Therapeutic Voicework which I have designed, trainees are encouraged to locate the spontaneous vocal expression of mood, affect, character and image in a Jungian model. An archetypal perception of the voice is thus interwoven into the training for the RSA diploma in Voice Movement Therapy.

Whilst, theoretically, there are implicit parallels between the precepts of Analytical Psychology and Therapeutic Voicework, practically, the methodology of Therapeutic Voicework which I have developed has an overt artistic dimension more comparable to the relationship between a performer and a theatre director and deviser or musical conductor than that between a psychotherapy patient and a reflective witness. The nature of Therapeutic Voicework thus has a lot in common with the performing arts. In fact it is within the field of theatre that the most consistent practical experimentation and investigation of Therapeutic Voicework has been undertaken and it is to this field that I shall now turn my attention.

Notes

1   Freud, S. (1953–74) *Standard Edition of the Complete Psychological Works of Sigmund Freud*, vol. 2, James Strachey in collaboration with Anna Freud, assisted by Alix Strachey and Alan Tyson. London: Hogarth Press and the Institute of Psychoanalysis, p.132.

2   Frey-Rohn, L. (1990) *From Freud to Jung: A Comparative Psychology of the Unconscious*. Boston: Shambhala.

3   Jung, C.G. (1953) *The Collected Works of C G Jung, vol. 2* (Bollingen Series XX). H. Read, M. Fordham, G. Adler and Wm McGuire (eds). Princeton, New Jersey: Princeton University Press and London: Routledge and Kegan Paul, p.322.

4   Jung, C.G. (1953) *The Collected Works of C G Jung, vol. 8* (Bollingen Series XX). H. Read, M. Fordham, G. Adler and Wm McGuire (eds). Princeton, New Jersey: Princeton University Press and London: Routledge and Kegan Paul, p.322–26.

5   Jung, C.G. (1953) *The Collected Works of C G Jung, vol. 3* (Bollingen Series XX). H. Read, M. Fordham, G. Adler and Wm McGuire (eds). Princeton, New Jersey: Princeton University Press and London: Routledge and Kegan Paul, p.40.

6   Jung, C.G. (1953) *The Collected Works of C G Jung, vol. 3* (Bollingen Series XX). H. Read, M. Fordham, G. Adler and Wm McGuire (eds). Princeton, New Jersey: Princeton University Press and London: Routledge and Kegan Paul, p.81.

7   Jung, C.G. (1953) *The Collected Works of C G Jung, vol. 8* (Bollingen Series XX). H. Read, M. Fordham, G. Adler and Wm McGuire (eds). Princeton, New Jersey: Princeton University Press and London: Routledge and Kegan Paul, pp.97–8.

8   Jung, C.G. (1953) *The Collected Works of C G Jung, vol. 2* (Bollingen Series XX). H. Read, M.
     Fordham, G. Adler and Wm McGuire (eds). Princeton, New Jersey: Princeton University
     Press and London: Routledge and Kegan Paul, p.601.

9   Jung, C.G. (1953) *The Collected Works of C G Jung, vol. 3* (Bollingen Series XX). H. Read, M.
     Fordham, G. Adler and Wm McGuire (eds). Princeton, New Jersey: Princeton University
     Press and London: Routledge and Kegan Paul, p.240.

10   Jung, C.G. (1953) *The Collected Works of C G Jung, vol. 1* (Bollingen Series XX). H. Read, M.
     Fordham, G. Adler and Wm McGuire (eds). Princeton, New Jersey: Princeton University
     Press and London: Routledge and Kegan Paul, p.47.

11   Jung, C.G. (1953) *The Collected Works of C G Jung, vol. 3* (Bollingen Series XX). H. Read, M.
     Fordham, G. Adler and Wm McGuire (eds). Princeton, New Jersey: Princeton University
     Press and London: Routledge and Kegan Paul, p.95.

12   Jung, C.G. (1953) *The Collected Works of C G Jung, vol. 3* (Bollingen Series XX). H. Read, M.
     Fordham, G. Adler and Wm McGuire (eds). Princeton, New Jersey: Princeton University
     Press and London: Routledge and Kegan Paul, p.95.

13   Jung, C.G. (1953) *The Collected Works of C G Jung, vol. 3* (Bollingen Series XX). H. Read, M.
     Fordham, G. Adler and Wm McGuire (eds). Princeton, New Jersey: Princeton University
     Press and London: Routledge and Kegan Paul, p.95.

14   Milligan, S. (1968) *Nonsense Rhymes.* London: Puffin.

15   Syd Barrett, *Barrett* CD (Capitol Records).

16   Campbell, J. (1991) *The Masks of God: Primitive Mythology.* London: Arkana, p.31.

17   Jung, C.G. (1953) *The Collected Works of C G Jung, vol. 8* (Bollingen Series XX). H. Read, M.
     Fordham, G. Adler and Wm McGuire (eds). Princeton, New Jersey: Princeton University
     Press and London: Routledge and Kegan Paul, pp.133–134.

18   Jung, C.G. (1953) *The Collected Works of C G Jung, vol. 8* (Bollingen Series XX). H. Read, M.
     Fordham, G. Adler and Wm McGuire (eds). Princeton, New Jersey: Princeton University
     Press and London: Routledge and Kegan Paul, p.174.

19   Jung, C.G. (1953) *The Collected Works of C G Jung, vol. 7* (Bollingen Series XX). H. Read, M.
     Fordham, G. Adler and Wm McGuire (eds). Princeton, New Jersey: Princeton University
     Press and London: Routledge and Kegan Paul, p.201.

20   Jung, C.G. (1953) *The Collected Works of C G Jung, vol. 9, pt. 1* (Bollingen Series XX). H.
     Read, M. Fordham, G. Adler and Wm McGuire (eds). Princeton, New Jersey: Princeton
     University Press and London: Routledge and Kegan Paul, pp.75–84.

21   Jung, C.G. (1953) *The Collected Works of C G Jung, vol. 9, pt. 1* (Bollingen Series XX). H.
     Read, M. Fordham, G. Adler and Wm McGuire (eds). Princeton, New Jersey: Princeton
     University Press and London: Routledge and Kegan Paul, p.152.

22   Jung, C.G. (1953) *The Collected Works of C G Jung, vol. 9, pt. 1* (Bollingen Series XX). H.
     Read, M. Fordham, G. Adler and Wm McGuire (eds). Princeton, New Jersey: Princeton
     University Press and London: Routledge and Kegan Paul, p.183.

23   Jung, C.G. (1953) *The Collected Works of C G Jung, vol. 5* (Bollingen Series XX). H. Read, M.
     Fordham, G. Adler and Wm McGuire (eds). Princeton, New Jersey: Princeton University
     Press and London: Routledge and Kegan Paul, p.292.

24   Jung, C.G. (1953) *The Collected Works of C G Jung, vol. 7* (Bollingen Series XX). H. Read, M.
     Fordham, G. Adler and Wm McGuire (eds). Princeton, New Jersey: Princeton University
     Press and London: Routledge and Kegan Paul, p.201.

25   Jung, C.G. (1953) *The Collected Works of C G Jung, vol. 8* (Bollingen Series XX). H. Read, M. Fordham, G. Adler and Wm McGuire (eds). Princeton, New Jersey: Princeton University Press and London: Routledge and Kegan Paul, pp.97–8.

26   Jung, C.G. (1953) *The Collected Works of C G Jung, vol. 5* (Bollingen Series XX). H. Read, M. Fordham, G. Adler and Wm McGuire (eds). Princeton, New Jersey: Princeton University Press and London: Routledge and Kegan Paul, p.368.

27   Jung, C.G. (1953) *The Collected Works of C G Jung, vol. 5* (Bollingen Series XX). H. Read, M. Fordham, G. Adler and Wm McGuire (eds). Princeton, New Jersey: Princeton University Press and London: Routledge and Kegan Paul, p.368.

28   Kopp, S. (1972) *If You Meet Budha on the Road, Kill Him : A Modern Pilgrimage Through Myth, Legend, Zen and Psychotherapy.* London: Sheldon Press.

29   Jung, C.G. (1953) *The Collected Works of C G Jung, vol. 7* (Bollingen Series XX). H. Read, M. Fordham, G. Adler and Wm McGuire (eds). Princeton, New Jersey: Princeton University Press and London: Routledge and Kegan Paul, p.238.

30   Jung, C.G. (1953) *The Collected Works of C G Jung, vol. 7* (Bollingen Series XX). H. Read, M. Fordham, G. Adler and Wm McGuire (eds). Princeton, New Jersey: Princeton University Press and London: Routledge and Kegan Paul, p.238.

31   Jung. C.G. (1968) cited in Miguel Serrano, *C. G. Jung and Herman Hesse: A Record Of Two Friendships.* Trans. by F MacShane. New York: Schocken, p.50.

32   Jung. C.G. (1968) cited in Miguel Serrano, *C. G. Jung and Herman Hesse: A Record Of Two Friendships,* trans. by F MacShane. New York: Schocken, p.50.

33   Fordham, M. (1985) 'Explorations into the self.' *Library of Analytical Psychology, 7.* London; Academic Press, pp.118–119.

34   Redfearn, J. (1985) 'My self, my many selves.' *Library of Analytical Psychology, 6.* London: Academic Press, p.131.

35   Hillman, J. (1977)*Re-Visioning Psychology.* New York: Harper & Row, p.88.

36   Hillman, J. (1977) *Re-Visioning Psychology.* New York: Harper & Row, p.32.

37   Hillman, J. (1977) *Re-Visioning Psychology.* New York: Harper & Row, p.24.

38   Aldridge-Morris, R. (1989) *Multiple Personality: An Exercise in Deception.* London: Erlbaum.

39   Redfearn, J. (1985) 'My self, my many selves.' *Library of Analytical Psychology, 6.* London: Academic Press, p.5.

40   Redfearn, J. (1985) 'My self, my many selves.' *Library of Analytical Psychology, 6.* London: Academic Press, p.117.

41   Samuels, A. (1985) *Jung and the Post-Jungians.* London: Routledge, p.12.

42   Hillman, J. (1978) 'Further notes on images.' *Spring: A Journal of Archetypal Psychology and Jungian Thought,* pp.152–82, (p.170).

43   Hillman, J. (1978) 'Further notes on images.' *Spring: A Journal of Archetypal Psychology and Jungian Thought,* pp.152–82, (p.165).

44   Hillman, J. (1978) 'Further notes on images.' *Spring: A Journal of Archetypal Psychology and Jungian Thought,* pp.152–82, (p.165).

45   Hillman, J. (1977) 'An inquiry into image.' *Spring: A Journal of Archetypal Psychology and Jungian Thought,*pp.62–88 (p.64).

46   Hillman, J. (1978) 'Further notes on images.' *Spring: A Journal of Archetypal Psychology and Jungian Thought,* pp.152–82, (pp.170–71).

47   Hillman, J. (1977) 'An enquiry into image.' *Spring: A Journal of Archetypal Psychology and Jungian Thought,* pp.62–88, (p.66).

48   Hillman, J. (1977) 'An enquiry into image.' *Spring: A Journal of Archetypal Psychology and Jungian Thought,* pp.62–88, (p.69).

49   Hillman, J. (1977) 'An enquiry into image.' *Spring: A Journal of Archetypal Psychology and Jungian Thought,* pp.62–88.

50   Moses, P.J. 'Letter to A Wolfsohn, 16 April 1961.' Repository: Alfred Wolfsohn Private Archives, Malerargues, France. © Marita Gunther. Reprinted by permission.

51   Wolfsohn, A. 'Orpheus or the way to a mask.' Trans. by M. Gunther (unpublished manuscript written Berlin, 1936–38). Repository: Alfred Wolfsohn Private Archives, Malerargues, France. © M. Gunther. Reprinted by permission.

52   Wolfsohn, A. 'The biography of an idea.' Trans. by M. Gunther (unpublished handwritten fragment written in Germany, undated). Repository: Alfred Wolfsohn Private Archives, Malerargues, France. © Marita Gunther. Reprinted by permission.

53   Wolfsohn, A. 'Notes on Orpheus.' Supplement to 'Orpheus or the way to a mask' , London, 1949. Posthumously published in *Spring: A Journal of Archetype and Culture,* 50 (1990), pp.76–79, (p.77).

54   Wolfsohn, A. 'Notes on Orpheus.' Supplement to 'Orpheus or the way to a mask.' London, 1949. Posthumously published in *Spring: A Journal of Archetype and Culture,* 50 (1990), pp.76–79, (p.77).

55   Wolfsohn, A. 'Orpheus or the way to a mask.' Trans. by M. Gunther (unpublished manuscript written Berlin, 1936–38. Repository: Alfred Wolfsohn Private Archives, Malerargues, France. © M. Gunther. Reprinted by permission.

56   Gunther, M. 'The human voice.' Paper read at the National Conference on Drama Therapy, Antioch University, San Francisco (November 1986). Published on audio tape by Roy Hart Theatre, Malerargues, France.

57   Jung, C.G. (1953) *The Collected Works of C G Jung, vol. 9, pt. 1* (Bollingen Series XX). H. Read, M. Fordham, G. Adler and Wm McGuire (eds). Princeton, New Jersey: Princeton University Press and London: Routledge and Kegan Paul, p.284.

58   Zweig, C. & Abrams, J. (eds.) (1991) *Meeting the Shadow: The Hidden Power of the Dark Side of Human Nature.* Los Angeles: Jeremy Tarcher.

59   Jung, C.G. (1953) *The Collected Works of C G Jung, vol. 9. pt. 2* (Bollingen Series XX). H. Read, M. Fordham, G. Adler and Wm McGuire (eds). Princeton, New Jersey: Princeton University Press and London: Routledge and Kegan Paul, pp.233–34.

60   Jung, C.G. (1953) *The Collected Works of C G Jung, vol. 9, pt. 2* (Bollingen Series XX). H. Read, M. Fordham, G. Adler and Wm McGuire (eds). Princeton, New Jersey: Princeton University Press and London: Routledge and Kegan Paul, pp.233–34.

61   Watson, L. (1995) *Dark Nature.* London: Hodder & Stoughton.

62   Gunther, M. (1990) 'The human voice: on Alfred Wolfsohn.' *Spring: A Journal of Archetype and Culture,* 50, pp.65–75, (p.71).

63   Gunther, M. (1990) 'The human voice: on Alfred Wolfsohn.' *Spring: A Journal of Archetype and Culture, 50,* pp.65–75, (p.71).

64   Gunther, M. (1990) 'The human voice: on Alfred Wolfsohn.' *Spring: A Journal of Archetype and Culture,* 50, pp.65–75, (p.71).

65   Pikes, N. (1993) 'Giving voice to Hell.' *Spring: A Journal of Archetype and Culture,* 55, pp.51–66.

66   Pikes, N. (1994) *The Whole Voice – The Creative Voice.* Publicity Pamphlet.

67   Pikes, N. (1994) *The Whole Voice – The Creative Voice.* Publicity Pamphlet.

68   Wolfsohn, A. cited in 'Stimme Ohne Fessel.' E. Weiser, *Die Weltwoche*, trans. by L. Halcrow. (30 September 1955).

69   Jung, C.G. (1953) *The Collected Works of C G Jung, vol. 9, pt. 1* (Bollingen Series XX). H. Read, M. Fordham, G. Adler and Wm McGuire (eds). Princeton, New Jersey: Princeton University Press and London: Routledge and Kegan Paul, p.284.

70   Luchsinger, R. and Dubois, C.L. (1956) 'Phonetische und Stroboskopische Untersuchungen an einem Stimmphanomen.' *Folia Phoniatrica*, 8, no. 4, pp.201–210.

71   Wolfsohn, A. (1955) cited in 'Stimme Ohne Fessel.' Eric Weiser, *Die Weltwoche*, trans. by L. Halcrow. (30 September 1955).

72   Weiser, E. (1955) 'Stimme Ohne Fessel', *Die Weltwoche*, September 30 1955.

73   Wolfsohn, A. (1955) cited in 'Stimme Ohne Fessel', by Eric Weiser, *Die Weltwoche*, trans. by L. Halcrow. (30 September 1955).

74   Newham, P. (1967) *The Prophet of Song: The Life and Work of Alfred Wolfsohn*. London: Tigers Eye Press.

75   Svenska Dagbladet, July 1982. cited in J. Martin (1991) *The Voice in Modern Theatre*. London: Routledge, p.67.

76   Pardo, E. (1984) 'Dis-membering Dionysus: image and theatre.' *Spring: A Journal of Archetypal Psychology and Jungian Thought*, p.163–179, (p.166).

CHAPTER 9

The Dramatic Voice
Therapeutic Voicework and Experimental Theatre

Introduction: Therapy in the Rehearsal Studio

Whilst Jungian psychotherapists discovered the inevitable performance component to imaginative expression within the therapeutic process, actors, directors and researchers within the field of the performing arts, particularly theatre, meanwhile, have discovered the psychological component to the creative process.

The history of Western theatre contains astoundingly rich and consistent investigations into the way vocal expression can communicate the nature of the psyche to an audience. Furthermore, probably no other subject has contributed more to the practical exploration of the vocal instrument.

In this chapter I will, therefore, outline this history, highlighting the connection between performance and psyche as revealed through the voice.

Elocution, Phonetics and Society

During the 18th century the hitherto prevailing neo-classic style of acting and vocal delivery, consisting of pantomimical and histrionic gesture, was challenged and reformed by the actor David Garrick, who introduced a simpler, more measured vocal delivery that focused on a precision of diction which sought to more properly represent the turns of thought underlying the text in the theatre. It was to Garrick's style that the elocution teachers Thomas Sheridan and John Walker turned in their search for models of vocal delivery which represented the art of elocution, which Sheridan defined as a 'just delivery' in a 'distinct articulation', 'pronounced in proper tones, suitably varied to the sense, and the emotions of the mind, with due observation of accent, of emphasis' and 'of rests or pauses of the voice', 'accompanied with expressive looks, and significant gesture'.[1] The elocutionists of the 18th century, like the scientists of their preceding era, believed the expressions of humankind to be governed by the same natural laws as those allegedly found in the order of the universe[2] and it was this philosophy which underpinned the writings of the Elocutionists.

Then, in the early 19th century, the American James Rush attempted to provide a scientific description of vocal physiology and a system for notating speech sounds, whilst simultaneously merging philosophy, biology and art in an attempt to explain the influence of the psyche on speech.[3] The American writer, actor and teacher James Murdoch, who was tutored by Rush, sought to carry on his work through his own teaching and, in so doing, became a leader of the American elocutionary movement for over fifty years. Moreover, a number of Murdoch's pupils went on to become influential teachers of the elocution movement in the American educational establishments of the 19th century, which formed the basis for the vocal delivery of America's great actors of the period – such as Charlotte Cushman, Mary Ann Duff and Edwin Booth, whose voices of orotund tones and pear-shaped vowels, consciously sculptured cadence and poetic rhythm suited the classic theatre popular at the time.

Towards the end of the nineteenth century, however, things began to change, partly due to Steele Mackaye, who was a devoted student of Delsarte and, in turn, passed the latter's work on to Hede Kallmeyer, who took it to Germany and passed it on to the American Silas Curry.

Curry rejected much of the mechanistic and didactic techniques which had descended from Rush's approach and became fascinated with deepening the connection between mind, body and voice, proclaiming that the inner motivations of the mind must be studied and trained in tandem with its outward expression through movement and sound.[4] This new approach to voice and speech lent itself to the emerging realism in the theatre. However, this focus on the inner truth behind the words was, in many ways, countermanded by a fresh force or emphasis on the outer mechanics of expression under the title of a new science: phonetics.

Phonetics is the study of speech sounds as formed by the mechanical movements of physiological components such as tongue, lips and teeth. It was the Briton, Henry Sweet, who, in the late nineteenth century first proclaimed the educational virtues of phonetics, pointing out its use in learning foreign languages and in creating a uniformity of pronunciation within a given language. When one of Sweet's students, William Tilly, went to America in 1918, he passed the science on to his pupils and it was to have a dramatic effect on the development of voice and speech training, particularly for actors.

The most renowned American proponent of this phonetic approach to standardising speech was Margaret Prendergast McClean, who influenced speech training in schools, universities and drama colleges. Her aim was to use phonetic science to remove the regional variation from speech and produce a standard American dialect called Transatlantic. This borrowed from standard British pronunciations and sought to provide a form of enunciation which did not reveal the ethnic, regional, geographical or cultural origins of the speaker. The influence of this training can be heard in the speech of a number of film actors, including Bette Davis, Katherine Hepburn and Tyrone Power. In Britain, the classic phonetic text for students is Clifford Turner's *Voice and Speech in the Theatre*.[5]

Both the Standard English, or Received Pronunciation, and the Transatlantic mode of speaking became associated, however, not with a neutral predicament but with the upper classes, the educated and the rich.

There are literally hundreds of so-called 'drill books' on the practical nature of speech training written during the 19th and 20th centuries. They include advisory prescriptions for vocal health by scientifically-orientated practitioners,[6] generalised and idiosyncratic approaches to vocal training propounded by voice coaches,[7] detailed descriptions of the significance of phonetics[8] and accessible texts combining instruction and explanation for student actors.[9] Some of these investigators of voice wrote in an inspiring and fluent manner and became minor legends in their own right, such as Caesari[10] and the maverick James Rush,[11] who treated the human voice as a scientific, philosophical, artistic and mystical phenomenon.[12] Many of these books perceived speech as a sociological phenomenon, that is to say the precision, diction and elocution of the spoken word was taken to be directly proportional to a person's intelligence, status and social worth. Probably the most well-known example of an equation between speech and social standing is revealed in the story of Eliza Doolittle, as told in Shaw's *Pygmalion*, and whose transformation from a 'sloppy speaker' to a 'posh speaker' is seen to be equivalent and directly related to her transformation from a member of a lower social class to a higher one. Such an understanding of the sociological function of speech is innately bound to a certain puritanical view of the English language where certain acoustic articulations are generated, inculcated and preserved by the privileged members of society who tend to be moneyed, physically able and educated. The perpetuation of this so-called superior etiquette in the manner of speaking has been the responsibility of elocution teachers in both England and America.

Melodrama

Most popular nineteenth century European theatre was prosaic in language, histrionic in gesture, decorative in scenic style and declamatory in utterance. This was a theatre which presented a world of exaggerated emotion, heightened atmospheres and a poetic inflation of mood, narrative and character. Such a theatre required a vocal style of delivery that could make audient the grandiose experience, the intense mood and the romantic sentiment of the world which it portrayed through the genre of theatre known as melodrama which was proliferate during this period.

Commonly, the word melodrama denotes a style of dramatic performance, extremely popular in the 19th century, where choreographically-stylised movement, graphic depiction of emotion and declamatory vocal enunciation portrayed sensational scenarios in which the good are ensnared by the clutches of evil as the audience await the inevitable and guaranteeable triumph of justice. The style of vocal delivery which served this theatre was somewhere between singing and speaking. It was a declaiming in which prosody and intonation drifted towards melodic composition and verbal intensities came close to musical crescendos.

The term 'melodrama', which to theatre practitioners refers to this style of drama, also denotes a musical genre in which a vocalist speaks or declaims a poem, text or libretto to the accompaniment of music, sometimes in silent pauses between melodic phrases and at others simultaneous with the music. Of course, dramatic action accompanied by music is as old as the theatre itself and melodrama may perhaps be best considered as a revivalist acknowledgement of a forgotten aspect of the great classic theatre of European antiquity, where the interrelationship between the music of the lyre and the declaimed poetry of the singer spun the stories of the Iliad and The Odyssey in a manner comparable to melodramatic declaiming.[13] However, melodrama as a named musical style is normally attributed to *Pygmalion* by Rousseau, the text of which was probably written by him in 1762 and was later set to music by Coignet. In the aftermath of Coignet's score a number of composers wrote new music to accompany Rousseau's dramatic text as others began to produce musical compositions for other poetic texts which were produced as melodramas.

In melodrama the words were not set to a musical score and the vocalist was, therefore, completely free from the demands of pitch, register, voice quality and note value and able to work as a declaimer, an orator or an actor but was not required to display the skills of a singer or musician.[14] Consequently, many composers simply laid text over a musical score and left it to the performer's discretion as to how to declaim it. One declaimer who enjoyed considerable repute was Yvette Guilbert, whose subtle art, which combined the sung and the spoken form of delivery, reaped the admiration of Sigmund Freud, with whom she sustained a long friendship.[15]

Later, this accompanied spoken text, which remained dissociated from the musical melody, was developed one step further towards singing where the speech was notated, dictating the note which words and syllables were to be spoken on. This was a pitch-controlled talking, something mid-way between speech and song known as 'Sprechgesang' or 'Sprechstimme'. This was first introduced in 1897 by Humperdinck in his opera *Königskinder*. However, the introduction of Sprechstimme is usually attributed to the piece *Pierrot lunaire* by Schoenberg, in the preface to which Schoenberg defines that he wants the pitch of each word to be exact but left to rise and fall in the manner of speech giving something unique resembling neither true singing nor talking.

The manner of declaiming used by the vocalist in musical melodrama is comparable to the form of vocal articulation used by actors on the theatrical stage during the 19th century.

There were a number of particularly renowned disseminators of this style, including France's great tragic actress Félix Rachel, the American Edwin Forrest and Edmund Keane, who made his sensational London debut as Shylock in 1814 and served the romantic poets so well, reaping the admiration of Byron. These performers were able to radiate intense emotion and larger-than-life behaviours and their voices rolled and curved like a song. Forrest's voice was described by one critic as 'tremendous in its sustained crescendo swell and crashing force of utterance' which 'surged and roared like the angry sea' as it 'reached its boiling, seething climax, in which the serpent hiss of hate was heard', 'it was like the falls of Niagara, in its tremendous down-sweeping cadence; it was a whirlwind, a tornado, a cataract of illimitable rage'.[16]

Therapeutic Voicework Methodology: Melodramatic Declamation

In the field of professional Therapeutic Voicework, where practitioners often find themselves working with artistically inexperienced clients who feel bereft of musical ability yet who desperately want to sing and give voice, the melodramatic form can provide a great inspiration and working model. In the tradition of classical Western European singing training the client is required to sing in tuneful alignment with the piano or other instrument, often whilst reading a musical score. The melodramatic model which I have found most useful, on the other hand, provides a client with an opportunity to give free reign to a natural but exaggerated speaking voice whilst the practitioner uses an instrument such as piano, guitar or concertina to underpin, illustrate and support the client's vocality dramatically rather than musically.

In addition, this work allows every person to transcend or delve beneath the articulatory aspects of speech which reveal educational or social status and experience the voice as an emissary for the deep archetypal sources of emotion which every human being hosts.

The Naturalistic Utterance

Towards the end of the 19th Century an avalanche of artistic sensibilities caused a pan-European and transatlantic shift in theatre away from declamatory romantic sensationalism towards an attempted more truthful replication of actual life behaviours which was instigated and compounded by a two-fold development within both the novel and dramatic literature.

First, the content of literature moved away from romantic and melodramatic scenarios towards the realism of sociopolitical reality. It was the French novelist Émile Zola, who, in the 1870s, first proclaimed the need for truthful representation in the literary arts, seeking to portray the realities of French social life, particularly the plight of the downtrodden peasant, which were also depicted by Leo Tolstoy. The second development in literature, which is the most pertinent to this study, was the development of a realistic dramatic text in which the style of dialogue moved towards the naturalism of everyday discourse without the hitherto dominance of poetic embellishment of verse, rhyme and metre. One of the effects of this development was to completely change the way the actor used the voice upon the stage.

In Norway the poet Henrik Ibsen, who had achieved great success with monumental verse plays, turned his pen to this new naturalistic style, which Henry James, after he had seen Ibsen's *Hedda Gabler*, described as portraying not an action but 'a condition', a 'state of nerves', of 'soul', 'of temper, of health, of chagrin, of despair'.[17] This portrayal of an inner condition rather than an outer circumstance required a subtlety of vocal delivery which could intimate the gentle pulse of an internal psychic reality. The plays of Ibsen, Turgenev and Chekhov, for example, also required a mode of delivery that did justice to writing which was conversational and akin to the way people speak in the garden, on the street and in the drawing room. Many of these plays relied on a kind of impressionistic build-up of effects from a multitude of minute details[18] in which 'stumblings and stammerings, grunts and sighs and sustained silences' drew attention to the psyche's inner ruminations. It required the audience to listen to a 'sub-text', an 'undertone', a hidden language of deeper desire that lay beneath that which the characters were able to express verbally in their social context, which was facilitated by various devices including the cadences of vocal expression.[19]

Because this style of dialogue and human representation usually went hand in hand with a realistic representation of society, with its hypocrisies and blemishes, the plays of the naturalistic school were often censored and reviewed harshly. In response to this, a number of private theatre clubs or societies were founded where new plays of the naturalistic style could be played to receptive audiences. One of the most famous of these was the French Théâtre Libre, where the naturalist experimenter André Antoine produced new plays by unknown writers using amateur actors, including an adaptation of a Zola novella about which the newspaper *République Francaise* said that 'if the naturalistic theatre has more such plays, it need not worry about its future'.[20]

Antoine broke with many of the presiding performance traditions which had been the very constitution of the actor's art, encouraged a simple undeclaimed vocal style of delivery and attempted to create for the audience the illusion of eavesdropping on someone's private affairs.

The Actor's Method of Naturalism

One of the famous private societies which produced naturalistic plays, censored in the main frame of conventional theatre, was the Moscow Art Theatre, where the Russian theatre director Constantin Stanislavski set himself the task of devising a methodological approach to training actors in how to manifest and embody the naturalistic vision of dramatic literature that elevated the elusive, implied, elliptical and obtuse.

To reflect the truth of human discourse and of the human condition meant allowing dialogue to retain its incompleteness, its manifold implications and dual meanings, its inherent conflicts of desire, its double-binds and ambivalences. Within Stanislavski's system careful attention was given to allowing the voice to contain both the text and the sub-text. He led the actor to the sub-textual dimension 'where the writer had concealed the motives which prompted him to create the play.'[21] To assist actors in imbuing vocal delivery with sub-textual information, Stanislavski taught actors to sing on open vowel sounds[22] for Stanislavski felt that it was in the subtle twists and turns of the vocal dimension to speech that the intricacy and ambiguity of meaning was communicable to an attentive audience.

In 1923 the Moscow Art Theatre toured America, exposing audiences and actors to the system of Stanislavski in action and in 1924 the principles of his method were taught by former members of the theatre at the American Laboratory theatre in New York. It was at these classes that Lee Strasberg first experienced the techniques, which he adapted to form the Strasberg Method which was to influence a generation of American actors, most notably Marlon Brando.

In the Americanised method approach, actors mumbled, spoke whilst eating and attempted to find the most naturalistic way of behaving, which meant letting the voice follow the reality of the inner life. With the elocutionist and phonetic approach no longer suited to the emerging school of realistic plays being written for the theatre, and with audiences seeking naturalism of enunciation even in the classic works of Shakespeare, a new approach to training the voice became necessary. In England it was Iris Warren, who, in the 1950s, whilst head of the London Academy of Music and Dramatic Art voice department, sought the means to releasing the actor's natural voice through relaxation and removing the blocks which prevent the voice from expressing inner feelings. And it was Iris Warren who passed this approach on to Kristin Linklater, a Scottish actress who went to the United States in the early 1960s to set up a voice studio.

Linklater continues to teach and claims that the voice is prevented from responding with spontaneity because 'most people have lost the ability, and, perhaps, the desire, to behave reflexively' except in moments 'beyond control', such as during the experience of extreme emotion. In the normal course of events, however, such 'reflex behaviour' is 'short-circuited by secondary impulses', which often tend to become 'so well developed that they blot out the impact of the primary, or reflex impulse' and thereby form a habit. Whilst some habits are useful, Linklater says that 'most mental and emotional habits' are constructed 'unconsciously and by people other than oneself, in childhood' and there is 'no choice attached to such conditioning'. As a result of such conditioning, 'the animal instinct level of emotional response to stimulus, deep in the unconscious mind, is largely conditioned out of us as we grow up'.[23] Linklater's reconditioning led her to lead workshops for non-actors and she contributed to the growth of the voice workshop movement.

In Britain it was Cicely Berry at the Royal Shakespeare Company who shifted the emphasis of the actor from the formal affectations of mannerism which had occupied the elocutionists for so long to amplifying the natural efficiency of the vocal mechanism and applying the consequent liberated voice to highlighting the overriding significance of meaning and emotion inherent in a text. Berry's approach has influenced many trainee actors as a result of her two books, *Voice and the Actor*[24] and *The Actor and his Text*,[25] which remain seminal reading for drama school students in the UK. She has also extended her work into the field of other forms of professional speaking with MPs, teachers and lecturers.[26]

The 'liberation' approach to voice has been further continued by one of Berry's students and colleagues, Patsy Rodenburg, who has, through her workshops and her two books, *The Right to Speak*[27] and *The Need for Words*,[28] contributed to a the notion of a voice workshop culture. In contradistinction to the underlying views of an earlier epoch, Rodenburg believes that the English language has been enlivened by 'its exposure to multiple linguistic habits' and her practical teaching works in opposition to the notion that there is 'only one right sound'.[29] Her aim is to free verbal facility from inhibition, self-consciousness and constriction in order that the musicality unique to its cultural base can be honoured, celebrated and conserved.

Berry makes only minimal and moderate reference to the psychological and emotional underpinnings of vocal use, stating, for example, that 'one's mood and state of being reflects in the voice – if you are tired or depressed you actually feel as though some part of your voice has cut out'.[30] Rodenburg, on the other hand, repeatedly reveals that she frequently deals with the residue of psychological operations, admitting that 'psychic trauma of any sort' can 'shut down the voice'.[31] Furthermore, she says that the voice teacher is 'in the front line of action' for the release of 'unexploded mines' of emotional material, such as grief, 'stored up over years' and which 'takes its toll' on the voice.[32] However, she states categorically that she 'would never claim that voice work is psychologically therapeutic'. In fact, she says 'that's one of the dangers to be avoided'. However, she proposes that 'as a kind of physiotherapy', vocal work does release hidden memories encased in the body' and therefore 'to that extent it is exceedingly therapeutic'.[33]

Indeed, throughout the field of speech teaching for actors there is some contradiction with regard to the role of the teacher in containing personal material, many of whom answer the problem with the attitude that although vocal training 'may lead to exploration and release of the actor's own thoughts and emotions, such exploration and release is a by product of the work not the aim of the work'.[34] At the other end of the spectrum, there are those who claim for voice teaching the potential for major life changes, comparing the vocal coaching session with psychotherapy without any serious consideration of the relationship between the two disciplines.[35]

Therapeutic Voicework Methodology: The Tiny Play

In professional Therapeutic Voicework subtle naturalistic theatre is occurring all the time. The client will inevitably experience the practitioner as a kind of audience, not only to the stylised Therapeutic Voicework, the singing and declaiming, but also to the gentle interruptive conversations and discussions which punctuate it. During a Therapeutic Voicework session the client moves back and forth like a pendulum between vocalising in response to the practitioner's guidance and talking about her experience. To facilitate a client in finding a voice, it is equally as important that the client can feel relaxed and safe enough to mumble, trip over words, stammer and struggle through her verbal descriptions of feelings, moods and ideas as it is that she can present or perform sculptured sound. The practitioner may be offering more to the client by listening compassionately and attentively to the client's verbal discourse than by providing inspirational instruction in how to release the voice.

This is particularly apposite to group work, where a client may feel able to be loud and sonorous when making non-verbal sound which is lost in the cacophony of fifteen other voices, yet she may feel nervous and timid about speaking individually before a listening group. The legacy of Stanislavski teaches us that the natural reticences, shyness, incompleteness and semi-structured nature of our verbal behaviour has an innate beauty, a truth and an authenticity which need not be eradicated and replaced with style and virtuosity to be of expressive and artistic value. The professional Therapeutic Voicework practitioner, therefore, should be able to abandon any idea of the perfect confident speaking voice and be prepared to perceive the exquisite vulnerability which occurs naturally in life.

Strindberg: From External Replication to Inner Truth

Whilst Stanislavski experimented in Moscow, news of Antoine's naturalistic experiments with the Théâtre Libre in France reached the Swedish writer August Strindberg, who formed his own society in Copenhagen which opened in 1889 with three short plays by himself. Strindberg believed that naturalism should show the 'richness of the soul-complex'[36] and, in presenting the human condition in its reality, Strindberg unwittingly became involved in portraying the nature of the inner psychic world. His characters were 'conglomerations of past and present stages of civilisation, bits from books and newspapers, scraps of humanity, rags and tatters of fine clothing, patched together as is the human soul'.[37] Strindberg wanted to avoid 'mathematically-constructed dialogue' and allow the characters' minds 'to work irregularly, as people's do in real life'. His dialogue, therefore, wandered and is 'worked upon, repeated, expanded and added to, like the theme in a musical composition'.[38]

This inevitable transient bridge from naturalism as a replication of life's behaviours to naturalism as a truthful portrayal of the way that life is experienced subjectively in Strindberg's writing symbolised a widespread move amongst writers to 'reach a deeper level of reality' than the 'deceptive appearances' of replicated discourse and to 'embody the inner nature of archetypal man in concrete symbols' rather than perpetrate the 'naturalistic depiction of socially defined individuals'.[39] Thus the notion of naturalism was broadened to include any form which represents the truth of 'the inner world' by tracing every nuance of the soul.[40] Thus naturalism carried the seeds of the future within it and led to a number of fresh waves or movements.

Therapeutic Voicework Methodology: From Tiny Play to Song Motif

The idea of distilling from naturalism the repeatable thematic and rhythmic components in such a way as to turn conversation into music, instigated by Strindberg,[41] is of great use in professional Therapeutic Voicework for it can help a client move from language to song without needing to substitute any personal authenticity for acquired virtuosity.

The Therapeutic Voiceworker listens astutely and acutely to all of the client's utterances, even the seeming asides, apologetic mumbles and 'throw-away lines'. From a state of open receptivity, the Therapeutic Voiceworker can ask the client to repeat one or more of these utterances, developing their musicality until a seemingly meaningless, but often repeated phrase, becomes the core element and motif of a musical song.

Symbolism and Silence

One of the fresh artistic waves which challenged the precepts of naturalism and realism was symbolism, embodied by the Belgian playwright Maurice Maeterlink, whose plays were first staged at the experimental Théâtre d'art in 1891. Maeterlink worked towards a theatre of silence, proclaiming that puppets make the ideal actors, and he sought to encourage his performers to abandon realistic expression for a 'musically structured gesture'.[42] Here the 'emphasis was placed on expressive tone and pitch in speaking rather than on the sense of what was said'.[43] This theatre of silence was in many ways a stripping away of superfluous verbal activity in an attempt to locate the central atmospheric essence of an image. It was a desire in keeping with the aims of the Symbolist poets Stéphane Mallarmé and Paul Valéry, who sought to abandon the embroidered Romantic lyricism of poetry which facilitated a declamatory style of reading. Valéry encapsulates this objective by saying that for a long time the human voice was the 'foundation and the condition' of all literature, 'until a day came when the reader could read with his eyes alone'.[44]

Mallarmé's thesis was that language had actually trespassed onto and invaded the land occupied by silence, a land which contains the material of true thought, true experience. He sought to reinstate this space by leaving blank spaces in the poetry, questioning and casting doubt over words by placing exclamation marks after them and dissolving all vestige of regular symmetrical rhythm. In so doing, Mallarmé showed great sensitivity for the phonaesthetic quality of words, indicating intonation, degree of emphasis and prosodic shape. The disruption of the intact lyric consequently drew attention to the acoustic sound of the words, and as their linguistic certainty of meaning was depleted, their musical value increased, moving poetry into a semiotic and non-discursive world beyond language.

One of the actors who had helped realise Maeterlink's vision was Aurelien Lugné Poë, who, following his success as an actor in Maeterlink's plays, launched his own company, the Théâtre de l'Œuvre, which he wanted to be a temple to Symbolist Drama and at which Alfred Jarry's infamous slapstick and absurd theatre production, Ubu roi, was performed in December 1896.

Futurism

Futurism was intitiated by the Italian poet Filippo Tommaso Marinetti, who established the new art of 'declamation' that was to be the trade mark of futurist performance.[45] This rally for a new style of vocal use was promulgated in one of the many other successive manifestos produced by the Futurists: *Dynamic and Synoptic Declamation.*[46] Marinetti claimed that the new form of declaiming should not be the 'nostalgic and pacifist' declaiming of theatre hitherto. He speaks of 'the deficiencies of declamation as it has been understood up to now'[47] and begs for a more dynamic, attacking kind which should be accompanied by declamatory movements of the arm and legs.[48] 'Gesticulate geometrically', the manifesto had advised, 'in a draughtsmanlike topological manner, synthetically creating in mid-air, cubes, cones, spirals and ellipses.'[49] He wanted the vocalist to 'completely dehumanise, systematically doing away with every modulation and nuance'.[50]

The first practical demonstration of Dynamic and Synoptic Declamation was in the performance of a free verse play written by Francesco Cangiullo, in which Marinetti performed early in 1914. The performers declaimed the words whilst the author played the piano. Concurrently, a number of home-made 'noise instruments' were played, including a saw with pieces of tin attached. The second performance, which also combined Marinetti's declamation with unmusical noise, was performed at the Dore Gallery in London in April 1914. Here Marinetti read from his play *Zang Tumb Tumb,* in which a General's orders were accompanied by banging of drums to simulate cannon fire rather than musical accompaniment.[51]

Marinetti wrote to the musician and experimentalist Luigi Russolo about this performance, describing the 'onomatopoetic gallery' and, after witnessing one of Pratella's concerts in Rome in March 1913, Luigi Russolo became convinced that mechanised noises were a viable form of music and wrote his manifesto *The Art of Noise.*[52] His intention was to combine the noises of trams, trains, shouting crowds and exploding motors and a futurist orchestra of specially constructed boxes which made such sounds at the turn of the handle were made. According to Russolo, at least thirty thousand diverse noises were possible. A performance of music composed of these noises was given in London at the Coliseum in June 1913 and was described by *The Times* as resembling 'the rigging of a channel-steamer during a bad crossing' as it played to the cries of 'no more' from the audience.[53]

Russolo's ideas had a significant effect on the later composer John Cage, who studied composition with Schoenberg in the mid-1930s. In Cage's 1937 publication *The Future of Music* he proposed that 'wherever we are, what we hear is mostly noise', such as 'the sound of a truck', or 'rain', or 'static between radio stations. Regardless of its origin', said Cage, 'we find noise fascinating'.[54] In his early performances his 'musicians' played beer bottles, flowerpots, cowbells and other found objects, expanding the musical frame-work to incorporate that which may, in other circumstance, be regarded as noise. To understand the sensibility behind this investigation, Cage advised interested parties to look at the writings of Russolo.[55]

The deconstruction of language and the broadening of the acoustic can-vas could also be witnessed in *Disconcerted States of Mind* by the futurist artist Giacomo Balla, in which four people recited together various sequences of numbers, vowels and consonants, and in Fortunato Deporo's performance called *Colours*, in which the characters were four cardboard objects and the live performers remained off-stage providing a vocal sound track consisting of nonsense sounds, such as 'bulubu bulu bulu bulu bulu bulu'.[56]

Futurism also took hold in Russia, where the deconstruction of language into a non-sense or sense-free use of verbality was encapsulated in the work of the poet Vladimir Mayakovsky, who provoked audiences with his readings and self-proclaimed genius and who sought through poetry a 'new linguistic element' which could 'extract poetry from the spoken language'.[57]

During the second two decades of the twentieth century a number of poets in Russia experimented with poetic language, among them was Viktor Sklovskij, whose *The Awakening of the Word* began: 'The oldest creative act of man was the creation of words. Now words are dead, and language resembles a cemetery'. The opera by Alexei Kruchenykh also attempted to disintegrate concept, words and musical harmony.[58] With similar intent, the poetry of Velemir Khlebnikov, in his poem 'Exorcism by Laughter', makes language 'perform extraordinary acrobatics' with a variety of 'different inflections' and 'build up' of non-existent words.[59] All of this futuristic work involved an 'attack on grammar and syntax' and placed the emphasis on 'sonic and picto-rial qualities of words'.[60] It aimed to enlarge the vocabulary of the people with factitious and fabricated words and 'declare boundless loathing for the language handed down to us'.[61]

Dada

Another radical and disruptive attack on artistic convention occurred in Zurich, where a group of artists presented spectacles designed to be anti-art. Their meeting place and platform was the Cabaret Voltaire, founded on 5 February 1916, and their movement was named 'Dada', out of which surreal-ism is said to have grown.

It was here, at the cabaret, that they experimented with the simultaneous poem in which 'three or more voices speak, sing, whistle' all at the same time[62] and where Huelsenbeck developed an identifiable reading style. Hugo Ball, meanwhile, invented a new species of 'verse without words' or 'sound poems' which he composed according to the acoustic properties of vowels and consonants to produce phrases such as 'glandridi glassala tuffm i zimbrabim'.[63] Ball acknowledged Marinetti as the initiator of the project to take the word out of the sentence 'nourish the emaciated big-city vocables with light and air and give them back their warmth, emotion and their original untroubled freedom'.[64] Ball said that 'language as a social organ can be destroyed without the creative process having to suffer. In fact, it seems that the creative process even benefits from it.'[65]

Meanwhile, in 1920s Paris, where Picasso was painting and Cocteau was experimenting with dream images in film and theatre, the composer Erik Satie, in the final years of his life, was experimenting with the potential musical noise of typewriters, sirens, aeroplane propellers and Morse tappers.

Therapeutic Voicework Methodology: From Prop to Instrument

Many clients feel a sense of regret, inadequacy and disappointment at not being able to 'play' an instrument. Yet all people make music in its broadest possible sense every day and a lot of this music is highly regular, rhythmical and, therefore, compositional because it is grounded in familiar domestic tasks: putting the kettle on, stirring tea, locking the front door.

Whilst clients may feel alienated by the presence of a musical instrument which they cannot play, many clients will feel comfortable with an object which has the capacity to make sound if it is presented as a dramatic prop for them to 'play with'.

In Therapeutic Voicework the practitioner can make use of this by introducing everyday objects which serve the theatre component of the work and by encouraging the client to utilise them as sound making objects.

The Experimental Pioneers

The vitality of the growing avant garde influenced the French poetic visionary Antonin Artaud, who spent the first half of the twentieth century oscillating between obsessional and pioneering ponderances on the potential of the theatre to provoke the most archetypal strata of the human condition and debilitating periods of mental illness.

Central to Artaud's quest was the search for a non-verbal use of the voice to communicate fundamental aspects of the human condition and the range of vocal delivery styles used in theatre groups since the 1960s, which used sounds rather than words and screams and cries rather than speech and owed much to the original impetus provided by his writings.[66]

Artaud, who admired the acting of Lugné Poë, being particularly fascinated by his 'surprising changes of voice' and 'his inflamed glances',[67] sought to liberate Western theatre from what he described as the 'exclusive dictatorship of words'[68] which, he believed, had arisen as a result of the dominance of the written text. Reacting against the great wave of realistic plays that had swept Europe, Artaud criticised the theatre for reducing what he regarded as the mysteriously unapproachable and evasive images of the human psyche to the level of everyday conversation and linguistic discourse.[69] For Artaud, the written text and the spoken word of the actor had turned theatre into an arena for 'psychological conflicts', a 'battlefield for moral passions',[70] containing nothing but stories about 'money troubles', 'social climbing', and 'sexuality sugar coated with eroticism yet shorn of mystery'.[71] Artaud believed that theatre should approach those subjects for which speech is inadequate or is unable to express, rediscovering 'the idea of figures and archetypal symbols'.[72] This theatre should not be verbal but vocal, utilising a 'genuine physical language, no longer based on words but on signs formed through the combination of objects, silence, shouts and rhythms'[73] which would be a 'powerful appeal through illustration to those powers which return the mind to the origins of its inner struggles'.[74] He thought that the theatre, in seeking to realise this, should return to 'the higher idea of poetry underlying the Myths told by the great tragedians of ancient times'.[75]

It was the focus on voice combined with the use of myth that influenced a chain of theatre practitioners who had studied and admired Artaud, including Peter Brook — for whom the twentieth century British theatre was restrained from dealing with such archetypal images by an unceasing adherence to the eloquent articulation of text. By the same token, Brook perceived the opera to be deprived of its potential potency by an overly scrutinising attention to the artificial formal structures of music.

Brook alleges that 'opera started fifty thousand years ago with people making noises as they came out of their caves' from which arose 'Verdi and Puccini and Wagner'. What was once 'a natural human expression' then 'turned into song' and later 'that process became codified, constructed, and turned into an art'. For Brook, 'the greatest challenge now' is to remind performers and audiences that opera is not artificial but natural'.[76] The means by which Brook sought to revive the natural expressive function of the human voice was to set up experimental theatre workshops at the Royal Shakespeare Company in the early 1960s, in which he required of his actors that they communicate to an audience without the use of words. It was here that Brook exercised his determination to investigate the degree to which Artaud's pleas might be fulfilled. Encouraged by his discoveries, Brook continued with his vocal experiments when he collaborated with the writer Ted Hughes to devise a production of *Oedipus* which used chants based on those uttered by the Maori peoples of New Zealand and irregular breathing rhythms derived from a recording of a medicine man in a trance.[77]

Brook became so intrigued by these experiments into the nature of vocal sound that he founded the International Theatre Research Centre in Paris, a company of actors of different nationalities, many of whom were prevented from talking to one another by a language barrier and where the theme of the first year's work was a study of structures of sounds.[78] The motivation was to discover vocal utterances, 'sounds and forms' which could communicate the essence of the great 'myths and archetypes' which 'touched the power beneath the surface', exposing the fabric of the 'the collective unconscious'.[79]

In a further collaboration with Ted Hughes, Brook created an entirely original language called 'Orghast' and with it the group of actors devised a play of the same name through which they discovered that 'the sound fabric of language' is an 'emotional code that bears witness to the passions that forged it'. Thus it is sufficient for an actor to speak syllables of another language, such as ancient Greek, 'to be lifted out of the emotional constriction of the twentieth-century city life into a fullness of passion which he never knew he possessed'.[80]

Later, in 1972, Brook set off with his actors to see if it was possible to communicate with people of the tribal communities of Africa through such a non-linguistic vocal code, seeking to 'create a work of theatre that could be accessible to everyone wherever it was played'[81] and 'discover whether the 'collective unconscious' 'can be tapped in sound'.[82]

During the African journey Brook's troupe encountered the Peuhl tribe and wondered how it would be possible for the actors and the local tribal members, who did not speak each other's language, to communicate and share a common experience. Brook's first idea was for the acting troop to sing a song but the Peuhls were not interested, so Brook tried asking the group to make an 'ah' sound 'that was to be extended and developed as far as it could possibly go'. In response, the Peuhls 'joined the sound' and, in exchange, 'sang their songs'. Brook 'knew at last that he was on the right road in the search for a universal language'.[83]

Whilst Peter Brook was searching for a universal language of sounds at Stratford, in Paris and in Africa, another theatre director called Jerzy Grotowski was researching a similar area in Poland.

In 1959 Grotowski became director of a tiny theatre in Opole, Poland called the Theatre of Thirteen Rows. In this theatre, in one of the poorest countries in Europe, a group of actors came together to explore the way in which the images of their own collective unconscious could be expressed through the body and the voice without recourse to the spoken word. They sought, like Artaud, to reach an audience, not through the narrative intrigues of everyday plots but through an expression of the archetypes which reflect the nature of every man and woman.

In the programme notes to their production of 'Akropolis', which premiered in October 1962, one of the members said that 'the means of verbal expression have been considerably enlarged because all means of vocal expression are used, starting from the confused babbling of the very small child' and including the most sophisticated oratorical recitation as well as 'inarticulate groans, animal roars, tender folksongs, liturgical chants, dialects, declamation of poetry' which 'brings back fleetingly the memory of all forms of language'.[84]

Above all else, Grotowski's group of devout actors became known for their revolutionary work on vocal expression and 'their voices reached from the smallest whisper to an astonishing, almost cavernous tone, an intoned declaiming, of a resonance and power' which some said had not been 'heard from actors before.'[85]

The use of non-verbal voice in these productions was part of Grotowski's investigation into the use of the actor's own psychological material as the substance of performance and his work was intricately and overtly bound up with a belief in the ability of a human being to physically and vocally express aspects of the psyche, including those aspects which are buried in the 'collective unconscious', without recourse to words. Grotowski said that in his theatre 'nothing is represented or shown, but we participate in a ceremonial which releases the collective unconscious'.[86] In Grotowski's scheme of things, the actor had to be able to draw from his psyche images of a personal and collective significance and give them form through the motion of the body and the sound of the voice.

Grotowski's ultimate aim was to effect in the actor change and growth, transformation and re-birth in order that the actor, in turn, could entice a similar development in the audience. He sought to bring actor and audience 'momentarily into contact with the deepest levels' within themselves, 'deeper than those engaged within the order of forms, through incarnate mythic confrontation', so that they may, 'through the shock of exposure, in touching those depths' be 'changed for ever'. The most 'significant factor to be born in mind is Grotowski's continual submission to the real possibility of *change* within the work and performance process' both 'for actor and spectator'.[87]

It was for this reason that Grotowski chose old master works based on timeless narratives as subjects for his productions, for he believed that they 'embodied myths and images powerful and universal enough to function as archetypes, which could penetrate beneath the apparently divisive and individual structure of the Western psyche, and evoke a spontaneous, collective, internal response.'[88] Grotowski said: 'in order that the spectator may be stimulated into self-analysis when confronted with the actor, there must be some common ground already existing in both of them, something they can either dismiss in one gesture or jointly worship'. For him, this common ground was provided by the myths, 'which are not an invention of the mind but are, so to speak, inherited through one's blood, religion, culture and climate'.[89] Grotowski 'saw that myth was both a primeval situation, and a complex model with an independent existence in the psychology of social groups'.[90] His actors thus drew images 'out from the depths of the unconscious with the aim of healing'.[91] What Grotowski asks of the actor, therefore, 'is not that he play the Lady from the Sea or Hamlet, but that he confront these characters within himself and offer the result of that encounter to an audience'.[92]

Grotowski, like Artaud, did not consider the text to be primary but believed that the text 'becomes theatre only through the actors' use of it – that is to say, thanks to intonations, to the association of sounds, to the musicality of language'.[93] Grotowski thus pursued the possibility of creating 'ideograms' made up of 'sounds and gestures' which 'evoke associations in the psyche of the audience'.[94] But, for Grotowski, there was, between the psychic image and the bodily and vocal expression, a series of inhibitions, resistances and blocks which prevent transformation from one to the other and it was these obstacles that his training of acting exercises set out to remove. Grotowski said that the 'education of an actor in our theatre is not a matter of teaching him something' but an 'attempt to eliminate his organism's resistance to this psychic process', the result being 'freedom from the time-lapse between inner impulse and outer reaction'. Training, for Grotowski, was 'not a collection of skills but an eradication of blocks',[95] which, he proposed, 'leads to a liberation from complexes in much the same way as psycho-analytic therapy'.[96] In rediscovering the power of mythical tales told not only through language but through the expressive power of the human voice, Grotowski reclaimed the therapeutic role of theatre which had been so fundamental to Greek tragedy and upon which Freud built his original cathartic method.

During the early 1960s Jerzy Grotowski had worked with an assistant called Eugenio Barba, who, in 1964, founded his own company in Denmark called Odin Theatre, using applicants who had been refused a place at traditional theatre school. The work of Odin now constitutes an internationally influential body of work, known as Theatre Anthropology, following the widespread influence of Barba's first book, *The Floating Islands.*[97] The aim of Theatre Anthropology is to study the cultural and technical foundations upon which different styles, traditions and genres of performance are based.[98] During his time in Poland, Barba helped Grotowski design the sound montage for a production which included 'varying vocal rhythms, of scored scraping and drumming on the set's metal pipes, and of different rhythms of marching and stamping made by the actors' wooden-soled boots'.[99] Barba thus took with him to Denmark an interest in sounds, particularly those made by the human voice.

Odin has drawn actors from many countries and the actors do not share a common mother tongue, which has led to experiments where, like Brook's group, they have devised pieces based upon the use of their own unique self-created language.[100] All of Barba's productions have a complex vocal score consisting of songs, naturalistic dialogue, languages from different countries, chants, incantations and 'vocables' in which the voice is used as a musical instrument.[101] Like the theatre of Grotowski, Barba's process is one in which the experience of the actor is revered as central and the dynamic relationships between company members is drawn upon in the rehearsal process.

Artaud and Grotowski also influenced the research of Richard Schechner, who founded the New York-based Performance Group in 1967 and has influenced the study of theatre in the West, initially through his seminal text *Performance Theory.*[102] Schechner wanted to develop a mode of theatre which mirrored participatory rituals indigenous to many non-western communities and in this envisioned theatre the established centrality of narrative and character was to be replaced by the ritual image.[103] Schechner's study of ritual uncovers an area of research and occurrence which he describes as existing between theatre and anthropology.[104] In this area he finds the occurrence of rituals in which the deepening of experience is often made possible by the transcending of verbal language into spontaneous vocal utterance.[105] The audience, for Schechner, was, therefore, not composed of audients who remain in a state of passive acoustic receptivity but active participants in the event. Schechner further believed that part of the power of such ritual theatre lay in a deep level of communication and expression that was beyond the realm of speech.[106]

Neither Artaud, Brook, Grotowski, Barba or Schechner were clinically trained or qualified as therapists yet their work on the human voice was deeply rooted in a respect for the intimate connection between vocal sound and soul. Their field of enquiry was not voice therapy but Voicework which had therapeutic implications. However, the implications of their work were equally relevant to the field of anthropology, performance, literature and mythology. In many ways they returned the notion of therapy to the arts from which it has been extracted. Such work is, therefore, significant, not only because of its content but because of its form: it reveals how the artistic process can be innately life enhancing without need for a clinical or thera-peutic context or explanation in order to qualify it or legitimate its value.

In this day, where there is an ever-increasing momentum towards what McNiff calls the 'obsessional concern with a clinification of the arts in order to validate their therapeutic application',[107] the work of these practitioners can provide inspiration. A Therapeutic Voiceworker is, perhaps, first and foremost, an artist who is prepared to acknowledge and respond to the very special responsibility which he has in composing form from the unformed substance of experience.

Augusto Boal and the Political Voice

Between 1922 and 1923 communist speech choirs came into existence in many Russian and East German cities, which engaged huge groups of work-ing people in the choral utterance of politicised poetry.[108] The speech choir movement spread to Britain, America, Czechoslovakia and Hungary and in the USA it was employed in schools.[109] Speech choirs, the original intention of which was to give the ordinary man a voice, both artistically and politi-cally, were an important symbol of the social, as opposed to the psychic, dimension to vocal expression for the voice is the means by which we assert our rights in the world, it is a metaphor for our democratic necessity and a medium of expression for our rightful demands. A contemporary theatre practitioner whose work belongs in the tradition of twentieth century avant garde, which was originally modelled on a sociopolitical approach to the voice and to whom the political concept of voice is still a central working component, is the Brazilian theatre director and workshop leader Augusto Boal.

Boal began developing a body of work known as *The Theatre of the Oppressed* in the 1950s when the aim of his work was to mobilise audiences and participants towards an activist stance against Brazil's widespread corruption and oppression of the poor. Central to the work was 'Forum Theatre', where scenes would be presented to an audience who would be permitted to intervene either by directing the actors or by acting themselves, thereby empowering one another to shape and direct the action. Brazil had a military coup in 1964 and again in 1968 and Boal used this theatre work to challenge the harsh conditions of dictatorship. He was then gaoled in 1971 where he was tortured and, on his release, he moved to Argentina, where he resided until 1976. It was here that Boal developed 'Image Theatre', where 'the human body is used as an expressive tool to represent, non-verbally, a wide repertoire of feelings, ideas, and attitudes'.[110] Forbidden to take part in activist theatre by the Argentinean regime, Boal developed 'Invisible Theatre'. These were scenes played out by actors in public spaces in such a way that the audience did not realise they were watching a performance. However, finding it impossible to work, Boal withdrew from theatre activity and wrote *Theatre of the Oppressed.*[111] From 1976 to 1986 Boal was in exile working in Europe.

In South America Boal's work was designed to mobilise people to stand up to what he termed the 'cop in the streets', that is the actual external social violence and pressure of social reality. However, in Europe workshop participants brought internal problems of psychic fragmentation, selflessness and a host of psychological struggles. At first Boal was frustrated by these oppressions, which seemed insignificant when compared to the social hardships he had been confronted with in South America. However, influenced somewhat by his wife, who later became a psychoanalyst in France, Boal began to conceive of the 'cop in the head' – that is the introjected and internal voices of oppression absorbed from society, parents, teachers and suspect moral values which continued to plague the adult. Boal's sociopolitical theatre techniques thus took on a therapeutic and psychoanalytic dimension and his workshops were presented, in many cases, as therapeutic processes. His work and its clinical validity was acknowledged when he was invited to give the keynote speech at the tenth convention of the International Association of Group Psychotherapy in Amsterdam in 1989, which led to the re-presentation of his theatre work within a therapeutic paradigm. In his subsequent book he describes the inner reality of introjected objects as being equally oppressing of an individual as the social realities of political tyranny. Boal describes his work as a 'psycho-theatre', a realm where theatre and therapy overlap[112] and this theatre catharsis, for Boal, means a purging of those 'detrimental blocks' which inhibit positive social and political action.[113]

Another practitioner who has investigated the inner psychic world of individuals and, at the same time, acted politically in giving marginalised individuals a central place upon the stage is Robert Wilson.

Robert Wilson was born in Texas in 1941 and, as a child, suffered from a severe speech impediment which made spoken language difficult to master because he felt 'tongue-tied', as though his 'tongue had been clipped' and 'tied to the bottom of' his mouth.[114] At the age of seventeen, Wilson met an elderly dance instructor, Bird Hoffman, who worked with him over a period of three months 'encouraging him to relax and release the tensions in his body through movement exercises,'[115] after which his speech impediment disappeared. Later, Wilson continued investigating the use of movement and performance with children and young people with varying kinds of disabilities, leading workshops where he worked 'with very simple exercises', such as 'crawling', 'pushing and pulling'.[116] In 1966 Wilson extended his clientele to adults and began facilitating 'psycho-somatic therapy work'[117] through workshops which he conducted with adults and with young, often handicapped children and which culminated in performances which were presented 'in construction sites', 'in churches', 'in garages or in vacant lots'.[118]

Influenced by his exposure to the dance work of Merce Cunningham and Martha Graham and the performance styles of the Judson Dance theatre – particularly the work of Kenneth King and Meredith Monk – as well as the theatrical 'Happenings' staged around New York, the artistic environment of east coast America in the early sixties 'shaped his tastes, interests and, ultimately, the aesthetics of his theatre'[119] as he began to create performances with adult friends and followers who were beginning to gather around him. The lessons learned from the special needs of those in the workshops, combined with the influence of other contemporaries, thus enabled Wilson to develop a non-narrative image-oriented theatre.

In 1970 Wilson became the artistic director of the Byrd Hoffman Foundation, named after the dance instructor who had saved him from his expressive restrictions. The aim of the foundation was to conduct workshops for children and adults, including those with disabilities and handicaps, using dance and theatre work and to mount performances which arose out of this process.[120] At the same time, the constituting members of the Foundation, known as the Byrds, became the performers in Wilson's own original performance pieces.

Wilson's rehearsals with the Byrds were very closely associated with his workshop activities, 'which have been consistently concerned with helping participants discover their own unique ways of moving'[121] and 'their own vocabulary of movement'.[122] In actuality, the 'workshops in psychosomatic therapy with grown-ups', designed to offer a healing process through participation in artistic process, 'did not differ greatly from his theatre workshops', which were designed to offer an audience an insight into the psychic reality of each performer, showing not a make-believe character 're-presented by an actor' but revealing the performers 'as themselves'.[123] In his therapeutic workshops Wilson provided movement exercises for participants and, at the same time, learned 'from their particular ways of expression, communication, and sensibility', which he then 'applied to his theatre workshops and performances', which, 'from the early stages', have been 'influenced to a great extent by his work with exceptional children'.[124]

Central to Wilson's investigations was his work with Raymond Andrews, a young boy who was almost totally deaf and had no command of language but who vocalised sounds and with whom Wilson achieved a 'radical integration of therapy into theatre'.[125] Wilson describes Andrews as possessing a 'special sensibility and unusual ways of communication' which 'provided a rich alternative and inspiration for the work' for 'in spite of his near total deafness and virtually no vocabulary', he became a 'communicative member of the group', 'demonstrating an ability to be exceedingly and exceptionally sensitive to the feelings of others' but perceiving and transmitting 'through kinetic, or kinesthetic awareness rather than through discursive, or verbal dialogue'. In children such as Andrews, Wilson 'sensed not only a deep, special talent but channels usually unknown for establishing lines of communication'.[126]

Wilson brought other performers into Andrews' world, constructing a secure nest inside which the young boy's 'own construction of reality could be played out'[127] and in which Wilson and the Byrds attempted to 'learn his language of sounds and gestures by imitating him'. Then, having acquired Andrews' language of non-verbal communication, the troupe constructed a theatre piece using it called *Deafman Glance*, first performed in 1970 with Andrews in the cast. The performance had hardly any words, it dealt almost entirely in images and in 'deaf sounds', like the ones Andrews made, and was the result of movements, gestures and drawings which Andrews had given Wilson.[128]

It has been said that 'a child stands in the foreground of most of Wilson's plays' like a figure of the disabled boy-child which was his youthful self.[129] Indeed, *Deafman Glance* presented a terrifying scenario in which little happens except that a woman pushes a knife into a boy's chest as Andrews screams 'the high-pitched, impotent utterance of a deaf mute'.[130] The piece was performed in such slow motion that it lasted one hour.

In later performances Wilson's use of his own voice aimed to show the way that the thoughts of the mind often flow 'in several directions at once,'[131] aiming to communicate the idea that 'verbal discourse cannot adequately provide or express insight'.[132] Wilson thus worked his voice through an array of sounds which included words and phrases which broke up into 'phonic abrogation',[133] 'wilfully distorted incantations',[134] a 'play of the vocal organs'[135] in which he allowed himself to become 'caught in a fandango' of his vocal cords, 'his tongue dancing in the rhythmic blast from his throat, twisting itself into the successive shapes of sounds next to one another'.[136]

In one production, which used thirty members of the Byrds and twenty Iranians, staged on the side of Haft Tan Mountain, Shiraz and which lasted 168 hours,[137] 'the vocal delivery incorporated a frequency of high-pitched screams, contributed by Wilson, which he alternated with odd phrases in a deep bass voice' combined with uses of falsetto voice, slowed-down pronunciation, lapses into chanting in gibberish, disjointed phrasing and experiments with staccato rhythm, whispering' and performers speaking 'past' each other.[138] This use of non-verbal voice also played a significant role in Wilson's most renowned production, *Einstein on the Beach*, born from a collaboration with the composer Phillip Glass, in which vocal elements included 'schizophrenic screaming', 'chattering nonsense language', 'laughter' and 'swearing'.[139]

Since his early work of the Seventies, Wilson has gone on to work collaboratively with some of the most prolific artists, including the German playwright Heiner Muller, American rock singer, lyricist and film-maker David Byrne, the soprano, Jessye Norman, musician, performer and visual

artist Laurie Anderson and the Beat poet Allen Ginsberg. Within the contemporary arts, Wilson has thus been held in high esteem and, in many ways, he
is an icon of late twentieth century post-modern performance. However, it is
important to remember that his work grew from therapeutic work with those
for whom the performance arts were, in the main, inaccessible. Wilson, in
effect, reminds us that therapy, particularly that which utilises voice, has been
conducted as much in the rehearsal rooms of experimental theatre as it has in
the consulting rooms of clinicians.

However, the therapeutic dimension to Wilson's activities were more
somatic than psychic. In many ways his approach drew from a physiological
model by which his clients were enabled to overcome certain physical obstacles in order to move, speak and express themselves. But, again, it is neither
appropriate nor necessary to identify Wilson's achievements as 'therapy' or to
align it with a clinical model. Wilson worked intuitively and sensitively and it
is, I believe, sufficient to acknowledge his investigations, and those of others
like him, as Voice-work, Body-work and Performance-work.

The Roy Hart Theatre

By far the most consistent, radical and significant contribution to vocal work
on the interface between therapy and theatre is that contributed by the members of the Roy Hart Theatre, a company which was founded upon the initial
research of Alfred Wolfsohn.

In the year following Wolfsohn's death, the group of students who had
studied with him, some of them for over 14 years, outlined the areas of investigation which their vocal work covered and which included psychology,
drama and music.[140] Wolfsohn's students had discovered that freeing the
voice 'also liberates other artistic aptitudes'[141] and that vocal malleability 'is a
great asset when it comes to dramatic production'.[142]

During the later period of his teaching, Wolfsohn had opened the studio
doors to the entire clientele of students at any time during the work so that
they were able to learn from both the experience of their own process and
also from the observation of others, which led to the organic emergence of a
working group. Among the group was a South African called Roy Hart, who
had come to England to study as an actor at the Royal Academy of Dramatic
Art.[143] Inspired by the performance quality of vocal demonstrations which
the pupils did for observers, Roy Hart was keen to develop the work beyond
presentations to invited guests for the purposes of demonstrating technique
towards theatre performances which utilised the extended vocal range in a

dramatic context and which stood in its own right as art. Thus he began performing poems and songs using an extended vocal range.[144]

With the death of Wolfsohn in 1962, Roy Hart announced clearly that it was his intention to further the work towards theatre and invited the group to join him in the pursuit of experiments in a new form vocal dramatics. Thus those who could not accept the shift into a performance-orientated ensemble headed by Roy Hart departed and as old people left, so new ones joined and between 1962 and 1967 a number of fresh people who had not known Wolfsohn began to take lessons with Roy Hart, who, as a result, became the leader of a new group. The 'Alfred Wolfsohn Voice Research Centre' now became the 'Roy Hart Actor Singers' and, eventually, the 'Roy Hart Theatre' and what 'had begun with small voice-demonstrations slowly took the shape of theatrical performances'.[145]

In 1967 the group began work towards its first theatrical production, which was based on *The Bacchae*. The rehearsal methodology involved a process which lasted over two years in which the troupe would 'read and re-read the text' as well as 'sing it, scream it and reduce it to gibberish'.[146] Among those who came to invited performances of *The Bacchae* were Peter Brook, Jerzy Grotowski, R. D. Laing, Irene Worth, Stockhausen and Jean Louis Barrault, the renowned avant garde theatre director and innovator who subsequently invited the group to present the piece at 'The World University Festival of Theatre' in France in 1969. In addition, the composer Peter Maxwell-Davies was also present at one of the initial presentations of *The Bacchae* and, in response to what he saw, he composed a full-length piece for Roy Hart called *Eight Songs for a Mad King*, with subsequent performances given internationally, and in response to which Hart was described as an artist who commands 'all the voices of the human register – ranging from the deepest bass to the highest soprano'.[147]

Indeed, *Eight Songs for a Mad King* has become the most frequently cited exemplification of the performance work which arose from Roy Hart's continuance of the research initiated by Wolfsohn. This composition is located in the context of increasing vocal experimentation by composers of the classical tradition in the mid-twentieth century. For example, in *Sequenza III* Luciano Berio created a portrait of a woman which was described by Berio's close collaborator and performer of the piece, Cathy Berberian, as 'like an X-ray of a woman's inner life'.[148] In this performance Berberian uses her voice in an untraditional way, combining extensive twists and turns of tone and timbre to animate the subject matter. The character is portrayed as though she is suffering from a severe mental disorder in which words are fractured and broken up and she sings using muttering, breathy whispering, whimpering, humming, laughter, changing intensity from very soft to very loud as well as freely combining combining syllables, vowels and consonants. Pursuing a similar process of investigation, in *Nouvelles Aventures* the composer György Ligeti presents a musicalised story told in an artificial language constructed by the composer but which presents an archetypal image 'as if it were the language of a newly discovered tribe'.[149] The piece begins with a mighty baritonal yell and involves, at one point, three voices breaking out into a rapid stammer, having been told by the composer that it should be 'as though one wanted by all means to explain something without being able to do so'.[150]

However, despite these other compositional contributions to a radical review of vocal performance, it was Roy Hart and his followers who made the most single-minded and determined effort to extend the boundaries of vocal expression in a performance context.

In 1969 Roy Hart performed a work composed especially for him by Karlheiz Stockhausen. In the same year the entire group performed their own devised piece, which used bodily movement and non-verbal sound but no language. This played for a week at the Roundhouse, London and the performers were described as people 'seeking to liberate their tensions' and those of the audience through 'a kind of abstract collage of sound and movement' which compares to 'a group therapy session in full cry' as the performers 'croak, scream, cry like seagulls, sing sweetly, and shout hoarsely'. This reviewer said that he had 'never seen actors giving quite so much of themselves'.[151] Another piece, entitled 'AND', provoked Catherine Backes-Clement to say that the performers revealed 'the meeting point of voice and myth' where 'the voice alone, apparently liberated from the constraint of rational meaning, finds meaning on the Other Stage; in the presence of the Unconscious'.[152]

Indeed, there was recognition of the psychological implications of the work not only from the theatre profession but from psychotherapeutic circles also. During the 1960s and early 1970s Hart and the company presented their research in the form of lectures and demonstrations at the Jung Institute in England[153] and at psychotherapy and arts therapy conferences all over the world, including London,[154] Wiesbaden,[155] Vienna,[156] Zagreb and the Seventh International Congress of Psychodrama. But, despite the psychological nature of the contexts in which he was invited to speak, a vocal theatre was still central to his aims and purposes.

In 1975 Roy Hart and two other members of the group – his wife, Dorothy Hart, and Vivienne Young – died in a car accident while on route from performances in Austria to a tour of Spain. Since then the group has expanded and diversified, with members teaching workshops all over the world, returning to their base at the Chateau du Malerargues in the South of France for an annual summer convention.

Central to the work of The Roy Hart Theatre has been the teaching of voice workshops based on the same philosophy as that initiated by Wolfsohn as early as 1933. Their performances and their approach to rehearsals, which utilise the human voice to animate the depths of the human soul, have not only astounded audiences world-wide but have had significant influence on the use of voice in the avant garde theatre. In particular, both Peter Brook and Jerzy Grotowski have acknowledged their debt to the work.

Many of the teachers who have graduated from the Roy Hart Theatre use the word 'therapy' to describe their approach and this has contributed both inspiration and confusion to the perception of Therapeutic Voicework. Many participants in Roy Hart Theatre workshops led by members of the network contact deep material with highly charged emotional resonance, however many of the workshop leaders are ambivalent regarding the degree to which they are able or willing to provide a therapeutic response, both within and after the workshop has finished. Consequently, whilst some participants have benefited from the approach, others have experienced a dearth of appropriate containment. Furthermore, different participants have had widely varying responses to different member teachers of the Roy Hart Theatre. Naturally, this reflects the general complexity inherent in the interface between theatre and therapy and the Roy Hart Theatre is probably the longest standing group of people who, despite ambiguity around the issue of therapy versus theatre, have nonetheless displayed unrivalled commitment to persevering with an investigation of this interface. Indeed, without the Roy Hart Theatre, the notion of an artistically orientated but therapeutic approach to voice would be severely impoverished.

Therapeutic Voicework Methodology: The Rehearsal

Rehearsal literally means 'to repeat' and is the method by which a raw and unsculptured emotional experience is crafted and wroughted until it has communicable form. In the theatre, during the early stages of preparation for production, the actor discharges the emotional expressions which seem appropriate to the character in great magnitude, often with gestures and motions which correlate. Then, through the process of rehearsal, the emotions and their expression are refined, plotted, scored, choreographed and inscribed so that they are repeatable with some degree of consistency. The price often paid for such security is the actor's loss of realism, of emotional authenticity, and many actors reach a stage in preparations where their original inspired performance seems staid, rigid and automatic. The final stage, before revealing all to an audience, is for the actor to rediscover and re-engender the original emotional fluidity within the contours of the rehearsed moves and choreographed interactions.

This process of rehearsal has great creative, therapeutic and pedagogical use in Therapeutic Voicework, particularly when a client brings to a session material which is highly charged with emotion to the point of being overwhelming, consuming and difficult to form and, therefore, to contain. For the practitioner, the process of requesting rehearsed repetition of the material can enable the client to shape an expressive container for intense affect. One project which has utilised this phenomenon is that arising from the collaborative work between Jungian analyst Marion Woodman and actress and voice teacher Michelle George, who was a member of Peter Brook's International Centre for Theatre Research for many years. Together, Woodman and George have provided workshops which enable participants to contact 'the well of untouched feeling in the belly' by opening the vocal folds which, metaphorically, says George, act as a 'cover to the well'.[157] Influenced by her theatre background, George asks participants to bring to the process written text to work on individually, witnessed by the group and the process of rehearsing and exploring this text, through speech and song, is a therapeutic process for the participant and for the witnessing group.[158]

In the methodological and integrated approach to Therapeutic Voicework I have found the rehearsal process one of the most liberating ways of relieving a client from the sense of being subjected to a clinical analysis and providing an opportunity to investigate the self through empowering artistic expression. Within the paradigm of the rehearsal, the wealth of insight and practical investigation which has been bequeathed by theatre practitoners such as those acknowledged in this chapter can be drawn upon.

Therapeutic Voicework Case Study: All the World's a Stage

James was 47 years old. He had been very happily married for 20 years before his wife left him to live with his best friend.

James' physical condition prior to his trauma had already been somewhat complicated. He was diabetic, had high blood pressure, had suffered from two stomach ulcers and one cardiac arrest. Since the divorce he had 'retrained' himself to live at a 'steadier pace' and, in fact, had been much healthier physically. However, at the time of his wife's departure, James described himself as having been extremely numb with shock, except for two excruciating sensations: a severe abdominal pain and a sticky lump in his throat. Moreover, these sensations, though they had decreased in intensity, had not fully receded.

James was an intelligent man and had, naturally, linked these conditions with feeling both gutted and choked by his trauma. Thus he had conceived that working through the voice may help him alleviate the sensations and resolve some of the emotional difficulties that had befallen him.

In taking James' history I noticed that he frequently referred to himself as a fool, often blaming himself for not seeing his 'wife's infidelity coming'. On reflection, he said, he should have known things could not go on as they were, yet he 'had avoided bringing the subject' of their marriage up with his wife. He had two grown daughters, of whom he was very fond, but they too considered him foolish. In many respects, James was consumed with regret, remorse and self-deprecation. As I listened to this man talk and looked at the splendid contours which life had etched on his weather-worn face, I could not help but think of Shakespeare's play *King Lear*.

As he knew this play, when we started to work I asked James to move and vocalise, first as Lear and then as Lear's fool. To the former he gave a modal voice in saxophone with lots of violin, ⟨⟩ M ⩒ , and the latter he portrayed in falsetto flute with lots of free air, ＞|＜ F . Taking pieces of the text from the play, James explored these two characters as aspects of himself, until they merged into a single figure which he characterised utilising two props which he took from the basket in my studio: a cap which he called 'a little man's cap' and a walking stick which he used to portray infirmity.

At a point towards the end of a session James suddenly became irate, his face flushing red and his breathing increasing in pace as he sat down with his head in his hands. When I asked him what he was feeling, he said: 'I am tired of feeling foolish and decrepit. I am mad, mad, mad.' He was, he said, furious with his wife and, as he rose from the chair, said: 'I should have killed her' and then immediately said: 'please God forgive me', as though he wished to withdraw the expression of his rageful and murderous feelings. As it was the end of the session I simply commented that perhaps Othello would be more appropriate than Lear.

At the beginning of the next session James was animated and excited, confessing that, as he had not known Othello, he had read the play in the interim and felt that he understood Othello's rage and his remorse. Thus he began to read excerpts from the text with a voice in saxophone timbre, deep in pitch with lots of vibrato and no violin, ⟨⟩ M ⊥⊥ ∧∧. The walking stick which he had used now became a sword and he exchanged the 'little man's cap' for a bowler hat.

When working with the piece of text which is uttered as Othello suffocates his wife, Desdemona, James began to cry and his voice moved to a falsetto sob in clarinet with lots of free air, ⟨▷ F, and he explained that he had made himself ill through over-working and had been 'completely blind' to the state of his marriage. He now felt foolish because he had always believed that his wife had not only supported him professionally but contributed to his ambition. In fact he said he had often secretly blamed her for 'driving him on', yet, 'as it turned out', she had left him as a result of circumstances initiated by what she felt to be James' obsessional 'marriage to his work'.

As James spoke of his illusion of being driven on by his wife, I naturally thought of Macbeth and the way in which he is driven by Lady Macbeth. James laughed when I intimated this connection and said: 'Oh yes I could play Macbeth with no trouble'.

By the next session James had isolated a scene in the play where Lady Macbeth persuades her husband to kill the king by questioning his resolve and his manhood. He began to utter Macbeth's words in clarinet timbre and in modal register, ⟨⟩ M. I then asked him to speak Lady Macbeth's part by staying in clarinet but allowing the vocal register to shift into falsetto with a moderate amount of violin, ⟨⟩ F ▷. As we worked, James played both characters, slipping and sliding in and out of Macbeth and Lady Macbeth. In rehearsing this transition James remarked that, on reflection, aspects of the relationship between him and his wife had been ridiculous and that they had been 'like the two characters on a weather clock' who pass in and out 'without ever meeting'. So we began to make the characters of Shakespeare's play into a bizarre king (Figure 9.1) and queen (Figure 9.2) who squabbled and

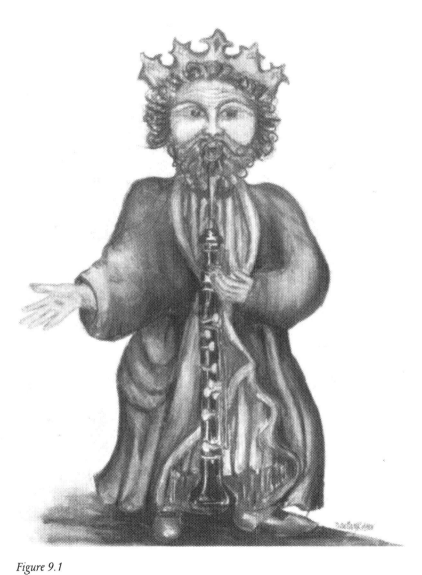

Figure 9.1

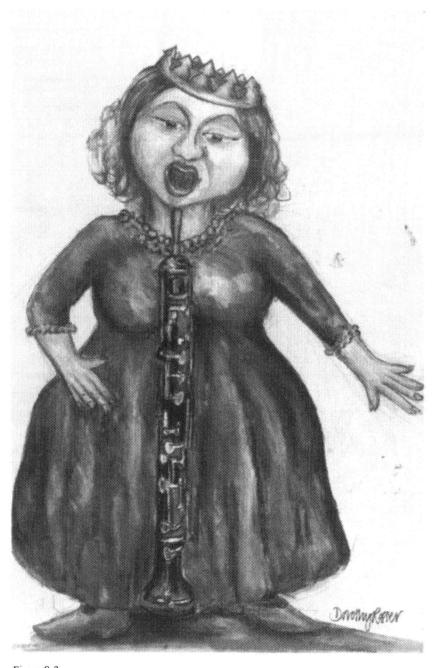

Figure 9.2

argued, failing to see each others point of view, allowing the vocal identity of each to become distinct only by way of register.

Because the change between the two vocalisations was so subtle, James felt just how close the two qualities of driving ambition, represented by the queen, and driven toil, represented by the king, were in himself. Because he had also slipped into falsetto when crying during the earlier work on Othello, he also felt the close proximity between his sorrow and his rage. Though he and his wife had never really met, the qualities in himself which had been separated and unacknowledged and projected out onto his wife, particularly his ambition and obsessional devotion to work, now met the other parts of himself. In a certain way he became whole by giving voice and dramatic character to different selves.

As James contemplated these dawning recognitions he began to use the characters of Shakespeare's texts as a container for his own voluminous rage, anguish, sorrow and regret. Pacing up and down the studio, he declaimed and sung, bellowing out an oratorio constructing a melodramatic amplification of four aspects of himself: the sorrowful remorse, the angry revenge, the driving ambition and the stressful toil. Without the characters, it is unlikely that he would have been able to sustain the mythic proportion of his feelings, which suited the amplified dimensions of Shakespeare's figures.

As a result of the work, the lump in James' throat and the pains in the abdomen disappeared and he developed a most malleable voice in singing and in speech. Encouraged by his progress, James put his work to use by working as a reader of plays and novels for blind people.

Conclusion: From the Therapy in Art to the Arts in Therapy

It is clearly apparent from the history of vocal work in the Western theatre throughout the twentieth century that a great deal of therapeutic investigation has occurred in the context of performance. Consequently, in seeking to create a working model for Therapeutic Voicework, the notion of the performing arts and their therapeutic potential seems to be an essential component.

Where the nature of performance and the process of psychotherapy meet quite deliberately and formally is within the field known as the expressive arts therapies: music therapy, dramatherapy and dance movement therapy. In seeking to deepen my investigation of Therapeutic Voicework, I shall, now turn my attention to these modalities in search of insight with regard to the therapeutic use of artistic vocal expression.

Notes

1   Sheridan, T. (1968) cited in R C Alston (ed) *Thomas Sheridan: A Course of Lectures on Elocution 1762.* Menston: Scolar Press, p.10.

2   Haberman, F. (1954) 'English sources of American elocution.' In K. Wallace (ed) *History of Speech Education in America.* New York: Appleton-Century-Crofts, pp.109–10.

3   Hale, L. (1954) 'Dr. James Rush' 'English sources of American elocution.' In K. Wallace (ed) *History of Speech Education in America.* New York: Appleton-Century-Crofts, p.223.

4   Coger, L. (1952) *A Comparison for the Oral Interpreter of the Teaching Methods of Curry and Stanislavski.* Ph.D. dissertation, NorthWestern University's School of Speech, p.111.

5   Clifford Turner, J. (1977) *Voice and Speech in the Theatre.* London: Pitman.

6   Brodnitz, F.S. (1988) *Keep Your Voice Healthy.* USA: College Hill.

7   Bunch, M. (1989) *Speak with Confidence.* London: Kogan Page.

8   Laver, J. (1980) *Phonetic Description of Voice.* Cambridge: Cambridge University Press.

9   McCallion, M. (1988) *The Voice Book.* London: Faber and Faber.

10   H Caesari, E. *The Alchemy of Voice.* London: Robert Hale, 1965) and *Vocal Truth.* London: Hale, 1969.

11   Rush, J. (1827) *The Philosophy of the Human Voice: Embracing its Physiological History; Together with a System of Principles, by which Criticism in the Art of Elocution may be Rendered Intelligible, and Instruction, Definite and Comprehensive. To which is Added a Brief Analysis of Song and Recitative.* Philadelphia.

12   Hale, L.L. (1949) 'Dr. James Rush - psychologist and voice scientist.' *Quarterly Journal of Speech, 35,* 4, pp.448–55.

13   Smith, J. (1973) *Melodrama.* London: Methuen.

14   Kravitt, E. (1976) 'The joining of words and music in late romantic melodrama.' *Music Quarterly,* lxii, p.571.

15   Guilbert, Y. (1929) *La Passante Emerveillée.* Paris: Bernard Grasset.

16   Booth, M. (1995) 'Nineteenth century theatre.' In J. Brown (ed) *The Oxford Illustrated History of Theatre.* Oxford: Oxford University Press, pp.299–340, (p.306).

17   James, H. 'On the Occasion of *Hedda Gabler,' New Review.* (June 1891).

18   Esslin, M. (1991) 'Modernist drama: Wedekind to Brecht.' In M. Bradbury and J. McFarlane (ed) *Modernism: A Guide to European Literature 1890-1930.* London: Penguin, pp.527–60.

19   Schlaf, J. (1906) *Maurice Maeterlink.* Berlin, p.31.

20   *République Francaise,* Review of work by Théâtre Libre, September 1896.

21   Stanislavski, C. (1983) *Creating a Role.* Trans. by E. Hapgood. London: Methuen, p.261.

22   Stanislavski, C. (1979) *Building a Character.* Trans. by E. Hapgood. London: Methuen, pp.82–108.

23   Linklater, K. (1976) *Freeing the Natural Voice.* New York: Drama Book: pp.11–12.

24   Berry,C. (1973) *Voice and the Actor.* London: Harrap.

25   Berry, C. (1987) *The Actor and his Text.* London: Harrap.

26   Berry, C. (1987) *Your Voice and How to Use it Successfully.* London: Harrap.

27   Rodenburg, P. (1992) *The Right to Speak: Working with the Voice.* London: Methuen Drama.

28   Rodenburg, P. (1993) *The Need for Words: Voice and the Text.* London: Methuen.

29   Rodenburg, P. (1992) *The Right to Speak: Working with the Voice.* London: Methuen Drama, p.107.

30   Berry,C. (1987) *Your Voice and How to Use it Successfully.* London: Harrap, p.37.

31   Rodenburg, P. (1992) *The Right to Speak: Working with the Voice.* London: Methuen Drama, p.86.

32   Rodenburg, P. (1992) *The Right to Speak: Working with the Voice.* London: Methuen Drama, p.87.

33   Rodenburg, P. (1992) *The Right to Speak: Working with the Voice.* London: Methuen Drama, pp.64–65.

34   Houseman, B. (1994) 'Voice and the release and exploration of emotion (from a theatre perspective).' *Dramatherapy, 16,* 2 and 3 (Autumn 1994), pp.25–27, (p.25).

35   Cooper, M. (1984) *Change Your Voice Change Your Life.* New York: Macmillan, p.96.

36   Strindberg, A. (1990) Introduction to *Miss Julie.* In *The Plays of Strindberg,* vol. 1. intro. and trans. by M. Meyer. London: Methuen, pp.99–112.

37   Strindberg, A. (1990) Introduction to *Miss Julie.* In *The Plays of Strindberg,* vol. 1. intro. and trans. by M. Meyer. London: Methuen, pp.99–112.

38   Strindberg, A. (1990) Introduction to *Miss Julie.* In *The Plays of Strindberg,* vol. 1. intro. and trans. by M. Meyer. London: Methuen, pp.99–112.

39   Innes, C. (1993) *Avant Garde Theatre 1892–1992.* London: Routledge, pp.19–20.

40   Fels, F.M. (1891) 'Die Moderne.' *Moderne Rundschau,* no. iv, pp.79–81.

41   Strindberg, A. (1990) Introduction to *Miss Julie.* In *The Plays of Strindberg,* vol. 1. intro. and trans. by M. Meyer. London: Methuen, pp.99–112.

42   Innes, C. (1993) *Avant Garde Theatre, 1892–1992.* London: Routledge, p.21.

43   Innes, C. (1981) *Holy Theatre: Ritual and the Avant Garde.* Cambridge: Cambridge University Press, p.18.

44   Valéry, P. (1958) *The Art of Poetry.* New York: Princeton, Bollingen Series, Volume VII, p.18.

45   De Maria, L. (ed) (1968) *Opere di F. Marinetti,* vol. 2. Verona.

46   Apollonio, U. (ed) (1973) *Futurist Manifestos.* London.

47   Flint, R. (1972) *Marinetti: Selected Writings.* New York: Straus and Giroux, p.142.

48   Flint, R. (1972) *Marinetti: Selected Writings.* New York: Straus and Giroux, p.143.

49   Marinetti, F.T. (1960) *Teatro F. T. Marinetti, vol 1.* Giovanni Calendoli (ed). Rome, p.50.

50   Flint, R. (1972) *Marinetti: Selected Writings.* New York: Straus and Giroux, p.144.

51   Kirby, M. (1971) *Futurist Performance.* New York: Dutton and Co.

52   Russolo, L. (1967) *The Art of Noise.* New York.

53   Author unknown, 'The Art of Noise', *The Times,* 30 June 1913.

54   Goldberg, R. (1995) *Performance Art: From Futurism to the Present.* London: Thames and Hudson, p.123–4.

55   Goldberg, R. (1995) *Performance Art: From Futurism to the Present.* London: Thames and Hudson, p.123–4.

56   Kirby, M. (1971) *Futurist Performance.* New York: Dutton and Co.

57   Mayakovsky, V. (1970) *How Are Verses Made?* Trans. G Hyde. London: Pluto Press, p.67.

58   Shklovsky, V. (1974) *Mayakovsky and his Circle.* London: Pluto Press.

59   Hyde, G. (1991) 'Russian futurism.' In M. Bradbury and J. McFarlane (eds) *Modernism: A Guide to European Literature, 1890–1930.* London: Penguin, pp.259–273, (p.264).

60   Hyde, G. (1991) 'Russian futurism.' In M. Bradbury and J. McFarlane (eds) *Modernism: A Guide to European Literature, 1890–1930.* London: Penguin, pp.259–273, (p.263).

61   Mayakovsky, V.I. et al, (1991) 'A slap in the face of public taste.' Cited in G. Hyde 'Russian Futurism.' In M. Bradbury and J. McFarlane (eds) *Modernism: A Guide to European Literature, 1890–1930.* London: Penguin, pp.259–273, (p.263).

62   Matthews, J. (1974) *Theatre in Dada and Surrealism.* Syracuse: Syracuse University Press.

63   Ball, H. (1974) *Flight out of Time.* New York: Viking Press, p.70.

64   Steinke, G. (1967) *The Life and Work of Hugo Ball.* The Hague: Mouton, p.88.

65   Ball, H. (1974) *Flight out of Time.* New York: Viking Press, p.76.

66   Martin, J. (1991) *Voice in Modern Theatre.* London and New York: Routledge, p.63.

67   Artaud, A. (1981) *The Theatre and Its Double.* Trans. by V. Corti. John Calder: London, p.11.

68   Artaud, A. (1981) *The Theatre and Its Double.* Trans. by V. Corti. John Calder: London, p.29.

69   Artaud, A. (1981) *The Theatre and Its Double.* Trans. by V. Corti. John Calder: London, p.58.

70   Artaud, A. (1981) *The Theatre and Its Double.* Trans. by V. Corti. John Calder: London, p.51.

71   Artaud, A. (1981) *The Theatre and Its Double.* Trans. by V. Corti. John Calder: London, p.58.

72   Artaud, A. (1981) *The Theatre and Its Double.* Trans. by V. Corti. John Calder: London, p.18.

73   Artaud, A. (1981) *The Theatre and Its Double.* Trans. by V. Corti. John Calder: London, p.83.

74   Artaud, A. (1981) *The Theatre and Its Double.* Trans. by V. Corti. John Calder: London, p.20.

75   Artaud, A. (1981) *The Theatre and Its Double.* Trans. by V. Corti. John Calder: London, p.60.

76   Brook, P. (1988) *The Shifting Point: Forty Years of Theatrical Exploration.* London: Methuen, p.169.

77   Innes, C. (1981) *Holy Theatre: Ritual and the Avant Garde.* Cambridge, Massachusetts: Harvard University Press, p.134.

78   Brook, P. (1988) *The Shifting Point: Forty Years of Theatrical Exploration.* London: Methuen, p.108.

79   Heilpern, J. (1989) *Conference of the Birds: The Story of Peter Brook in Africa.* London, Methuen, p.191.

80   Brook, P. (1988) *The Shifting Point: Forty Years of Theatrical Exploration.* London: Methuen, p.130.

81   Roose-Evans, J. (1989) *Experimental Theatre: From Stanislavski to Peter Brook,* 4th edn. London: Routledge, p.175.

82   Roose-Evans, J. (1989) *Experimental Theatre: From Stanislavski to Peter Brook,* 4th edn. London: Routledge, p.177.

83   Heilpern, J. (1989) *Conference of the Birds: The Story of Peter Brook in Africa.* London, Methuen, pp.143–144.

84   Flaszen, L. (1975) 'Akropolis – treatment of the text.' In J. Grotowski (ed) *Towards a Poor Theatre.* London: Methuen, 61–70, (p.69).

85   Seymour, A. (1987) 'Revelations in Poland.' *Plays and Players,* (October 1963), pp.33–34. Cited in J. Kumiega, *The Theatre of Grotowski.* London: Methuen, p.69.

86   Grotowski, J. (1961) 'Dziady jako model teatru nowoczesnego.' *Wspolczesnosc,* 21, p.8. Cited in J. Kumiega, *The Theatre of Grotowski.* London: Methuen, 1987, p.36.

87 Kumiega, J. (1987) *The Theatre of Grotowski.* London: Methuen, p.97.

88 Kumiega, J. (1987) *The Theatre of Grotowski.* London: Methuen, p.130.

89 Grotowski, J. (1975) 'Theatre is an encounter.' In J. Grotowski (ed) *Towards a Poor Theatre,* ed. by. London: Methuen, pp.55–60, (p.56).

90 Grotowski, J. 'Towards a poor theatre.' In J. Grotowski (ed) *Towards a Poor Theatre.* London: Methuen, pp.15–26, (p.22).

91 Flaszen, L. (1987) 'Studium o Hamlecie', (Opole, March 1964). Cited in J. Kumiega, *The Theatre of Grotowski.* London: Methuen, p.73.

92 Roose-Evans, J. (1989) *Experimental Theatre: From Stanislavski to Peter Brook,* 4th edn. London: Routledge, p.166.

93 Grotowski, J. (1975) 'Towards a poor theatre.' In J. Grotowski (ed) *Towards a Poor Theatre.* London: Methuen, pp.15–26, (p.21).

94 Grotowski, J. (1975) 'The theatre's new testament.' In J. Grotowski (ed) *Towards a Poor Theatre.* London: Methuen, pp.27–54, (p.39).

95 Grotowski, J. (1975) 'Towards a poor theatre.' In J. Grotowski (ed) *Towards a Poor Theatre.* London: Methuen, (pp.15–26, (pp.16–17).

96 Grotowski, J. (1975) 'The Theatre's New Testament' in *Towards a Poor Theatre,* ed. by J. Grotowski. London: Methuen, pp.27–54, (p.46).

97 Barba, E. (1979) *The Floating Islands.* Holstebro: Odin Teatret Forlag.

98 Barba, E. (1995) *The Paper Canoe: A Guide to Theatre Anthropology.* London: Routledge, p.9.

99 Watson, I. (1993) *Towards a Third Theatre: Eugenio Barber and the Third Theatre.* London: Routledge, p.14.

100 Watson, I. (1993) *Towards a Third Theatre: Eugenio Barber and the Third Theatre.* London: Routledge, p.3.

101 Watson, I. (1993) *Towards a Third Theatre: Eugenio Barber and the Third Theatre.* London: Routledge, p.86.

102 Schechner, R. (1994) *Performance Theory.* London: Routledge.

103 Schechner, (1982) *The End of Humanism: Writings on Performance.* New York: Performance Arts Journal Press, p.98.

104 Schechner, R. (1985) *Between Theatre and Anthropology.* Philadelphia: University of Pennsylvania Press.

105 Schechner, R. (1995) *The Future of Ritual : Writings on Culture and Performance.* London: Routledge.

106 Innes, C. (1981) *Holy Theatre: Ritual and the Avant Garde.* Cambridge: Cambridge University Press, p.57.

107 McNiff, S. (1996) Interview with P. Newham at Endicott College, Mass. USA (June, 1996).

108 Hoffman, L. and Hoffman-Ostwald, D. (1961) *Deutsches Arbeitertheatre 1918–1933.* Berlin: Henschelverlag.

109 Gullan, M. (1929) *Speech Training in the School.* London: Evans Brothers.

110 Schutzman, M. and Cohen-Cruz, J. (eds) (1994) *Playing Boal: Theatre, Therapy, Activism.* London: Routledge, p.3.

111 Augusto Boal, (1993) *Theatre of the Oppressed.* London: Pluto.

112 Augusto Boal, (1990) *Méthode Boal de Théâtre et de Thérapie: l'Arc-en-ciel du Désir.* Paris: Ramsay, p.17.

113 Augusto Boal, (1995) *The Rainbow of Desire*. London: Routledge, p.69–70.

114 Wilson, R. (1994) cited in S. Brecht, *The Theatre of Visions: Robert Wilson*. London, Methuen, p.14.

115 Shyer, L. (1989) *Robert Wilson and his Collaborators*. New York: Theatre Communications, p.xvi.

116 Wilson, R. (1994) cited in S. Brecht, *The Theatre of Visions: Robert Wilson*. London, Methuen, p.17.

117 Wilson, R. (1994) cited in S. Brecht, *The Theatre of Visions: Robert Wilson*. London, Methuen, p.30.

118 Wilson, R. (1994) cited in S. Brecht, *The Theatre of Visions: Robert Wilson*. London, Methuen, p.15.

119 Shyer, L. (1989) *Robert Wilson and his Collaborators*. New York: Theatre Communications, p.xiv.

120 Wilson, R. (1994) cited in S. Brecht, *The Theatre of Visions: Robert Wilson*. London, Methuen, p.31.

121 Martin, J. (1991) *Voice in Modern Theatre*. London and New York: Routledge, p.145.

122 Simmer, B. (1976) 'Robert Wilson and Therapy.' *Drama Review*, T69, vol. 21, no. 1, p.103.

123 Martin, J. (1991) *Voice in Modern Theatre*. London and New York: Routledge, p.144.

124 Deak, F. 'Robert Wilson', *The Drama Review*, 18 (2), June 1974, pp.67–73, (p.69.).

125 Schechner, R. (1994) *Performance Theory*. London: Routledge, p.217.

126 Wilson, R. *Production notes to The King of Spain*, cited in F. Deak, 'Robert Wilson.' *The Drama Review*, 18 (2), pp.67–73, (p.69).

127 Schechner, R. (1994) *Performance Theory*. London: Routledge, p.217.

128 Martin, J. (1991) *Voice in Modern Theatre*. London and New York: Routledge, p.147.

129 Shyer, L. (1989) *Robert Wilson and his Collaborators*. New York: Theatre Communications, p.xix.

130 Shyer, L. (1989) *Robert Wilson and his Collaborators*. New York: Theatre Communications, p.6.

131 Brecht, S. (1994) *The Theatre of Visions: Robert Wilson*. London, Methuen, p.157.

132 Brecht, S. (1994) *The Theatre of Visions: Robert Wilson*. London, Methuen, p.159.

133 Brecht, S. (1994) *The Theatre of Visions: Robert Wilson*. London, Methuen, p.157.

134 Brecht, S. (1994) *The Theatre of Visions: Robert Wilson*. London, Methuen, p.159.

135 Brecht, S. (1994) *The Theatre of Visions: Robert Wilson*. London, Methuen, p.159.

136 Brecht, S. (1994) *The Theatre of Visions: Robert Wilson*. London, Methuen, pp.157–59.

137 Trilling, O. (1973) 'Robert Wilson's Ka Mountain and Guardenia Terrace.' *Drama Review*, T58, 17, 2, p.34.

138 Martin, J. (1991) *Voice in Modern Theatre*. London and New York: Routledge, p.147.

139 Martin, J. (1991) *Voice in Modern Theatre*. London and New York: Routledge, p.151.

140 Hart, R. and members of the Alfred Wolfsohn Voice Research Centre, 'An outline of the work of the Alfred Wolfsohn Voice Research Centre.' Subsequently published in 'The Roy Hart Theatre: documentation and interviews.' David Williams (ed) *Dartington Theatre Papers*, Fifth Series, 14, 1985. Series ed. by Peter Hulton. (Pub. by Dartington College of Arts. ISSN 0309 - 8036), pp.2–7.

141 Sheppard, L. 'An empirical therapy based on an extension of vocal range and expression in singing and drama.' Unpublished paper read at the Sixth International Congress of Psychotherapy, London, August 1964. Repository: Leslie Sheppard, private collection of papers and recordings.

142 Hart, R. and members of the Alfred Wolfsohn Voice Research Centre, 'An outline of the work of the Alfred Wolfsohn Voice Research Centre.' Subsequently published in 'The Roy Hart Theatre: documentation and interviews.' David Williams (ed) *Dartington Theatre Papers*, Fifth Series, 14, 1985. Series ed. by Peter Hulton. (Pub. by Dartington College of Arts. ISSN 0309 - 8036), pp.4–5. (pp.2–7).

143 Hart, R. 'How voice gave me a conscience.' Unpublished paper read at the Seventh International Congress for Psychotherapy, Wiesbaden, 1967. Repository: Roy Hart Theatre Archives, Malerargues, France.

144 Hart, R. Unpublished phonograph recordings, 1957–1960 .

145 Gunther, M. (1990) 'The human voice: On Alfred Wolfsohn.' *Spring: A Journal of Archetype and Culture*, 50 (pp.65–75), p.73.

146 Gunther, M. (1985) Interview with David Williams, Malerargues, France, February 1985, cited in 'The Roy Hart Theatre: Documentation and Interviews.' David Williams (ed) *Dartington Theatre Papers*, Fifth Series, No. 14. Series ed. by Peter Hulton. (Pub. by Dartington College of Arts), pp26–27.

147 Jochaim, H. *Die Welt*, 20 (October 1969).

148 Berberian, C. (1984) cited in I. Anhalt, *Alternative Voices: Essays on Contemporary Vocal and Choral Composition*. Toronto: University of Toronto Press, p.41.

149 Anhalt, I. (1984) *Alternative Voices: Essays on Contemporary Vocal and Choral Composition*. Toronto: University of Toronto Press, p.41.

150 Anhalt, I. (1984) *Alternative Voices: Essays on Contemporary Vocal and Choral Composition*. Toronto: University of Toronto Press, p.41.

151 Kretzmer, H. (1979) 'Stunning – this trip with the human voice.' *Daily Express*. Cited in 'Roy Hart Theatre.' Unpublished anthology of reviews, extracts from articles and other material, compiled by Barrie Coghlan with assistance from Noah Pikes in 1979.

152 Backes-Clement, C. (1979) 'Voice and madness; echo of the origin of man.' *Lettres Francaises*. Cited in 'Roy Hart Theatre.' Unpublished anthology of reviews, extracts from articles and other material, compiled by Barrie Coghlan with assistance from Noah Pikes in 1979.

153 Hart, R. (1968) 'Context.' Paper read at the Third International Congress of Psychodrama, Vienna.

154 Sheppard, L. (1964) 'An empirical therapy based on an extension of vocal range and expression in singing and drama.' Unpublished paper read at the Sixth International Congress of Psychotherapy, London, August 1964.

155 Hart, R. (1967) 'How voice gave me a conscience.' Unpublished paper read at the Seventh International Congress for Psychotherapy, Wiesbaden, .

156 Hart, R. (1968) 'Context.' Paper read at the Third International Congress of Psychodrama', Vienna.

157 George, M. *Drink from the Well*. Cassette. (Boulder, Colorado: Sounds True Audio).

158 Conference series notes and information leaflets to Giving Voice, four annual conferences held at Cardiff, Centre for Performance Research, 1993–96.

CHAPTER 10

Voice, Art and Psyche
Therapeutic Voicework and the Arts Therapies

Introduction: Looking for Voice in the Expressive Arts Therapies

Therapeutic Voicework as a strategy with psychotherapeutic implications may find its most apposite and comparable model in the expressive arts therapies, which utilise various creative media as a channel for the expression of psychic contents.

Whilst for Jung the pursuit of fine art was a welcome ancillary and complimentary contribution to the process of verbal therapy, the therapeutic and analytic use of painting has since become a strategy in itself and over half of the registered art therapists in Britain work in the remaining public sector provision of a National Health Service.[1] Furthermore, therapeutic use of the other arts in clinical institutions is increasingly widespread. In order to further ascertain the relevance of the expressive arts therapies to a methodological and integrated approach to Therapeutic Voicework, I will, in this chapter, outline some of the relevant components of music therapy, dance movement therapy and dramatherapy, extracting that which may be used as a basis for future work within a vocal modality.

There are a number of seminal books which overview the combined use of various arts in therapy, including texts by Fleshman and Fryrear,[2] Robbins,[3] Warren[4] and McNiff.[5] In addition, a professional journal for the use of the arts in psychotherapy has been published quarterly in the USA since the early 1970s.[6] However, nowhere in any of these publications is it possible to find anything more than a cursory reference to the psychotherapeutic value and application of singing and non-verbal sound making. Furthermore, when such mention is made, Therapeutic Voicework is invariably seen as an adjunctive component of either dramatherapy or music therapy.

Strangely enough, it is in the field of dance movement therapy, where one would perhaps least expect to find models of Therapeutic Voicework, that the majority, yet small, amount of research has been conducted. It would perhaps seem more reasonable to expect dramatherapy to be forthcoming with both research and methodology in the field of psychotherapeutic Voicework, given the lively history of vocal experimentation in the avant garde theatre, as documented in Chapter Nine, combined with the long established use of drama as a psychotherapeutic medium in hospitals on both sides of the Atlantic. However, there is a disappointing lack of research and application in the field of dramatherapy. It is within the field of music therapy that one might reasonably expect to find the most consistent and developed application of singing and non-verbal Therapeutic Voicework but, 'as a number of senior clinicians have pointed out, serious use of voice within music therapy is tragically lacking and nobody seems to want to investigate it in any depth'.[7] Thus, music therapists continue to find their voice through an instrument and this modelling is implicitly communicated to their clients. There has, however, been some valuable investigation of the use of singing and vocalisation pursued by a number of key individuals within the field of music therapy and it is with this work that I shall begin.

Music Therapy

Music therapy is now a formally recognised procedure by which to facilitate the personal well-being and psychosocial development of people with widely differing needs. Both art and music therapy have in common a lengthy history of use in mental hospitals throughout the USA, Britain and Europe but the transition from providing background music, reminiscent sing-songs and a box of paints to detract confined patients from boredom to the analytically creative use of musical and artistic processes is one which has occurred only in the last forty years.[8]

In northern America music was used frequently to calm the sufferings of the hospitalised throughout the 18th, 19th and 20th centuries, with a surge of animated activity in the aftermath of the First World War when the hospitals were full of soldiers. The discovery of the positive effect of music on shell-shocked soldiers continued to influence psychiatric procedures and was again increased after the Second World War. Recognising the need for training in this area, the first course, a four-years full-time bachelors degree in music therapy, was implemented in 1944 at Michigan State College and the American National Association for Music Therapy was founded in 1950.

The mainstream use of music therapy in Britain is represented by the The British Society of Music Therapy, which was formed in 1958 by Juliette

The mainstream use of music therapy in Britain is represented by the The British Society of Music Therapy, which was formed in 1958 by Juliette Alvin, author of *Music Therapy*,[9] in the aftermath of an increasingly successful application of music in psychiatric hospitals and day centres for those with so-called handicaps during the 1950s. Alvin defined music therapy as 'the clinical and remedial use of music in the treatment, education and rehabilitation of children and adults suffering from emotional, physical or mental handicap'.[10] For the first ten years of the Society's existence there was no formal training for music therapists and the society acted as a forum for diverse groups of musicians utilising their skills in a clinical context. In many of these contexts the musicians were often perceived as incoming entertainers offering both clients and staff a break from the monotony of institutionalised regularity. As Meigs says, in these early days music therapy 'was often more akin to entertainment and diversion', what she describes as a 'cheer-up' period for patients.[11] There are many expressive therapists, however, who still feel that in a great deal of music therapy the 'entertainment function' remains more developed than the therapeutic and analytic application.[12]

In the early 1950s one of the key contexts in which music therapy had its birth was St Bernard's Psychiatric Wing of Ealing Hospital, London. In the early seventies Peter Wright and Mary Priestly, authors of *Music Therapy in Action*,[13] came into this context and shifted the emphasis away from entertainment and play towards analysis of the patient's inner world through improvisation. Parallel to this development of music therapy, Paul Nordoff and Clive Robbins, who began working together in 1959 at Sunfield Children's Home in Worcestershire, developed an approach to the therapeutic use of music which they believed was highly suitable for children, particularly those with handicaps. Their research was presented through the book *Therapy in Music for Handicapped Children*,[14] first published in 1971. A decade later, the Nordoff-Robbins Music Therapy Centre opened in London, which houses the second of the three main music therapy training courses in the UK. The first formal training in music therapy opened in 1968 at the Guildhall School of Music, a course which continues to run under its licentiate. In the UK music therapy is now a paramedical discipline recognised by the department of health and has a third main training course at Roehampton Institute of Higher Education.

Nordoff and Robbins

Nordoff and Robbins made a minor inroad into the therapeutic use of voice by recognising that 'a child can improvise a song in which the words and the specific melodic idiom express her feelings'. Noticing the innate musical value of 'therapeutically instigated singing', they said that 'such singing out of an emotional need can have the character of an aria'.[15] Nordoff and Robbins also perceived that tonal, rhythmic, or exclamatory sounds are made by children with severe or total speech handicaps', often in response to 'improvised music which the therapist finds to be emotionally significant for the child', the melodic and rhythmic structure of which 'both evoke the form of the vocalization and support it.'[16] They asserted that 'the singing of a child's name', and 'the improvising of special songs' or other 'vocal material' induces 'changes of behaviour'. For example, they perceived that 'a child who is initially unable to be either rhythmically or vocally active can respond emotionally to the therapist's singing' and 'out of the character of the relationship this creates, he can move or be led into outwardly active experiences'.[17] Exemplifying such a process, Nordoff and Robbins describe their work with a 'young, speechless, hyperactive girl' who, they say, 'could beat only a very slow, compulsive beat' which would 'remain in its regular metronomic tempo, no matter what music was played'. However, 'eventually, by using a counter-rhythm' the therapists were able to 'break' the child's 'fixed beat'. As a result, 'she speeded up her tempo' and, 'at about the same time', the little girl began to speak, repeating the 'rhythmic phrase of the song' which consisted of the words 'Pif-Paf-Poltrie and Fair Katie', at first 'rhythmically uttering the vowels' and later 'approximating the words.' A short while following this 'she began to sing it and by degrees her enunciation improved'. Nordoff and Robbins say that within two months of this experience 'she went on to sing other songs' and 'subsequently she learned to speak'.[18]

Through their use of music, Nordoff and Robbins highlighted cases of misdiagnosis and consequently provided for a more positive prognosis. For example, children labelled as autistic were subsequently revealed to be aphasic due to brain injury with additional emotional disturbance. Because music and sound making provided an alternative to speech, by which the client could express previously dammed up thoughts and feelings, the emotional disturbance often lessened and the symptoms which had attracted the diagnosis of autism receded.

Since the early research of Nordoff and Robins, scientific medical research has made some headway in verifying that the capacity for speech conception and articulation is processed in a distinctly localised area of the brain separate from that which composes and initiates the utterance of non-verbal musical phrases. Yet the discovery made by Nordoff and Robbins that non-verbal singing nonetheless has the potential to assist in the development of speech activity is beginning to be rediscovered in centres which combine artistic and clinical approaches to communication difficulties and disorders.

The Need for Singers Who Can Help Children Speak

An example of contemporary work which has shown how non-verbal vocali-sation can assist in the development of spoken communication is the research of the music therapist Julie Sutton in Northern Ireland, who has combined the use of an expressive arts therapy modality in tandem with the co-operative assistance of a speech and language therapist working with chil-dren who have speech impairments. Sutton provides insight into this process through her complete case study of Paul, a boy with Lexical Syntactic Deficit Syndrome, which causes a patient to experience problems with the rules gov-erning sentence building and retention of vocabulary. Sutton found that as a result of his 'anxiety in understanding and being understood in a world of words', the boy 'rarely vocalised during music making'. However, she says that when she brought a kazoo to the session Paul organised them with one each and they 'held prolonged conversations of expressive babble, accompa-nied by exaggerated gesture'. Stunned by the ease with which he entered into this interaction, Sutton wondered whether 'he had the opportunity to play vocally and explore at any other time' outside the therapy sessions. Sutton says that the patient's experience of vocal play seemed to directly facilitate the articulation of expanded phrases in talking when assisted by the work of his speech therapist. In general, from her research so far, Sutton is convinced that 'the experience of spontaneously expressing themselves through the non-verbal medium of music' can 'at least partially' result in 'increased confi-dence to communicate through words'.[19]

Sutton's work is emblematic of research in the area of Therapeutic Voice-work long overdue within music therapy and is made possible not only by the collaborative relationship between her and the speech and language therapist but by her willingness to utilise her own voice as an instrument of play, crea-tion and communication with patients. Unfortunately, such willingness is often stifled by embarrassment or reticence on the part of therapists, includ-

ing those working in music therapy. The situation is summed up perfectly by
Gianluigi di Franco, a psychiatrist, vocalist, Freudian Group Psychoanalyst
and the Italian representative for the European Music Therapy Committee,
who points out that 'there are many music therapists' who have 'a great fluency' when communicating through the playing of instruments but 'have a
great difficulty' or 'resistance' to 'expressing themselves through the use of
their voices.'[20] Di Franco highlights this as a rather unfortunate gap which
leaves music therapy bereft of a primary channel of investigation. He says
that birth is essentially 'a primary trauma where the fetus, now becoming a
baby', loses the 'containment' or 'protection' he had when in the womb,
'where communication occurred through filtering membranes'. Therefore, at
birth 'there is a need to express the whole affective sense resulting from this
trauma to the external world', which is almost always 'characterised by the
use of the voice, which screams to the world its own tragedy'.[21] Because of
the primacy of voice in development, di Franco proclaims that 'therapy developed through a sound medium has to include vocal intervention at a vocal
level, as the voice is always involved at the first moment of the expressive and,
therefore, communicative life of each of us'.[22] The reticence of music therapists to use their voice as a primary instrument and the lack of training in the
means to do so is, consequently, from di Franco's perspective, a serious hindrance to the development of therapeutic efficacy.

Within the field of the methodological approach to Therapeutic Voicework which I have founded, Mary Law has been investigating the use of
singing as a modality auxiliary to psychotherapy, psychology and psychiatry
with patients at the Mental Health wing of the Lister Hospital, under the
supervision of Cressida Pryor, a speech and language therapist, dramatherapist and head of arts therapies at the wing. Two other graduates, Paddy
Holden and Jane McDermott, both utilise music and singing work with those
who are described as having 'special needs' in residential and educational day
centres, working without clinical implications but within an educational and
remedial framework. Whilst both Holden and McDermott are trained classical musicians, Law has no musical training and, through the supervision
meetings of *The International Association for Voice Movement Therapy*, it has been
possible to investigate the advantages and disadvantages of previous musical
training when working through a vocal modality with different client
groups.

In addition to having no formal musical training, Law is also not a trained
clinician. However, the case conference team at the Lister Hospital have

found it expedient and beneficial to refer some clients to Law for individual Therapeutic Voicework, which has been conducted at the Mental Health wing with clients receiving the work as part of the public sector provision of mental health resources. In addition, the speech and language therapists of the main hospital have referred clients with voice production problems to Law, whom she sees privately on a fee-paying basis at her own consulting room. Though it is early days of professional Therapeutic Voicework, these small measures set the precedent and the hope that non-clinical practitioners, such as those of Voice Movement Therapy, will work effectively and collaboratively with allopathic and clinical professionals for the benefit of the client. Moreover, by offering the professional Voice Movement Therapy training to those who, like Law, are exempted from other creative and therapeutic music courses, it is possible to focus on identifying the precise area of skill and expertise which is distinct to working with the voice specifically, rather than music generally.

Of course, there is a healthy population of music therapists who belong to a profession with a substantial history, each of whom undergo a rigorous training enabling them to contribute clinical work to a variety of settings. In contrast, there are only a small number of practitioners who have graduated from the professional training in Voice Movement Therapy which I direct. In addition, the notion of Therapeutic Voicework as a distinct discipline is very new. However, it is my hope that the future will graduate a pool of competent practitioners who will be able to liaise with music therapists, seeking to understand how the voice can be used to aid the objective of the expressive arts therapies.

Dance and Movement Therapy

Dance movement therapy rests upon the employment of physical movement as a medium through which to express and analyse psychological material and contains within its spectrum of approaches a number of analytic frameworks.[23] Among those using a Jungian approach, which is the analytic framework I have found most suitable to expressive Therapeutic Voicework, are Mary Stark Whitehouse,[24] Joan Chodorow,[25] and Amelie Noack,[26] all of whom seek to give physical form to unconscious contents through shape, rhythm, gesture, pose and kinetic geometric configurations. A number of dance movement therapists have accommodated the intrinsic relationship between dance and song by nurturing collective singing,[27] but the use of the voice has remained peripheral to the therapeutic procedures employed by

most practitioners. Nonetheless, of all the arts therapies, it is within the therapeutic application of dance and movement that the most extensive, consistent
and serious investigation into Therapeutic Voicework has been conducted.

The fundamental idea that the principles of human movement may systematically express the nature of the human soul is probably most eloquently
described through the work of Rudolf von Laban, who was born in 1879 in
Bratislava, which was then a part of the Austro-Hungarian empire and who
became a prolific teacher and innovating educator in the field of dance,
movement and theatre. Laban's premise was that 'movement satisfies a need',
which can be a purely practical one of moving from one place to another, a
psychosomatic need to discharge energy or a need to make the inner attitudes
of the mind and its deeper and less conscious feelings palpable through
action. For Laban, therefore, 'understanding movements and their functions'
was a way of 'understanding people'.[28] According to Hodgson and Preston-
Dunlop, Laban 'recognised that it was through movement that feelings,
moods and ideas were conveyed and that voice was part of the whole, simply
another manifestation of movement'.[29]

Laban encountered the work of Delsarte in Paris during the early 1900s
through one of the latter's pupils and found that Delsarte's understanding of
vocal expression as being composed of word, tone and gesture, as well as his
vision of the body being composed of torso, head and limbs as three distinct
units of expression, mirrored his own research. In addition, during the years
of the First World War, Laban encountered the work of Analytical Psychology and found that Jung's 'extroverted' and 'introverted' personality
delineations were analogous to and expressed through his own physical and
energetic 'inward flow' and 'outward flow' categories of motion. Furthermore, Laban had formed the theoretical and analytical paradigm which
perceived all movement as a combination in varying proportion of the
dimensions of space, flow, weight and time which he believed to mirror
Jung's personality characteristics of thinking, feeling, sensation and intuition
respectively.[30] Moreover, Jung's notion of the shadow was also, according to
Laban, visible in unconscious movement patterns.

Laban's four functions were each composed of a spectrum between two
extreme qualities: the movement quality of space could be direct or indirect.
This is observable by watching the degree to which a person moves directly
to the object of relationship and the degree to which he or she circumvents it.
The quality of flow can be free or bound, observable in the amount of muscle
tension and resistance to physical action; the quality of weight can be light or

heavy, observable in the gravitational presence with which a person moves; and the quality of time can be quick or slow, observable through the dimension of kinetic tempo. Laban's work in the therapeutic arena came to fruition through the research pursued by those of his students who went on to apply his paradigm in the field of dance and movement therapy. In the USA the most notable of these figures are Trudi Schoop[31] and Irmgard Bartenieff.[32]

Irmgard Bartenieff, a German refugee, brought Laban's work to New York, where she applied it to helping children with Poliomylitis to increase their movement potential. As a result, she found herself in dialogue with psychiatrists and medical doctors and began to discover the ways in which Laban's approach to physical movement yielded to a psychological interpretation of the human condition in keeping with the language of her fellow colleagues. By the early 1960s she was using dance as a therapy for a variety of children and adults with both mental and physical difficulties and her work has influenced the development of dance therapy across the east coast of northern America.[33]

In addition to Schoop and Bartenieff, many students of the prolific dancer Mary Wigman, whom Laban trained, have also made contributions to therapeutic practice. Whilst in England, Warren Lamb, who had worked with Laban in his later years, used his method to form what he called 'Action Profiling', which was applied to such everyday processes as enabling executives to select the appropriate person for a specific job based on an analysis of their movement patterns.[34]

Laban did not, judging from the various biographical accounts, bequeath any applicable or practicable specific vocal methodology. However, his system of profile and analysis has been extended to analysing and training the voice by a number people, including Lamb. In *Posture and Gesture* Lamb continues Laban's view of the voice as a motor function and a physical action, stating that 'the voice is itself is produced by physical actions of a number of parts of the body'.[35] Lamb's main focus, therefore, is the way 'throat and mouth' gestures merge with or extend into posture and body movement. However, only one example of a therapeutic application of such a view is offered by Lamb and comprises a description of how a man with a stammer was allegedly cured by retraining the energetic and choreographic nature of the body movements which invariably accompanied the speech impediment.[36]

Laban's work was also applied to the training of the singing voice by the renowned British folk singer Ewan McColl, who was born in 1915 and

raised in Salford. As a young man, McColl was a fiery working-class intellectual who gravitated to street theatre, which led to his first marriage to Joan
Littlewood, founder of the Theatre Workshop for which McColl wrote some
of the plays during the 1940s. These dramas, which were heavily political
and highly innovative in the use of stage space, scenic design and actors'
physical movement, were an extension of McColl's socialist politics. It was
here that both Littlewood and McColl discovered the work of Laban which
influenced both in their work.[37] However, McColl departed from the Workshop when it established a permanent base in London and no longer
accommodated his overt political preoccupations. McColl felt that the
'trouble with theatre', including his own, 'was that it had failed to find a
language embedded in working-class experience'.[38] McColl's answer to this
was to move from a literary theatre to a musical one and he began experimenting with vocal renditions of biographical folk ballads which he felt
spoke about and to the common experience of the common people. Furthermore, McColl 'claimed that many British folk-song styles were part of an
Indo-European tradition' and he cited the work of ethnomusicologist Alan
Lomax to verify his belief. Part of McColl's political agenda was, therefore, to
acknowledge the roots of folk ballad; and it has been suggested that he is primarily responsible for what is now the widespread availability and
dissemination of the genre known as 'world music'.[39]

McColl was not a trained musician but, through his singing, drew on the
acting techniques which were familiar to him. His later professional partnership and marriage to the singer and musician Peggy Seeger thus provided a
strength which he lacked whilst, in compliment, his theatrical nature balanced her introverted personality and performance reticence. Together,
McColl and Seeger not only sang but trained a new generation of young
poets, vocalists, writers and political activists to use song as a dramatic means
to express political conviction. In so doing McColl drew on the work of
Stanislavski, helping singers to analyse texts and inviting them to 'identify
closely with characters in the narrative', to know 'who they were in a song'
and to be cognizant of why they were singing a particular story. For McColl,
'the most acceptable reasons were often political'.[40] In his attempt to bring
dramtic authenticity to a singer's rendition, McColl 'transposed Rudolf
Laban's theory' from 'movement to vocal sound' by using Laban's framework
to analyse the underlying psychological and emotional depth beneath the
vocal expression.[41]

Laban's attempt to understand the connection between inner psychic processes and their expression in both physical movement and the motion of the voice was the subject of a manuscript which he worked on with William Carpenter in 1954. This manuscript passed to one of Laban's students, Yat Malgrem, who further developed the ideas contained therein, deepening the comparability with a Jungian analysis of human character.[42] Malgrem taught this work to trainee actors, first at the Central School of Speech and Drama and later at Drama Centre, where he still teaches. Malgrem was especially sensitive to Laban's belief that 'movements of the body, including movements of the voice-producing organs', are 'indispensable' to authentic performance on the stage.[43] It was under the tutorship of Malgrem at Drama Centre, where I initially trained as an actor, that I began to understand the links between voice and physical action which now form part of the Therapeutic Voicework methodology which I teach.

Therapeutic Voicework Methodology: The Illusion of Acoustic Physicality

From my training with Malgrem at Drama Centre I realised that there is a certain muscularity to the voice which gives it a quality analogous to physical movement and which operates through the illusion of kinetic activity. For example, words can appear to punch, poke, pierce and cut; words can stroke, squeeze and envelop. Words can be made to caress, pat and fondle or they can be uttered with a tone which throttles, pelts and tears. If the voice had no relation to physical intent, then Freud would not have been led to discover that words become a 'substitute for deeds'.[44] Of course, this physical nature of the voice is, in part, illusory, for the words uttered do not make kinetic impact with the listener except for contact of the sound wave with the ear drum. However, common experience of both speaker and listener will testify to the seeming reality of such an illusion.

In the Therapeutic Voicework methodology which I am disseminating, I utilise an exercise which explores this illusion of physicality. The client takes a simple piece of text, either from an authored publication or from her own utterance or journal of spontaneous writing. This text is then uttered a number of times, each with a specifically chosen physical intent, which the client mirrors with appropriate bodily action. For example, the text may be spoken six times consecutively with intent to stroke, shake, nuzzle, prod, ruffle and smear, a few of the several hundred actions developed from Laban by Malmgrem and Carpenter. With each utterance, the client performs stroking, shaking, nuzzling, prodding, ruffling and smearing movements with the body as she speaks.

Many clients who come into Therapeutic Voicework find it hard to imbue the voice with certain emotions. For example, a client may find it impossible to vocalise anger or assertiveness. This presents the practitioner with the task of finding ways to enable the client to access the peripheralised emotions and express them vocally.

One way of meeting this problem is to bypass a direct engagement with emotion and to transpose affective contents onto physical actions. Thus, instead of asking the client to vocalise the text with anger, the practitioner asks the client to speak the text whilst physically miming an action with a shaking quality to it, such as vigorously shaking out a duvet, or to speak the text whilst enacting a movement with a prodding quality, such as digging with a trowel. Because such physical actions effect the muscular kinesis of the voice, the client finds that the vocal expression takes on a punching or prodding quality which brings underlying psychological punching and prodding, in this case connected to anger and assertiveness, to the surface.

Thus, through a Laban-based approach, emotional material can be accessed, vocalised and integrated through somatic activity.

Creative Movement and Psychoanalysis

Whilst the approach to the physicality of vocal utterance and analysis which first inspired my own work emanates from Laban's interest in Jung's Analytical Psychology, as taught by Malmgrem at Drama Centre, there is another framework of vocal analysis which descends from the Psychoanalytic tradition of equal significance to the practice of Therapeutic Voicework, within which the most relevant contribution is the Kestenberg Movement Profile.

The Kestenberg Movement Profile was initiated by the psychiatrist and psychoanalyst Judith Kestenberg, who drew ideas from two of her teachers, Irmgard Bartenieff and Warren Lamb, who, in turn, had been deeply influenced by the approach to the inner psychological motivations revealed through human movement and its notation developed by Rudolf Laban. Kestenberg herself admired Laban's work, setting herself a similar task as he had done in 'trying to find the epistemology which underpins the thinking which stimulates movement'[45] and originally borrowed a number of terms from Laban. However, unlike the Jungian orientation of Laban's work pursued by Schoop and Bartenieff and the Action Profiling of Lamb, the Kestenberg Movement Profile observes and analyses human movement from a Freudian Drive Theory and Object Relations perspective on developmental psychology, drawing on the work of Anna Freud[46] and Margaret Mahler,[47] both of whom assessed infant development in terms of movement patterns.

Kestenberg's concern was the way motor apparatus is 'put into the service of developing mental structures' and she observed in infant development the way sophisticated movement evolves from rhythmic alterations of muscular tension and body shape in the same way that 'speech evolves from the infant's cry and vocalizations to the formation of words and sentences'.[48] Kestenberg took from Laban the notion of 'free' and 'bound' flow and related it to the development of muscular 'tension' and 'relaxation' gradually acquired by the developing infant in order to control primary actions such as suckling, defecating, holding, throwing and chewing. Laban had observed that the body acts like a swelling and shrinking amoeba, extending and retracting during movement.[49] Kestenberg linked this both to the process of inhalation and exhalation and to the acts of ingestion and defecation, both of which, she believed, compound the body's tendency to 'swell and shrink' in the way conceived by Laban.[50]

Within the Kestenberg Movement Profile, the history of infant development and its determination of psychic disturbance are seen to be present in the client's somatic manifestation of body rhythm, muscular tension and the general choreographic shape of pedestrian movement.[51] In the object relations approach to infant development, fundamental body parts and their physical actions are a dominant analytic factor, particularly areas which provide a locus for intense early infantile experience, such as the anal sphincter and the mouth. It is the action of these body parts which provide the locus around which basic psychic experience and components are formed. The Kestenberg Movement Profile considers such primal physical actions as squeezing, holding, expelling, biting and chewing to be composed of definable rhythmic and tensile movements which are not only localised in orificial body parts but become distributed throughout the somatic musculature. Thus they continue to be expressed by the skeletal choreography in adult life in the same way that the alleged underlying psychic meaning of developmental physicality continues to effect the grown mind and its patterns of experience.[52] Flowing movements of arms and legs which seem to be uncontained, squeezing movements of fingers which seem to be seeking to expel and regular masticatory movements of the torso during walking, sitting or speaking which seem to be comparable with biting are sought in the body's natural dance and traced to primary actions and the psychic disposition which they are supposed to reveal within a psychoanalytic framework.

The clinical application of the Kestenberg Movement Profile has been extended for use in combination with a Jungian-orientated dance therapy by Penny Lewis, one of the leading authorities in the field of dance movement therapy.[53] Lewis has been instrumental in developing a cogent clinical and interpretative framework within which the practice of dance movement therapy can be located. This has enabled dance and creative movement to be perceived both as the medium through which transformation of psychic material can be achieved and as an expressive dimension which will withstand analysis and interpretation from a number of varying clinical perspectives.[54] Lewis originally trained with Marion Chace, who encouraged psychiatric patients to support postural and gestural expressive movements with breath and sound. Later, Lewis found the expression of 'authentic sound' to be 'central to the transformative process'.[55] In investigating the vocal medium, Lewis has collaborated with Anne Brownell, a mental health counsellor and expressive arts therapist who trained with Norma Canner on the Intermodal Expressive Therapy training programme implemented by Canner, Shaun McNif, Paulo Knill and Mariagnese Knill Cattaneo at Lesley College, Massachusetts. Brownell was also the first north American graduate of the professional training programme in Voice Movement Therapy which I direct in London. Together, Brownell and Lewis have sought to investigate whether the Kestenberg Movement Profile can be applied to qualities of the spoken voice.[56] Listening to the voices of a range of clients, they sought to discover whether primary physical tensile expressions, such as those which accompany the control of the sphincters in early life, also effect laryngeal motility and can be heard in the acoustic timbre of the voice. Thus squeezing, biting, throwing and holding qualities, for example, are listened for in the combination of rythm, prosody and timbre within the vocal expression and analysed within a psychoanalytic paradigm.[57]

Voice and Psychomuscularity

Brownell was influenced by the dance movement therapist Norma Canner who was in turn a student of the dance educationalist Barbara Mettler, to whom the intimate and essential necessity of the voice as a natural extension of bodily movement has been an ongoing focus of investigation.[58]

In the early days of her dance class teaching, Mettler thought that she needed a pianist to accompany her classes, but could not afford one.[59] She therefore experimented with allowing the dancers to accompany themselves with percussion instruments. Later, after all such instruments had been destroyed in a fire, her dance students began to 'use sounds of voice, hands and feet and ordinary objects',[60] from which Mettler began to realise that 'at their source within us dance and music are one'.[61] Consequently, Mettler broke with the tradition of dance teaching and encouraged her students to allow the voice to sound of its own accord as an integral part of the movement. Her premise was that 'the feeling of a movement is sometimes more easily expressed if we let the sound of the voice be a part of it'.[62] Mettler points out that many natural expressions in life are equally both movements and sounds, such as yawning, sobbing and laughing.[63] Furthermore, like the work descending from Laban, Mettler points out that 'tactile qualities such as rough, smooth, oily, sticky, prickly, watery' can be expressed through the sounds of the voice as well as through bodily movements.[64]

More than any other dance teacher, Mettler has implemented the often forgotten connection between sound and movement, reminding that 'sound is an outgrowth of movement, and the quality of a sound expresses to some extent the quality of the movement which produces the sound'.[65] Mettler's approach has little time for the spectator and relegates the audience to a subordinate role. Her aim is to facilitate free creative dance for the participant.[66] This makes her work entirely process-orientated, yet, at the same time, she is an aesthete and openly confesses her disinterest in any kind of therapeutic process.

Inspired by Mettler, but frustrated by the aesthetic emphasis, Brownell found the seeds for a fusion of voice and movement within the therapeutic context from which Mettler absconded in the work of Norma Canner, a movement therapist who encourages clients to vocalise whilst dancing[67] and who stimulates spontaneous vocalisation in combination with movement with children in therapy.[68]

As a therapist, Canner's innovation was the introduction of vocal sound making to her work with developmentally delayed children, enabling them 'to connect to their whole selves' as it emerged 'in authentic movement and sound'.[69] Drawing on Bernfield's theory regarding 'the roots of fascination', which asserts that a child will mimic and emulate the appearance of intense stimuli in order to master it,[70] Canner amplified her own facial expressions and body movements which accompanied the sounds she made, encouraging children to emulate both the acoustic and the kinetic component.[71] Inspired by Canner and Kestenberg, Brownell, in collaboration with Penny Lewis, found that spontaneous sound making 'allows for a sense of self and other' and increases the 'capacity to integrate split-off parts of the self'.[72] Like the music therapist Sutton, the work of Canner, Brownell and Lewis also found the use of vocalization therapeutically applicable to children with organic speech impairments and encouraged them 'to explore specific body movements, sounds and rhythms that can stimulate and facilitate the development of language and expression'.[73] Brownell is now co-teacher on the USA professional training in Voice Movement Therapy.

Through my studies of dance movement therapy, particularly of Lewis' multi-modelled interpretation of human movement, I began to investigate the use of expressive movement combined with vocalisation, developing something which I refer to as a Voice Movement Journey.

Therapeutic Voicework Methodology: The Voice Movement Journey

Therapeutic Voicework in its therapeutic capacity, as I conceive of it, seeks to employ the acoustic emissions of phonation as the primary channel through which to allure ostracised and expropriated images and de-integrates of the psyche into consciousness. It is active imagination and amplification through vocal sound and singing and may perhaps best be described as psychophonic, a term which I first used in 1992.[74]

Psychophonics may be defined as the process of conveying authentic psychological information in the form of non-verbal vocal sound. Such sounds may be called psychophonic when they contain qualities which are the audible manifestation of affect and image according to the intuitive perception of the vocalist which may also be witnessed by a listener or audient. Such sounds do not translate logically into a discursive schema but yield to metaphorical amplification, that is they may be described as expressing certain psychic components which comprise mood, character, emotion, image, essence and instinct and which have a semiotic or ontological presence.

One of the contexts in which such psychophonic amplification can be explored is in what I have named the Voice Movement Journey and which is among the most popular strategies practised by graduates of the professional training in Voice Movement Therapy because, in Penny Lewis' words, 'it affords the client a maximum degree of self determination in the process'.[75]

During a Voice Movement Journey session the client or group of clients moves and vocalises, allowing the body and voice to embody images, animals, characters and feelings as they arise, discovering parts of the self which have for a long time remained unvisited. The little lost girl and the devouring wolf thus emerge from the larynx in sounds which are numinous and charismatic, tear provoking, terrifying, affecting and arresting and always genuinely expressive of the de-integrates, sub-personalities, complexes and networks of images, moods and emotions that constitute the fabric of the singer's psyche. As with the other artistically-orientated therapies, the integrity of these sounds is not measured by their entertainment value, their musical eloquence or their formal virtuosity, but by their depth of genuineness and authenticity, the degree to which the client can be incontrovertibly heard to express something which, in Gilligan's terms, rears up from the depths of the psyche.[76]

As the clients move through spherical space, with recourse to the vocal timbral parameters and the physical and postural body work which I have outlined, they allow the skeletal musculature to create shapes which embody, amplify and choreograph the psychophonic material. This may mean direct empathy with a figure or animal which moves improvisationally through space in tandem with vocalisation or it may mean the repetitious rehearsal of a single gestural movement accompanied by the rhythmic staccato utterance of an accompanying sound.

As the clients follow what I first described as a 'voicedance',[77] they allow themselves to experience and vocalise the emotionality as it arises, connecting an inner world of affect with an outer and tangible dimension of voice and movement. During this Voice Movement Journey the practitioner watches, listens and records observations of the client's vocal and physical expressions and, at the end of the journey, feeds back to them what was observed with advice as to how areas which appeared rigid, fixed and resistant to transformation might be assisted in loosening and changing.

A Voice Movement Journey usually has a starting point provided by the practitioner in response to the presenting issues of the clients. This may be a psychokinetic idea, such as a journey involving throwing, grasping, gathering and expelling, which provides an opportunity for primary developmental material to be expressed and worked through. It may be an emotional staring point, such as a journey through sorrow, longing, discovery and celebration, offering a chance for elemental passions to be reclaimed and integrated.

Regardless of the starting point, the aim remains the same: to experience the authenticity of the Self and its constituents through the immutable power of voice and movement in a safe and non-judgmental container.

Dramatherapy

There are now enough dramatherapists to be able to discern a spectrum of approaches almost extensive as those which constitute the psychotherapies, not least because those practising dramatherapy have been influenced by widely differing analytic frameworks.[78] However, dramatherapy, which is also now a recognised therapeutic strategy in Britain, Europe and the USA, cannot claim such a long established presence in the field of mental health as can painting and music. We do know plays to have been performed by the inmates of certain French asylums during the eighteenth century and this is epitomised, dramatised and idealised nowhere more captivatingly than in the film of Peter Brook's Royal Shakespeare Company production of the *Marat/Sade Play* by Peter Weiss. This tells the fictional tale of the Marquis de Sade's attempt to control his fellow inmates of the asylum Charendon by producing a play based on the assassination of the French revolution's political hero, Jean Paul Marat, by Charlotte Corday. In fact, the Weiss play was produced with actual patients of a psychiatric hospital in the USA during the early 1970s.[79]

Indeed, dramatherapy may be seen as descending from the mounting of theatre productions, first for psychiatric patients and later with them, in hospitals on both sides of the Atlantic. In the USA particularly, the use of drama was, in the early part of the twentieth century, an extension of 'recreational therapy', in turn a substrata of occupational therapy which included the provision of crafts, gardening, sports, exercise and play rehearsal within a single framework. During the 1950s, however, a number of theatre groups, influenced by the methodological and psychological approach of Stanislavski, began to take performances with accompanying workshops into community settings, including psychiatric hospitals. Here the emphasis was on the use of improvisation to engage the participants in self reflection. Among the key figures in this development was Eleanor Irwin, who developed the use of therapeutic drama at the Pittsburgh Child Guidance Centre, and Gertrud Schattner, one time director of a dramatherapy training programme at at Turtle Bay Music School in New York and who has edited a collection of essays by practitioners of this approach.[80]

The serious investigatory and analytical research of people like Irwin and Schattner highlighted the difference between the use of drama as recreation and its therapeutic application, with the consequence that, in 1978, after 25 years of diverse activity across northern America, a team of practitioners, including Irwin and Schattner, formed the American National Association

for Dramatherapists. This was one year after the Association for Dramatherapists had been formed in the UK, arising out of work which took shape in
Britain during the 1960s and 1970s pioneered by Sue Jennings, among others.

Dramatherapy in Britain began as an attempt to consolidate the principles
which had, for some time, informed the practice of Remedial Drama: theatre
games, trust exercises, improvisation classes and a host of activities which had
their history in the various methodological elements of an actor's training
and rehearsal. Dramatherapy sought to apply such practices to the educational and social development of those with divergent physical and
emotional needs. There are a number of trainings in dramatherapy, resulting
from the initial impetus which came from the Remedial Drama Centre, now
known as Playspace, set up by Sue Jennings, Roy Shuttleworth and Gordon
Weisman in 1964 with the accreditation of the Polytechnic of Central London and which offered courses in the use of drama for health professionals,
special needs teachers and others. There is also a second strand to the British
dramatherapy movement, known as the Sesame approach, which was
founded by Marion Lindkvist.[81] This approach is rooted not in textual discourse or the analytic interpretation of improvisation, but in movement,
mime and story telling.[82]

At the heart of all dramatherapy practice is the fundamental belief that
aspects of the unconscious can be admitted to consciousness through the act
of performing. Dramatherapy owes its origin, in conception at least, to the
work of Jacob Moreno, who developed what he called Psychodrama in the
1920s and 1930s. Psychodrama was a process by which a person acted out
various roles in improvised situations taken from his or her life and which
provided an opportunity to complete an action or ventilate an emotion that
had been inhibited during its actual occurrence. Its philosophy was primarily
a cathartic one, the talking cure became the acting cure.[83] It also offered an
opportunity for the patient to become the actor, not only in notion but in
action, by which she assumed the role of other people in her own life or the
lives of other patients in the psychodrama group. This encouraged the patient's 'sense of I' not only to recognise the different roles it played in the face
of certain situations but also to empathise with the feelings of others by acting in their shoes. It was through this process of entering the character of
another person that the patients of Moreno's therapeutic theatre were
encouraged to recognise their problems as arising from an essentially social
cause. For Moreno, psychological degeneration originates in our inability to
comprehend and appropriately respond to the complex social dynamics in

which human behaviour is contextualised and, in order for progress to be made in this direction, the dynamics of familial and societal situations have to be recreated. It was from this game of role playing that the Gestalt Therapy of Fritz Perls grew.[84]

Perls encouraged patients not only to use other actors as representative of significant persons but to use objects such as chairs, pillows and curtains. A patient could scream at a chair in order to express the unventilated revenge he felt towards his mother for dying when he was a child or crawl across the floor to demonstrate and physicalise the way he felt hindered in his ambitions, staggering towards his future without reward. Perls' therapeutic procedure was predominantly dramatic, employing props, scenes and role-playing. By setting up synthetic conversations between the significant characters of the participant's life or between different parts of the self, represented by inanimate objects, Perls was continuing in a dramatic model of therapy initiated by Moreno and to which the now widely established practice of dramatherapy owes a considerable part of its origin.[85]

But, whilst Moreno focused on the social, Perls was concerned with the individual and internal. Two of these innermost parts, which Perls was keen to prove to be aspects of all people, was the 'top dog' and the 'under dog'. The top dog is the role we play when we are in charge, dominant and leading the way. The underdog is our frightened subservient response to danger or authority. In addition, Perls also encouraged patients to view parts of their body as personalities: they could speak to the chair as if it was their penis or their legs or their acne. In fact, this process of relating to body parts as indubitable psychic facets of the self was not an invention of Perls but had occupied the attention of a number of therapists, including post-Freudian analysts, among whom the most renowned is Melanie Klein.[86]

One of the results of this work was that, in embodying different characters or aspects of the self, the client would give specific voices to each person or aspect represented. Yet neither Perls nor the practitioners of psychodrama have developed a methodology for working dramatically with the voice as a specific and delineated medium of expression.

Dramatherapy's Plea for Voice

A small number of dramatherapists have been keen to encourage non-verbal vocal expression as part of their approach. For example, Steve Mitchell, influenced primarily by his work with member's of Grotowski's Theatre Laboratory, includes vocal exercises in his group sessions.[87] However, despite the broad and expansive investigation into Therapeutic Voicework and its psychological overtones in the avant garde theatre, within the field of dramatherapy, meanwhile, clinical models for vocal work are completely absent and the number of practitioners investigating Therapeutic Voicework is startlingly small.

In the 1994 edition of *Dramatherapy*, the journal which represents the profession in Britain, the dramatherapist Luisa Passalacqua stated that 'the literature about the voice is wide and yet it is rarely possible to find a comprehensive theory about vocal phenomena within a multi-disciplinary frame'. She points out that it is either 'dealt with scientifically', as in 'voice therapy, phonology, laryngology, physiology', or it is approached in an 'artistic or mystical' way, as in 'the field of singing, religion and the martial arts'. The voice, she says, 'is therefore a borderline area.'[88] Passalacqua points out that, even in specialist fields of human communication, the vocal element of the acoustic message is often confused with the verbal and, indeed, in dramatherapy voice and speech are often not differentiated.

As a dramatherapist, Passalacqua is concerned not 'with how dramatherapy can help clients with speech or voice disorders' but rather with how drama 'can help clients get in touch with their inner reality and bring it out in a constructive, balanced way' through the voice.[89] However, she also says that the client group suitable to the dramatherapist focusing on the voice 'may be most effectively composed of those who would like to make a different use of their voices and, maybe, also, those who have minor functional voice disorders', such as stammering.[90]

Passalacqua reveals a lack of clarity with regard to the level of functional voice disorder which may, potentially, be alleviated by a vocally-orientated dramatherapy. It would seem reasonable to expect that functional voice disorders which are verifiably psychogenic in origin may be best suited to such a modality. However, since most functional voice disorders become somatically sustained through habitual muscle misuse, a degree of knowledge regarding the physiology of voice function and dysfunction would be needed by a dramatherapist employing vocal work. Any future vision of a vocally-orientated dramatherapy would, therefore, benefit from a broadening of the dramatherapist's training to incorporate both technical and experiential Therapeutic Voicework. At the moment, such a component of the training is lacking in Britain.

Despite the lack of a coherent model for dramatherapeutic Voicework highlighted by Passalacqua, there have been a number of individual practitioners in the field of dramatherapy who have made modest contributions to the notion of a vocal modality. Morrant claims that within the first few seconds of meeting a new client, the dramatherapist can form an initial impression of the likely difficulties, based upon the vocal clues present in the voice.[91] Piers Partridge, meanwhile, a gestalt Psychotherapist, published his recommendations in the journal *Dramatherapy,* which consist of a 'toolkit' of certain specific 'clues' which can allegedly be heard in the voice. First, he suggests listening to the tone of the client's voice whilst considering whether it is one which 'is bass or treble', 'rich' or 'thin', 'pleasant to listen to or harsh and jarring', carrying 'a clear emotional tone' or 'devoid of any feeling at all.' Next, Partridge suggests hearing the voice in terms of a spectrum between 'hot and cold' and encourages the dramatherapist to ask whether clients are 'warm and easy with contact', whether they are 'carrying some difficulty that makes them keep a cool distance', whether they are 'hot to the point of being uncontained, like a pot of overflowing metal' or 'cold to the point that no one talks to them in tea breaks'. Then, Partridge suggests, the dramatherapist should listen for energy as an acoustic dimension and ask whether the client has 'a sense of authentic vitality or of forced power', whilst listening to 'where in the body the voice appears to come from'. Additionally, Partridge proposes that both 'the slowness and speed of speech', the accent and the 'oldness or youngness' of the voice also provide clues for therapeutic assessment.[92]

Partridge's system is predicated upon a highly subjective and countertransferential interpretation of vocal quality and is, perhaps, more useful as a reminder of the inescapable nature of the therapist's own idiosyncratic and intuitive responses to the client's expressions. Consequently, any arts therapy seeking to use Therapeutic Voicework should, perhaps, be built on a model which makes provision for the conscious recognition of the therapist's counter transference in response to vocal quality.

Therapeutic Voicework Methodology: Dramatising the Voices Within

In the approach to Therapeutic Voicework which I have developed, the reader will be aware that use of the ideokinetic tube is of central importance. One of the ways this system of vocal timbral analysis can be applied towards both a creative and therapeutic end is in the vocalisation of distinct characters. In fact, dramatic casting for stage, screen and radio makes use of such a process constantly, where performers are chosen for the particular impression given by their voice.

For the client of Therapeutic Voicework these equations between certain vocal parameters and specific figures, characters or caricatures open For the client of Therapeutic Voicework these equations between certain vocal parameters and specific figures, characters or caricatures open the way to a process of experimentation by which the client passes through the vocal spectrum, assuming the physicality and the inner attitude of fleeting characters as they arise. Indeed, for most people it is impossible to play with combinations of the various vocal parameters without experiencing changes in self-image which feel comparable to acting various characters.

This process can be assisted by taking a single piece of text, perhaps from a client's dream or journal of spontaneous writing, and repeating the utterance of the text in a variety of timbral combinations. A combination is chosen from the parameters of free air, violin, disruption, modal, falsetto and vibrato within different pitch ranges in flute, clarinet and saxophone to sculpt and define an aspect of the Self through characterisation. The client then notices the change in self-image which occurs as a result of the vocalisation and amplifies this new image to form a figure in the manner of a dramatic rehearsal. This also provides a means to enabling clients to excavate characteristics which may lay just beyond their reach. I have taught this work at a number of British drama schools and to actors during rehearsal in repertory theatre, where they have found it extremely useful as a means to creating an increased flexibility and sense of choice regarding vocal embodiment of character.

Application of this field of Therapeutic Voicework with actors in rehearsal has been developed by Bernadette O'Brien, a graduate of the professional training in Voice Movement Therapy, who applies the systematic methodology of timbral parameters to help actors connect the authenticity of their performance with the malleability of their vocal range. Though O'Brien presents her work as training in the context of rehearsal, she has found that the use of the system inevitably provokes intimate and emotional responses from the actors, who invariably present issues of fear, anxiety and embarrassment regarding their voice. O'Brien has, therefore, come to believe that the 'vocal therapeutic process takes place within the creative activity of theatre-making', whether or not the procedure is directly named as 'therapeutic'. By the same token, in her private one-to-one consultations, which are acknowledged as containing a therapeutic dimension, she has found that the rehearsal process by which the client vocalises characters or sub-personalities is equally present. From this she deduces that 'the rehearsal is also present in the therapeutic consulting room'.[93]

Because O'Brien is also keenly devoted to encouraging theatre which combines use of both the physicality of the actor's body and the use of song as part of a theatre performance, she also finds herself utilising processes which originate in the field of dance and music. Her work thus reminds us that vocal expression is indeed an aspect of all expressive arts and therefore has a place within all the expressive arts therapies.

Having looked in some detail at the Therapeutic Voicework component of some of the individual arts therapies, it will, therefore, be useful to consider the notion of an integrated expressive arts therapy.

Voice as the Bridge: Integrated Arts Therapy and Vocal Expression

Voice is a musical phenomenon and can serve the precepts and objectives of music therapy; voice is a dramatic process and is central to the medium of expression used by the client of dramatherapy; and voice and breath also figure in the natural release of feeling in the field of dance therapy. Despite this, no integrated model of Therapeutic Voicework exists which synthesises the approach of the various arts therapies – primarily because there are few projects which fuse the various arts in a single therapeutic training or application. It is in response to this dearth that I have ensured that the professional training in Voice Movement Therapy integrates use of all the arts within a single coherent paradigm. There are a number of other exceptions to this dearth of what we may call an integrated expressive arts therapy, among which is the work of innovator Arthur Robbins, who developed a way of working therapeutically which moved between the use of art, theatre, movement and music. In his early work Robbins also attempted to facilitate Therapeutic Voicework in a psychotherapeutic context and the book which he co-wrote with colleagues, *Expressive Therapy*, bequeaths a number of passages on the subject.

Arthur Robbins

Robbins says that 'singing is potentially more threatening than playing an instrument' because it emerges from the human body, which is 'exactly where psychic reality is located'. Therefore, for Robbins, 'the connection between one's feelings and one's voice can seem dangerously direct'. Citing Winnicott, he says that singing 'becomes a transitional phenomenon' as it is rooted 'in the infant's early babbling and the older child's singing of his repertory of songs while preparing for sleep'.[94] With the primacy of the voice in mind, he says that 'it is generally accepted among professional singers that there are at least two basic registers in the voice', which are called 'head register' and 'chest register'. Applying these registers analytically, Robbins says that, 'based on clinical experience', the head register, which 'is experienced as resonating above the mouth in the cavities of the head, psychodynamically represents vulnerability, or the ability to be receptive', whilst the 'chest register, which 'is experienced as resonating in the chest and throat, psychodynamically represents the ability to be aggressive'. Furthermore, he states that 'the head register generally represents the female imago, and the chest register the male imago'. Given that the aim of therapeutic work is to achieve greater integration and wholeness, Robbins says that 'a patient whose speaking or singing voice is harsh and chest-register-dominated would need to work on opening up the head register, whereas one whose voice is delicate and head-register-dominated would need to work on developing the chest'.[95]

Robbins here predicates his insight on certain intuitive and non-empirical equations between the acoustic properties of registration, that is the falsetto and modal or head and chest register, on the one hand and specific psychological or personality traits, such as 'delicate' and 'female' or 'aggressive' and 'male', on the other. This is very common within the extant literature on psychotherapeutic Voicework and it should be remembered that whilst such intuitive assumptions can be appropriate, they can also serve to perpetuate a faulty analysis which emanates more from culturally established and projected stereotypes than from authentic individual expression. For example, it is true that in the European classical tradition of singing it is the women who sing in falsetto or head register whilst the men sing in modal, with the exception of the male counter tenor. However, in many other cultures men and women use both registers. The equation between falsetto or head register and the female imago is, therefore, an interpretation constructed and compounded by cultural and political circumstances and may have little relevance to the therapeutic analysis of voice quality in a broader context. Again, however, the flaws in these assumptions should not be used to fuel criticism of Robbins' work but rather should remind us of the widespread lack of applicable and reliable information about the voice available to therapists who are struggling to include vocal expression in their work with clients.

Robbins goes on to describe the work with one of his clients in which he makes use of an equation between register and gender-based psychic contents. The patient, a forty-year-old social worker, came to work with Robbins 'as an auxiliary to her verbal psychoanalysis' and asked to work through singing. As a child, her mother, who wrote books, was 'pushy and controlling and attempted to define her feelings and needs for her', whilst her father, who was a minister, 'did not relate to her or anyone else in the family, hardly ever spoke, and never knew what was going on'. Robbins says that 'at the beginning of music therapy she sang in a 'sweet', 'head-register' voice of a 'latency-aged child', which in general, 'lacked discipline' and which, 'regardless of the differing affects of the texts, had a hollow sadness in it because of a lack of high frequencies in her voice, and a feeling of fragility because of the relatively low overall volume'. The patient declared that she needed to be more in touch with 'anger, nastiness, and sexiness'.[95] Robbins interprets that the patient's 'head-register-dominated voice indicates a certain lack of discipline' and that she needs help to 'focus her singing with a mixture of chest register'. Robbins says that the patient's 'voice problems vividly symbolise' both 'regressive wishes' and 'frustrations of her early family relationships' in that 'her voice, on the one hand, yearned for some type of mothering softness, while on the other ruled out feelings of domination, aggression, or control', that is to say 'the voice represented an imbalance of mother, father, and child'.[96]

Here Robbins perceives fundamental components of the client's personality, including historic autobiographical details, reflected in the timbral quality of the voice. In so doing he raises a vital question with regard to vocal quality, as to whether the interpreted content emanates from the client or from the therapist's own associations. For example, when Robbins describes the client's voice as 'sweet', possessing a 'hollow sadness' and a 'feeling of fragility', is this an admission of the way the voice effects him – which may effect other therapists quite differently – or does the sound genuinely emanate from the client's contemporaneous feeling of sweetness, sadness and fragility which initiates and is further compounded by the sound? Naturally, one method of establishing the appropriate reality of the therapist's experience is to ask the client to verbally describe her emotion, and, indeed, Robbins asserts that the client herself wished to express more anger, nastiness and sexiness. However, in many instances the therapeutic procedure is mobilised with such speed and fluidity that the therapist is literally forced to act or refrain from acting purely on the basis of his own intuition or counter transference. Furthermore, there is a thesaurus of terminology which may be used to simultaneously signify both vocal parameters as well as human properties, yet this simultaneity can be as confusing and demeaning as it can be useful and enlightening. For example, to what precisely does Robbins refer when he describes the client's voice as lacking in precision, structure and discipline? In music this may refer to an inability to sustain a constant tone or a difficulty in refining a melodic motif. But what, if anything, does it mean in the context of a psychotherapeutic analysis of the voice?

Robbins proceeds to speak of a further session with the aforementioned client which begins with her singing a 'short melody in head register'.[98] When the therapist asked her to add chest register, the patient 'vocalized upwards until a very high chest register was reached', which, he says, 'naturally brought about an intensification in the energy of the high frequencies, quite different from the diffuse, gentle sound with which she began the improvisation'.[99] The therapist then noticed 'a particular hooded, heavy-lidded look that had suddenly come into the patient's eyes during the singing' and asked the patient to watch herself in the mirror while singing. The therapist interpreted the gaze as revealing anger and asked the patient to focus her gaze 'very carefully on one eye in the mirror and sing', at which point he heard an increase in anger in the patient. He then asked her to 'put the sound farther forward', 'by the front teeth', and suggested that the patient attempted a 'biting on the bottom note'. As the patient sang, the therapist experienced yet a further increase in the patient's expression of anger and encouraged her to sing 'in and out of the angry-feeling lower register'. Afterwards, the patient said that she thought she sounded like a male tenor.[100]

The patient went on to use this quality of voice to sing a folk song written in the words and from the perspective of a man who, in the patient's view of the song's narrative, was 'nasty' and who was blaming a woman unjustly. The therapist consequently encouraged the patient to sing as though she were the man, exaggerating his posture and mannerisms as well as vocal tone and timbre, from which he posited that the patient, 'instead of denying and dissociating herself from a threatening male introject, 're-experienced it' and 'acted it out' and, by so doing, 'gained some mastery over the figure'.[101] As the patient continued to work, the therapist found moments of the song where she could mix the head register and chest register, the latter of which had become associated with the male character, facilitating a process which Robbins describes as aiming for 'a sphere of male-female wholeness in her voice'.[102] Robbins thereby describes a way in which a simple equation between an identifiable acoustic property of the voice with a specific matrix of personal characteristics can be established and investigated through the singing voice, leading to psychological integration via vocal re-composition.

In addition to the issue of the therapist's own responses, a further area of contention is raised through Robbins' work, which is that of the training component of a vocally-orientated arts therapist. This issue is exemplified through Robbins' description of a further case, a 'forty-five-year-old German-born business woman with two grown children' who, at the beginning of therapy, sang in 'a constricted, chest-dominated voice, which was overly focused with too many high frequencies and not enough head-tone'. The author says that 'regardless of the text, she sang with a harsh, forced quality, which, although piercing, gave the impression of instability, due to breath being supported by extreme muscular tension'. Robbins' interpretation was simply that she needed to 'be more in touch with the gentle, vulnerable parts of herself' and that 'her basic psychological responses are of the ego-orientated sphere, which cruelly represses warm affects'.[103]

Because of the excess muscular tension which Robbins identifies, the therapy begins with 'some voice training, emphasizing a relaxed throat and jaw'.[104] Thus Robbins implicitly assumes the role of vocal trainer and draws upon the knowledge with which to encourage healthy somatic vocal functioning.

A highly pertinent issue raised by a study of Robbins work is that concerning how much physiological and somatic understanding an arts therapy practitioner needs to be able to physically prepare the vocal instrument for psychological expression. In this case, Robbins chooses to prepare the client for the expression of gentle affects. However, another therapist may, with equal viability, have decided to amplify the client's existing voice, intensifying what Robbins hears as 'harshness'. Often, in therapy it can be as useful to amplify and magnify what is present as to seek that which, in the ears of the therapist and client, is missing. In cases where this involves the vocalisation of extremely non-gentle material, such as fury and rage, the voice may, however, not be able to withstand its expression without tissue damage unless it is trained in voice production techniques which facilitate healthy ways of making extreme sounds. Consequently, the arts therapist may need a greater understanding of physiology than is offered to student therapists in order to provide the client with such vocal training. Perhaps, in order to deepen the vocal component of expressive arts therapies, it is necessary to encourage research into the fascinating borderland where the physiology of the expressive instrument meets the psychology of the material which the medium communicates.

McNiff and Knill: An Intermodal Expressive Arts Therapy

Despite the fact that Robbins utilised a number of arts in his work with clients, he did not fuse them into a single strategy but rather selected what he or the client felt was appropriate at any given time, enabling him to respond effectively to a range of client needs. There is, however, a body of work which seeks to take a step further than this in trying to combine a number of different artistic modalities within a common therapeutic procedure simultaneously and which originates in the collaboration between Shaun McNiff, Norma Canner, Mariagnese Knill-Cattaneo and Paulo Knill.

During the late 1970s and throughout the 1980s, The Lesley College Graduate School, in Cambridge, Massachusetts, under the innovative guidance of McNiff, Canner, Knill-Cattaneo and Knill, developed an approach to the use of arts in psychotherapy known as 'Intermodal Expressive Therapy'. This model attempts to integrate the various arts therapies – art therapy, music therapy, dance movement therapy, psychodrama and dramatherapy – into an interdisciplinary framework and the approach was explored in Knill's self-published book, *Intermodal Learning in Education and Therapy*, first printed in 1978.[105] In addition to the continuation of this approach at Lesley College, a programme based on the techniques is also run in Toronto at the Canada branch of the International School for Interdisciplinary Studies, taught by Steven Levine[106] and Ellen Levine[107] who also edit the *Journal of the Creative and Expressive Arts Therapies Exchange*. Neither McNiff or Knill have any more connection with Lesley College, which, like many institutions founded upon the vision of pioneers, seems to have diluted its approach. Paulo Knill is now working primarily in Europe, where he directs a multidisciplinary arts therapy training at the recently formed European Graduate School, a state-approved University in Switzerland; Shaun McNiff, meanwhile, implements programmes at Endicott College, Massachusetts.

Whilst Knill has remained lesser known to the wider field of expressive therapies, his original collaborator, Shaun McNiff, who is probably the single most significant contributor to this field, has sustained a higher profile, originally through his first book, *The Arts in Psychotherapy*,[108] and sustained through his later works, which include *Educating the Creative Arts Therapist*[109] and *Art As Medicine*.[110]

Both the written works of Knill and McNiff, and the Intermodal Expressive Arts Therapy training at Cambridge and Toronto, where I have had the privilege of making a contribution to the programme, are, however, incomplete in that they do not offer a study of, or a model for, Therapeutic Voicework as an artistic and therapeutic modality. Levine and McNiff, with whom I have discussed the nature of Therapeutic Voicework, both believe in the necessity of forging a means to incorporate voice into an integrated modality of arts therapy, yet, like many trainers, they are regretfully cognizant of the sparsity of research and practical investigation in the field. Indeed, McNiff asserts that it 'is crucial to ask why so little attention has been paid to the expressive use of the voice within the field of the arts therapies'.[111]

In McNiff's early writing he does draw attention to the voice, beginning from the premise that 'art orders emotion at the deepest levels of consciousness'[112] and acknowledging that the use of voice 'allows for a primal and very direct expression of the emotions'.[113] It is here that McNiff briefly describes his own use of Therapeutic Voicework, an approach that he names 'Sound Enactments and Therapeutic Opera' and which constitutes one of the few descriptions of applied Therapeutic Voicework in an artistically-orientated psychotherapeutic context by an experienced expressive therapist.

McNiff describes 'a sound improvisation session' which he conducted with a group of 'severely disturbed' young children, amongst which there was a boy of about nine years old who consistently interrupted 'the group process with angry gestures'. With a view to allowing the child to 'musically express his anger and thus get it out of his system', McNiff gave the child some long sticks with which he started to bang a series of objects. Then the young boy 'let lose' a number of 'shockingly loud' 'primal screams' and 'began to lose control'. McNiff says that 'in listening to this particular child's screaming', he 'encountered the depth and power of his pain'.

The session was being conducted in a museum where some rooms had been set aside for expressive therapy work. However, McNiff felt that though the 'museum staff were supportive' of the work, nevertheless 'the kind of sound' that the child made 'was not appropriate within the museum setting'. McNiff states that 'the screams not only frightened the other children' but threw him and the other therapist working him 'off balance'. In order to 'stop the child's screaming', McNiff says that he 'had to pick him up and hold him, all the while speaking to him in a gentle voice'.

From this experience, McNiff concluded that 'primal expressions of this kind might be perfectly appropriate in a private, one-to-one session in a soundproof room', where the aim of the therapeutic process would be 'to help the child express primal rage within a setting where it will be acknowledged and supported'. But, says McNiff, 'with this particular case', the environment was 'incapable of supporting this kind of expression'. Furthermore, 'it was questionable whether or not the child was capable' of 'purging' himself of 'his angry feelings' because they were 'so all-encompassing' that he 'completely lost control whenever he began to express' them directly, such that no amount of screams were capable of 'venting his feelings'. In fact, 'they only served to stir up more conflictual emotion'.

In leading 'sound enactments' and 'operatic musical dramas', what is needed, says McNiff, is an 'ability on the part of the therapist to provide a 'safe and orderly environment over which control is maintained'. However, 'at the same time, the therapeutic space should also encourage spontaneous and free expression'. The problem, he acknowledges, however, is that 'primal sound expression has a unique ability to disrupt social situations' whilst the same 'is not true for painting and poetry', where primal emotions 'can be expressed within more highly controlled and private structures'.[114]

The trepidation which McNiff experiences and describes in response to the vocal expression initially made by the child in the public gallery could well typify a certain fear which therapists experience on encountering the raw and inarticulate quality of the human voice. Of course, with a small child who is swamped in undifferentiated affect with an aggressive component is, as McNiff implies, probably not the kind of client most suitable to Therapeutic Voicework. However, many people will, at some stage, express highly intensified emotions during Therapeutic Voicework and there are many clients who would benefit from such a modality for whom there is little provision and McNiff cautiously wonders whether it is fear that underlies the reason why so few therapists have wanted to expand upon the use of Therapeutic Voicework, given the way that the voice can express the deepest affect with an intensity which is unparalleled in any other channel of human expression.[115]

Shaping the Cathartic Clay

As with many descriptions of vocal expression in a therapeutic context, McNiff identifies in the client a need to 'purge', 'exhaust' or 'rid' an emotional experience from 'the system'. It is partly McNiff's observation that no amount of screaming would have achieved such a catharsis for the child that causes him to conclude that the context is inappropriate. In response to the inescapable volatility of the voice, McNiff concludes that 'as harmful as primal vocal expression might be for a person who is immersed in the chaos of anger and rage', it might, on the other hand, be a 'positive therapeutic objective' for the 'inhibited and tightly controlled person who is afraid and severely blocked in relation to expressing fundamental feelings'.[116]

In response to McNiff's comments, I am led to ask whether 'primal vocal expression' is harmful for such clients or whether it is rather that the therapist is often without resources with which to contain it. Furthermore, I believe it is of equal importance to seriously ponder whether inarticulate or non-verbal sound making necessarily denotes 'primal vocal expression' or whether vocal sounds can be inarticulate without being primal. In my experience the term 'primal', when used in relation to sound, usually indicates the utterance of extremely loud emotionally charged sounds emanating from pain and suffering. Furthermore, such sounds are usually immediately perceived as being part of a cathartic process in which the underlying emotions are imagined to be an expendable energetic quantity which can be purged or exorcised. In my view, if highly affective sounds are to be worked with in a way that is helpful to the client, it is necessary to depart from a purely cathartic view of therapeutic procedure, which stems from Freud's original abreactive work and was developed in the field of voice by those such as Reich[117], Lowen[118], Grof[119], and Orr[120]. In its place, I believe, it is necessary to recognise and utilise the innate therapeutic and containing function of artistic compositional structure.

Nonetheless, McNiff's beliefs and questions regarding the appropriate use of, and context for, Therapeutic Voicework are predicated on his own passionate commitment to a convergence between artistic freedom of investigation and therapeutic responsibility to the consequences of such a process, for which I have the greatest respect. The regrettable fact is, perhaps, that for such therapists there has never been a reliable methodology for containing, directing and intervening during a client's vocal expression, which, as McNiff says, understandably threatens the therapist who can often feel without resources and thus unable to provide the safety necessary for the client's continued expressions. One of the results of this lack of methodology is a deficit of procedural methods of informed professional intervention during vocally expressed affective experiences. Most clients, when working through the voice with deep feelings, will give the appearance of being involved in an infinite and inexhaustible emotional tirade and, for inexperienced therapists, it may well appear frightening because it seems to have no end. It is for this reason that the notion of working cathartically and working artistically must be differentiated. Therapeutic Voicework should, in my view, involve the compositional and artistic shaping of the material, no matter how intense, as it appears. For, in most cases, the fantasy of a catharsis through which emotional trauma can be expelled from the so-called system is of questionable therapeutic efficacy, particularly for the purposes of long-term recovery. Of greater benefit is to facilitate the client in a shaping of the sound into a form which can be contained and repeatedly revisited and rehearsed, leading to greater containment.

For the therapist, this entails intervening and dialoguing with the client during vocal sound making. Often, however, the intensity of vocal emission seems to create a wall of sound which the therapist cannot penetrate other than to bring the sound to a halt. Alternatively, a therapist may feel that there is no choice but to await the natural exhaustion of the voice and the emotions which lie behind it, by which time emotional distress may have manifested as physical distress, resulting in unnecessary psychic pain and tissue damage. Of course, what is desperately required is a means to intervene during vocalisation which respects the need for continuity and unrestrained emotional and acoustic intensity but which, at the same time, can shape it without depleting its potency but also without either client or therapist being paralysed by its power.

It was my own sense of inadequacy and lack of resources in the face of intense vocal expression, first that of my own parents and later that displayed by severely handicapped young adults, which led me towards my attempt at laying the foundations for a methodological Therapeutic Voicework which can offer such intervention.

Therapeutic Voicework Methodology: Expressive Arts Analysis and Intervention

During the Therapeutic Voicework session, as I conceive of it, practice it and train others to do likewise, the client's expressions, no matter how intense, highly charged and disturbing, are perceived on a number of levels, which include the technical, the artistic and the psychological. When a client is consumed, involved in or overwhelmed by highly affective material – perhaps screaming or wailing, perhaps yelling and hollering, perhaps bemoaning a tragic cacophony – the practitioner should not only identify and empathise with them. This is not enough. In fact, on its own it often paralyses the practitioner and hinders positive intervention. The Therapeutic Voiceworker must, rather, simultaneously perceive the client's expressions as a drama, as a song and as a dance, that is as a piece of choreography and as a piece of musical and dramatic composition, as though the client is rehearsing. In addition, the practitioner must notice the technicality of the voice within the system which I have described, comprehending the breathing pattern, the configuration of the vocal tract, the pitch and its fluctuation, the loudness, glottal attack, degree of free air, the presence or absence of disruption, the register and the degree of violin. This enables the practitioner to intervene on levels which remain separate from the emotional field or content. Thus the Therapeutic Voiceworker can, without disturbing the emotional experience, intervene as an artist, requesting that the client develops the choreographic, musical or dramatic components in the same way a choreographer, conductor and theatre director may guide a rehearsal as the performers work without bringing them to a stand-still.

The Therapeutic Voiceworker asks the client to repeat particular units of expression again, in the manner of rehearsal, offering kinetic, dramatic and musical ideas which help the client develop and transform the experience and the expression of it. Second, the practitioner may also give technical instructions, asking the client to, for example, increase the degree of free air, lower the pitch and decrease the vibrato whilst focusing the breathing pattern on slow abdominal displacement. Here the practitioner works in the manner of a voice coach and singing teacher, enabling the client to authenticate the expression whilst simultaneously bringing the experience under conscious creative control.

This process, to those unfamiliar with Therapeutic Voicework, may sound rather strange for, indeed, I am proposing that, whilst in the midst of an intense affective experience, the practitioner speaks to the client on a technical and creative level, almost as though to ignore the authentic, and possibly painful nature, of the client's predicament. It is as though someone comes into a room, clearly disturbed and painfully effected by a tragedy, explaining the story which has led to the overwhelming state of anxiety, only to have the listener ask her to repeat a section of the story again with more free air, lower in pitch with less vibrato and more amplified abdominal displacement. On one level it may seem as an insult to emotion. However, it is the creative and technical intervention and its ability to facilitate rehearsal which authenticates and contains the experience as well as providing the grounds for transformation. This is what every performer knows.

In order to work in such a manner, I train practitioners to perceive that everyday human expression can be seen as a conglomerate of certain expressive dimensions. First, there is a physical dimension as the body gesticulates and moves through space. Second, there is a textual dimension as the linguistic apparatus articulates words with distinct meaning. Third, there is a vocal dimension which underscores these words with intonation, prosody, stress, rhythm and timbre. Fourth, there is the musical dimension which is the melody inherent in this vocal score and which would be revealed if the words were sung rather than spoken.

These dimensions, when witnessed from the outside by an observer and audient, can be seen as artistic delineations. As we watch the body move, we can perceive it as a choreography. As we listen to the speech, we can hear it as a text, a poem, prose or monologue. As we listen to the voice, we can hear the dramatic, the theatrical, that is the particular attitudinal and emotional source of the text and the sense of a character or caricature who utters it. Finally, we can also listen to the prosody as though we were hearing a concert, attuning ourselves to the melodic composition. In the approach to work which I am disseminating, the expressions of the client are perceived simultaneously through the windows of these dimensions. Consequently, the practitioner can intervene and shape the client's work with specific attention to a particular dimension. He may intervene as choreographer, as writing editor, as theatre director, as vocal coach or as musical composer without necessarily needing to encumber the process by interrupting the perceived emotional content of the expressions with his interpretations, which, in any case, are inevitably an extension of his own subjective personal associations and counter transference. This multi-disciplinary focus is highly demanding but I am finding it an increasingly significant technique which I am developing with students.

Therapeutic Voicework Case Study: Getting the Colour Back in the Cheeks

Catalina was part Irish and part African and had built a very successful career as a singer, drawing on a number of different musical styles which she performed throughout Europe. However, following a long tour she had become extremely ill, first with chickenpox, then with a kidney infection and finally with recurring laryngitis.

When she began working, she described herself as feeling 'frail', 'thin', 'emaciated' and 'at death's door'. She also said that, in a way, she felt it was

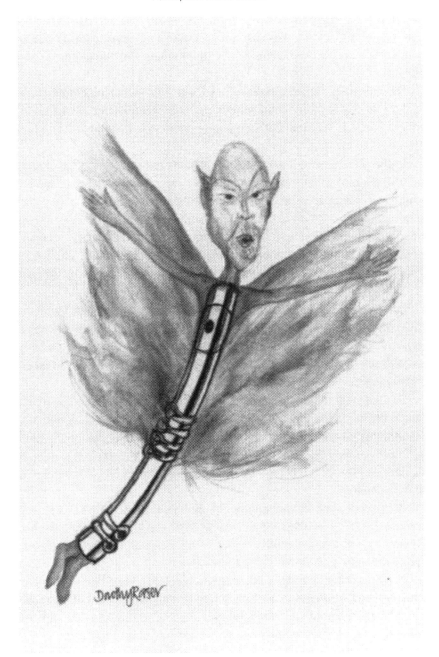

Figure 10.1

THERAPEUTIC VOICEWORK

pointless coming to work because 'she had no voice'. She was also quite worried because she had, on two separate occasions some years ago, had nodules on her vocal folds which had receded with prolonged rest but left her feeling anxious.

On vocalising, Catalina produced a voice in flute, with hard glottal attack, high in pitch with a moderate vibrato and a constant frictional disruption, which, she said, was part of her singing style, $>< 2$| ᴨ ᴧᴧ $\approx\approx$ which reminded me of Bonnie Tyler.

Rather than placing fresh demands on someone who seemed as though she had been over-demanded of in the first place, I suggested that Catalina amplify the image of feeling emaciated whilst sustaining high, falsetto, free air notes in flute, **F ᴨ >|<**. As she did so, her feet started to lift off the floor as she moved on to 'tiptoe' and her eyes fluttered. I suggested that she exaggerate this and, in time, her arms began to stretch out like wings. On asking Catalina to describe this image, she said she felt like a 'sick angel' (Figure 10.1). Then she began to cry.

I made a gentle sound with my own voice on the consonants 'mmm' to offer empathy and acknowledgement and placed one hand upon her upper back and another on her abdomen, encouraging her to deepen her breathing. As I did this, her sobbing intensified and the studio filled with her incessant and passionate wailing.

Catalina's sister had died at the age of eleven of a blood disease, at which time Catalina was sixteen years old. Whenever Catalina fell ill, she was reminded of her sister and it provoked 'mixed feelings'. She felt guilty that it had not been her that died, she felt bereaved at the loss, she felt a sense of shame that she was achieving success and she felt that maybe she was going to die as well.

Her parents had divorced after the death of her sister and both had seemed to show much less interest in Catalina than before. In fact, she had felt in some way that her childhood and her relationship with her parents had ended abruptly with the death of her sister.

As she continued to cry, I asked her to repeat the third line of a lullaby which she had written in an earlier session: 'It was never black and white and Mummy isn't always right'. Each time she did this I asked her to develop the choreography of her arm movements, sometimes hitting and striking out, sometimes stroking, sometimes punching the air and sometimes enacting gathering movements. She performed these movements with incredible force and intensity, like a wild creature tearing its way out of captivity. I was still in contact with her body and, as she became more emotionally charged, she asked me to keep hold of her, as though she was frightened.

As I noticed that she was still on tiptoe, I suggested that she develop a rhythmic dance and percussive composition with her heels on the floor. Her work now became like flamenco and her sobbing rung out in tones of pathos. I began to let her go and asked her to drop the pitch of the voice and take out some of the free air. With this, her tears turned to laughter in an instant. When I looked at her, she said: 'I have always wanted to dance'.

In the interim period until the next session I asked Catalina to write a Family Song about her sister, which she did with commitment but open trepidation. The song, which she sang at the next session, began: 'Sorry for the tyrant that I was; don't tell me that it killed you in the end'. As Catalina sang these words, both her eyes and mine filled with tears. What she described as her 'rasping', 'scraping', 'don't mess with me sunshine' voice suddenly revealed itself in a different light. It was like the voice of someone who had been up all night crying after a death, which, in fact, is what the family did the night her sister died.

It was shortly after this that Catalina had begun to sing in bands and she soon found that her disrupted and muscularly-constricted voice attracted warm responses from listeners. Despite the fact that it had provided her with a career, it was, in fact, causing sore throats, laryngitis and a host of other difficulties.

On asking Catalina about her song, she said that she had consistently 'tormented' her sister as a child and they had been rivals more than companions. Though she felt it to be 'ridiculous', nonetheless there was part of Catalina that felt responsible for her sister's death.

Catalina now returned to the image of the sick angel and sang her song with the accompanying movements. As we worked, we realised that this sick angel was in some way also her sister, that Catalina had begun to get recurring illnesses after her sister's death and that Catalina felt 'sick' with herself for having not treated her sister better when she was alive.

On teaching Catalina to enter into primate and expand pharyngeal dimensions, she became concerned because as the vocal tract expanded and the pressure between the vocal folds decreased, so the disruption in her voice became less severe. Catalina was worried that she was going to lose the singing voice which earned her living and which she felt expressed her 'very being'. In addition, she felt the sound to be 'ugly' and, indeed, her primary

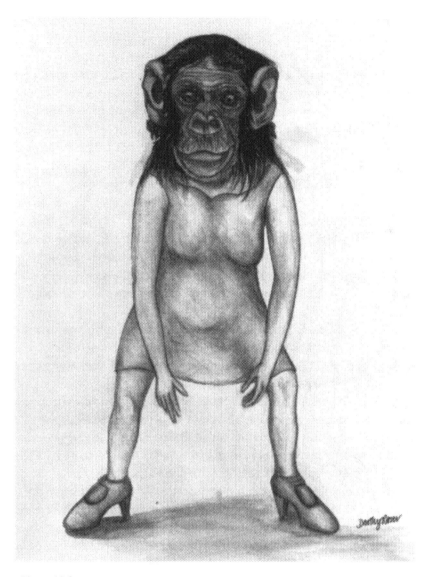

Figure 10.2

sensate experience of the Primate position was focused around her face. She said she didn't like 'looking like a monkey' (Figure 10.2).

On investigating this, it was revealed that Catalina's sister had been very dark of skin, whilst Catalina said that God had 'dished out' to her 'a mixture of two pigments', which left her 'neither one thing nor the other', neither black nor white. Catalina had experienced extreme difficulty at school. Neither black nor white, she had been ridiculed as a 'half-caste'. Furthermore, she resented her sister for having a clear visual identity. As Catalina described this, she looked up to heaven and sarcastically said: 'Thanks very much God'.

It was in that moment, as she spoke those words, that I heard her vocal tract open and a new quality of clarinet emerge, **<>**. It was still mildly disrupted but more resonant and with much less pressure on the vocal folds. The voice had arisen out of what Catalina described as her 'desire to be black' like her sister and yet she felt somewhat guilty about this, as though she was a 'fraud' and a 'fake'.

As we returned to primate she now began to cry again for she remembered that when she was at school, she had also been called 'monkey face' and that one of the ways she had defended herself was by 'growling' in a loud disrupted voice which made them run away screaming. This had become a repetitive process, whereby children called her monkey face in order to hear her make this extraordinary noise, which she demonstrated for me and which compared to her original singing voice.

With these realisations regarding the connection between the particular quality of voice which she had developed as a singer and her personal history, Catalina seemed to become more relaxed, as though letting go of something which was causing her tension.

At the next session Catalina arrived wearing a fantastic long, flowing dress. As she walked into the room she said: 'I have decided. I may be no angel but I am black and I am beautiful and I want to sing'.

We now took the primate work one stage further and opened out the vocal tract into saxophone configuration. The disruption was still present but the tissue structures surrounding the vocal folds were pulled back, the muscular tension and compression was decreased and, in consequence, the pitch was slightly lower, **() ～～ |ᴿ ++**. Because of the increased vocal tract dimensions, Catalina gained a richness of harmonic resonance in return for losing the 'squeezed', 'slightly anguished', 'crying sound'(Figure 10.3).

As she left the session, she said: 'Maybe I should try some gospel' and again looked to the ceiling and, without sarcasm, said: 'Gee, thanks God'.

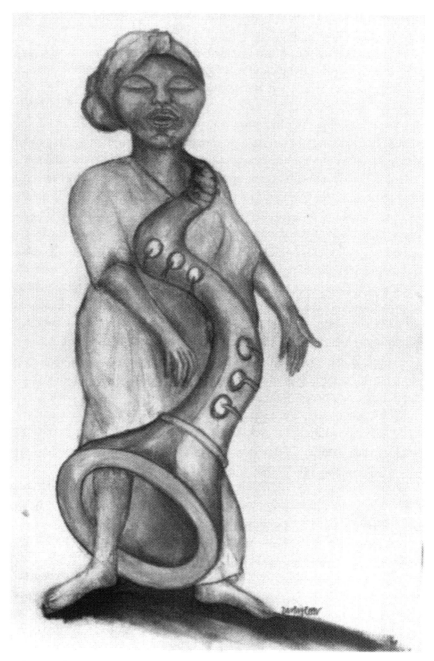

Figure 10.3

The Therapeutic Voicework process for Catalina included a certain claiming of her ethnicity, her race and her colour, divorcing it from the disgraceful and historically established equations between being black and being 'primitive', 'bad', 'instinctive' and 'ape-like'. In addition, she had learned to overcome a method of voice production which was causing her physiological problems. Furthermore, this had influenced her artistic style.

It seemed that the anger at other children at calling her 'monkey face' was used to confront the audience, as though in some ways they were also an enemy. As we begn to work, the new voice led to the possibility of a different relationship with her audience, which perceived them as those who were there because they wanted to hear her, not to persecute her. Catalina had not had this relationship to her parents and they had not helped her overcome her guilt at her sister's death. By changing the voice quality she was able to release the sorrow which underpinned the anger contained by the frictional disruption and her singing concerts continued with a different repertoire but with no less success.

Conclusion: Body, Art and Politics

In the pioneering and much needed work of psychotherapist Michael Vannoy Adams, it is asserted that we can no longer ignore the complexities of 'race', 'skin colour' and ethnicity' in the psychotherapeutic process,[121] and the previous case study exemplifies an example of a racial component to the Therapeutic Voicework process.

However, it also reveals the inescapable physiological component to Therapeutic Voicework. If Catalina had not sought help, she may well have contracted nodules again and possibly, eventually, seriously damaged her voice and lost her career.

This means that although the Therapeutic Voicework modality compares to the arts therapies, it also necessitates a level of physiological and physical understanding. Thus it is to the field of physical and physiological vocal work that I shall now turn my attention.

Notes

1   Case, C. and Dalley, T. (1992) *The Handbook of Art Therapy*. London: Routledge, p.6.

2   Fleshman, B. & Fryrear, J. (1981) *The Arts in Therapy*. Chicago: Nelson-Hall.

3   Robbins, A. (1986) *Expressive Therapy: A Creative Arts Approach to Depth-Orientated Treatment*. New York: Human Sciences Press.

4   Warren, B. (1993) *Using the Creative Arts in Therapy: A Practical Introduction.* London: Routledge.

5   McNiff, S. (1981) *The Arts in Psychotherapy.* Springfield Ill: Charles C. Thomas.

6   *Journal of the Arts in Psychotherapy.* Pergamon: New York.

7   McNiff, S. Interview with P. Newham at Endicott College, June 1996.

8   Walker, D. (1991) *Becoming a Profession: The History of Art Therapy in Britain 1940–82.* London: Tavistock/Routledge and J Alvin, Music Therapy London: Stainer and Bell.

9   Alvin, J. (1991) *Music Therapy.* London: Stainer and Bell.

10   Alvin, J. (1991) *Music Therapy.* London: Stainer and Bell.

11   Moore Meigs, M. (1991) 'Introduction to music therapy.' *Self and Society,* XVIX, 1 (Jan/Feb. 1991), pp.10–12, (p.11).

12   McNiff, S. Interview with P. Newham at Endicott College, (June, 1996).

13   Wright, P. and Priestly, M. (1975) *Music Therapy in Action.* London: Constable.

14   Nordoff, P. & Robbins, C. (1992) *Therapy in Music for Handicapped Children.* London: Victor Gollancz.

15   Nordoff, P. and Robbins, C. (1992) *Therapy in Music for Handicapped Children.* London: Victor Gollancz, p.68.

16   Nordoff, P. and Robbins, C. (1992) *Therapy in Music for Handicapped Children.* London: Victor Gollancz, p.68.

17   Nordoff, P. and Robbins, C. (1992) *Therapy in Music for Handicapped Children.* London: Victor Gollancz, p.68–70.

18   Nordoff, P. and Robbins, C. (1992) *Therapy in Music for Handicapped Children.* London: Victor Gollancz, pp.30–31.

19   Sutton, J. (1993) 'The guitar doesn't know this song: an investigation into parallel development in speech/language and music therapy.' In M. Heal and T. Wigram (eds) *Music Therapy in Health and Education.* London: Jessica Kingsley, pp.264–72.

20   di Franco, G. (1993) 'Music therapy: a methodological approach in the mental health field.' In M. Heal and T. Wigram (eds) *Music Therapy in Health and Education.* London: Jessica Kingsley, pp.82–90, (p.85).

21   di Franco, G. (1993) 'Music therapy: a methodological approach in the mental health field.' In M. Heal and T. Wigram (eds) *Music Therapy in Health and Education.* London: Jessica Kingsley, pp.82–90, (p.85).

22   di Franco, G. (1993) 'Music therapy: a methodological approach in the mental health field.' In M. Heal and T. Wigram (eds) *Music Therapy in Health and Education.* London: Jessica Kingsley, pp.82–90, (p.85).

23   Payne, H. (ed) (1992) *Dance Movement Therapy: Theory and Practice.* London: Tavistock/Routledge.

24   Whitehouse, M.S. (1979) 'C G Jung and dance therapy: two major principles.' In P. L. Bernstein (ed) *Eight Theoretical Approaches in Dance-Movement Therapy.* Dubuque: Kendall/Hunt, pp.51–70.

25   Chodorow, J. (1991) *Dance Therapy and Depth Psychology.* London: Routledge.

26   Noack, A. (1992) 'On a Jungian approach to dance movement therapy.' In Helen Payne (ed) *Dance Movement Therapy: Theory and Practice.* London: Tavistock/ Routledge, pp.182–201.

27   Meekums, B. (1992) 'Dance movement therapy in a family service unit,' and Monika Steiner (1992) 'Alternatives in psychiatry: dance movement therapy in the community.' In

Helen Payne (ed) *Dance Movement Therapy: Theory and Practice*. London: Tavistock/Routledge.

28   Hodgson, J. and Preston-Dunlop, V. (1990) *Rudolf Laban: An Introduction to his Work and Influence*. Plymouth: Northcote House, p.17.

29   Hodgson, J. and Preston-Dunlop, V. (1990) *Rudolf Laban: An Introduction to his Work and Influence*. Plymouth: Northcote House, p.25.

30   Hodgson, J. and Preston-Dunlop, V. (1990) *Rudolf Laban: An Introduction to his Work and Influence*. Plymouth: Northcote House, p.56.

31   Schoop, T. and Mitchell, P. (1979) 'Reflections and projections: the schoop approach to dance therapy.' In P. Bernstein (ed) *Eight Theoretical Approaches to Dance-Movement-Therapy*. Dubuque: Kendall Hunt.

32   Bartenieff, I. (1975) 'Dance therapy: a new profession of rediscovery of an ancient role of the dance?' In H. Chaiklin (ed) *Marian Chace: Her Papers*. Maryland: American Dance Therapy Association.

33   Rubenfield, I. (1995) 'Interview with Irmgard Bartenieff.' In D. Johnson (ed) *Bone, Breath and Gesture: Practises of Embodiment*. Berkeley: North Atlantic Books, pp.222–237.

34   Lamb, W. and Watson, E. (1987) *Body Code: The Meaning in Movement*. Princeton: Princeton.
     Lamb, W. (1965) *Posture and Gesture: An Introduction to the Study of Physical Behaviour*. London: Duckworth.

35   Lamb, W. (1965) *Posture and Gesture: An Introduction to the Study of Physical Behaviour*. London: Duckworth, p.41.

36   Lamb, W. (1965) *Posture and Gesture: An Introduction to the Study of Physical Behaviour*. London: Duckworth, p.117.

37   Hodgson, J. and Preston-Dunlop, V. (1990) *Rudolf Laban: An Introduction to his Work and Influence*. Plymouth: Northcote House, p.41.

38   McColl, C., (1992) cited in S. Richards, *Sonic Harvest: Towards Musical Democracy*. Oxford: Amber Lane, p.90.

39   Richards, S. (1992) *Sonic Harvest: Towards Musical Democracy*. Oxford: Amber Lane, p.91.

40   Richards, S. (1992) *Sonic Harvest: Towards Musical Democracy*. Oxford: Amber Lane, p.91.

41   Richards, S. (1992) *Sonic Harvest: Towards Musical Democracy*. Oxford: Amber Lane, p.91.

42   Malmgrem, Y. and Carpenter, W. (1954) *Movement Psychology*. Unpublished manuscript.

43   Hodgson, J. and Preston-Dunlop, V. (1990) *Rudolf Laban: An Introduction to his work and Influence*. Plymouth: Northcote House, p.42.

44   Freud, S. (1953–74) *Standard Edition of The Complete Psychological Works of Sigmund Freud*, vol. 3. James Strachey (ed) in collaboration with Anna Freud, assisted by Alix Strachey and Alan Tyson. London: Hogarth Press, p.36.

45   Laban, R. (1960) *The Mastery of Movement*, 2nd edn. London: McDonald and Evans, p.19.

46   Freud, A. (1965) *Normality and Pathology in Childhood: Assessment of Development*. New York: International University Press.

47   Mahler, M. (1968) *On Human Symbiosis and the Vicissitudes of Individuation*. New York: International University Press.

48   Kestenberg, J. (1995) *Sexuality, Body Movement, and the Rhythms of Development*. Northval, New Jersey: Aronson, pp.189–190.

49   Laban, R. (1960) *The Mastery of Movement*, 2nd edn. London: McDonald and Evans.

50   Kestenberg, J. (1995) *Sexuality, Body Movement, and the Rhythms of Development*. Northval, New Jersey: Aronson.

51   Kestenberg, J. (1995) *Sexuality, Body Movement, and the Rhythms of Development.* Northval, New Jersey: Aronson.

52   Kestenberg, J. (1995) *Sexuality, Body Movement, and the Rhythms of Development.* Northval, New Jersey: Aronson.

53   Lewis, P. (1994) 'The clinical interpretation of the kestenberg movement profile.' Unpublished thesis.

54   Lewis, P. (1986) *Theoretical Approaches in Dance Movement Therapy,* vols. 1 and 2. Dubque: Kendall Hunt.

55   Brownell, A. and Lewis, P. (1990) 'The Kestenberg movement profile in assessment of vocalization.' In P. Lewis and S. Loman (eds) *The Kestenberg Movement Profile: Its Past, Present Applications and Future Directions.* Keene: Antioch New England Graduate School, pp.139–154, (p.141).

56   Brownell, A. and Lewis, P. (1990) 'The Kestenberg movement profile in assessment of vocalization.' In P. Lewis and S. Loman (eds) *The Kestenberg Movement Profile: Its Past, Present Applications and Future Directions.* Keene: Antioch New England Graduate School, pp.139–154.

57   Brownell, A. and Lewis, P. (1990) 'The Kestenberg movement profile in assessment of vocalization.' In P. Lewis and S. Loman (eds) *The Kestenberg Movement Profile: Its Past, Present Applications and Future Directions.* Keene: Antioch New England Graduate School, pp.139–154, (p.141).

58   Brownell, A. (1987) 'The singing self.' Unpublished Masters Thesis, Lesley College, Cambridge, Mass.

59   Mettler, B. (1985) *Dance as an Element of Life.* Tuscon, Arizona: Mettler Studios Inc., p.13.

60   Mettler, B. (1985) *Dance as an Element of Life.* Tuscon, Arizona: Mettler Studios Inc., p.16.

61   Mettler, B. (1985) *Dance as an Element of Life.* Tuscon, Arizona: Mettler Studios Inc., p.12.

62   Mettler, B. (1985) *Dance as an Element of Life.* Tuscon, Arizona: Mettler Studios Inc., p.55.

63   Mettler, B. (1985) *Dance as an Element of Life.* Tuscon, Arizona: Mettler Studios Inc., p.55.

64   Mettler, B. (1985) *Dance as an Element of Life.* Tuscon, Arizona: Mettler Studios Inc., p.55.

65   Mettler, B. (1979) *Materials of Dance as a Creative Activity.* Tuscon, Arizona: Mettler Studios Inc., p.266.

66   Mettler, B. (1985) *Dance as an Element of Life.* Tuscon, Arizona: Mettler Studios Inc., p.35.

67   Canner, N. (1968) *And a Time to Dance.* Boston: Plays Inc.

68   Canner, N. (1972) 'Stimulating sounds and vocalization through body movement and rhythm with hospitalized children.' In *Writings on Body Movement and Communication.* Columbia, MD: American Dance Therapy Association.

69   Brownell, A. and Lewis, P. (1990) 'The Kestenberg movement profile in assessment of vocalization.' In P. Lewis and S. Loman (eds) *The Kestenberg Movement Profile: Its Past, Present Applications and Future Directions.* Keene: Antioch New England Graduate School, pp.139–154, (pp.140–141).

70   Bernfeld, S. (1954) cited in P. Moses, *The Voice of Neurosis.* New York: Grune & Stratton, p.11.

71   Brownell, A. (1989) 'The voice and dance movement therapy.' Unpublished paper.

72   Brownell, A. and Lewis, P. (1990) 'The Kestenberg movement profile in assessment of vocalization.' In P. Lewis and S. Loman (eds) *The Kestenberg Movement Profile: Its Past, Present Applications and Future Directions.* Keene: Antioch New England Graduate School, pp.139–154, (p.142).

73   Brownell, A. and Lewis, P. (1990) 'The kestenberg movement profile in assessment of vocalization.' In P. Lewis and S. Loman (eds) *The Kestenberg Movement Profile: Its Past, Present Applications and Future Directions.* Keene: Antioch New England Graduate School, pp.139–154, (p.142).

74   Newham, P. (1992) 'Jung and Alfred Wolfsohn: analytical psychology and the singing voice.' *Journal of Analytical Psychology*, 37, pp.323–6, (p.335).

75   Lewis, P. (1995) Personal communication with the author, Boston, November.

76   Gilligan, C. (1993) *In a Different Voice: Psychological Theory and Women's Development.* Cambridge: Harvard University Press.

77   Newham, P. (1993) *The Singing Cure: An Introduction to Voice Movement Therapy.* Boston: Shambhala.

78   Jennings, S. (ed) (1987) *Dramatherapy: Theory and Practice for Teachers and Clinicians.* London: Routledge.

79   Brookes, J. (1975) 'Producing Marat/Sade: theatre in a psychiatric hospital.' *Hospital and Community Psychiatry*, 26, no. 7, pp.429–35.

80   Schattner, G. and Courtney, R. (eds) (1980) *Drama in Therapy*, vols. 1 and 2. New York: Drama Book.

81   Pearson, J. (1996) *Discovering the Self through Movement and Drama.* London: Jessica Kingsley.

82   Wethered, A. (1973) *Drama and Movement in Therapy.* London: MacDonald and Evans.

83   Moreno, J.L. (1946) *Psychodrama*, vol. 1 and 2. New York: Beacon House.

84   Perls, F. (1969) *Gestalt Therapy Verbatim* Utah: Real People Press.

85   Davies, M.H. (1987) 'Drama therapy and psychodrama.' In S. Jennings (ed) *Dramatherapy: Theory and Practice for Teachers and Clinicians.* London: Routledge, pp.104–123.

86   Klein, M. (1948) *Contributions to Psychoanalysis.* London: Hogarth Press.

87   Mitchell, S. (1992) 'Therapeutic theatre: a para-theatrical model of dramatherapy.' In Sue Jennings (ed) *Dramatherapy: Theory and Practice*, 2. London: Routledge, pp.51–67.

88   Passalacqua, L. (1995/96) 'Voice work in dramatherapy.' *Dramatherapy*, 17, 3 , pp.17–24, (p.17).

89   Passalacqua, L. (1995/96) 'Voice work in dramatherapy.' *Dramatherapy*, 17, 3, pp.17–24, (p.17).

90   Passalacqua, L. (1995/96) 'Voice work in dramatherapy.' *Dramatherapy*, 17, 3, pp.17–24, (p.18).

91   Morrant, J. (1981) 'The first few minutes.' *Canadian Journal of Psychiatry*, 26, 6, pp.432–34.

92   Partridge, P. (1994) 'The voice as a clue.' *Dramatherapy*, 16, 2 and 3, 34–37.

93   O'Brien, B. (1996) 'Rehearsal, character, voice and self: the actor's experience of emotion and character when working through the voice.' Unpublished paper presented to the International Association for Voice Movement Therapy, October.

94   Robbins, A. (1986) *Expressive Therapy: A Creative Arts Approach to Depth-Orientated Treatment.* New York: Human Sciences Press, p.242.

95   Robbins, A. (1986) *Expressive Therapy: A Creative Arts Approach to Depth-Orientated Treatment.* New York: Human Sciences Press, p.244.

96   Robbins, A. (1986) *Expressive Therapy: A Creative Arts Approach to Depth-Orientated Treatment.* New York: Human Sciences Press, p.245.

97   Robbins, A. (1986) *Expressive Therapy: A Creative Arts Approach to Depth-Orientated Treatment.* New York: Human Sciences Press, p.246.

98   Robbins, A. (1986) *Expressive Therapy: A Creative Arts Approach to Depth-Orientated Treatment.* New York: Human Sciences Press, p.246.

99   Robbins, A. (1986) *Expressive Therapy: A Creative Arts Approach to Depth-Orientated Treatment.* New York: Human Sciences Press, p.247.

100   Robbins, A. (1986) *Expressive Therapy: A Creative Arts Approach to Depth-Orientated Treatment.* New York: Human Sciences Press, p.247.

101   Robbins, A. (1986) *Expressive Therapy: A Creative Arts Approach to Depth-Orientated Treatment.* New York: Human Sciences Press, p.248.

102   Robbins, A. (1986) *Expressive Therapy: A Creative Arts Approach to Depth-Orientated Treatment.* New York: Human Sciences Press, p.248.

103   Robbins, A. (1986) *Expressive Therapy: A Creative Arts Approach to Depth-Orientated Treatment.* New York: Human Sciences Press, p.253.

104   Robbins, A. (1986) *Expressive Therapy: A Creative Arts Approach to Depth-Orientated Treatment.* New York: Human Sciences Press, pp.254–55.

105   Knill, P. (1978) 'Intermodal learning in education and therapy.' Unpublished manuscript.

106   Levine, S. (1992) *Poesis: The Language of Psychology and the Speech of the Soul.* Toronto: Palmerston Press.

107   Levine, E. (1995) *Tending the Fire: Studies in Art, Therapy and Creativity.* Toronto: Palmerston Press.

108   McNiff, S. (1981) *The Arts in Psychotherapy.* Springfield Ill: Charles C. Thomas.

109   McNiff, S. (1986) *Educating the Creative Arts Therapist: A profile of the Profession.* Springfield Ill: Charles C Thomas.

110   McNiff, S. (1992) *Art as Medicine: Creating a Therapy of the Imagination.* Boston: Shambhala.

111   McNiff, S. Interview with P. Newham at Endicott College, June, 1996.

112   McNiff, S. (1981) *The Arts in Psychotherapy.* Springfield Ill: Charles C. Thomas, p.xv.

113   McNiff, S. (1981) *The Arts in Psychotherapy.* Springfield Ill: Charles C. Thomas, p.143.

114   McNiff, S. (1981) *The Arts in Psychotherapy.* Springfield Ill: Charles C. Thomas, pp.143–44.

115   McNiff, S. Interview with P. Newham at Endicott College, June, 1996.

116   McNiff, S. (1981) *The Arts in Psychotherapy.* Springfield Ill: Charles C Thomas, p.144.

117   Reich, W. (1948) *Character Analysis.* London: Vision Press, 32d edn.

118   Lowen, A. (1976) *Bioenergetics.* London: Penguin.

119   Grof, S. (1985) *Beyond the Brain: Birth, Death and Transcendence in Psychotherapy.* New York: State University of New York Press.

120   Orr, L. (1983) *Rebirthing in the New Age.* Berkeley: Celestial Arts.

121   Adams, M. (1996) *The Multicultural Imagination: Race, Colour and the Unconscious.* London: Routledge.

CHAPTER II

Voice, Breath and Body
A Physical Approach to Therapeutic Voicework

Introduction: Back to Bone and Basics

Having toured the various psychological and creative terrains of vocal work, I will, in this chapter, remind the reader that the voice is also a somatic phenomenon which requires a physiological and physical understanding.

As in Chapter One, I will try to speak clearly but hopefully without demeaning the complexity of physiological function and dysfunction. For more detailed understanding, the reader is referred to those seminal texts which are informative yet comprehendible.

The nature and varieties of dysfunction and disease with appropriate clinical therapeutic procedures for voice problems has been presented most clearly by Aronson;[1] by Greene and Mathieson;[2] by Boone and McFarlane;[3] and by Fawcus.[4] In addition, a collection of photographs of the vocal folds in health and disease, with accompanying explanation, diagnosis and exemplified treatment, is provided by Hirano and Bless.[5]

The Voice as Flesh and Blood

The human voice is, at one level, a muscular phenomenon. The fine movements of the vocal folds which phonate to create the sound source of the human voice are instigated by neuromuscular activity which creates a precisely controlled interchange of varying tensions throughout a loom of woven muscles. The larynx, which holds the vocal folds, is suspended like a trapeze, hung and drawn from all corners, from above and below, by the tensile filaments of muscles which form a labyrinthian terrain stretching across and throughout the entire body. Consequently, Therapeutic Voicework is interwoven with work on the body.

During the acquisition of a motor activity a person often continually instigates more volitional nervous impulses and, therefore, stimulates contraction of more muscle fibres than is necessary to effectively execute the action and when this motor activity becomes habitual and unconscious, the unnecessary level of neuromuscular activity continues of its own accord. The proverbial and unnecessary muscle tension thus becomes integral to a motor activity to such a degree that it becomes impossible even to imagine executing that action without the familiar use of tension.

A kinetic activity is controlled not only by the motor nerves, whose task it is to instigate and maintain the precise settings of tension in the various muscle fibres, but also by other nerves, which have a sensing function. The sensory nerve messages travel in the opposite direction to those of the motor nerves, and are sent towards the brain, which, as a result, is able to respond appropriately with a motor response, such as withdrawing the hand from a hot fire. It is the receipt of nerve stimulus by the sensory cortex that enables the brain to be aware that a particular motor task has been achieved. It does this by measuring the degree of fibre contraction in the muscle groups apposite to that action. If, therefore, a particular action is repeatedly performed with an excess of muscle fibre tension beyond that which is expedient to perform the task, the brain may not register that the task has been achieved unless the usual, but unnecessary, amount of tension is activated. For example, if someone has been walking or turning, cycling or eating for many years with a high amount of muscle tension, the sensory cortex associates the feedback of that tension with the satisfactory achievement of the task. To attempt the tasks with less tension is, consequently, enormously difficult because the brain, poetically speaking, cannot believe the task has been achieved.

The sensing nerves are receptive to both physical and psychological phenomena because both somatic and psychic operations are, at one level, neurological processes. The nerves are equally receptive to touch upon the skin or a change in temperature as they are to a swiping insult or shocking news. At the level of sensory nerve impulses there is no division between psyche and soma, between mind and matter. Indeed, many of the chemicals which act as stimulators for muscle action are also those released in response to emotions such as fear and sorrow, joy and anger. Therefore, if the acquisition of a motor activity, such as learning to walk, is continually accompanied by an undesirable emotional state, such as anxiety, then the increased nervous stimulation instigates a higher degree of tension in a higher quantity of muscle fibres than is either necessary or optimal. Unfortunately, many of us are or have been subject to impinging emotional conditions at the period of our lives during which we are acquiring new muscular patterns, and these take their toll in the form of muscle fibre tension in excess of that required for efficient, healthy and comfortable action.[6]

One of the most difficult, enduring and demanding of these acquired motor activities is learning to speak, which requires a complexity of neurological signalling more sophisticated than almost any other acquired human activity. Moreover, the acquisition of speech is a learning experience more consistently couched in an emotional environment of punishment and reward, success and failure than any other. The act of phonation and speaking, as much as any other acquired habit, is, therefore, prone to incorporate unnecessary degrees of tension within an excess of muscle fibres. Moreover, because the use of the voice is couched in so many fears and anxieties and is so intimately connected to our sense of well-being, our sense of worth and our communicative efficiency, it is probably more prone to accumulation of the muscular ramifications of negative emotionality than any other expressive faculty and these muscular patterns can continue to operate unconsciously long after the specific events which instigated the stress have disappeared.

This is made more potent by the fact that in addition to the predominance of muscle tissue throughout the voice apparatus, the vocal folds also connect to the thyroid cartilage, a dominant station on the endocrine circuit which distributes hormones throughout the body. Because hormonal release is such an integral component to emotional experience, the voice is doubly susceptible to psychophysical events.

The healthy development of the boy's larynx at puberty, as with all masculine gender characteristics, is dependent on the release of these hormones by the endocrine glands which cause physical changes to the larynx, including a shift in position of the thyroid cartilage, resulting in a change of voice quality. The hormonal secretions of the thyroid also effect a woman's voice, not specifically at puberty but throughout life, particularly during menstruation, pregnancy and menopause, all of which can be accompanied by changes in the audible qualities of the voice.[7] There is also some evidence to suggest that the hormonal activity stimulated by sexual excitement causes changes in vocal timbre and pitch and there may, therefore, be some scientific basis for the popular conception of a stereotypical 'sexy voice' accompanying a highly-developed sexual appetite.[8]

Because the quality of the voice depends, in part, upon the chemical processes of the endocrine system, any hormonal transformation can potentially cause a change in vocal timbre. Moreover, because hormonal alterations can occur as a result of our emotional reactions to events and circumstances, anything which effects the psyche can influence chemical, neurological and physical operations which, in turn, will affect the voice.[9]

Voice, Body and Breath

Just as vocalisation is impossible without neuromuscular activity, it is equally dependent upon breathing. It is the passage of air from the lungs through the vocal tract which creates the sound of the human voice and Therapeutic Voicework is, therefore, not really possible without implicit or explicit work on the breath. But, as with the physicality of voice, the kinetics of breath are intimately connected to emotional influences. In fact, the Greek word '*psyche*', meaning 'soul', has the same root as the word '*psychein*', meaning 'to breathe' and the Greek word '*pneuma*', meaning 'spirit' also means 'wind'. Furthermore, the Latin words '*animus*', meaning 'spirit' and '*anima*', meaning 'soul', come from the Greek '*anemos*', which is another word for 'wind'. Similar connections also exist in Arabic and German and they remind us that in many cultures the notions of psyche, spirit and soul have been related to the idea of moving air. Furthermore, in the practice of Therapeutic Voicework the connection between breath and psyche is made consistently palpable in the way that attention to the process of breathing often moves people to experience and express intense emotions. Indeed, in the everyday occurrences of life, it is often the sounds of the expired and inspired breath which reveal the undercurrent of emotional experience: the sighs of despair, the gasps of shock, the blows of relief and the huffs and puffs of fury. Therapeutic Voicework is thus intimately related to work on the breath.

Therapeutic Voicework, Bodywork and Breathwork

Through careful and informed work with a proficient practitioner, the potential and optimal capacity for liberated muscular voice use and breathing patterns can be facilitated. However, this inevitably provokes disturbance on a psychological and emotional level as the muscular patterns are so intimately linked with the psychological patterns by which the Self is aligned to a familiar, yet often limiting, identity. To release the muscular patterning from negative effects involves retraining the neuromuscular system and such de-patterning can only be achieved through the same process by which the neuromuscular patterns were originally instilled, that is through movement.

Everything that we achieve with our muscles we have learned through movement. We intend through imitation, which stimulates a motor nerve message, which, in turn, instigates muscular movement and knowledge of the execution of this movement is established in the brain by the return message of the sensing nerves. One use of movement in a therapeutic and educational context is to satisfy the brain with a different neurological message which reports that a motor action has been achieved with less demand upon the tensile condition of muscle tissue.

A poignant example which serves to crystallise this concept is that provided by the use of movement and dance with the blind and partially sighted, for whom contact with an object often spells the potential for injury and consequently compounds an unconscious muscular withdrawal.[10] The effect this has upon the general neuromuscular state of the body is one which causes permanent predisposal to extreme contraction of fibres within muscles which activate movements of retreat. Simultaneously, in contradistinction to this, the visually challenged person also relies to a great extent upon touch as a source of information and sensory stimulation and, therefore, has a need for tactile affirmation. These two opposing and equally potent relationships to sensory contact encase the significance of touch in an ambiguous framework for the visually impaired. In order to retrain the muscles of such a person to sustain contact where the natural tendency is to withdraw requires a process rooted in the body and its movement patterns which facilitates positive experience of sustained contact. Recognition of this has provided the initial impetus for a number of movement projects in the UK through which blind people have been able to retrain muscle response through a dance form known as 'Contact Improvisation' founded by Steve Paxton, with whom I have trained and from whom I have acquired some of the techniques which constitute my physical approach to Therapeutic Voicework.[11]

Connective Tissue

The contraction or tension of muscle fibres requires nutrients and oxygen, both of which are supplied by blood which absorbs these essential ingredients from the lungs and digestive system respectively and which is pumped around the body by the heart. As a result of the muscle fibre's consumption of oxygen and nutrients, there is a continual accumulation of carbon dioxide and other toxic waste matter, some of which is absorbed by the lymph vessels

– which break down toxins before they are expelled in expired air, sweat and urine.

Muscle work, then, involves a continual exchange of great volumes of fluid which has to pass through the connective tissue that keeps the body's internal parts supported. Connective tissue surrounds every nerve, every bone and every organ. For blood, waste or any other gas or liquid to move from one place to another, it must pass through connective tissue. Given that physical or physiological processes are not possible without the movement of gas or fluid, connective tissue plays a highly significant role and is being constantly impregnated, drenched and infused with liquids and gases which are on their way out or else on their way in.

Connective tissue, like gelatin, is capable of hardening and softening depending on its temperature and the degree to which it is kept moving. Physical activity which generates muscle movement and, in turn, creates heat disturbs the static complacency of the connective tissue and causes it to become more molten and fluid. Stasis, cold temperature and lack of exercise, meanwhile, allows the connective tissue to become solidified. Chemical and gaseous substances move more easily and more rapidly through a substance the more fluid it is. Therefore, the more pliable and supple the connective tissue, the more easily and efficiently substances pass through it and so the more the muscles can be assisted in their work. If the connective tissue becomes too set, then many of the toxic wastes do not pass through but are retained by it.

One of the ways solidified connective tissue can be made pliable is through massage, which has the effect of softening and warming it, reviving its suppleness and thereby assisting the free flow of substances through it, which, as Ida Rolf discovered, can have profound effects on the structure of the body[12] and which, more recently, has been researched by Chaitrow.[13]

The use of movement in the model of Therapeutic Voicework which I have developed aims to reverse unnecessary habits relating to vocalisation by giving the body a new sensory experience. The purpose is to bring the client to experience that it is possible to communicate effective vocal signals without the habitual accompaniment of a vastly distributed high degree of muscle fibre tension throughout the whole body, particularly the neck and upper back. The use of massage in this model aims to further facilitate fluid and expedient muscle use by encouraging pliability of the connective tissue.

A Background to Voice, Breath and Body Work

The use of retraining muscular patterns to assist vocal function was researched in depth by W. M. Alexander who, whilst working as an actor, found that on many occasions he would begin to lose his voice half-way through a recital and, despite numerous medical consultations, he could not find the cause. In a search for his own answers, he erected mirrors in which he watched himself recite, noticing the physical movements which accompanied the use of his voice and observed particularly that he pulled his head backwards and downwards whenever he came to speak. Eventually Alexander realised that these movements had a direct influence and effect on all the other muscles of his body and developed a technique for resisting these and other habitual movements and of relearning a more natural use of the musculature.[14]

In recent years a number of practitioners have reappropriated the Alexander technique into a vocally-orientated framework. In the UK these include Ron Murdoch, who combines breathwork with Alexander technique in his role as voice teacher at various London drama schools[15] and in independent workshops,[16] and Alan Mars, who combines the technique with Neuro-Linguistic Programming in workshops and one-to-one consultations.[17]

There are a number of other independent practitioners who have developed a keen awareness of the relationship between voice production and muscle use in their practice as teachers, facilitators or therapists. These include Darien Prichard, partner and co-worker with Frankie Armstrong, who utilises the Feldenkrais technique to increase the body's potential for fluid unhindered movement which directly enhances the capacity of the body to resonate in response to vocalisation.[18] The workshop leader Henk Kooij also practises a combination of voice work, massage, body work and movement, 'using the body as a sounding board to voice the history it contains'.[19] In addition, a psychotherapeutically-orientated approach to the voice through body and breath is employed by Carolyn Braddock in the USA. By enabling clients to move, vocalise and amplify their manner of breathing, Braddock assists them in releasing body, breath and voice from the constriction which has developed in response to negative experience and she specialises in issues of sexual trauma.[20]

Another approach to vocal work which is predicated on an understanding of the connection between body and voice is Functional Voice Training, a pedagogic modality originating in the Voice Research Project founded in 1980 by Gisela Rohmert, Eugene Rabine and Peter Jacoby in West Germany.

Functional Voice Training begins from the starting point that each voice sound is a 'vocal movement' which results from a bodily action or gesture of those anatomical parts which constitute the vocal apparatus, such as the tongue, lips, pharynx and jaw. This approach acknowledges that these anatomical components are connected to the entire skeletal musculature and the task of the Functional Voice Trainer is to impart exercises which return to each component a functional independence, freeing the voice from the unnecessary influence of muscular habits.[21] Furthermore, the interrelationship of psyche and soma, the way muscles of vocalisation respond to emotional experience, is integral to the techniques used.[22]

Another significant pioneer who has contributed important insights to the relationship between movement and vocalisation is Emile Jaques-Dalcroze, a Swiss musician, artist and educator born in 1875, for whom music generally, and vocalisation specifically, is rooted in the rhythm of bodily movement. Music, he said, 'is composed of sound and movement' and, moreover, sound itself 'is a form of movement'. Dalcroze connected this with the etymology of the word 'emotion', meaning to 'move outwards', and adhered this to his notion of thought, which he saw as the mobility of ideas.[23] He believed, therefore, that 'music is not heard by the ear alone but by the whole of the body'[24] and his aim was to 'transform the whole organism' into what he called an 'inner ear'.[25] The name which Dalcroze gave to his work was Eurythmics and its purpose was to lift music from the notated score into the muscular action of the body.

Dalcroze assisted musicians with physical problems due to the postures demanded by playing, he worked with young children whose innate musical aptitude was uncovered by extending their natural tendency to move the body rhythmically in response to music and he remedied psycho-motor disabilities in many people. Today, the therapeutic application of Dalcrozian Eurythmics is one of the modalities accepted by the French clinical mainstream and there are professional training courses in Eurythmics throughout the world with graduates working in a variety of settings, including special schools for handicapped children, music colleges and infant schools.

Because many habitual forms of muscle use created patterns of movement which become unconscious, the process of muscular retraining often involves making something of which we are unaware consciously apprehensible. Such a process is extremely apparent in working with breath because during normal daily activity, the process of breathing is for the most part unconscious and occurs as a result of involuntary muscle action. As soon as one introduces the notion of 'working on the breath', however, this unconscious process is observed, analysed and brought to a level of awareness not normally experienced.

In cultures where spiritual belief is intimately connected to the physical practice of expressive movement forms, there is a widespread deliberate use of consciously-controlled breathing patterns for healing purposes, a pursuit which originates in the ancient religious practices of the East and which has always been particularly dominant in Hindu Yoga. In more recent years the tenets of this discipline have been published in English and the so-called 'Science of Breath'[26] and the Hindu Yogic breathing exercises[27] have become available to contemporary readers.

In addition to the Yogic breathing methods originating in India, the ancient Chinese also bequeathed treatises on the use of breathing to prolong life and sustain health which were recorded in the Taoist Canon, the Tao Tsang, and have also been translated into English.[28] Among Chinese traditions is the art of Qi Gong, which involves the practice of regulating the pattern of breathing to alleviate symptoms of ill health and which has recently become an increasingly popular pursuit in the UK and the USA.[29]

One result of the influx and availability of Eastern breathing practices in the West has been a rapid emergence of workshop leaders who have pieced together their own eclectic programmes which combine consciously-controlled breathing exercises with a variety of other pursuits originating in non-Western spiritual and healing practice. Some of these group leaders have published books which extol the virtues of breathing as an art of self-awareness,[30] a way to preserve health[31] and as a means to discovering 'personal power' and 'energy'.[32] There have also been attempts to explain the relationship between the science of the respiratory process and the tenets of yogic breathing.[33]

Interest in breathing in the West was first pursued during the second half of the nineteenth century in Paris by Francois Delsarte, who, due to poor instruction, lost his voice and in seeking to reclaim it turned to the exploration of movement and breathing. Delsarte noticed that the breath, voice and body tends to select from a spectral set of possibilities definite parameters of vocal and physical expression when, for example, experiencing joy, which are never used in expressing another affect, such as grief. It was this recognition of an equation between breathing pattern, physical movement and vocal intonation on the outside and the matrix of thoughts and feelings on the inside which led to the reduction and bastardisation of his system to a simplified chart of signifying gestures and sounds which allegedly designated certain emotions.[34] However, the integrity of his work was imported to the United States by his devoted student Steele Mackay, where he passed it on to the German teacher Hede Kallmeyer, who was to have significant influence in the field of breathwork.

Another influential figure within the development of what we might call breathwork was the Austrian Leo Kofler, who, in 1860, was afflicted by tuberculosis, which had killed three of his sisters. In 1886 he emigrated to the United States and took a position as choirmaster at St Paul's Church in Manhattan. Inspired by his own illness, and the death of many of his relatives from respiratory disease, Kofler dedicated himself to the study of breath from the standpoint of anatomical studies and practical physical exercises. It was his own research that culminated in his cure and it was this that led him to teach others how to make use of his discoveries in what he called the 'art of breathing'.[35]

Two German women, Clara Schlaffhorst and Hedwig Anderson, came to New York to study with Kofler and on returning to their home country began teaching classes and programmes based on Kofler's system, which became the basis for the Rottenburg Breathing School which they formed and which is still active in Germany today. Among the students of this School was Elsa Gindler, who also had a long history of tuberculosis as motivation for her study. In addition to studying at the Rottenburg School, Gindler had become familiar with Delsarte's work through her studies with Hede Kallmeyer and, by synthesising these approaches, she became central to a movement in Germany in the aftermath of the First World War which re-visioned traditional physical education.[36]

Gindler's work was, in turn, passed on to a number of students, including her assistant Carola Speads, Marion Rosen and Charlotte Selver, all of whom were refugees who went to America from Germany in the 1930s and all of whom have continued teaching methods based on Gindler's work in the United States. Selver, in her teaching, has focused on the general bodywork and its application to improving physical sensation and function. Among her early students were Fritz Perls, Alan Watts and Erich Fromm.[37] Speads has focused exclusively on the breathing aspect and its ability to improve the quality of life.[38] Marion Rosen, meanwhile, has gone on to develop a method of bodywork influenced by Analytical Psychology.

Before leaving Germany, Rosen worked with the masseuse and dancer Lucy Heyer and her husband Gustav Heyer, Jung's student and colleague who had also trained with Gindler. The Heyers ran regular therapeutic groups, many of which Rosen attended, innovatively combining the principles of Jung's Analytical Psychology with breathing exercises. This experience convinced Rosen that breathing was an essential area of investigation for the future development of bodywork and that both breath and bodily movement were connected to emotional constructs. When Rosen went to the Unites States to develop her work these two tenets of belief became central to her investigation.[39] The Rosen Method is now widely practised in Northern America.[40]

Another German practitioner influenced by the work of Delsarte and further inspired by Gindler was Ilse Middendorf, who began her life working in the field of gymnastics and movement teaching early in the twentieth century. On discovering a fascination with the nature of breath she developed what she described as a 'breathing science'[41] and implemented a school of research and teaching to pass on a methodological approach to the educative and healing potential of breathing practices which she called 'the perceptible breath'[42] and which she believed provided a therapy as well as a pedagogical system of training.

Middendorf identifies three methods of breathing: the unconscious breathing which occurs involuntarily as we go about our daily business, the conscious breathing which occurs when we deliberately, through cognitive volition, engage the musculature in an interference of our usual breathing pattern to enhance gymnastic or artistic performance or to execute such expressions as a sigh or cough and a third form, which Middendorf extols, which she calls 'the perceptible breath', by which breathing is allowed its unconscious intuitive manner but is simultaneously consciously sensed and allowed to change and move through the most subtle of muscular patterns.[43] Middendorf also associated the vocalisation of specific phonetic sounds with defined movements and alleged that intoning on certain vowels assists in the healthy functioning of specific body parts,[44] a belief most adamantly disseminated by Rudolf Steiner.

Steiner was an Austrian visionary mystic, born in 1861, who developed a mutual flair for science and the arts coupled with a keen interest in social reform and spiritual reflection.[45] Steiner became a prolific teacher, influencing and contributing to fields as diverse as medicine, architecture, farming, children's education, religion and philosophy and his sphere of influence forms an international movement known as Anthroposophy. In addition, there are children's schools all over the world founded upon his name and upon his understanding of child development where 'teachers work with the natural grace and creative powers present in children'.[46] Steiner also lectured on the subject of therapy and developed a number of techniques and exercises with spiritual, curative and educational objectives.[47]

Within Steiner's vision and model of education and human development, music, movement and speech play a significant role and he developed an entire field of investigation known as Eurythmy, which is, in simple terms, speech made visible through movement.

For Steiner, speech is an act of physical movement utilising the lungs, larynx and lips. For the sound 'O' or 'P' to be made, for example, these parts of the body have to move and co-ordinate in a very particular way and only a specific physical gesture will give rise to these particular sounds. Steiner extended these speech gestures into movement which utilised the whole body, creating a vocabulary which, like the vocabulary of phonetics, is fixed with definite movements assigned to specific speech sounds.

Curative Eurythmy consists of a network of exercises which can allegedly help with a variety of dysfunctions, diseases and disorders – such as asthma, allergies, migraines, multiple-sclerosis, cancer, depression and phobias. Eurythmy therapy is claimed to be particularly effective in treating children with mental or physical disabilities.[48] The therapy exercises are 'often introduced by using images which give rise to the particular qualities required' and 'accompanied by sounds of speech which are spoken by the therapist as the movement is made', each sound having its 'own unique dynamic and quality' which 'helps to support the gesture'.[49] In Eurythmy specific vowel sounds and their accompanying movements or gestures are believed to alleviate certain dysfunctions. For example, 'N' is used for diarrhoea, 'F' for bed-wetting in children and 'U' for those who 'cannot stand properly'.[50]

Agathe Lorenz-Poschmann, a renowned German actress who gave up her career to study Eurythmy, says that through the activity of 'forming speech on the out breath', 'man becomes a sculpture of the outer air but at the same time he works back upon his soul-spiritual as well as his physical aspect'. For her, as for all Steiner practitioners, speech is, therefore, both a mystical and a physical act and neglect of the speech apparatus can lead to spiritual as well as physical problems which 'can develop into all kinds of illnesses'.[51]

A significant therapeutic tangent to Eurythmy is Chirophonetics, a body of work developed by the Austrian Speech Pathologist and Anthroposophian Alfred Baur, who founded his work whilst working in a clinic for children with profound speech problems, many of whom could not articulate any speech sounds and others who had not progressed beyond the babbling stage. Seeking for ways to facilitate some speech function, Baur hit upon the simple idea of using his hands and fingers to stroke shapes on the childrens' backs as he articulated accompanying sounds.[52] The allegedly non-arbitrary patterns specific to each speech sound which Baur transcribed into designated hand strokes relate to the vision of the human body developed by Steiner and the gestural choreography used in Eurythmy.

Whilst the clinical application of Steiner's initiations have been developed by Baur, the artistic development of Steiner-based singing pedagogy is the area represented by Valborg Werbeck-Svärdström, whose starting point is that the human voice 'needs no training' because 'it is already there, finished and perfect as an entity sounding in the ideal world'. What the voice requires is 'liberation' or 'uncovering'.[53] Thus, says Werbeck-Svärdström, 'no teaching and art of singing can be appropriate for our times without a science capable of penetrating into its inner realm'.[54] Werbeck-Svärdström does not only denounce scientific discovery in the field of voice in favour of a spiritual approach but she somewhat weakens her arguments by making scientific claims about the physiology of the body which are incorrect.[55] Furthermore, the quasi-spiritual language and pretensions inherent in much Anthroposophical writing tends to obscure the more grounded, creative and practical applications of Steiner's Eurythmy vision detracting from any communicable clinical or educational efficacy which the work may certainly have.

A key figure of the Steiner musical tradition in England who has managed to locate his work in a clearer language is Michael Deason-Barrow, who originally trained to be a boy soprano and became a national figure but who, after his pubertal voice change, did not sing publicly again. His interest in and passion for the voice, however, remained and he is now a trainer of music teachers at Emerson College in Sussex, where he founded Tonalis, the Centre for the Study and Development of Music.[56]

Thus, though little known, there is a rich history of Voicework which is grounded in the act of bodily motion and respiratory process.

Catharsis Through Breath

Distinct from both the pedagogic approach of the German breathing schools and the mystical approach of Steiner is a further field of breathwork which draws support from equating itself with the tenets of psychotherapy. Among such work is that of Stanislav Grof.

Grof's thesis proposes that perinatal and prenatal traumas can be remembered and their negative effects overcome through intense breathing, a process which he calls Pneumocatharsis. He says that 'profound changes in consciousness can be induced by both extremes in the breathing rate – hyperventilation and prolonged withholding of breath – or a combination of both'.[57]

Grof's 'Holotropic Breath Work' may be seen as a historical extension of the respiratory work pursued by Wilhelm Reich, whom Grof acknowledges as having discovered that psychological resistances and defences are compounded through restricted breathing. His own work began, however, with the development of using psychedelic drugs, primarily LSD, as a psychotherapeutic tool and his more recent work with breathing still echoes the search for extreme and intensified experiences.[58]

Grof's approach to working with clients is to intensify the amplitude and increase the rapidity of the breathing volume and rate, inducing a condition which may be clinically identified as hyperventilation. However, Grof proclaims that the clinical 'understanding of the effects of hyperventilation', which are 'usually seen in a pathological context', are incorrect. Extolling the virtues of hyperventilation, Grof says that having 'conducted the breathing sessions with many thousands of persons', he believes that 'there exist many individuals in whom even dramatic hyperventilation carried over a long period of time does not lead to classic hyperventilation syndrome, but to progressive relaxation, intense sexual feelings, or even mystical experiences'. Furthermore, although he acknowledges that during breathing sessions some people 'develop tensions in various parts of their bodies', 'continued hyperventilation does not lead to progressive increase of these tensions, but to their climactic culmination followed by a profound relaxation', in a manner 'resembling sexual orgasm.'[59]

Grof's work is predicated on a cathartic paradigm where, in his view, muscular tension and spasm followed by relaxation and relief serves to eliminate or reduce 'pent-up energy'. Because of this pneumatic release, which is inherent in his approach, the expressive and spontaneous utterances of the human voice often contribute to the cathartic process. A Holotropic breath session often involves 'tremors, twitches, dramatic body movements, coughing, gagging, vomiting, screaming and other types of vocal expression'.[60] In such a session music is often used to assist the client's process, who is encouraged to 'give full expression to whatever the music is triggering – crying or laughing, grimacing, shaking, various contortions of the body, sensual pelvic movements, and any other emotional, vocal, and motor manifestations.'[61]

Central to Grof's model of the mind is something he calls a Coex System, which he defines as 'a specific constellation of memories consisting of condensed experiences' and 'related fantasies from different periods of the individual' and which 'are associated with a strong emotional charge of the same quality'.[62] Grof's notion of the Coex system, which is comparable to Jung's notion of the complex, includes provision for the possibility of intra-uterine experiences. Grof's interest in the foetal experience and his belief that such experiences could be relived through therapeutic modalities originated during his work with the use of LSD. He proclaimed that, during the use of LSD, 'concrete episodes that appear to be memories of specific events from an individual's intrauterine development are rather common' and of which many 'involve instances of psychotraumatization resulting from various noxious and disturbing stimuli of a mechanical, physical, biological, or biochemical nature'. Those clients 'reporting these relivings seem to be convinced that the fetus can subjectively experience not only gross disturbances of its existence, such as attempted abortions, penetrating and loud sounds, intense vibrations, and mechanical concussions, but also the distress associated with the mother's somatic condition when she is ill, exhausted, or intoxicated'. Grof goes on to claim that he has heard 'numerous independent claims that the foetus is aware of or shares its mother's affective states', such as 'anxiety attacks, emotional shocks, outbursts of aggression or hate, depressive moods, and sexual arousal' as well as 'feelings of relaxation, satisfaction, love and happiness'. Equally frequent among the reports of clients, says Grof, 'are episodes of positive oceanic feelings and blissful unity with the mother, accompanied by a nourishing exchange of physical, emotional, and spiritual energies as well as comforting thoughts and insights'.[63]

One of the aims of Grof's therapy, initially through the use of psychedelic drugs and latterly through intense breathing exercises, is to provide a context in which true or imagined recapitulation of intrauterine, perinatal, post-natal and early infant experiences can be relived in order that they may be related to neurotic or psychotic conditions experienced in current adult life. However, Grof is clear that 'the authenticity of recaptured intra-uterine events is an open question' and, for him, 'it seems, therefore, more appropriate to refer to them as experiences rather than memories'.[64]

This aspect of Grof's work brings him into alignment with the work initiated by Leonard Orr in America during the early 1970s, which is now known mainly as Rebirthing but also as Conscious Breathing, Conscious Connected Breathing and Spiritual Breathing.[65]

Like the work of Grof, the work initiated by Orr also relies upon the use of breathing techniques with some peripheral attendance to vocalisation. Orr's inspiration came whilst sitting in the bath one day. Finding himself numb, apparently paralysed and unable to leave the tub, his mind began to enter into a trance-like state where he noticed the varying patterns of breathing which seemed to inspire 'insights into infancy'.[66] Later, he noticed that consciously altering the rhythm and patterns of breathing produced dramatic and bizarre experiences, including memories of the birth trauma.

Orr mused that, for most people, birth is traumatic and therefore, therapeutically speaking, needs to be revisited if the scars inscribed by prenatal and neonatal experience are to heal. He asserts that 'all too often, the ideal birth situation is not achieved and the child is forced to rely on its own resources', which he compares 'to having a severe accident in a remote place where, regardless of mental anxiety and physical exhaustion, the person must save himself' and which inevitably leaves 'a traumatic scar.'[67]

The fundamental tenet of Rebirthing, which has recently been described as 'not in itself psychotherapy' but a process which can be 'used as a psychotherapeutic tool',[68] is that this physical trauma of birth 'acts like a severe shock on the nervous system and the brain, and may lead to life-long tensions throughout the system'.[69] In the true cathartic tradition, the conclusion is that such a trauma must be relived in order for its effects to be abreacted. But, unlike abreactions associated with the traumatic effects of specific infantile experiences which release the adult from the neurosis generated by it, according to Orr the birth experience can, when revisited, sweep the adult free of all the major neurosis which stem from it. Orr declaims that 'for all of you who have ever dreamed of being reborn and starting life all over again, you can now make it possible'[70] through the method of Rebirthing, which 'occurs when people feel they are in an environment safe enough to re-experience their birth'.[71] Like Grof before him, Orr claims that hyperventilation is not a pathology but 'a cure for subventilation', which he describes as the shallow and insubstantial breathing that is instilled as a result of the birth trauma.[72]

Since Orr's publications and orginal work, he has, it is reported, given up utilising the techniques and revised his beliefs. However, the line of inquiry which he initiated continues to be practised by those who enthusiastically accept him as their forefather.

Over-Breathing or Hyperventilation

Hyperventilation means over-breathing. It usually occurs when a person increases the amount of air inspired in a given amount of time, usually measured in litres per minute. As a result of over-breathing, too much oxygen is absorbed and too much carbon dioxide is released. Consequently, carbon dioxide levels in the blood start to drop, upsetting its acid-alkaline base.

Lowered levels of carbon dioxide in the blood strengthen the bond between the haemoglobin and oxygen making it more difficult for the haemoglobin to give the oxygen up to the tissue of the brain and other organs which need it. This state, called hypoxia, can cause increased pressure in the arteries, known as hypertension. In addition, the lowered oxygen level in tissue cells results in a lowered level of oxygen in the veins, which leads to dilation of the venous blood vessels, which can, in turn, cause varicose veins and haemorrhoids. The sufferer is also likely to experience exhaustion, tiredness, increased heart rate and there can occur a cut in oxygen rate to the brain by up to 50 per cent. Now, caught in a vicous catch-22, the brain's response to this condition is to stimulate and excite the breathing mechanism even more, which further increases the over-breathing, leading to a progressive reduction of carbon dioxide. The body, though, has various mechanisms of defence against the loss of carbon dioxide, which include spasm of the bronchi and blood vessels, increased levels of cholesterol production in the liver and lowering of the arterial pressure. However, this, in turn, causes hypotension, increased mucus and phlegm production, increased production of lactic acid and, in consequence, causes metabolism to suffer.

Because the respiratory process serves to oxygenate all tissue, not a single part of the body is exempt from the potential problems resulting from hyperventilation. In fact, people with Hyperventilation Syndrome are frequently misdiagnosed as having a variety of disorders, including multiple-sclerosis, peripheral neuropathy, epilepsy and mental illness.[73] The decreased carbon dioxide levels which mark the onset of hyperventilation, in combination with the body's defence against it, effect the central neurovascular system, causing faintness, dizziness, unsteadiness, impairment of concentration and memory, feelings of unreality and, sometimes, loss of consciousness. It effects the peripheral neurovascular pathways causing numbness, coldness of the fingers and toes and tingling in the limbs and face. It effects the skeletal muscles causing tremors and spasms. It effects the respiratory system causing shortness of breath, tightness in the chest and effects the heart causing palpitations.

During hyperventilation a variable degree of slowing in the frequency of the brain waves occurs, which correlates with alterations in the level of consciousness. When mean electroencephalographic frequency falls below 5 cycles per second, conscious awareness is markedly reduced. Of course, the body, being innately wise, takes advantage of this lack of consciousness and returns to a more normal breathing rate. However, if hyperventilation is immediately reinstated, the person swings back and forth between different brain-wave frequencies, the overall effect being one of an ecstatic state for it is, indeed, an altered state of consciousness.

There is a school of thought which proposes that Hyperventilation is such a common symptom of many stress-related disorders, as well as being potentially a cause of anxiety, and that the aim of any therapeutic modality should be to decrease the frequency of its occurrence and eventually eradicate it.[74] By decreasing hyperventilation, the symptoms associated with it can allegedly be alleviated.

One of the more developed therapeutic techniques aiming to deal specifically with the eradication of hyperventilation is the Buteyko Method of Breathing Reconditioning. Buteyko recognised that a vast majority of asthmatics suffered from prolonged Hyperventilation Syndrome, as did those with a feast of other disorders, and he developed a method of retraining the breathing pattern, rectifying short-falls of carbon dioxide in the blood.[75] A number of similar programmes are now offered, both by physiotherapists, allopathic clinicians and practitioners within the field of alternative modalities, to control Hyperventilation Syndrome. There are also a number of self-help manuals written for sufferers of Hyperventilation.[76]

Despite the dangers of hyperventilation, therapeutic modalities which extol its virtues, such as those descending from the work of Grof and Orr, are extremely popular, as are practices which draw on the spiritual disciplines of the East. However, neither sources form part of the work which I have developed and which I teach to practitioners. Rather, my work draws on a Western history of scientific investigation, physical exercise and psychotherapeutic inquiry which seeks to facilitate conscious understanding of and methodical transformation of the client's expressivity without deliberate instigation of an ecstatic experience which relies upon an unsustainable physiological condition such as hyperventilation and without deliberate recourse to culturally contextualised spiritual phenomenon.

The Mechanics of Breathing

The integrated methodology of Breathwork which I have originated is rooted in physiological principles and I will therefore begin by introducing the rudimentary mechanics of breathing.

The thorax, or thoracic cavity, which constitutes the upper half of the trunk, houses the lungs – two spongy, curvilinear, balloon-like organs which are composed of over three hundred million minuscule air sacs or alveoli. The blood, pumped by the semi-spherical heart, circulates through the alveoli, absorbing oxygen from the air, which is inspired from the external atmosphere, and releasing carbon-dioxide, which is expired into the same exterior environment. This oxygen, which the blood absorbs, is circulated throughout the body through a labyrinth of tubes and is released into the body of the organs and tissue structures which require it to function.

As a result of the inward passage of air through the respiratory pathway when we breathe in, the lungs inflate. When we breathe out, the lungs deflate and air is expelled. This process is crucial to the maintenance of life. If it ceases for more than four to five minutes, death is inevitable.

In order for the lungs to expand when we breathe in, increased volume has to be created in the torso for when the lungs are inflated they occupy more space than when they are deflated. This can be achieved in a number of ways.

As the reader will now be fully aware, central to the methodological approach to Therapeutic Voicework which I have developed is the simple yet profound ideokinetic image of the tube or cylinder as a major anatomical template for a variety of components. It is again the image of the tube upon which I have based my approach to Breathwork.

The torso itself, like the respiratory tract, may be perceived as a cylinder or a large tube (Figure 11.1a). Consequently, in seeking to increase its volume to accommodate or instigate lung expansion, there are, by the laws of geometry and mechanics, three motions which can be effected. First, the cylinder can be dilated to possess an increased diameter by expanding its walls outwards (Figure 11.1b). Second, the floor of the cylinder can be lowered, moving the base of the cylinder downwards, making it deeper from the bottom (Figure 11.1c). Third, the lid of the cylinder can be raised, moving the top of the cylinder upwards, making it higher from the top (Figure 11.1d). In fact, these are the three mechanical and muscular means which the body employs to expand the torso, creating increased volume in which the lungs may expand for the purposes of inspiration.

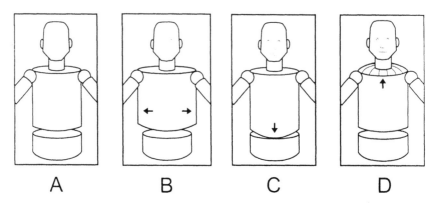

Figure 11.1

The diametrical expansion of the cylinder walls, often referred to as 'thoracic breathing', is achieved in the following way. The lungs are housed by a scaffolding of bones, known as the rib cage, which are curved in shape, ten pairs of which are attached to the back bone or vertebrae behind and to the breast bone or sternum at the front. The lower two pairs of ribs are shorter than the others and are attached only to the vertebrae with their other end protruding; these are known as the floating ribs. Although the top ten pairs of ribs are attached front and back, they are not fused solidly but are joined by cartilage and joints so as to be able to move.

Between the ribs, inside and outside the cage which they form, there are two sets of intercostal muscles, the expansion and contraction of which causes the ribs to be pulled upwards and outwards, increasing the size of the thoracic cavity. This causes the chest to rise and protrude at the front, back and sides creating a cylindrical dilation around the upper torso (Figure 11.2).

The lowering of the cylinder floor is achieved in the following way. Underneath the lungs there is a long muscle called the diaphragm, which is stretched out from one side of the trunk to the other separating the thorax from the abdomen. When the diaphragm relaxes it bends upwards against the floor of the lungs, assuming a shape similar to an upside down salad bowl, decreasing thoracic space but increasing the volume of the abdomen (Figure 11.3a). When it contracts, however, it is pulled downwards and flattened and because it is joined to a layer of tissue, known as the pleura, which is in turn joined to the floor of the lungs, it literally pulls the lungs down with it, expanding them from the bottom so that inspired air fills the freshly created

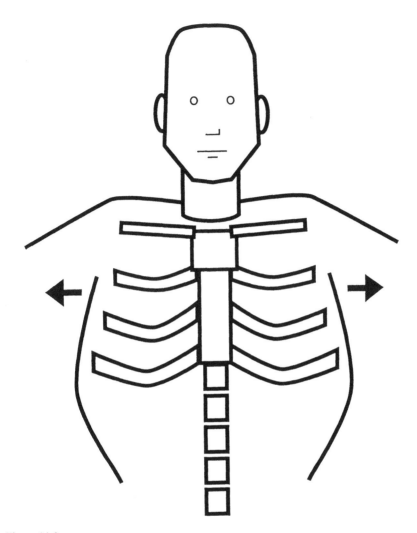

Figure 11.2

space (Figure 11.3b). When the diaphragm relaxes, it returns to its vertical curvature, assisting in the expulsion of air from the lungs (Figure 11.3a).

Due to the laws of gravity and the morphological distribution of the air sacs or alveoli, there is a greater concentration of blood cells in the lower portion of the lungs. Consequently, the most efficient absorption of oxygen can occur when fresh inspired air finds its way to the bottom of the lungs. This is the main reason why maximum displacement of the diaphragm during

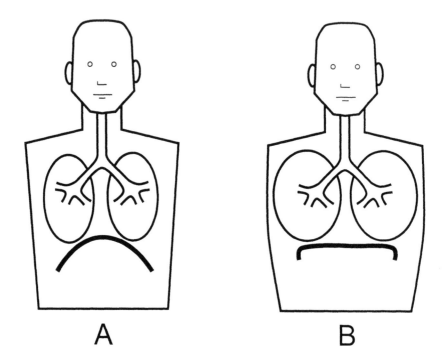

A   B

Figure 11.3

breathing, often referred to as 'diaphragmatic breathing', is believed by some to be most advantageous to health. This displacement of the diaphragm is the method of expansion and contraction which infants spontaneously employ to breathe until they have learned to effect the dilation of the torso walls.

During optimal breathing the movement of the diaphragm occurs in tandem with intercostal muscle motility, simultaneously expanding and contracting the cylindrical walls of the torso and lowering and raising the diaphragmatic floor, by which the entire torso is inflated and deflated.

The raising of the cylinder's roof is achieved by muscular contraction across the top of the back and shoulders, which has the effect of elevating the clavicles, or collar bones, creating increased space around the top of the lungs (Figure 11.4). This method of expansion, often referred to as 'clavicular breathing', is frequently employed in the service of exercise or extreme activity when extra quantities of air are required.

The distribution of muscular displacement or palpable movement of the body in these three areas of chest, abdomen and the clavicular region consti-

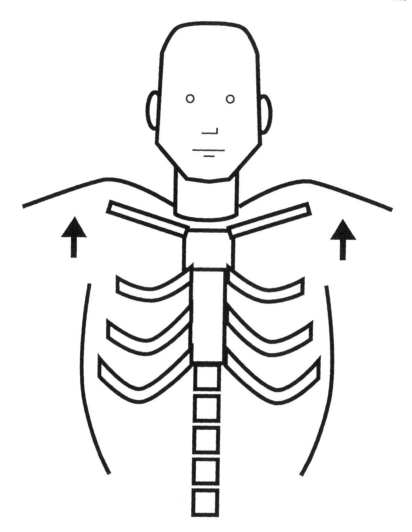

Figure 11.4

tute part of what we may call a Breathing Pattern, which may be more or less in service of optimal functioning.

BREATHING PATTERN COMPONENT ONE: MUSCULAR DISPLACEMENT

The first component dimension to a Breathing Pattern is, therefore, the distribution of what we shall call Muscular Displacement, that is the observable or palpable muscle action accompanying respiration and its distribution across the torso, which may show greater or lesser motility around the chest and the back to achieve diametrical expansion of the torso's walls, may show greater or lesser movement in the muscles of the abdominal wall and lower back, revealing the motion of the diaphragm which expands the floor of the cylindrical torso downwards, and may show greater or lesser muscle action across the shoulders to raise the clavicles and expand the torso upwards.

BREATHING PATTERN COMPONENT TWO: FORCE AND PRESSURE

In addition to the expandability, elasticity or degree of displacement in the muscles of the torso which assist respiration, this musculature also acts within a certain spectrum of force or pressure by which it decreases the internal volume of the thorax, assisting the deflation of the lungs and the expiration of breath. In assessing the way in which someone breathes, we may, therefore, observe the power, force, pressure or strength with which the respiratory musculature compresses and contracts the body. This, in turn, increases subglottal air pressure in the vocal tract with the effect of creating a louder sound.

The second component to the Breathing Pattern is, therefore, the contractile force in the muscles responsible for expiration.

BREATHING PATTERN COMPONENT THREE: RESPIRATORY FREQUENCY

Naturally, respiration takes place in time and, therefore, within a continuum between faster and slower. The third component to the breathing pattern is, therefore, the amount of respiratory cycles, or combined inspirations and expirations, which take place in a given unit of time.

BREATHING PATTERN COMPONENT FOUR: TIDAL VOLUME

The combination of these three aforementioned dimensions to the breathing pattern naturally influence the quantity of air that is exchanged with each respiratory cycle. This amount of air breathed may, therefore, be identified as a fourth dimension to the breathing pattern and may be defined as the volume of air which passes into the lungs with each inspiration and out of the lungs with each expiration. This may be called the tidal volume of air and the quantity of air which a person is able to exchange may be called their tidal capacity.

BREATHING PATTERN COMPONENT FIVE: SENSATION OF DEPTH AND SHALLOWNESS

The breathing pattern is also composed of what is often described as the degree of depth or shallowness which a person experiences during the breathing process. For the most part, the depth or shallowness of breathing is a subjective sensation arising from the combination of the other dimensions. For example, fast respiratory frequency combined with maximum thoracic displacement, a degree of clavicular displacement and minimal abdominal movement would create the sensation of shallowness. Low respiratory frequency combined with enhanced abdominal displacement would, conversely, create the sensation of depth. This subjective sensation is underpinned by the objective depth to which the inspired air in the lungs descends. Because increased amplitude or displacement of the diaphragm pulls the tissue floor of the lungs downwards, drawing air deeply into the lungs, it creates a sensation of depth greater than that experienced with minimal diaphragmatic movement and increased thoracic expansion, which tends to concentrate the exchange of air at the top of the lungs.

The positive sense which many people derive from abdominal displacement may, therefore, also be due to the ability of the body to sense that more efficient gaseous exchange takes place in the lower regions of the lungs.

BREATHING PATTERN COMPONENT SIX: DIMENSIONS OF THE UPPER AIRWAY

The stream of breath which is inspired and expired passes through a tube or tract which dilates and constricts, lengthens and shortens and, during vocalisation, this gives rise to distinct timbres. However, the dimensions of the upper respiratory tract also effect the experience of breathing. For example, when we blow someone a kiss or cool down hot food, the airway is narrow and short, that is in flute configuration; when we steam up a pair of spectacles to clean them, the airway is more dilated and lengthened, that is in clarinet configuration; and if we then open the oral and pharyngeal cavities, lower the larynx and yawn, the tract is in saxophone configuration.

The sixth component dimension to the Breathing Pattern is, therefore, the configuration of the upper respiratory tract or tube, which is identical with the vocal tract.

Sensations of Breathing

By comprehending the process of breathing, in simple terms, as being made up of these six components, it is possible to both empathise with and to understand some of the commonly occurring and different patterns of breathing and, therefore, of vocalisation.

For example, a driven passage of air expelled from the lungs during expiration may be maintained at constant pressure by consistent contractile muscle action, but if the tube through which this air passes is dilated and constricted, it will decrease and increase the pressure respectively. Therefore, the smaller the diameter of the airway, the greater the sensation of air pressure in the tube when the amount and force of air expelled from the lugs remains constant. Many people, as a result of habitual muscle use, have a narrow tract with a particularly squeezed pharyngeal space. If such clients also have a large lung capacity with breath expelled under high pressure due to strong contractile force of the respiratory musculature, there is an enormous pressure of breath which has to be bottle-necked through a very small opening. Such a client may have the sensation of breath being damned up under great force and, consequently, may feel emotionally pent-up and pressurised, about to burst, forever waiting release but never able to express or depress the pressure. When someone feels exasperated or furious and would like to shout but is refrained by the circumstances, it is common to make a flute configuration and blow air through its narrow dimensions; people also often suck air in audibly through a flute-shaped vocal tract when expecting bad news or experiencing sustained suspense. The experience of shallowness is also often instigated by a narrow and short airway through which a limited volume of tidal air can pass, whilst depth can be facilitated by increased airway dimensions. Conversely, the same contractile muscle power expelling air from the lungs through a vocal tract which is dilated and lengthened so that a greater volume of air passes out in a given unit of time can create the sensation of slippage, a lack of control or depleted containment and a sense of not being able to store or restore any breath and, therefore, energy. These are just a few of the voluminous variety of possible problems and conditions which it is possible to perceive by investigating the breath according to the systematic framework of six breathing pattern components which I have outlined.

Therapeutic Voicework Methodology: Enhancing the Breathing Pattern

The work on breath which I have developed consists of a series of exercises and guided experiential processes which enable the client to become conscious of the components of her breathing pattern and make changes to its employment, which facilitate physical and psychological well-being.

To enable the client to experience potential for the three areas of displacement, the practitioner places his hands over the relevant areas and, utilising a little pressure, amplifies and exaggerates the natural movement of the appropriate muscles, increasing sensation of natural motility. By varying the amount of pressure which the practitioner uses, the client can experience a spectral range of contractile and expiratory pressures and, where there is muscle damage, fatigue or disability, alternative muscle groups can be trained to assume the contractile work (Photograph 11.1).

Further to this, the aim of the work is to facilitate an experience of the airway and a sense of its elasticity. To this end, the Therapeutic Voiceworker encourages clients to experience its potential for dilation and contraction, lengthening and shortening, by which they are enabled to acquire an increased malleability of the tract, thereby enhancing respiratory sensation (Photograph 11.2).

During the process of investigation and intervention, the practitioner observes the volume of air that is exchanged and the frequency with which cycles of inspiration and expiration occur, encouraging component combinations which facilitate optimal functioning and a positive sense of well-being.

Naturally, as with all Therapeutic Voicework, the practitioner must be cognizant of any respiratory illness or dysfunction, past and present, in order to ascertain whether it is safe and within the limits of Therapeutic Voicework to work with the client. Again, training is absolutely essential.

Therapeutic Voicework Methodology: Voice Movement Massage

Within the therapeutic field, many of the manipulatory and massage-based techniques are employed quite separately and often by different practitioners to those utilising dance and expressive movement. Moreover, attendance to the client's vocalisation is rarely incorporated into either of these two approaches. In the massage modality which descends from the Swedish tradition and in manipulatory therapies such as osteopathy, physiotherapy and chiropractic, the silent client is usually passive, often laying on a table where she is mobilised by the practitioner. In expressive movement, such as dance movement therapy, meanwhile, the silent client is often untouched by the practitioner and is free to explore her own movement patterns before an analytic and interpretive witness. Both approaches, naturally, have different uses and provide equally necessary services for diverse problems. However, the

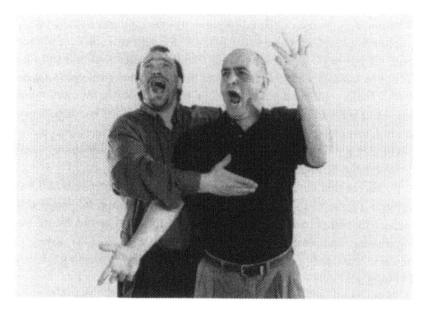

Photograph 11.1

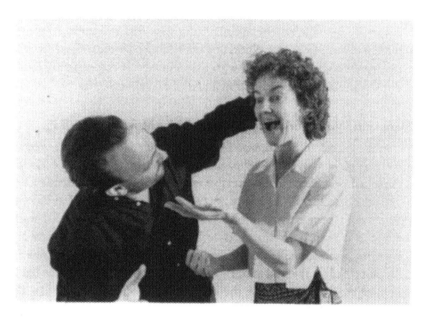

Photograph 11.2

separation of the two approaches also denies clients of the benefits of an inte-grated approach. The work which I have developed seeks to synthesise tenets of expressive movement with those of massage and manipulation in combi-nation with vocalisation. I have called this strategy 'Voice Movement Massage'.

In Voice Movement Massage the client moves according to an expressive dance, authenticating her own impulses and experiences artistically. At the same time, the Therapeutic Voiceworker maintains physical contact, moving as an improvisational dance partner whilst simultaneously massaging and manipulating the body, releasing tension in areas where excess stress is appar-ent, softening tissue where excess solidity can be felt and enhancing sensation of the breathing pattern and method of voice production.

During this process the client is leader of the dance and can depart from contact or move towards the practitioner or otherwise influence the spatial and physical relationship with him at any time. This technique enables the practitioner to respond to the body as it is in motion, building a picture of the skeletal distribution of tension based on a direct experience of kinetic expres-sion. Furthermore, because the client's dance is rooted in the experience and expression of affect, the respiratory pattern, as well as the voice, paints a col-lage within which is revealed an emotionality which, in some way, contributes to the body's muscular state. It is, therefore, possible to experi-ence palpably the way that the psyche influences the body.

I have developed this strategy from my training with Steve Paxton, founder of Contact Improvisation, with whom I trained at Dartington Col-lege of Arts over a period of four years. Paxton's work aims to utilise the gravitational relationship between two partners in constant contact as the starting point for an improvised dance which is conducted in silence. Because the form requires a relaxed responsivity, training sessions in Contact Improvisation are often preceded by periods in which participants provide each other with exploratory massage. My appropriation of this technique has involved animating the acoustic component, combining it with simultaneous massage and utilising it to a therapeutic and educational end.

This technique of Voice Movement Massage involves attendance to spe-cific parts of the body which relate to the process of breathing and voice production, the most significant of which are the neck, the chest and the abdomen.

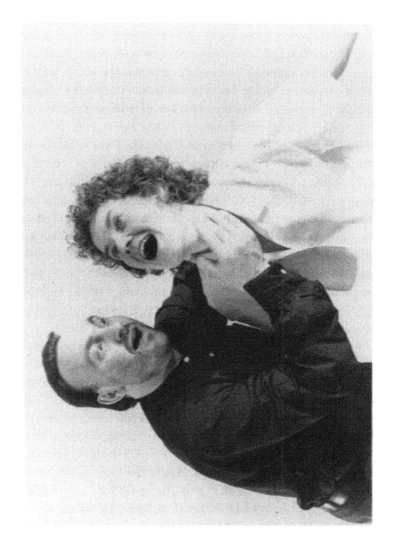

Photograph 11.3

The Neck

The neck is the host of that mysterious area called the throat, which, for many, is the locus of conflict and ambivalence. It seems as if the throat is like a bottle neck and a point of convergence for two pathways: one being the flow of cognitive thoughts which, in terms of somatic sensation feel as though they descend from the head to be expelled from the mouth as words, and the other being the flow of feelings which feel as though they rise up from the heart and the belly to emerge from the mouth as unformed sounds. For some people these two pathways are incongruent or in conflict and the thoughts which descend from the head act to critically suppress the feelings which rise from the depths. Consequently, there is a war in the neck which neither party wins and which culminates in a suicide of feeling and thought ending in silence.

In facilitating the breach of this silence and encouraging free vocalisation, a common problem is one of unpleasant physical sensations in the neck, or, more specifically, the throat, which seem to somatise that inner part of the client which is determined not to let the voice out. It is, therefore, not uncommon for a client to cough or gag, placing her hands around the neck and describing a feeling of constriction. The dimension of the vocal tract in such a situation is normally short and narrow and the sound is usually, therefore, one of disrupted flute. In order to enable the client to overcome this suppression of the voice, and to expand the expressive range, it is necessary to encourage the vocal tract to lengthen and dilate, moving first into clarinet and then into the saxophone configuration. The purpose of aiming to fully lengthen and dilate into saxophone is that it prevents the constriction of the tissue structures which can cause friction between the vocal folds. At the same time, it keeps the acoustic resonating tube open so that the sound can be amplified rather than dampened or quashed.

One way to achieve this is through direct massage and manipulation, by which the practitioner takes hold of the client's larynx encouraging it to move vertically up and down, freeing it from the constraints of solidified connective tissue, increasing malleability in the laryngeal musculature, facilitating the ability to lower the floor of the vocal tract and thus increasing timbral resonance (Photograph 11.3). This can be combined with expressive movement which helps to create sensations of descent, such as passing through the Developmental Postural Cycles.

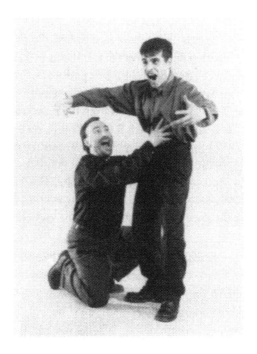

Photograph 11.4

For certain clients with heightened sensitivity to the connotations of contact with the neck, this can provoke fears of being throttled or strangled. The practitioner must have been trained to know exactly where to place the fingers and how much pressure to use; the muscles of this region are attached to a freely suspended hyoid bone which can easily be broken and, indeed, usually is snapped when someone is strangled.

As the practitioner massages the neck he can begin to work across the shoulder and down to the scapulas, meeting the area which is worked on through contact with the chest.

The Chest

Contact with the chest enables the practitioner to positively enhance the movement and breathing pattern and thus the efficacy of voice production and the respiratory processes. Like most of the physical movement methodologies which I have found to be effective, this operates around a spherical conception of space which moves the body through convex and concave configurations. To begin, the practitioner places one hand in the centre of the torso, just below the sternum, and the other hand in the middle of the back. Using pressure alternately between the two hands, the client is moved back and forth between a position in which the spine is curled forwards, creating a concave implosion at the front and a convex curve at the back of the body, and a position in which the spine is arched back, forming a concave curve at the back and a convex arch at the front (Photograph 11.4 and 11.5). During these movements the practitioner uses manipulation to elongate and stretch the spine, discouraging vertebral compression. As the pendulum-like movements proceed, the practitioner combines manipulative pressure and massage so as to assist in the liberation of the breathing pattern from ineffective habitual activity.

One of the areas which, when expanded and released from compressive solidification, can assist an expanded respiratory capacity is the space beneath the scapulas. By working the hands under the bone and massaging the tissue therein, the client can experience an increase in magnitude and breathing volume as well as feeling released from tension.

During contact with the chest it is helpful to use guided imagery by which the client can focus upon the organs which are housed by the chest and develop a positive emotional relationship to them. The practitioner, may for example, speak to the client about the heart as a seat of courage, of bravery and of love. The client may consider how her heart has been broken and how she bears the scars of heart-ache but also how she has the heartful courage to love again. The practitioner may ask the client to consider when she wears her heart on the sleeve, when her heart goes out to someone. The client may also consider when she is hard of heart, perhaps in order to protect herself from exploitation. The heart is also divided, separated into two halves, one for oxygenated blood and the other for de-oxygenated blood, and this poeticises that universal human experience of being divided against oneself or feeling pulled in two directions, which the client may focus on during the guided journey. In addition, the client may experience the heart as being able to take one emotion in whilst releasing another, which mirrors the breathing process.

As the pratitioner works, so the client may focus on an imaginative exploration of the images conjured by focusing on the inner terrain of the torso.

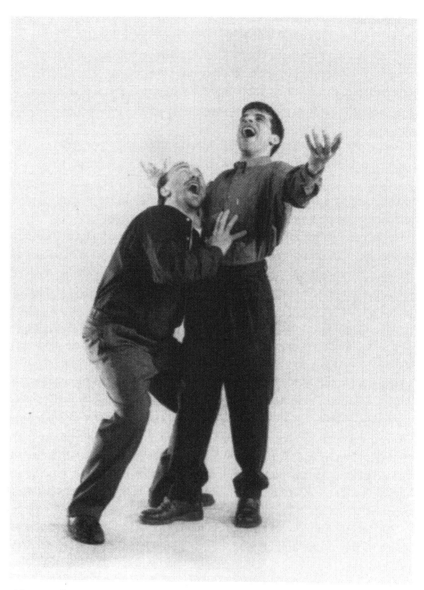

Photograph 11.5

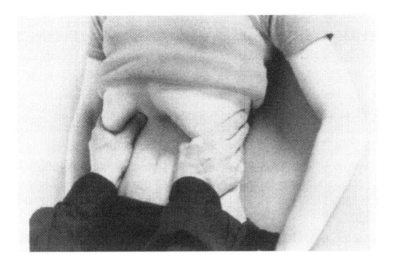

Photograph 11.6

The Abdomen

When the diaphragm moves downwards it puts pressure on the abdominal organs, instigating a gentle squeeze or compression of the blood vessels and serving to increase circulation. This is a positive force, up to a certain limit, and excess pressure on the organs is prevented by the expansion of the abdominal wall, which displaces outwards to form an unfashionable but essential paunch or belly, re-establishing the space for the abdominal contents. If the muscles of this wall are too taught, however, such displacement is hindered and optimal lung expansion depleted. Through Voice Movement Massage, the practitioner can enable to client to release the abdominal wall from excess tension and facilitate enhanced breathing (Photograph 11.6).

When the practitioner makes physical contact with the abdominal area, it highlights the psychophysical relationship between the vocal tract and the stomach and bowels. The mouth and the oropharynx are multi-functional, serving as the respiratory tract through which gas passes during breathing, the digestive tract through which food is ingested and vomited and the vocal tract out of which sounds emerge. In the brain, neurological pathways are organised to mirror the spatial organisation of the body – that is to say that two parts of the body which are in close spatial proximity, such as the nose and lips, have their nerve endings close together in the brain. The region of the pharynx and larynx is highly innervated with nerves and the various constituting structures are so close together that it is almost impossible for the brain to distinguish between sensations of the upper trachea and sensations which emanate from the oesophagus. Consequently, any uncomfortable sensation in that region becomes generalised as a sore throat. Furthermore, because of the close proximity of the oesophagus and the trachea, and because the same tract serves to accommodate food and voice, sensations or sensory memories associated with one can become equated with the other. In Therapeutic Voicework this is commonly observed when a client is attempting to open the vocal tract to its widest gauge, that is to saxophone. During such a process, physical sensations and emotional experiences connected to digestion, and, therefore, to intestinal processes, can be vivified, which often tends to cause the client to silence herself for fear of regurgitating intestinal contents.

Indeed, there is widespread occurrence of psychogenic selective mutism in combination with eating problems which is particularly prevalent in children and young people, where it occurs more frequently in girls than in boys.[77] Selective mutism, or aphonia, denotes a syndrome in which a client refrains from vocalising in specific contexts whilst reassuming voice in others. Recorded examples include its occurrence in response to bereavement accompanied by a dislike for for food,[78] or a complete refusal to eat whilst in the company of parents,[79] foster parents,[80] whilst at school[81] or whilst in the presence of any other person.[82] Mutism can accompany anorexia[83] or can occur in the aftermath of vomiting following the intake of food[84] – in such cases the mutism is usually constant but with successive short intensive periods without eating.[85] Often, children who are selectively mute when outside the family context are later discovered to be containing a secret and a number of cases have been reported where taboo or stigmatised subjects, such as the prevalence of mental illness[87] or violence[88] in the family, had to be kept undeclared and the pressure on the child to say nothing led to mutism.

The potential therapeutic value of the methodological approach to Therapeutic Voicework which I have founded is being applied in work with women suffering from eating disorders by psychotherapist and musician Irene Kessler in Florida, USA, as part of her doctoral research by which the specific indications and contra-indications of the work with such a clientele will hopefully be made clear.

Contact with the abdomen also stimulates in the client the sensation of the stomach as a seat of primary affects, a notion which is found in many cultures world-wide and which for centuries has been part of the vernacular vocabulary in many European languages which are full of metaphors pointing to the stomach as an emotional centre. The physiological evidence for this was revealed in 1895 when a nine-year-old Irish American boy destroyed his oesophagus by drinking a scalding bowl of clam chowder and had a permanent hole made in his stomach into which his meals could be poured. By regularly looking through this hole into the stomach, his doctor was able to note how emotional experiences such as fear, anxiety, excitement, trepidation and joy, as well as 'mere conversation about an unpleasant event', sent his stomach 'into a rage of activity', and, in extreme situations, actually 'made his stomach bleed'. From this and subsequent biofeedback research we can safely conclude that 'the stomach reveals that humans conceal an enormous amount of emotion, which churns in their insides'.[87]

This relationship between the movement of substance in the stomach and intestines and related psychological or emotional movement forms the basis for a body of work known as 'Biodynamic Psychology and Psychotherapy', developed by Gerda Boysen.[89] This is predicated on the belief that psychological trauma negatively influences the digestion of ingested food material in the stomach, as well as giving rise to hindered movement of waste matter through the intestines.[90] For Boysen, the excretion of faecal matter through diarrhoea can be perceived as comparable to a vocal catharsis achieved through affective talking, whilst constipation is a retentive process synonymous with mutism or hindered verbal release. Based on such deductions, her work involves intervention through the act of massage, with particular attention played to the abdominal wall, where attempts are made to loosen fixed, retained and solidified matter and, by association, have the same effect on emotional and psychological material which has become 'stuck', rigid and immobilised.[91]

During Voice Movement Massage the practitioner can assist in the therapeutic exploration of the abdomen and its psychosomatic nature through guided imagery. For example, the client may be asked to consider the stomach and to focus on that which, metaphorically, she has stomached or swallowed. Such awareness often mobilises the will to work towards a more assured sense of self, which can deflect negativity which has hitherto been accepted. In like fashion the client may focus on the guts and the gall as a metaphor for audacity and strength in the face of fear. Such a process may remind the client of times when she has felt gutted, as well as times when stoicism has prevailed.

The belly is the reservoir of the deeper, less frequently accessed emotions such as grief. Rarely do we reach to touch our chest when in bereavement; frequently the hands clutch the abdominal cavity, which is often experienced not as a compartmentalised composition of intestines, bladder, stomach, liver and womb but of a single mass of psycho-physical experience which we may call the belly.

The belly is also a seat of our deepest laughter, the belly laugh. It is not the giggles of a heart in love but the guttural roar of extreme humour. The belly is also a container for our wisdom, all of those insights which we have acquired as a result of experience and which formulate the things we know instinctively down in the belly: our gut instincts. The belly as a combined container for laughter and wisdom is deliciously symbolised in the great laughing Buddha.

These exemplify just some of the issues which can be explored by poeticising the significance of bodily organs as the practitioner works upon the abdomen.

Amplified Sensation

The process of breathing serves the process of respiration, which infuses the blood with oxygen, which is then carried and delivered to all the organs and tissue structures of the body. In order to understand the nature of Breathwork, it must be appreciated that because breathing oxygenates all body parts, it therefore has the capacity to increase sensation throughout the somatic container. Often, during enhanced breathing, a niggling ache will become an excruciating pain and a slightly stiff neck will become extreme hyperkinetic rigidity. Facilitating change in the pattern of breathing may, therefore, stimulate unpleasant sensations within the body as well as providing the means to establishing greater comfort and ease for oxygen is like a sense enhancer which magnifies and amplifies that which is already there.

Furthermore, as a result of this work, most clients will experience emotional volatility and animation. The client's expression of emotion will often be through the sounds arising from the audible breath. Gasps, sobs, shivers, exasperations, exultant jubilations, melancholy whimpers and a whole spectrum of feelings may be heard within the breath sounds. At all times it is vital that the practitioner affirms, encourages and supports the client with an open heart and an objective mind. Providing procedures are followed and the practitioner is trained, combining this hands-on manipulative work with vocal investigations can enable the tonal and timbral range of the client's voice to be remarkably increased.

Physical Dysfunction and Disease

There have been a number of clients with whom I have worked whose muscular condition, breathing pattern and vocal expression has been hindered by an extreme physical condition. One of the most challenging problems which I have encountered is partial paralysis of the intercostal muscles, which forces the client to depend heavily on diaphragmatic displacement and thus abdominal expansion. The decreased or disabled capacity for thoracic expansion puts pressure on the muscles responsible for abdominal expansion to work more quickly than they would if sharing responsibility for the respiratory cycle with the intercostal muscles responsible for thoracic expansion. In order to maintain conversations at a speed equivalent with that used by an able-bodied person, the client will often be seen to gasp air in sudden convulsive movements, visible in the abdominal region, which leave her exhausted. This is made more excruciating if the sufferer is bound to a wheelchair for the sitting position tends to implode and fold the belly wall, hindering liberated abdominal expansion.

I have also worked with a number of people with severe psychomotor dysfunctions, a common condition amongst whom is an expanded oral cavity but an extremely narrowed and constricted sub-oral tract. Though this is rarely seen for more than the briefest moment in able-bodied human beings, in certain kinds of handicaps, however, such radical opening of the vocal tract combined with hyperkinetic contraction of the pharynx is quite common, particularly where neuro-muscular control and dexterity is depleted and perseverative movement or spasm is consistently concurrent with vocalisation. For the client this is very frustrating as it feels as though the mouth is wide open yet the sound will not come out.

Disorders of the voice are also manifold and may be divided into two kinds: organic and functional. Organic voice disorders are those in which the constituting tissue of the voice apparatus, such as the vocal folds, laryngeal musculature, oral palates, nerve endings or nasal passages, become structurally altered, deformed or diseased. Organic disorders include inflammation of the larynx or laryngitis, scars, cysts, polyps or other growths on the folds, cleft palate and benign or malignant tumours. These conditions all exemplify physical dysfunction of the voice which requires medical and allopathic treatment and ministration.

Functional voice disorders, meanwhile, are conditions which prohibit effective and optimal voice production, usually as a result of misuse, without causing mutational changes in the tissue structures. Such disorders include excess of muscle tension, excess of breath released during vocalisation and erratic pitch contours or prosody. However, there is not a tidy boundary between the fields of organic and functional, for the use of the voice effects the way it functions, which, in turn, can effect its structure. For example, someone may use their voice at a very high pitch at levels of intensity or loudness, which, in turn, causes friction between the vocal folds. Consequently, this may cause a haemorrhage in the blood vessels of the folds, which may then harden to become protrusions, known as nodes or polyps, which make it impossible for the speaker to produce a voice with a clear sound. Here the use of the voice effects its function, which, in turn, changes its structure. Such somatic voice disorders which are not, in origin, based on an inherent structural laryngeal pathology, account for between one-third and one-half of all cases seen by the speech and language therapist[92] and House and Andrews have contributed much insight into the way clinicians can understand the effect of the psyche on voice function and dysfunction.[93] Furthermore, many of these disorders are caused through hypertension, that is excess muscle tension in the larynx and related area, which, in turn, is often the result of psychological factors.[94] Indeed, a vast range of vocal problems, functional and organic, are psychogenic in origin.[95]

The connection between the psychological and emotional condition of a vocalist and the resulting voice use, which can cause actual organic damage, began to be recognised by allopathic clinicians in the 1950s, when an increasing number of medical professionals became interested in a holistic approach to vocal treatment.

In 1958, Heaver, a doctor of medicine, called for 'a holistic consideration of all laryngeal disease', asserting that 'vocal abuse which results in nodes and polyps appears in patients who use their voice for the expression of their excessive hostility and aggressive impulses'. Thus he believed that the 'entire laryngologic profession' should be guided by the 'axiom of a holistic consideration of all laryngeal disease' within which the 'larynx should always be judged by the voice it produces, and the voice should always be interpreted as a relentless expression of the speaker's personality'.[96]

Since these remarks, a number of laryngologists have noted similarities in the personality components of those who display nodes and polyps and who have been described as 'ambitious', 'aggressive', 'highly motivated', 'hardworking' and 'perfectionist'.[97] But polyps and nodules constitute only two examples of the ways in which vocal ill-health can result from the misuse of the voice which, in turn, arises from the expression of a psychological state or emotional attitude. There are many other less specific manifestations of the same process which give rise to discomfort, inflammation or strain, all of which impair vocal function.

The Holistic Voice

In recognition of this, Bloch, a medical phoniatrist, made a continual plea in the early 1960s for doctors to incorporate into their practice more of a psychological interpretation and analysis of vocal disorders, stating that 'we cannot examine a voice by itself, we cannot separate it from the speaker, we must examine the entire person,'[98] for very often the vocal problem 'does not even pertain to the larynx' but originates in an emotional difficulty which has been 'channelled' into vocal expression. Medical specialists in the field of voice have, said Bloch, been too occupied with 'the movement of the vocal cords which are so much less important that the emotional cords'.[99] In 1962, Friedrich Brodnitz, one of the most world-famous voice clinicians, referred to the importance of understanding the voice as a 'holistic' phenomenon, pleading with all specialists to consider 'the relationship between the voice he hears and the total personality of the individual who produces it'.[100] In 1955, Weiss,[101] a speech and language therapist, analysed the effect the voice has, not on the listener but on the speaker, and dealt with 'the rather neglected relationship of the speaker or singer to his own voice.'[102] Drawing from his clinical experience in the consulting room, Weiss proposed that 'a successful therapy of the voice might be equivalent to the effects of a thoroughgoing psychotherapy.'[103] He stated that 'the voice and the psychological make-up of an individual mutually influence each other. If a person is psychologically disturbed, the voice suffers, and in turn the deterioration of the voice exerts a negative influence upon the psyche'. For Weiss this meant that it was possible to 'approach this viscous circle from either the psychological or the vocal angle'. However, for Weiss, psychotherapy was often a 'hazardous and always lengthy procedure' and, moreover, 'the voice would have to be treated in any case'. On the other hand, in the treatment of the voice he felt on 'pretty firm ground' and thus sought to attack 'the formerly vicious circle from this point of view' and believed that by 'improving the phonation' it was possible to 'influence the psyche in a favourable manner', which, in turn, created 'more favourable conditions for the voice itself'. Thus 'the vicious circle was converted into a "virtuous" one'.[104]

Teacher or Therapist?

Many people, though they may not possess symptoms of great enough magnitude to attract a diagnosis of pathology and thereby receive allopathic treatment, nonetheless are not reaping the rewards of an optimally functioning voice but are living in constant toleration of a restricted and impeded vocal expressivity. Thus, although we define a voice disorder as 'something that has to be treated by a specialist', an estimated 25 per cent of the adult population, although they do not have real voice disorders, 'are displeased with the way they sound and with the way their voices affect their careers and social lives'.[105]

However, such a person may not know whether they have a voice disorder which requires clinical ministration or a voice production problem which requires re-education. Consequently, they may not know whether to seek a voice teacher or a speech and language therapist. For this reason, speech and language therapists often find themselves confronted with a patient who needs voice teaching whilst voice teachers may, knowingly or not, be working with someone who requires the skills of the speech and language therapist. It is, therefore, in the client's most urgent interest that communication between the two disciplines and some understanding of the two fields is understood by practitioners in both professions.

Christina Shewell, lecturer at the National Hospitals' College of Speech Sciences in London, defines a voice therapist as 'a speech and language therapist who specialises in the treatment of voice disorders'[106] and notes that although 'speech and language therapists work with voice disorders, and voice teachers work with voice problems', there is, nonetheless, a 'cross over' area,[107] for both voice teachers and voice therapists 'work at different but overlapping points along the continuum of vocal use, to enable their clients, patients or students to produce healthy, free and flexible voices'.[108] Consequently, she says that 'in the practices of voice teachers and voice therapists, problems and disorders will often merge into one another' and thus 'we need to know not only the scope of each other's work, but how to refer on'. It is from this move towards a multi-disciplinary humility that she believes Voiceworkers from all fields 'can work together in a mutually beneficial way that will provide our clients with the best possible help, and enrich our own understanding and techniques of voice work.'[109]

Shewell also asserts the centrality of emotional issues to any kind of Therapeutic Voicework, including that pursued by both speech and language therapists and voice teachers, both of whom know, she says, that 'because our voices are the link between our inner and outer worlds, we cannot work on the voice without expecting feelings to come out' as though 'in the prolonged, intoned, open-throated, sung note one's very soul may become visible'. The speech and language therapist and the voice teacher should, therefore, know that 'they may have to incorporate the role of emotional support or counsellor into their work.'[110]

Shewell is, however, clear about a certain distinction between the speech and language therapist and the voice teacher: 'voice therapy', she says, 'seeks to mend a voice problem, whilst voice teaching takes a normal voice and aims to strengthen and train it into an instrument of aesthetic power and flexibility'. In addition, she also proposes that one of the components which differs between the therapist's and the teacher's approach is the use of imagery, believing that the teacher will make far more use of images than will the therapist.[111]

I hold Shewell's opinions in high regard and I believe that all professional Therapeutic Voiceworkers should to understand the limits to their role and how to effectively refer a client who requires clinical ministration.

Therapeutic Voicework Case Study: Martha and the Giant Cyclops

Martha had suffered severe spinal injury in a road traffic accident, which had left her paralysed in both legs and one arm, blind in one eye and permanently scarred across her face. The accident occurred when she was 36 years old. She was 43 when she came to work with me. At the time of the accident she lived with her husband, who had since divorced her and their two children had gone to live with Martha's sister.

Martha had suffered from asthma since childhood and, on occasions, the attacks, from which she still suffered, would cause her to experience muscle spasm throughout the torso, instigate blurred vision in her healthy eye and leave her feeling exhausted.

Before I even began working with Martha my attention was drawn to her propriety and sense of correctness. In her discussion with me during the initial taking of her history she was polite, punctilious with detail, succinct and extremely perceptive. I was also struck by the way she dressed: tightly fitting blouse, jacket and trousers.

On asking Martha to create a sense of a containing sphere, she proceeded to steer herself in her wheel-chair, tracing an area only slightly larger than herself, and I could not help feeling that she had made something to hem her in, comparable to the same way as she seemed to be hemmed in to her clothes, her wheel-chair and her manner of discourse.

On introducing Martha to some physical movements involving guiding the torso back and forth from convex to concave, I pointed out to her that the spherical space which she had created was not big enough to accommodate her in stretching her arms out. Having made a larger sphere, Martha began to pursue the physical exercises with enthusiasm. However, now that she was animated it was clear to me that her clothing also restricted her movement, so, at my suggestion, we loosened the top button of her blouse, took off her jacket and adjusted the belt that passed around her waist and strapped her into the chair. As she did this she said that she had trouble keeping herself in her wheelchair because if she stooped forwards she did not have the muscular strength to stop herself from falling out of the chair completely. I thought it seemed ironic that she should be strapped into a chair, given that after the accident the seat belt had entwined about her neck and kept her from escaping the wreckage until the emergency team had cut her out.

When we came to explore the breathing pattern it seemed logical to imagine that her internal experience was comparable to her sense of a compressing and stifling outer space which kept her strapped in with no room to move. Indeed, in listening to the breath it appeared that the vocal tract was quite tightly constricted in the flute configuration and the morphology of her tissue around the neck and shoulders seemed extremely dense and tightly packed to the touch. I therefore suggested to Martha that we attempt to do the same with the inner tubes as we had done with her outer sphere and enlarge them. I thus began to massage her neck and shoulders whilst simultaneously guiding her with gentle pressure through spherical movements, teaching her how to lengthen and dilate the vocal tract to the saxophone configuration. At one point she stopped and looked a little worried and said: 'I keep expecting that I am going to have a spasm but I don't think I am'. As a result of this work, Martha began to feel that she was gaining 'room to move' as well as 'room to breathe'. Now she wanted to find her voice.

Martha had been aphasic, that is unable to speak, for nearly a year following the accident. Indeed, it is common for major shock to silence the voice and one of the many skills of a speech and language therapist is being able to help a client regain it.[112] Indeed, speech therapy had refound Martha's voice but, on rediscovering it, she experienced it to be 'weak', 'frail' and 'pathetic'. To my ears, her voice was in clarinet, high in pitch with a great amount of free air and with a very limited range of prosody, $<\flat\ \pi$.

During the Therapeutic Voicework, however, I observed that though predominantly quiet and softened by a high degree of free air, her voice seemed to spontaneously switch into low-pitched soft growls which lasted only momentarily, $\underline{\underline{\sqcup}}$ $\overline{\sim\!\sim}$. Second, the fingers of her active hand seemed to be making repetitive and rhythmical gripping movements, causing an alternating hypertension and relaxation throughout the entire torso. I began working with this by asking her to amplify, exaggerate and intensify both the vocal switches between high, light soft, airy, wispy sounds and low, guttural, soft growling sounds, $<\flat\ \pi/\underline{\underline{\sqcup}}$ $\overline{\sim\!\sim}$, as well as the physical switches between tense gripping movements and released relaxation of the fingers. As she proceeded to rehearse this instruction, I began to imagine her to be climbing a mountain and suggested that she try to use this image to give specificity and substance to her work. Her reply, to my surprise and amusement, was that prior to the accident, one of her hobbies had been rock climbing.

As we worked the scenario, I suggested that she imagine that the softer sounds were gasps and sighs of satisfaction as she reached various resting plateaus during the ascent of the mountain and that the lower more assertive voice qualities were ambitious and driven sounds of toil and determination accompanying the difficult and effortful climb. As she rehearsed, her body and voice took on epic proportion, her muscles bulged and her vocal sounds swung and sung. As I watched and listened, my eyes and ears saw and heard a multitude of images, which I relayed to Martha in words as she worked. I witnessed and described an ape, a savage Neanderthal, a grumbling bear, a giant, an avid explorer, a prowling leopard, a great bovine – part buffalo, part mule – and, as I spoke and she worked, I felt a certain increase in aggressive instincts radiate from this quiet and morose woman.

Seeking to enable the client to sense her aggression in a creative framework, I guided her through an imaginary journey where she conceived of herself as a prehistoric mythical creature, part leopard, part bear and part bull. The driving force for this animal's movement was extreme hunger and her actions were hindered by an injury, a wound. I asked the client to experience the fateful combination of hunger, anger and extreme vulnerability due to injury. The sounds which she released were both terrifying and tear-provoking as her body clamoured and careened.

It should be remembered that people who have been disabled are not hindered in their dreams but run, jump, twist and turn unimpeded by the damaged frame which they confront when the waking hour comes. In exploring the Self through Therapeutic Voicework, disabled people can capitalise on the dream time by exploring the able and unimpeded body of the dream through the vocal and choreographic waking imagination.

All the time during my work with Martha I was in close physical contact with her, helping her feel safe enough and secure enough to know that she would not fall out of the chair and hurt herself, yet free enough within the chair to fully investigate the journey. I held her around the abdomen, hugged her shoulders, sat on one arm of the wheel-chair with one ankle on each of the foot-rests as we danced together in intimate, yet task-orientated, proximity. Then I noticed her eyes; they were closed.

On asking Martha to speak a little of her sight, she explained that her sight had always been poor, even as a child, but mentioned that when mountaineering she rarely wore glasses but did most of the work 'by feel'; she would only put her glasses on when she stopped and wanted to view the landscape. I therefore suggested that she now remove the glasses, which she still wore, in order to assist the eye that had not been blinded in the accident and continue to rehearse. When she took them off I could sense the fabric of her vulnerability; indeed, the off-centre and asymmetrical set of her eyes, to me, gave Martha the appearance of timidity and defencelessness. However, the moment she began again the choreographic gripping and the vocal transformations, her eyes became electrified, deliberate, concentrated and bold as she became totally absorbed in the climb. It was then that, for some reason, I thought of the Cyclops, the mythical one-eyed giant who captured Jason and his crew. I suggested the image of the Cyclops to this now energised woman who seemed to be discovering such vitality and potency through the work and she placed herself at the opening of a great cave and began leaping and calling, yodelling and booming. As the session proceeded, her body became more animated and her voice loud and rich until, sweating, tired and somewhat amazed at herself, she came to rest with the words: 'I can't believe that was me'.

When I asked her what she had been imagining during the journey involving the cave, she said that she was protecting her young 'monster cubs' from being taken from her. As she said this she burst into tears, sobbing and crying on the words 'what happened to my children'.

The depth and severity of the pain which a woman such as Martha suffers is, for most of us, simply unimaginable and such pain can leave a person dumb, mute and exhausted. Yet, no matter how terrifying or overwhelming, this pain is better voiced. Nothing can enable Martha to mother her children, or walk, or drive a car or go rock climbing again but that does not mean that she needs to silence the magnitude of her feelings in response to what has befallen her.

Working through body, breath, voice and image can, therefore, provide a way of contextualising and containing such expressions, whilst at the same time make some small contribution to the alleviation of physical constraint.

Conclusion: Back to the Body and the Mind

A study of the physical nature of voice and Therapeutic Voicework in some way brings us full circle to how this book began: with the muscle and bone of an elastic tube rooted in a complex neuromuscular terrain. Yet it is also evident that vocal expression through the use of this physical instrument inevitably stimulates emotional and psychological experience. Consequently, the Therapeutic Voiceworker operates at the interface between the psychic and the somatic. In addition, the Therapeutic Voiceworker is also utilising creative and artistic strategies, as vocal expression often yields the fruit of music and theatre as well as accompanying the dance of the body.

In the next chapter I will, therefore, attempt to address some of the core principles which unite these disparate components of Therapeutic Voicework into a working model, whilst at the same time interrogating more deeply the proposal and the assumption that Therapeutic Voicework can provide a means of travelling down the royal road to the soul.

Notes

1   Aronson, A. (1990) *Clinical Voice Disorders*. New York: Thieme.

2   Greene, M. and Mathieson, L. (1991) *The Voice and its Disorders*. London: Whurr.

3   Boone, D. and McFarlane, S. (1988) in *The Voice and Voice Therapy*. New Jersey: Simon and Schuster.

4   Fawcus, M. (1991) (ed) *Voice Disorders and their Management*. London: Chapman and Hall.

5   Hirano, M. and Bless, D. (1993) *Video Stroboscopic Examination of the Larynx*. London: Whurr.

6   Carlson, N. (1991) *Physiology of Behaviour*. Boston: Allyn and Bacon.

7   Greene, M. and Mathieson, L. (1989) *The Voice and its Disorders*, 5th edn. London: Whurr, pp.197–98.

8   Greene, M. and Mathieson, L. (1989) *The Voice and its Disorders*, 5th edn. London: Whurr, p.197.

9   Becker, J., Breedlove, M. and Crews, D. (eds) (1992) *Behavioural Endocrinology*. Cambridge: MIT Press.

10   Kilcoyne, A. (1991) 'Common sense: making use of the sense of touch.' *The British Journal of Visual Impairment*, 9, 2, pp.47–49.

11   Paxton, S. (1981–82) *Contact Improvisation. Dartington Theatre Papers*, Fourth Series.

12   Rolf, I. (1990) *Rolfing and Physical Reality*. Rochester: Healing Arts Press.

13   Chaitrow, L. (1988) *Soft-Tissue Manipulation*. Rochester: Healing Arts Press.

14   Alexander, F.M. (1987) *The Use of the Self*. London: Victor Gollancz.

15   Law, M. (1996) 'Interviews with contemporary voice practitioners.' Unpublished research papers prepared for the International Association for Voice Movement Therapy.

16   Conference series notes and information leaflet to *Giving Voice*, four annual conferences held at Cardiff, Centre for Performance Research,1993–96.

17   Information leaflet, Rosehill Hospital, (September 1996).

18   Law, M. (1996) 'The practice of voice: an investigation into the diversity of approaches to vocal work as exemplified by current practitioners.' Unpublished research project prepared for the International Association for Voice Movement Therapy.

19   Law, M. (1996) 'The practice of voice: an investigation into the diversity of approaches to vocal work as exemplified by current practitioners.' Unpublished research project prepared for the International Association for Voice Movement Therapy.

20   Braddock, C. (1995) *Body Voices: Using the Power of Breath, Sound and Movement to Heal and Create New Boundaries*. Berkeley: Page Mill Press.

21   Rohmert, G. (1991) *Der Sänger auf dem Weg zum Klang*. Köln: Die Deutsche Bibliothek.

22   Apel, D. (1989) 'The interrelationship of psyche and soma in functional voice training.' Masters Thesis submitted to Antioch University.

23   Dalcroze, J. (1965) 'L'Initiation au rythme.' In *Le Rythme, la Musique et l'Education*. Lausanne: Foetische, pp.37–44, 43.

24   Mothersole, A. (1920) 'La Rythmique est-elle une Lubie?' *La Rythme*, 5, p.23.

25   Dalcroze, J. (1965) 'Les Etudes Musicales et l'Education de l'Oreille', in *Le Rythme, la Musique et l'Education*. Lausanne: Foetische, pp.9–12, (p.10).

26   Ramacharaka, Y. (1905) *The Science of Breath : A Complete Manual of the Oriental Breathing Philosophy*. Chicago: Yogi Publication Society.

27   Ramacharaka, Y. *The Hindu-Yogi Breathing Exercises: A System of Physical, Mental and Soul Development*. Chicago: Yogi Publication Society, date not given.

28   Huang, (1993) *The Primordial Breath: An Ancient Chinese Way of Prolonging Life Through Breath Control*, vols. 1 and 2. California: Original Books, Newcastle Publishing.

29   Ellis, G. (1993) *The Breath of Life: Mastering the Breathing Techniques of Pranayama and Qi Gong*. North Hollywood,California: Newcastle Publishing.

30   Zi, N. (1994) *The Art of Breathing: A Course of Six Simple Lessons to Improve Performance and Well-Being*. Glendale, California: Vivi Coo.

31   Feils, R. (1988) *Breathing Alive: A Guide to Conscious Living*. Shaftesbury: Element.

32 Sky, M. (1990) *Breathing: Expanding Your Power & Energy*. New Mexico: Bear and Company.

33 Rama, S., Ballentine, R. and Hymes, A. (1990) *The Science of Breath*. Pennsylvania: The Himalayan International Institute.

34 Shawn, T. (1954) *Every Little Movement*. New York: Whitmark and Sons.

35 Kofler, L. (1893) *The Art of Breathing as the Basis of Tone Production*. New York: Edgar S. Werner.

36 Gindler, E. (1995) 'Gymnastik for people whose lives are full of activity.' In D. Johnson (ed) *Bone, Breath and Gesture: Practises of Embodiment*. Berkeley: North Atlantic Books, pp.3–14.

37 Schick, J. (1995) 'Interview with Charlotte Selver.' In D. Johnson (ed) *Bone, Breath and Gesture: Practises of Embodiment*. Berkeley: North Atlantic Books, pp.16–21.

38 Speads, C. (1992) *Ways to Better Breathing.* Vermont: Healing Arts Press.

39 Mayland, E. (1995) 'The Rosen method.' In D. Johnson (ed) *Bone, Breath and Gesture: Practises of Embodiment*. Berkeley: North Atlantic Books, pp.52–64.

40 Rosen, M. and Brenner, S. (1991) *The Rosen Method of Movement*. Berkeley: North Atlantic Books.

41 Middendorf, I. (1990) *The Perceptible Breath: A Breathing Science*. Paderborn: Junfermann-Verlag.

42 Middendorf, I. (1990) *The Perceptible Breath: A Breathing Science*. Paderborn: Junfermann-Verlag.

43 Middendorf, I. (1990) *The Perceptible Breath: A Breathing Science*. Paderborn: Junfermann-Verlag, pp.23–30.

44 Middendorf, I. (1990) *The Perceptible Breath: A Breathing Science*. Paderborn: Junfermann-Verlag, pp.63–64.

45 Lissau, R. (1987) *Rudolf Steiner: Life, Work, Inner Path and Social Initiatives*. Stroud: Hawthorn Press.

46 Stoehr, S. (1983) *Eurythmy: An Art of Movement for Our Time*. Stourbridge: Robinswood Press.

47 Steiner, R. and Wegman, I. (1967) *Fundamentals of Therapy*. London: Rudolf Steiner Press.

48 Steiner, R. (1983) *Curative Eurythmy*. London: Rudolf Steiner Press.

49 Stoehr, S. (1983) *Eurythmy: An Art of Movement for Our Time*. Stourbridge: Robinswood Press.

50 Kirchner-Bockholt, M. (1922) *Fundamental Principles of Curative Eurythmy*. London: Temple Lodge, pp.129–30.

51 Lorenz-Poschmann, A. (1982) *Breath, Speech and Therapy*. New York: Mercury Press, pp.7–12.

52 Baur, A. (1993) *Healing Sounds: Fundamentals of Chirophonetics*. Fair Oaks, California: Rudolf Steiner College Press, pp.xi–xii.

53 Werbeck-Svärdström, V. (1985) *Uncovering the Voice*. London: Rudolf Steiner Press, p. 32.

54 Werbeck-Svärdström, V. (1985) *Uncovering the Voice*. London: Rudolf Steiner Press, p.37.

55 Werbeck-Svärdström, V. (1985) *Uncovering the Voice*. London: Rudolf Steiner Press, p.54.

56 Deason-Barrow, M. Lecture given at Songs of Heaven and Earth Conference, (Findhorn Foundation, Forres, 30 March–6 April 1996).

57 Grof, S. (1988) *The Adventure in Self Discovery: Dimensions of Consciousness and New Perspectives in Psychotherapy and Inner Exploration*. New York: State University of New York, p.170.

58   Grof, S. (1975) *Realms of the Human Unconscious: Observations from LSD Research*. New York: Viking Press.

59   Grof, S. (1988) *The Adventure in Self Discovery: Dimensions of consciousness and New Perspectives in Psychotherapy and Inner Exploration*. New York: State University of New York, p.172.

60   Grof, S. (1988) *The Adventure in Self Discovery: Dimensions of Consciousness and New Perspectives in Psychotherapy and Inner Exploration*. New York: State University of New York, p.173.

61   Grof, S. (1988) *The Adventure in Self Discovery: Dimensions of Consciousness and New Perspectives in Psychotherapy and Inner Exploration*. New York: State University of New York, p.186.

62   Grof, S. (1993) *Realms of the Human Unconscious: Observations from LSD Research*. London: Souvenir Press, p.46.

63   Grof, S. (1993) *Realms of the Human Unconscious: Observations from LSD Research*. London: Souvenir Press, p.158–9.

64   Grof, S. (1993) *Realms of the Human Unconscious: Observations from LSD Research*. London: Souvenir Press, p.159.

65   Minett, G. (1994) *Breath and Spirit: Rebirthing as a Healing Technique*. London: Harper Collins, p.23.

66   Orr, L. and Ray, S. (1983) *Rebirthing in the New Age*. Berkeley: Celestial Arts, p.75.

67   Minett, G. (1994) *Breath and Spirit: Rebirthing as a Healing Technique*. London: Harper Collins, p.107.

68   Minett, G. (1994) *Breath and Spirit: Rebirthing as a Healing Technique*. London: Harper Collins, p.91.

69   Minett, G. (1994) *Breath and Spirit: Rebirthing as a Healing Technique*. London: Harper Collins, p.107.

70   Orr, L. and Ray, S. (1983) *Rebirthing in the New Age*. Berkeley: Celestial Arts, p.76.

71   Orr, L. and Ray, S. (1983) *Rebirthing in the New Age*. Berkeley: Celestial Arts, p.76.

72   Orr, L. and Ray, S. (1983) *Rebirthing in the New Age*. Berkeley: Celestial Arts, pp.80–81.

73   Hough, A. (1994) *Physiotherapy in Respiratory Care*. London: Chapman and Hall.

74   Bradley, D. (1992) *Hyper Ventilation Syndrome: A Handbook for Bad Breathers*. Berkeley, California: Celestial Arts.

75   Unpublished papers on the Buteyko method.

76   Freid, R. (1990) *The Breath Connection : How to Reduce Psychosomatic and Stress Related Disorders with Easy to do Breathing Exercises*. New York: Plenum Press.

77   Lebrun, Y. (1990) *Mutism*. London:Whurr, p.20.

78   Russell, J. (1864) 'A case of hysteric aphonia.' *British Medical Journal*, 2, pp.619–21.

79   Youngerman, J. (1979) 'The syntax of silence: electively mutetherapy.' *International Review of Psycho-Analysis*, 6, pp.283–95.

80   Goll, K. (1979) 'Role structure and subculture in families of elective mutism.' *Family Proceedings*, 18, pp.55–68.

81   Wright, H., Miller, D., Cook, M. and Littman, J. (1985) 'Early identification and intervention with children who refuse to speak.' *Journal of the American Academy of Child Psychiatry*, 24, pp.739–46.

82   Wallace, M. (1987) *The Silent Twins*. London: Penguin.

83   Blotcky, M. and Looney, J. (1980) 'A psychotherapeutic approach to silent children.' *American Journal of Psychotherapy*, 24, pp.487–95.

84 Kaplan, S. and Escoll, P. (1973) 'Treatment of two silent adolescent girls.' *Journal of the American Academy of Child Psychiatry,* 12, pp.59–72.

85 Chethik, M. (1990) 'Amy: the intensive treatment of an elective mute.' In J. Macdermott and S. Harrison (ed) *Psychiatric treatment of the Child.* New York: Aronson, pp.117–36.

86 Pusrom, E. and Speers, R. (1964) 'Elective mutism in children.' *Journal of the American Academy of Child Psychiatry,* 9, pp.287–97.

87 Lesser-Katz, M. (1986) 'Stranger reaction and elective mutism in children.' *American Journal of Orthopsychiatry,* 56, pp.458–69.

88 Zeldin, T. (1994) *An Intimate History of Humanity.* London: Sinclair-Stevenson, pp.177–8.

89 Boysen, G. (1987) *Über den Körper die Seele Heilen: Biodynamische Psychologie and Psychotherapie.* München: Kösel-Verlag.

90 Boysen, G. (1995) *Von der Lust am Heilen.* München: Kösel-Verlag.

91 Boysen, G. and Boysen, M. (1987) *Biodynamik, des Lebens: Die Gerda Boysen Methode.* Essen: Synthesis Verlag Gerken.

92 House, A. and Andrews, H. (1988) 'Life events and difficulties preceding the onset of functional disruption.' *Journal of Psychosomatic Research.*

93 House, A. and Andrews, H. (1987) *The Psychiatric and Social Characteristics of Patients with Functional Disruption.*

94 Aronson, A. (1990) *Clinical Voice Disorders.* New York: Thieme.

95 Butcher, P., Elias, A. and Raven, R. (1993) *Psychogenic Voice Disorders and Cognitive-Behaviour Therapy.* London: Whurr.

96 Heaver, L. (1958) 'Psychiatric observations on the personality structure of patients with habitual disruption.' *Logos,* 1–21. Cited in P. Bloch, 'New limits of vocal analysis.' *Folia Phoniatrica,* 12 (1960), pp.291–297, (p.294).

97 Arnold, G. (1962) 'Vocal nodules and polyps: laryngeal tissue reaction to habitual hyperkinetic disruption.' *Journal of Speech Disorders,* 27, p.205.
Luchsinger, R. and Arnold, G. (Eds.) (1965) *Voice, Speech and Language.* London: Constable.
Morrison, M.D., Nichol, H. and Rammage, L.A. (1986) 'Diagnostic Criteria in Functional Disruption.' *Laryngoscope,* 94, p.1.

98 Bloch, P. (1960) 'New limits of vocal analysis.' *Folia Phoniatrica,* 12, pp.291–297, (p.292).

99 Bloch, P. (1960) 'New limits of vocal analysis.' *Folia Phoniatrica,* 12, pp.291–297, (p.294).

100 Brodnitz, F.S. (1962) 'The holistic study of the voice.' *Quarterly Journal of Speech,* 48, no. 3, pp.280–84, (pp.283–84).

101 Weiss, D.A. (1955) 'The psychological relations to one's own voice.' *Folia Phoniatrica,* 7, pp.209–222.

102 Weiss, D.A. (1955) 'The psychological relations to one's own voice.' *Folia Phoniatrica,* 7, pp.209–222, (p.209).

103 Weiss, D.A. (1955) 'The psychological relations to one's own voice.' *Folia Phoniatrica,* 7, pp.209–222, (p.215).

104 Weiss, D.A. (1955) 'The psychological relations to one's own voice.' *Folia Phoniatrica,* 7, pp.209–222, (p.215).

105 Boone, D. and McFarlane, S. in (1988) *The Voice and Voice Therapy.* New Jersey: Simon and Schuster.

106 Shewell, C. (1991) 'A lack of understanding about two professions.' *Human Communication.* (November 1991), pp.8–10, (p.8).

107 Shewell, C. 'Voice problems and disorders: voice disorders 2.' Unpublished teaching pamphlet C4-CMS-C404, National Hospital's College of Speech Sciences.

108 Shewell, C. (1991) 'A lack of understanding about two professions.' *Human Communication.* (November 1991), pp.8–10, (p.8).

109 Shewell, C. (1991) 'A lack of understanding about two professions.' *Human Communication.* (November 1991), pp.8–10, (p.8).

110 Shewell, C. (1991) 'A lack of understanding about two professions.' *Human Communication.* (November 1991), pp.8–10, (p.9).

111 Shewell, C. (1991) 'A lack of understanding about two professions.' *Human Communication.* (November 1991), pp.8–10, (p.9).

112 Rose, R., Whurr, R. and Wyke, M. (1993) *Aphasia.* London: Whurr.

CHAPTER 12

Imagination and Intervention
Towards an Integrated Psychophysical Methodology of Therapeutic Voicework

Introduction: Towards Integration and Intersection

In this book I have, so far, proposed and consistently assumed that the human voice reflects the nature of the human psyche. Furthermore, I have implied that diverse fields of enquiry, within the arts and sciences, can provide the foundations for a methodology of Therapeutic Voicework which I have called Voice Movement Therapy.

In this chapter I will subject this to an analysis and offer some insight into the way that the physical, the psychological and the artistic intersect at a common point.

Voice, Speech and Incongruence

Communication between human adults is a holistic phenomenon. It is comprised of the simultaneous operation of a number of communication channels: eye movements, facial expression, the body language of gesture and motion and the sounds emitted by the voice. When we witness someone communicating, we attend to all of these channels to form a whole by which we believe ourselves to appreciate what the person means, understand who they are and comprehend what they feel.

However, although the body language of gestural movements, facial expressions and eye contact contributes to the messages which are conveyed by each of us in everyday expression, it is the sophistication of the acoustic signals activated by the vocal instrument that separates humans from animals. Of all the dimensions to communication, the oral channel is the most widely used in day-to-day interaction between homo sapiens and this oral channel is itself composed of two levels: the vocal and the verbal, or voice and speech.[1]

Most people are quite aware that the same verbal phrase can be uttered in such a variety of ways as to communicate significantly different meanings. That is to say, in the words of a common but wise adage, 'it is not what you say but the way that you say it'. The speech component of oral communication has been defined as 'conveyance of the facts',[2] whilst 'voice' relates to the way in which this is uttered through use of the component parameters of vocal sounds[3] – which are allegedly the emissary for our state of mind, moods, emotions and inner attitudes.[4]

Skinner proposed that the emotional aspect of speech communicated through the voice is not just a dispensable embellishment but that the verbal aspect of oral communication can only be used effectively when the vocal dimension implies to the listener the way in which the words are intended to be interpreted.[5] Sullivan also described the vocal channel as 'sound accompaniments' to speech which suggest what is to be made of the verbal propositions stated.[6] This sound accompaniment to language has been named 'paralanguage'[7] and consists primarily of the colour of the voice, that is a composite of harmonic resonance, pitch and its fluctuation, loudness, glottal attack, free air, disruption, register and nasal resonance, or violin, which 'transmit the emotional tone of the message.'[8]

Although the voice may give speech its meaning, particularly emotional implication, it does not necessarily simply enforce the meaning of the verbal content. For example, if the speaker is in some kind of personal conflict, the two channels may carry conflicting information, a phenomenon that has been called 'incongruence'[9] and which often occurs, for instance, when the words we choose paint the public face behind which an undeclared emotion brews. We say that we are willing to do something for a friend with a tone of voice which, to the attentive listener, reveals a reluctance to help; we say that we are 'doing fine' whilst we are actually choked with sadness. Sarcasm relies upon such incongruence in which we verbally affirm one message whilst simultaneously denying it in our tone of voice. In cases of mental illness these incongruities are present to a heightened degree and are a highly significant source of information for the psychotherapist or psychiatrist, whose diagnostic conclusions have long-lasting and often irreversible effects on the patient. Moses asserted that when such an incongruence between the vocal and verbal message occurs, 'the voice is more likely to reveal the truth about the personality'[10] than the speech and that 'before attempting to analyse the voice, one must divorce it from the message it seeks to convey'.[11]

A common kind of incongruence can often be heard in the acoustic messages conveyed to children by their parents and which demands of the listeners a sophistication of interpretation often in excess of their years. An exasperated mother seeking to stop her child from running out of her sight whilst waiting for a train may pick him up, sit him firmly on a bench and say: 'You just move from there once more'. Of course, the mother actually intends her message to be decoded to mean 'do *not* move from there again'. In a situation like this, the melodic stress or prosodic intonation of her voice is likely to leave the child in no doubt as to what she really means. However, there are other less overt cases of incongruence which can often confront children with an impenetrable ambivalence as to what the message intends. Gregory Bateson has carried out considerable research into the unwitting transmission of ambiguous or contradictory signals by parents to their children through an incongruence between the phonic and linguistic dimensions of speech, hypothesising that a high frequency of such 'double binds' sets up fertile ground for the genesis of schizophrenic disturbance.[12] But it is not only in cases of schizophrenia that the negative psychological effect of such ambiguous parental messages can be witnessed: many functional adults have been so treated and, in consequence, repeat such a form of communication with those they relate to. Having been denied consistent single messages themselves, they too find it hard to convey a single intention or feeling and instead paint one picture with the words they speak and another with their vocal intonation.

For the purpose of analysis then, the vocally produced acoustic signals of communication in the human species can be divided into the phonic and the linguistic, or voice and speech. Phonic expression occurs as a result of the vibration of the vocal folds, which we call phonation. Linguistic communication, or speech, is born from the co-ordinated articulation of the tongue, mouth, lips and jaw. The term '*linguistic*', in fact, comes from '*lingua*', the Latin word for tongue, and indeed the articulation of the tongue is the first essential prerequisite in the production of speech. The linguist Lotz has pointed out that if you were to make a quantitative analysis of the acoustic signals emitted by the adult human voice, only 1 per cent would prove to be of linguistic use and purpose, the remainder being entirely vocal or phonic.[13]

It is vocal or phonic communication which occurs first in the development of the individual and which, it seems reasonable to speculate, accompanied the early development of the human species. Language is, and probably was, acquired subsequently, although, as we accrue proficiency and dexterity in verbal language, the instinctive phonic sound making becomes subservient to linguistics but retains a certain importance in giving speech its stress, emotional colour and melody. The importance of this vocal quality in communication cannot be overestimated.

The phonic quality of a voice independent of the words it utters reveals much about the personality of the speaker and a change in phonic characteristics can completely alter the meaning of the same verbal sentence, imbuing it with passivity or ferocity, triumph or defeat. In the quality of a voice you can hear the vales of depression and the peaks of excitement, you can hear the lulls of concern and self-reflection and the sharp points of provocation and attack. In it you can hear the calm tone of age and wisdom and the effervescent innocence and enthusiasm of youth. In the voice you can hear resignation, indignation, hope and despair. In short, in the voice you can hear the psyche, or so we believe.

Our intuitive and subjective interpretation of the underlying acoustic properties of the voice are often sensory. For example, we frequently hear the voice as though we are perceiving it through the sense of touch. We feel pinched, slapped, compressed, pierced, hammered, stroked, tickled or shaken by the voice of a speaker. This physicality of the voice is only one amongst a number of ideosensory dimensions contained within our perception of vocal communication. We also respond as though we taste a voice, hearing the despondent bitterness, the citrus tang of jealousy or the sugary sweet sycophanticism. In addition, we hear the colour of a voice, the deep blue of melancholia, the green of envy and the red of retaliation. Temperature too is used to describe the quality of a voice, which can be experienced as warm, cool, burning hot or ice cold. This process of borrowing a term which applies to one sense, such as sight, taste or touch, and applying it to another, in this case hearing, is called 'synaesthesia', which is not an objective framework of analysis but a description of a listener's subjective experience, in this case the experience of hearing the voice of another person. A person's voice may also stimulate the impression of a particular character, conjuring the impression of a certain face, walk, dress and attitude. In addition, a voice can stimulate personal associations, reminding us of someone we have known.

All of these qualities that we believe to be present in the voice of another, and the associations which they provoke, are subjective interpretations. They are, in many ways, descriptions of the way the listener feels they have been influenced by the vocalist. And the constituting units of this sensory, intuitive experience of a voice are images: images of colour, of taste, of touch and of character.

But we should not confuse the notion of image with an optical construct for, as Hillman has said, to 'talk about images as if they were pictures' is a 'mix up' which ignores the image as body and as sound.[14] For Hillman, image is a function which combines all the senses and is, at the same time, independent of them.[15] Hillman's collaborator, Paul Kugler, an aesthetician with a keen interest in archetypal psychology and linguistics, proposes that 'vocal sounds stimulate images in the mind of listener independent of their linguistic signification and semantic context'.[16] This occurs through what he calls a 'phonetic imagination'.[17] This phonetic imagination is a highly sensitive alchemical laboratory which transforms an acoustic signal generated by someone's vocal apparatus into a pantheon of images which arise from our subjective associations but which we often attribute to the actual disposition of the vocalist.

The question that a Therapeutic Voiceworker must ask is whether there is a direct relationship between these subjective images which are conjured in the listener's phonetic imagination and the vocalist's actual character, emotional experience or intention. Does the voice of an individual distort or reflect his or her so-called true nature? Do we hear what is uttered or only what we are prepared to amplify within the subjective auditory canal of our own ears? Concisely: does the voice truly reveal the soul?

Voice and Psyche: The Research and Evidence

In 1985 I conducted an academic inquiry, based at Exeter University with the financial support of the British Academy, to discover what historical empirical evidence there was to support the claim that the non-verbal sounds of the human voice accurately convey information which truly reflect the vocalist's personality and emotional experience. The personal objective for this research was to substantiate my practical work on developing a grounded strategy for the practice of Therapeutic Voicework. However, the results of my investigations were extremely humbling.

In 1925 Wagoner suggested that there was a relationship between the temperament of an individual and his or her vocal qualities.[18] Later, in 1931, Rieffert proposed that dimensions of voice such as 'prosody, rhythm, pitch and tempo' are expressive of 'temperamental traits' and devised a characterological vocal typology which compartmentalised voices into certain categories which were also alleged to reflect types of personality.[19] Since then, and continuing throughout the twentieth century, there has been a great deal of research into the degree to which identifiable components of a speaker's personality and aspects of his or her emotional intent can be communicated to listeners through the vocal channel alone. This research, undertaken primarily by experimental psychologists working in the field of empirical and statistical studies, involved the assembly of volunteer listeners from a variety of contexts. These volunteers were gathered together and asked to listen to a series of carefully chosen speakers or vocalists, each of whom would, in most cases, speak an identical piece of text, very often from behind a screen or onto a tape recorder or phonograph or over the radio or a public address system so that the volunteer listeners had no visual picture of the speaker. Because each speaker spoke the same words and could not be seen, the listeners had only the vocal channel of expression from which to draw conclusions about the speaker's personality. With the advent of technological advancement, it became possible to remove the verbal coherence of spoken sentences with electronic filters which left the vocal prosody and all other voice features in tact. Some experimenters asked actors or teachers to simulate emotions while others took a series of emotionally charged word samples, sometimes from mentally ill people[20] and sometimes from the from actual life situations of healthy individuals.[21] They then subjected these to electronic filtering, reducing the degree to which the verbal content could be recognised. Researchers thus began to investigate the degree to which the voice could communicate 'psychological properties'[22] and the term 'content free speech' came into play.[23]

The most renowned of these experiments into the psychology of the human voice was initiated by an English professor of Psychology who placed an advertisement in the *Radio Times* announcing an experiment in which he selected nine people to read an identical passage of text over the radio.[24] In the advertisement he asked radio listeners to guess each speaker's age, sex, profession or occupation, the location of birth, the location affecting speech and whether the speaker was accustomed to leading others. Over 4000 reports were sent in and, although many of them were accurate, Pear recorded that 'a person's voice often conforms to a stereotype'[25] in the minds of listeners. In other words, certain vocal qualities which are evident in the voice of a speaker tend to conjure up the same notions of personality in many listeners, even though the speaker may not conform to that disposition in real life.

These modest experiments hailed an era of widespread testing to discover which properties of personality, character, disposition and social status could be accurately ascertained from vocal qualities such as pitch, loudness, free air and other timbral vocal components. Experiments were conducted to see whether the sound of a person's voice, independent of the words uttered, could accurately convey the person's dominant personality traits,[26] their intelligence[27] or IQ,[28] their weight, height and sex, their occupation, their political orientation, their social status,[29] their level of nervousness and aggressiveness,[30] the degree to which the person was introverted or extroverted,[31] the degree to which they were submissive or dominant and whether they were accustomed to leadership,[32] how tired or rested they were, how sociable someone was[33] and whether they were telling the truth or lying.[34] Other experiments sought to discover if listeners could correctly match a person's voice with their handwriting,[35] with photographs of their faces and bodies[36] and with the speaker's own description of their personality.[37] One experiment investigated whether listeners could write an accurate free description of the personality behind the voice which they heard.[38] In others, experimenters sought to discover whether listeners could correctly match voices with the six Spranger,[39] personality types of theoretic, social, aesthetic, economic, political and religious[40] and whether listeners could correctly match voices with the Kretschmerian constitutional types of pyknic, leptosomatic and athletic.[41] One experiment tried to ascertain whether people could identify correctly a voice which they had heard from a vocal identity parade at time intervals ranging from one day to five months.[42] Other enquiries sought to find out whether emotion can be determined from the pitch of the voice[43] and whether listeners associate certain pitch changes with particular emotions,[44] such as happiness or sadness,[45] as well as seeking to find which other vocal components convey emotion.[46] Others investigated whether pitch range influences the perception of the personality[47] and the personal attributes vocalists are attributed with.[48] Other experiments sought to find whether there was an equation between how 'socially adjusted someone is' and the qualities of pitch and force in their voice,[49] whether pitch can indicate anxiety and depression,[50] whether there was a relationship between certain personality traits and other voice qualities in addition to pitch, such as as 'breathiness, 'whine' and 'harshness',[51] and whether such qualities influence the interpretation of verbal communication.

In other investigations, experimenters tried discover whether the voice quality of nasal resonance, or violin, 'interferes with effective verbal communication'[53] and whether hypernasalty, or high degree of violin, interferes more than hyponasality, or lack of violin.[54] One experiment tried to ascertain whether listeners could hear changes between a 'conserved voice' and a 'released voice' when the voice was used under the influence of different moods.[55] There were also experiments which sought to discover whether the emotions of anger, fear, happiness, jealousy, love, nervousness, pride, sadness, satisfaction and sympathy could be heard in the voice[56] and whether these qualities could be ascertained from spoken letters of the alphabet[57] and from numerals[58] when spoken with the deliberate simulation of various feelings. Others sought to discover whether isolated letters[59] or phonetic sounds[60] convey any accurate psychological information about the vocalist, whether deaf people draw the same emotional inferences from reading such phonetic sounds as those gained by hearing people when listening to them uttered,[61] whether the vocal sound of laughter conveys psychological information[62] and whether certain vocal sounds convey the feeling of joy.[63]

In order to ascertain whether listeners could judge accurately the personality of a person from their voice alone, the experimenters obviously had to have an allegedly accurate profile of the personality against which to compare listener's assessments. To formulate this, the experimenters subjected vocalists to a series of psychological tests which were believed to produce an accurate personality description. These included such famous tests as the Maslow Social Personality Inventory,[64] the Bell Adjustment Inventory,[65] the Bernreuter Personality Inventory,[66] the Turstone Intelligence Test, the Heidbreder Personal Traits Rating Scale, the Allport A-S Reaction Study,[67] the Allport and Vernon Study of Values,[68] the Wisconsin Scale of Personality,[69] the Flanagan Sociability Scale and the Hollingshead Two Factor Index of Status Position.[70] However, McKelvey[71] and Tyler[72] have pointed out how many of these personality tests have problems which render their use as the objective criteria in experiments questionable. Campbell also pointed out that no 'criterion is available as a perfect measure or defining operation against which to check listeners' assessment of the personality behind a voice.[73] In the light of this, it was suggested that the existence of stereotypes across 4000 listeners in experiments conducted by Pear may be of more importance than findings wrongly conceived as objective within fewer judges.[74]

But the most consistent discovery, and the most overwhelming deduction, which researchers extracted from these experiments was that the degree to which listeners agreed with one another about the imagined personality or emotion behind the voice was always far in excess of the degree to which their imaginings corresponded to the actual personality and condition of the vocalist. That is to say that many of the volunteer listeners colluded in hearing within the voices established stereotypes rather than correctly ascertaining the vocalist's nature.[75] Thus whilst certain aspects of personality may be expressed by the voice, the widespread stereotypical judgments far exceed the reliable ability to accurately perceive the person through the voice.[76] Therefore, the only accurate general conclusion to such experimentation is that 'all correlations need to be verified before we have any reason for believing that there is a relationship between voice and personality of predicative value'.[77]

Stereotype and Projection

The psychological experiments of the twentieth century have shown how the conclusion we draw about someone based upon their voice often has little to do with the person's actual personality and much more to do with a stereotype or a subjective association in the form of an image.

For example, one stereotype is predicated on the assumption that breathiness or a high degree of free air in a woman's voice reveals a high sexual appetite. Consequently, many listeners may perceive a vocalist with high free air as erotically stimulating or as intending to be so. Moreover, some women may consciously or subconsciously increase or decrease free air depending on the image they want to present, thereby manipulating a known stereotype with their voice.[78] In fact, there is evidence to show that identifiable changes in voice quality do occur in women when they are with intimate companions[79] and particular vocal qualities are often utilised in combination with certain clothing, gestures and facial expressions to communicate attractiveness.[80] However, the presence of free air in the voice by no means always indicates libidinous factors.

In addition to the sensual voice, another common pair of stereotypes is what has been called the 'childish'[81] or 'babyish'[82] voice on the one hand and the 'wise' or 'mature' voice on the other.[83] This reflects the two sides of an archetypal construct composed of the puer and senex, that is the eternal youth, or *Puer Aeternus*,[84] and the wise old figure, or *Senex*,[85] respectively. Both old and young age are usually asociated with a voice with a high degree of violin but, again, the images of infant and sage may well reside in the ear of the beholder.

However, it is, nonetheless, by way of stereotypical assumptions based upon the sound of our voice that people make judgments about our character and upon which they make their decisions with regard to how to treat us. It seems that 'as soon as we open our mouths and speak we are judged' in such a way that 'assumptions are made' about 'our intelligence', 'background, class, race', 'education' and other qualities and abilities'.[86] Consequently, changing the sound of the voice tends to change the way we are received.

Among the researchers of psychological experiments with voice there were those who were enthused by the prospect that certain 'personality mal-adjustments' could be resolved by changing the sound of the person's voice.[87] It was also said that the voice teacher 'must take into consideration' the fact that often a 'vocal habit results from a general style or pattern of social adjustment' and that 'correction' of such a voice 'may involve psychological procedures, since in order to make fundamental changes in voice, readjust-ments may have to be made in related characteristics of personality'.[88]

But the actual findings of the research imply more that 'certain kinds of voices which are not definitely defective, but which carry to listeners the inference of an unpleasant personality' may be changed through Therapeutic Voicework in such a way as to provoke change in the 'attitude of listeners' in response to the person's speech, rather than effecting change in the vocalist's personality.[89]

Indeed, in my experience, many people come for Therapeutic Voicework not because they wish to effect change of their Self through the voice but because they wish to alter the misconceived and stereotypical perception which others have of them, based upon the sound of their voice.

Self-Image and Self-Perception

Often, the presence of a particular vocal quality influences not only the way a listener perceives the personality but the way the vocalist perceives herself and can enforce a certain image through 'vocal self perception'.[90] Changing this voice, therefore, has the potential to change the way one perceives one-self.[91] This quality that gives a voice its unique image serves an important function in maintaining a sense of identity for the sound of our voice reminds us of who we are, it affirms and reinforces our sense of Self. In the same way that our sense of identity is continually reaffirmed by the visual reflection provided by a mirror, so too the sound of our voice enables us to hear reflected an audible expression of our own image, our own sense of Self.

As time passes, we often become over-identified with a single image of ourselves. This monocentric self-image is revealed physically in our habitual body language: the way we walk, sit, turn, the way we eat, drink, indeed all of our kinetic activities. It is also revealed in the quality of our voice. This becomes particularly apparent when a person has been informed and effected by a more or less severe set of experiences. In such cases a person's thinking, feeling and behaviour, indeed their whole psyche, may come to be dominated and saturated with a particular emotional tone such as bitterness, defeat, anxiety, fear or rage and all of these emotional tones find their expression in the acoustic tones of the voice.

In addition, a person's psyche may become dominated by a single image of itself as a particular character. A person may become 'stuck' in a childlike image, in a dominating and bombastic image, in a kindly and self-effacing image – often because of an over-identification with a particularly influential person. These character images also find expression through the quality of vocal tones. Often, this vocal manifestation of identification can be heard in young children, who, whilst playing with their peers, assume tones of voice and turns of phrases which are obviously a direct inheritance from their parents and which sit uneasily in their young mouths.

Because the echo of the tone of our own voice in our own ears is so important in reaffirming our own image, we become caught in a vicious circle by which the bitterness or anxiety which we hear in our voice serves only to reinforce the image of ourselves as bitter or anxious, by which the childlikeness or aggressiveness which we hear in our voice reinforces our idea of our self as a child or an aggressor. If a person's psyche becomes saturated with a single emotional tone, it may become difficult for that person to communicate and the voice can, without warning, simply let them down. They may wish to express a particular emotion or image, such as anger or authority, or they may need to instil confidence or calm, but their voice has become so identified with a particular aspect of themselves that it cannot move. Often, this can cause the person some distress, it is as though their voice has become a rigid mask which they are unable to remove, reminding us of the original meaning of the word 'personality' which referred to the sound passing through the mouth hole in the mask worn in ancient Greek theatre. A person with such a mask may feel mature but sound childlike, may feel enraged but sound intimidated, may feel saddened but sound unmoved, they seek help but their voice signals self-certainty, they seek warmth and affection but their voice signals guarded detachment, they seek respect but their voice attracts belittlement. What Therapeutic Voicework can offer is an opportunity to step outside the fixity of accustomed vocal masks and reanimate a vocal malleability.[92] Psychologically, this can enable a person to visit and express those parts of herself which have hitherto remained undercover.

It was Weiss who first stated that the voice creates a certain image in the ears of the vocalist and that Voicework could, by transforming this voice, also effect changes in the sense of self.[93] It is this process that is crucial to Therapeutic Voicework.

In Therapeutic Voicework the practitioner is not exempt from projecting an array of stereotypical judgements onto the client, which may well not represent her actual personality. All of the practitioner's stereotypical judgments, idiosyncratic perceptions and unique interpretations are consequently bound to effect the way the process unfolds. Therefore, a viable model of Therapeutic Voicework can only be predicated on an understanding and a use of the practitioner's own perceptions of what he hears, or what he thinks he hears. Therapeutic Voicework, as I conceive of it, emanates from the practitioner's willingness to engage with his own intuitive and subjective responses to the client's voice on the assumption that they may well not necessarily reflect the so-called true personality of the client. In other words, Therapeutic Voicework takes place within the transference and counter-transference between practitioner and client.

Transference and Counter-Transference

Singing and non-verbal sound making provides an immediate expression of affect in a form of utmost vitality. As the Therapeutic Voiceworker witnesses the process, the client, meanwhile, exposes and reveals a grand pantheon of emotion through sounds which may range from the expression of grief to extreme joy. Consequently, the Therapeutic Voiceworker's subjective associations will often be highly intense, exposed as he or she is to a continuously highly charged affective field sustained by the client's vocalisations.

At times, these feelings which the Therapeutic Voiceworker may have can be frightening because they may lead him or her to all kinds of imaginings with regard to the client's experience, which often take the form of vivid imagery. The Therapeutic Voiceworker may look at and listen to the client and imagine the vocalist as a dying swan, a raging bull, a sweet maiden, a bitter witch, a king or queen. The Therapeutic Voiceworker may also be reminded of images from their own life; the client may seem to compare to the Therapeutic Voiceworker's aunt or uncle, sister or friend. But, far from being an intrusion or unwanted occurrence, these imaginative experiences and emotional responses which the professional therapist or Therapeutic Voiceworker has in response to the client are, as Heimann says, 'the most important tools for his work' because they are 'an instrument of research into the patient's unconscious' and 'if we try to work without consulting such feelings and experiences' our work 'can only be poor'.[94] In psychotherapy, these associations, images, feelings and experiences which a therapist has in response to a client are called the counter-transference.

Sigmund Freud proposed that the patient in psychoanalysis uses the analyst and her relationship to him as the means by which to reactivate and revisit strong feelings and patterns of response which originate in childhood experiences of early relationships. By observing the emotive patterns by which the patient responded to the analyst, Freud believed he could see mirrored the same patterns which the patient had learned to use in order to cope with earlier relationships, particularly those with the parents. Freud called this transfer of feelings and responses from the relationship with early primary figures to the relationship with the analyst the 'transference' and defined it as being composed of 'facsimiles' of 'feelings', 'tendencies', 'phantasies' and 'a whole series of psychological experiences' which were originally experienced towards a figure of the past but which are 'revived', 'aroused' and 'made conscious during the progress of the analysis' where they are re-experienced towards the analyst in 'the present moment' as though he were a conglomeration of those original primary people.[95]

Just as the patient revives past experiences in the form of behavioural responses to the analyst, so too the analyst, by nature of being human, is predisposed to transfer his feelings and habitual patterns of retort onto the relationship with the patient. This is called counter-transference. Racker has clarified the meaning of counter-transference, describing it as 'the totality of the analyst's psychological response' to the patient which is composed of a 'fusion of present and past, the continuous and intimate connection of reality and phantasy, of external and internal, conscious and unconscious'.[96]

Though transference and counter-transference were originally conceived as dynamics central to the psychoanalytic consultation, they are also operative in many other professional, social and intimate arenas. Transference and counter-transference may be observed between actor and director, between lovers, between chiropractor and client and between singing teacher and student. The transferential dimension is also highly active within the Therapeutic Voicework session.

In fact, it is from the Therapeutic Voiceworker's counter transference that he or she draws ideas and interpretations which provide the ground for positive work. Such a process is of great value providing that the practitioner can sustain a sense of difference between the counter-transference and objective factors.

In the training of psychotherapists this is achieved by two means. First, the therapist becomes the patient in their own therapy where they discover those incentives and persuasions which they hold most dear, in order that they may refrain from interpreting their patient's text according to their want. By undergoing their own therapy, the practitioner can come to a level of insight regarding the idiosyncratic sources upon which their interpretations are based. Second, when they begin to work with their own clients, they attend supervision where they can discuss their client case load. Both of these processes serve to make the practitioner aware of their own patterns of emotive interlocution in order that they may refrain from projecting them onto the patient and seeing them where they do not really exist, other than as a reflection of themselves. This leaves the therapist free to receive the transference of the client, so that he or she may trust that the experiences which he or she undergoes in response to the client's expressions are in some measure a result of their effect upon him or her.

The importance of the psychotherapist's ability to refrain from projecting his own psychological material onto the patient's expressions applies equally to the art therapist's analysis of the visual image. It also applies no less to the dramatherapist's analytic scrutiny of the psychological dynamics expressed through dramatic action. Most apposite to this study, moreover, is that it particularly applies to the voice because, as we saw from the data previously presented, the qualities which most listeners believe they hear in the voice usually have no relationship to the personality of the vocalist at all but reveal only the listener's counter-transference.

Transference and Art

It was Melanie Klein, whose particular contribution to psychoanalysis was that she pioneered the means to analyse children, and who resultingly instigated an understanding of the transference within an artistic context. Because a detailed fluency of verbal discourse was not the most available form of communication with her young patients, she introduced another element: play. Klein invited children to play with toys, to paint or to draw and to talk to her simultaneously so she might understand what the child was displaying with pen and paper or with a particular arrangement of dolls. Klein observed how inanimate objects came to represent parts of the child's own body as well as other people and the child's relationship to them and it was the interpretation of the nature, structure and intentions inherent in play that yielded the analysis.

This introduction of a new element to the therapeutic procedure also generated new channels of communication. Now there was not only the verbal disclosure between patient and therapist but also the active relating between patient and play object, between therapist and play object and the therapist's interpretive analysis of that dynamic.

Klein's pioneering work with children's play and the psychodynamics therein is highly relevant to the operational framework of art therapy, where there are also three lines of communication: 'between therapist and client, client and painting, therapist and painting'.[97] In art therapy the canvas acts as the blank screen upon which the contents of psychological functioning may be given visual representation and the therapist's analytical conclusions regarding the patient's predicament come as much from an interpretation of the visual image as they do from the decoding of the patient's text about the painting.

The demands upon the art therapist's faculties of interpretation therefore differ from those which are placed upon the psychotherapist. The former must be familiar with the non-discursive characteristics of visual imagery whilst the latter is continually drenched in the discursive nature of linguistic dialogue.

One of the first art therapists to be influenced by psychoanalytic principles, Margaret Naumberg, said that the 'process of art therapy is based on the recognition that man's most fundamental thoughts and feelings, derived from the unconscious, reach expression in images rather than words'[98] and the skill of the analytically-orientated art therapist rests in the ability to interpret the psychological significance of these images without projecting onto the canvas aspects of his or her own pathology – that is without a negative counter-transference. For Hillman, the insight necessary to highlight the multitudinous resonances of the images requires of the therapist a special kind of perceptive faculty that has more to do with artistic erudition and aesthetics than with clinical proficiency in the analytic scrutiny of words. He says that in seeking for a training for therapists who work with image, 'we are forced toward the field of those who are specialists in images – the field of aesthetics in its broadest sense'.[99] For those training in Therapeutic Voicework, therefore, perhaps the most significant aspect of their own therapeutic process consists of their work on their own voice with another Therapeutic Voiceworker, where they can experience their own psyche expressed through acoustic images.

The Politics of Transference

These issues relating to the therapist's counter-transference with an artistic object are also pertinent to any voice practitioner's response to a client's artistic expressions through voice and song, in as much as a client of Voicework paints through vocal sound. The socially endorsed stereotypes according to which we hear voices are also present in the way we listen to music, which makes the music therapist equally vulnerable to an interfering counter-transference for 'we may never be sure that the description of the client's music which the therapist suggests is the same as given by the client himself'.[100]

In music the differing cultural perceptions of instrumentation and song styles is particularly informed by the ethnicity of the context. For example, the use of falsetto may, for many, imply a feminisation within the confines of a Western European and classical perception of music, yet it would have no such connotations in other cultural environments. Ruth Bright has pointed to the necessity of remembering such cultural aspects of music therapy and asserts that the particular tastes of the therapist are informed by cultural mores and reflect class, ethnic origin and other factors.[101] Admitting the presence and influence of a cultural, and, therefore, political, dimension to the therapist's responses transposes the counter-transference, and, therefore, the entire therapeutic encounter, from an allegedly apolitical framework and replaces it in a highly politicised structure.

The political nature of the counter-transference, and of psychotherapy generally, is investigated in the work of British psychotherapist Andrew Samuels, who challenges Jung on his neglect of 'economic, social, political and historical factors' in the formation of individual psychological predicaments. Samuels also challenges contemporary Jungian psychotherapists, many of whom, he says, maintain 'the tendency to see all outer events in terms of inner, usually archetypal dynamics' without recourse to sociopolitical factors as a separate and influential reality which has a bearing upon psychic reality.[102]

A common tendency in contemporary writing in the tradition of Jung is to use fairy-tales and legends taken from every conceivable culture, the characters and images of which are proposed to be reflections of the inner workings of the psyche. Yet, as Zipes points out, even the seemingly apolitical European fairy-tales by Grimm and Hans Anderson have a societal origination, a political motif and therefore deserve a sociopolitical analysis if their psychological meaning is to be appreciated in a viable context of holistic reality[103] for fairy-tales have been used to control, subjugate and delude as much as they have inspired and reflected psychic reality.[104] Marina Warner also draws attention to the political significance of fairy-tales and their tellers, pointing to the way in which they serve as hidden messages in times of censorship and as verbal weapons and curses of the disenfranchised and disarmed, particularly for women.[105]

One of the reasons that artistic and therapeutic expression should be allowed their political nature is that it is often the divestment and evaporation of political issues that facilitates a restricting and inaccurate analysis of issues relating to gender. For example, in the realm of classical European singing, the nature of beauty dominates the standards by which vocal quality is judged and the politics of beauty always make themselves visible through Therapeutic Voicework. Particularly for women, the conception of beauty perpetuated by media culture and consisting of a specific optical image, usually white-skinned, thin and blonde, is associated with a specific acoustic tone and timbre, usually high in pitch with a lot of free air in falsetto. This 'beauty myth' is, as Naomi Wolf has pointed out, often a stifling form of political and psychological oppression.[106] Therefore, any therapeutic process aiming to facilitate liberation should presumably be both a political and psychological process in which the professional practitioner refrains from imposing any set of aesthetic, social or attitudinal precepts.

Working with Image

Because in the Therapeutic Voicework session we must, in my view, have the humility to remember that we are in the realm of the transference and not of objective diagnostics, the practitioner requires a mode of discourse, a dimension of experience which turns this into a positive and openly acknowledged investigation of subjective perception. And, in my view, the language of this interaction is constituted of images.

Jung paid particular attention to the way in which no bodily action or mental thought can be brought to consciousness unless it takes the form of an image by which it can be represented in the psyche.[107] Jung did not make any distinction between a psychic content and an image, neither did he differentiate between psychological processes and the faculty of imagination because, for Jung, 'every psychic process is an image' and an 'imagining', otherwise 'no consciousness could exist' for 'imagination is itself a psychic process'[108] and 'the psyche consists essentially of images', that is to say that 'it is a picturing of vital activity'.[109]

The prime example of the appearance of these images is the dream, where they take the form of optical impressions seemingly etched upon the inner surface of our eyes and recaptured the following day through our verbal recollections. This process of dreaming is not only a psychological function but a creative process of the imagination. Because images are the language of the psyche, any process of imaginative creativity is by nature also a process of psychological investigation. This is the hub of Jung's Analytical Psychology. For Jung, 'not the artist alone, but every creative individual whatsoever owes all that is greatest in his life to fantasy' and, furthermore, 'the dynamic principle of fantasy is play' without which 'no creative work has ever yet come to birth'. For Jung, it is, therefore, 'in the imagination that a man's highest value may lie'.[110]

The function of the strategic relationship between therapist and patient in Jung's view of psychotherapy is to stimulate this 'creative work' by which the imagination may be encouraged to fantasise, actively imagining and amplifying the contents of the psyche in words, as an artist is wont to do with paint upon the canvas. There is, therefore, an aspect of this relationship which is fundamentally akin to playing. As Winnicott has said: 'psychotherapy has to do with two people playing together'[111] and the materials of this play are images. It is this aspect of the therapeutic relationship that has been deliberately intensified in art therapy, where the interaction between client and therapist is essentially playful and in which imagery is given optical and plastic representation in two or three dimensional colour.[112] In Therapeutic Voicework we are working with images through sound.

Image and Body, Feeling and Voice

One of the most inspiring fields of research to have altered the face of therapeutic and medicinal procedures in the twentieth century is the use of image and imagination to alter the client's state of physical and mental health and one of the crucial modalities from which we are able to draw support for the curative function of imagination is that of biofeedback.

In biofeedback the client is subjected to a number of objective measurement procedures, such as pulse, heart rate, pupil dilation, muscle tension, blood glucose, salivation, adrenalin, thyroxine release and respiratory pattern, whilst he or she is asked to imagine certain positive or negative situations, occurrences or experiences. What such experiments show is that imagined phenomenon have exactly the same effect on the body as one would expect of the real event, only in variously lesser proportion.

As early as 1929, Jacobsen discovered that if a person simply thinks intensely about a particular movement, the motor neurons appropriate to that action are fired but to a lesser intensity than would accompany the movement if it were mechanically enacted.[113] Similarly, it was discovered that imagining the eating of a lemon, for example, increases the activity of the saliva glands.[114] Because of this relationship between imagined experience and body reaction, the imagination can be positively exploited to assist in the healing process by deliberately calling into mind images of occurrences, phenomena or experiences which deplete the strength of the illness and foster the immune system's deterring abilities.[115] Furthermore, because the patient can witness changes in physiology as recorded on technological devices, they can actually train the body to adjust a web of neurological activities for the purpose of healing and such methods have been used effectively to treat a wide spectrum of dysfunctions, including migraine, circulatory disorders, asthma, arthritis, menstrual difficulties and diabetes, all of which are recorded in the *Quarterly Journal of Biofeedback and Self Regulation*.[116] This process of self-training by the patient has been given the modern term 'Autogenic Training'[117] but, in fact, originates in the shamanic practices of indigenous non-Western communities.[118]

The use of image has also had an increasing clinical role in the alleviation of neuroses within the psychotherapies,[119] where the research shows an impressively successful application in the alleviation of a number of problems, including phobias, anxieties, sexual problems, depression, drug and alcohol abuse.[120] Within this field, the general nomenclature used to cover the application of image is 'Guided Affective Imagery', a term first used in 1954 by Leuner[121], whose work instigated the augmentation of an International Society for Guided Affective Imagery. Here the therapists asks the client to close his eyes and imagine himself in an environment populated by certain elemental pictures, such as a meadow, a house or a river. The patient describes the particular details which characterise his or her particular idiosyncratic vision of the elemental image and the therapist may suggest certain events or obstacles, arrivals or departures which the patient visualises and imagines confronting.

Such therapeutic use of imagery in Europe may be traced back to a sequence of therapists beginning with Janet, who, in the 1890s, discovered that images which Freud later referred to as 'hysterical symptoms' could be changed through suggestion.[122] Following Janet, Freud himself evoked images in patients whilst pressing their forehead with his thumb and took advantage of the client's imagistic thinking by allowing them to spontaneously verbalise their inner imaginings. In the footsteps of Freud, Jung further developed techniques which encouraged the client's spontaneous articulation of imagery. More recently, Joseph Reyher[123] and Joseph Shorr[124] have both elaborated upon these classic techniques. In addition, Alfred Binet, famous for his intelligence tests, encouraged patients to converse with their visual images whilst in a semi-hypnotic state which he called 'provoked introspection', believing that the images revealed deep unconscious propensities. Binet's technique was further developed during the 1920s in Germany by Carl Happich, who introduced meditation, muscular relaxation and breathwork, moving Binet's Provoked Introspection into a deeper state of unconscious processing which Happich called a 'meditative zone'.[125] In France, meanwhile, Eugene Caslant used imagery to help his clients replace habitual fixations and mental constraints with images which could assist in personal growth[126] and, after the Second World War, Robert Desoille developed his '*le rêve éveillé dirigé* 'or 'directed daydream' method, which drew on the earlier work of Freud, Jung and Caslant.[127] In addition, Eugene Gendlin developed a method which uses image to move a general problem to a stage where the core of it can be perceived via representative images, a process which Gendlin calls 'Focusing'.[128] It was thus from quite a rich tradition of fantasy and imagery work that Hans Leuner emerged with Guided Affective Imagery. It is from the same tradition that the image-based technique known as 'Eidetic Psychotherapy' was developed by Anees Sheikh[129] and Akhter Ashen[130] and it is against the background of this tradition that Roberto Assagioli[131] founded the psychotherapeutic modality known as 'Psychosynthesis' and whose work on imagery influenced the development of Transpersonal Psychology.

In addition to the use of image in psychotherapy, however, imagery has been used by singing teachers to effect positive changes in the use of voice for hundreds of years and probably constitutes the singing teacher's most frequently used tool and a number of practitioners have investigated its use specifically within the context of Therapeutic Voicework.

Voice, Image and Ideokinetics

In 1942 William Faulkner discovered that suggesting imaginary situations of a pleasant or unpleasant quality affected the activity of the oesophagus, the diaphragm, the nature of the breathing and the audible characteristics of the voice. He proposed that the 'range of diaphragmatic movement in patients can be altered by suggesting situations which arouse strong emotions. If these emotions are pleasant they cause increased amplitude of diaphragmatic movement; while the unpleasant type restrict it.'[132]

Jellineck also used guided imagery in which 'the subject closes his eyes and reports aloud to a listener what he sees as it appears before him'. Using this technique, he enabled singers to hold in mind 'vivid pictures' of their 'ideal of perfect singing' and found that 'when these pictures are recalled before a later performance', the singer's function is at its best.'[133] Jellineck also found some success in relieving vocal disorders, such as stammering and improving voice quality, through the use of imagery by which he observed 'the psychotherapeutic effect inherent in the success of vocal rehabilitation', stating that 'rehabilitation of the voice' through 'correction of the faulty vocal technique' and 'reestablishment of technical competence' is 'often sufficient to relieve the subject's anxiety' and 'frequently brings back the patient's self confidence and equilibrium'.[134]

The most widespread type of imagery used in training the voice is ideokinetic, which means the images are mechanical and structural rather than emotional or figurative. Ideokinesis is an educational method by which kinesthetic imagery, that is images of the body in motion, are used to stimulate specific muscular responses. The purpose of ideokinesis is to encourage a client to use the body in a way synonymous with the organic and healthy functioning of anatomical mechanics. Given the complexity and inconceivability of these mechanical processes to many clients, ideokinesis translates them into pictures based on everyday experience. Ideokinesis, therefore, denotes the 'psycho-physical process in which imagery and kinesthetic sense stimulate bodily change.'[135]

Ideokinesis has been most widely used in the teaching of dance and originates in the work of Mabel Todd, who proposed that the teacher should come to understand the precise mechanical operations of the muscular and skeletal system and then be able to translate these complex operations into simple kinetic images.[136] Her premise was that 'concentration upon a picture involving movement results in responses in the neuromusculature as necessary to carry out specific movements with the least effort'.[137] Todd called this process 'psychophysical and psychophysiological'.

The legacy of Todd's work gave rise to a new generation of dancers and movement teachers, including Barbara Clark[138] and Lulu Sweigard,[139] as well as being used by music and voice teachers,[140] amongst whom the term ideokinesis became the accepted one to describe this process of using anatomically grounded images to cultivate healthy human movement.

One of the contemporary leaders in the field of ideokinetic dance education, who trained many of the British Post-modern dancers of the 1980s and early 1990s, is Mary Fulkerson, with whom I studied for four years.[141] Taking Fulkerson's techniques of enabling the dancer to conceive of the skeleton in motion through strong mental images, I was led to investigate the use of imagination to focus on the physical movements of the vocal tract. It was this work which led me to identify the vocal tract configurations of flute, clarinet and saxophone and their consequent acoustic timbres which form the methodological approach to Therapeutic Voicework which I have implemented. The discovery of this system was also made possible because I was able to observe the movements of the larynx and pharynx as I vocalised by way of a fibre optic camera.[142]

Of course, most voice workers instinctively know the value of ideokinesis and understand that the most essential key to extricating the voice from constriction is the ability to use images which the client can translate into liberated vocal activity. However, the problem has been that in the absence of knowledge with regard to the physiological operation of the vocal instrument, many voice teachers throughout history have constructed ideokinetic images on their illusion of physiology, with the result of confusing students and mitigating against a shared understanding of vocal function.

There is, consequently, a widespread terminology used by vocal practitioners of all orientations which bears no relation to objective analysis and often originates in a subjective interpretation of voice quality and 'the terms used to describe voice quality vary not only between professions' but also within 'the medical profession' and 'amongst clinicians of the same discipline'.[143] Voice teachers have, therefore, stumbled along in the dark, unaided by the internal terminological conflicts of physiology. Such teachers have become highly imaginative in their intuitions, by which they, 'like medical clinicians themselves', have 'become very adept at handling processes' of which they have little objective understanding.[144]

Often, the images used by voice and singing teachers take poetic liberties with physiological evidence. They translate the discursive language of science into the non-discursive symbols of colour, shape, form, mood, action and, above all, sensation. One medical doctor has pointed out that 'the semantics of singing have used descriptions of the sensations a sound gives the vocalist', which are purely subjective and which 'may mean one action to one pupil but something different to another'. However, she states that 'the effect is real in producing physiological adjustments'. She points out that 'scientific appraisal has often taken singing terms literally and discredited them as not meaning what they say', the best known example being the idea of 'singing from the diaphragm', which is physiologically meaningless 'but often a good term to convey an action to a pupil'. The 'brain takes instructions in terms of collections of actions it recognises from experience and not individually, muscle by muscle, like an anatomy book'. Therefore, 'teaching phrases cannot use direct physiological jargon' for 'what pupil could respond to requests' which ask him, for example, to 'alter the opening quotient of your larynx please'. The fact that 'the languages of vocal training and science are not the same does not invalidate methods of teaching singing but the differences may lead to a mutual suspicion between disciplines'.[145] In my view, this suspicion between disciplines can only be dissolved through collaboration and inter-professional co-operation and by a compromise of language between disciplines which describes vocal function in terms comprehensible by all.

As a result of interdisciplinary communication, some voice teachers are beginning to model their teaching style on an ideokinetic model, such as the work of Arthur Samuel Joseph in the USA, who believes that an understanding of the physiological processes which govern voice production 'helps us design efficient methods of training the voice'[146] and that the subtle semantics of voice teaching are crucial to good instruction.[147] Joseph also exemplifies a teacher who works within a system which accepts that Voicework 'brings up a whole panoply of psychological barriers' based on issues such as 'voice and sexuality' and 'voice and identity'.[148] He says that 'if the eyes are the windows of the soul, then the voice opens that window'. Like many contemporary practitioners, he believes that 'vocal work enriches our understanding of ourselves' by unearthing 'hidden feelings' revealing fully 'our moods, our fears, our tensions and our emotions'.[149]

The difference between ideokinesis and the application of a wide range of imagistic suggestions, such as those used by Faulkner, Jellineck, Assagioli and others, is that Ideokinesis, as Todd and her students conceived of it, utilises images of a strictly mechanical nature. It is a non-emotive process. But ideokinesis is only one type or genre of imagery, that which is based in anatomy and mechanical movement. The work of Faulkner and Jellineck took the principles of Ideokinesis beyond the realms of anatomy and drew upon images of all kinds, emotional, figurative and sensory, to influence vocal function, suggesting to the client an environment populated by objects, characters and animals and often attempting to provoke in the client particular emotions.

The hypothesis which I assert is that ideokinetic and mechanical imagery based upon physiological function *stimulates* emotional reaction because it is through the motion of the physiology that feelings are expressed. Muscular activity is the physical result of feeling activity and, simultaneously, feelings are stimulated by physical movement; motion and emotion are conjoined.[150] Moreover, nowhere is the convergence of muscularity and emotionality so apparent as in the mechanism of singing, where feeling gives rise to muscular action which, in turn, expresses feeling.[151]

The aim of the work which I have developed is to synthesise ideokinetic work with a careful use of images drawn from the practitioner's counter-transference which help the client unfix the mask of rigid self-image and facilitate the development of a flexible sense of Self comprising different elements through the acquisition of a malleable vocal range. At the core of this synthesis is the principle of the inseparable inter-connection between ideokinetic image, the mechanical operation of the voice, the expression of emotion and the sense or perception of the Self.

Therapeutic Voicework Methodology:
Affective and Figurative Ideokinetic Process

Affective and Figurative Ideokinetic Process is the core and most important methodological principle which I have discovered.

The central component to the work which I have developed is the simple notion of the vocal tract as an expandable elastic tube which can be arbitrarily conceived as having three configurations: flute, clarinet and saxophone. The various configurations of the vocal tract, combined with the transience of other vocal component parameters, naturally changes the acoustic quality of the human voice. Because this acoustic quality contributes to the sense of Self, or self-perception, developing the malleabilty of vocal expression also expands the sense of Self. Because it is through the vocal sound that emotion is expressed, diversifying vocal quality also creates a sense of expressing a broader emotional field. Finally, because the nature of voice quality influences the way we are perceived, according to the subjective experience of those who listen to us, creating vocal malleabilty liberates the the vocalist from the confines of receiving constant stereotypical judgement.

Because the voice provokes such strong counter-transference in the practitioner, the ideokinetic tube and the other component vocal parameters offer the Therapeutic Voiceworker a reliable way of utilising the voice to probe and investigate the client's sense of Self and his perception of it through the realm of imagination, without the dangers of predicating the work on an unacknowledged counter-transference or inaccurate and inappropriate associations which are mistakenly assumed to be objective diagnostics.

For example, the client is not asked to sound less childlike but to sing with less free air or the client is not asked to increase aggression but to sing disruptively with high force of glottal attack. Of course, such requests which the practitioner makes of the client may well be based on his own counter-transference which perceives infantile regression or resistance and repression of anger. But the translation of these responses into ideokinetic activity offers a way of enabling him to draw from such counter-transference but to prevent them from acting directly on the client before they have been tested and related to the client's own self-perception.

As the work progresses, the client is invited to identify for herself the sense of character and emotional experience which she has during the vocalisation, which may or may not be connected to childishness or to lack of aggressive expression. When the practitioner is certain to have gained insight into the nature of the client's imagination, he can then furnish the client with details that flesh out, magnify and amplify the work, drawing from his own associative imagistic thinking, asking the client to imbue the sounds with certain figurative, emotive, physical, and synaesthetic images.

Based on my experience to date, I would say that this method of working has proved extremely useful for a number of different professionals who work with the voice.

Conclusion: Therapeutic Voicework, Voice Movement Therapy and Dissemination

In this chapter I have tried to outline the way that somatic, psychological and political issues intersect through the practice of Therapeutic Voicework and the way the practitioner can draw upon his or her own subjectivity and intuition to facilitate authentic self-expression.

In many ways, this completes the scope of this book, in which I have attempted to draw out the various dimensions to Therapeutic Voicework and locate them in a historical, theoretical and practical framework. There is, however, a subject which I have not covered: the issue of ethics.

Therapeutic Voicework is practised in the context of social processes and is, or should be, subject to the same scrutiny as any process of human interaction. Therapeutic Voicework needs to be predicated on ethical grounds and disseminated according to moral principles in keeping with compassion and integrity. Though such a subject is vast, I will, in the first Appendix, briefly outline some of the issues central to the subject of ethical dissemination in order, at least, to remind the reader of its importance.

Notes

1   Soskin, W.F. 'Some aspects of communication and interpretation in psychotherapy.' Paper read at American Psychological Association, panel on 'Communication in the Counselling Situation' (Cleveland: September, 1953).

2   Buhler, K. (1934) *Sprachtheorie.* Jena.

3   Sapir, E. (1927) 'Speech as a personality trait.' *American Journal of Sociology,* 32, 892–905.

4   Soskin, W.F. (1953) 'Some aspects of communication and interpretation in psychotherapy.' Paper read at American Psychological Association. Panel on Communication in the Counselling Situation. (Cleveland: September, 1953).

5   Skinner, B.F. (1957) *Verbal Behaviour.* New York: Appleton-Century-Crofts.

6   Sullivan, H.S. (1954) *The Psychiatric Interview.* New York: Norton, p.7.

7   Trager, G.L. (1958) 'Paralanguage: a first approximation.' *Studies in Linguistics,* 13, 1–12.

8   Ostwald, P.F. (1960) 'Human sounds.' In D. A. Barbara (ed) *Psychological and Psychiatric Aspects of Speech and Hearing.* Springfield, Illinois: Charles C Thomas.

9   Kauffman, P.E. (1954) 'An investigation of some psychological stimulus properties of speech behaviour.' Unpublished doctoral thesis, University of Chicago.

10   Moses, P.J. (1954) *The Voice of Neurosis.* New York: Grune and Stratton, p.5.

11   Moses, P.J. (1954) *The Voice of Neurosis.* New York: Grune and Stratton, p.8.

12   Bateson, G. (1987) *Steps to an Ecology of Mind.* USA: Aronson.

13   Lotz, J. (1955) *Linguistics: Symbols Make Humans* New York: Language and Communication Research Centre, Columbia University.

14   Hillman, J. (1978) 'Further notes on images.' *Spring: A Journal of Archetypal Psychology and Jungian Thought,* pp.152–82, (pp.158–59).

15   Hillman, J. (1977) 'An inquiry into image.' *Spring: A Journal of Archetypal Psychology and Jungian Thought,* pp.62–88, (p.82).

16   Kugler, P. (1978) 'Image and sound: an archetypal approach to language.' *Spring : A Journal of Archetypal Psychology and Jungian Thought,* pp.136–151.

17   Kugler, P. (1979) 'The phonetic imagination.' *Spring : A Journal of Archetypal Psychology and Jungian Thought,* pp.118–129.

18 Wagoner, L.C. (1925) 'Speech as an indication of temperamental traits.' *Quarterly Journal of Speech Education*, 2, pp.237–242.

19 Rieffert, J.B. (1931) 'Sprechtypen.' *12th Kongr. Ges. Psychol.*, pp.409–413.

20 Ostwald, P.F. (1973) *The Semiotics of Human Sound.* The Hague and Paris: Mouton.

21 Soskin, W.F. and Kauffman, P.E. (1961) 'Judgment of emotion in word-free voice samples.' *Journal of Communication*, 11, 2, pp.73–80.

22 Kauffman, P.E. (1954) 'An investigation of some psychological stimulus properties of speech behaviour.' Unpublished doctoral thesis, University of Chicago.

23 Starkweather, J.A. (1956) 'The communication value of content-free speech.' *American Journal of Psychology*, 69, pp.121–123.
Starkweather, J.A. (1956) 'Content-free speech as a source of information about the speaker.' *Journal of Abnormal Psychology*, 52, pp.394–402.

24 Pear, T.H. *Radio Times.* 14 January 1927.

25 Pear, T.H. (1931) *Voice and Personality.* New York: Wiley, p.28.

26 Eisenberg, P. and Zalowitz, E. (1938) 'Judging expressive movement: iii. judgments of dominance-feeling from phonograph records of voice.' *Journal of Applied Psychology*, 22, pp.620–31.

27 Michael, W. and Crawford, C.C. (1927) 'An experiment in judging intelligence by the voice.' *Journal of Educational Psychology*, 18, pp.107–114.

28 Fay, P.J. and Middleton, W.C. (1940) 'Judgment of intelligence from the voice as transmitted over a public address system.' *Sociometry*, 3, pp.186–91.

29 Harms, L.S. (1961) 'Listener judgments of status cues in speech.' *Quarterly Journal of Speech*, 47, no.2, pp.164–168.

30 Stagner, R. (1936) 'Judgments of voice and personality.' *Journal of Educational Psychology*, 27, pp.272–277, (p.276).

31 Fay, P.J. and Middleton, W.C. (1942) 'Judgment of introversion from the transcribed voice as transmitted over a public address system.' *Quarterly Journal of Speech*, 28, no.2, pp.226–28.

32 Fay, P.J. and Middleton, W.C. (1943) 'Judgment of leadership from the transcribed voice.' *Journal of Social Psychology*, 17, pp.99–102.

33 Fay, P.J. and Middleton, W.C. (1941) 'The ability to judge sociability from the voice as transmitted over a public address system.' *Journal of Social Psychology*, 13, pp.303–309.

34 Fay, P.J. and Middleton, W.C. (1941) 'The ability to judge truth-telling or lying from the voice as transmitted over a public address system.' *Journal of General Psychology*, 24, pp.211–215.

35 Wolff, W. (1930) 'Ueber faktoren characterologischen urteilsbildung.' *Zsch. F. Angrew. Psychol.*, 35, pp.385–446.

36 Bonaventura, M. (1935) 'Ausdruck der personlichkeit in der sprechtstimme und im photogramm.' *Arch. Gen. Psychol.*, 94, pp.501–570.

37 Taylor, H.C. (1934) 'Social agreement on personality traits as judged from speech.' *Journal of Social Psychology*, 5, pp.244–248.

38 Wolff, W. (1950) 'Voice and personality.' In *The Expression of Personality.* New York: Hermitage House, pp.43–58, (p.55).

39 Spranger, E. (1928) *Types of Men.* Halle (Saale): Niemeyer, p.402.

40 Fay, P.J. and Middleton, W.C. (1939) 'Judgment of Spranger personality types from the voice as transmitted over a public address system.' *Character & Personality*, 8, pp.144–155.

41   Kretschmer, E. (1925) *Physique and Character*. New York: Harcourt and Brace, p.266.

42   McGehee, F. (1937) 'The reliability of the identification of the human voice.' *Journal of General Psychology*, 17, pp.249–271.

43   Fairbanks, G. and Pronovost, W. (1938) 'Vocal pitch during simulated emotion.' (Preliminary report), *Science*, 8, pp.382–383.

44   Lynch, G.E. (1934) 'A phonophotographic study of trained and untrained voices reading factual and dramatic material.' *Archives of Speech*, 1, pp.9–25, (p18).

45   Skinner, E.R. (1935) 'A calibrated recording and analysis of the pitch, force and quality of vocal tones expressing happiness and sadness.' *Speech Monograph*, MIZ vol. 2.

46   Costanzo, F., Markel, N. and Costanzo, P. (1969) 'Voice quality profile and perceived emotion.' *Journal of Counselling Psychology*, 16, pp.267–70.

47   Addington, D. (1968) 'The relationship of selected vocal characteristics to personality perception.' *Speech Monographs*, 35, pp.492–503.

48   Apple, W., Streeter, L. and Krauss, R. (1979) 'Effects of pitch and speech rate on personal attributions.' *Journal of Personality and Social Psychology*, 37, pp.715–27.

49   Duncan, M.H. (1945) 'An experimental study of some of the relationships between voice and personality among students of speech.' *Speech Monograph*, M107, 12, pp.47–60, (p.59).

50   Eldred, S.H. and Price, D.B. (1958) 'A linguistic evaluation of feeling states in psychotherapy.' *Psychiatry*, 21, pp.115–21.

51   Moore, W.E. (1939) 'Personality traits and voice quality deficiencies.' *Journal of Speech Disorders*, 4, pp.33–36.

52   Glasgow, G.M. (1944) 'The effects of nasality on oral communication.' *Quarterly Journal of Speech*, 30, pp.337–340.

53   Moser, H.M., Dreher, J.J. and Adler, S. (1955) 'Comparison of hyponasality, hypernasality, and normal voice quality on the intelligibility of two digit numbers.' *Journal of Acoustical Society of America*, 27, pp.872–874.

54   Trojan, F. (1959) 'Die ausdruckstheorie der sprechtstimme.' *Phonetica*, 4, p.121.

55   Davitz, J.R. and Davitz, L.J. (1959) 'The communication of feelings by content-free speech.' *Journal of Communication*, 9, pp.6–13

56   Dusenbury, D. and Knower, F.H. (1939) 'Experimental studies of the symbolism of action and voice ii: a study of the specificity of meaning in abstract tonal symbols.' *Quarterly Journal of Speech*, 25, part 1, pp.67–75.

57   Pfaff, P.L. (1954) 'An experimental study of the communication of feeling without contextual material.' *Speech Monograph*, 21, pp.155–156.

58   Moore, C.E. (1938) 'A preliminary study of the emotional effects of letter sounds.' *Quarterly Journal of Speech*, 24, part 1, pp.134–149.

59   Moore, C.E. (1938) 'A preliminary study of the emotional effects of letter sounds.' *Quarterly Journal of Speech*, 24, part 1, pp.134–149.

60   Eisenson, J., Sucher, S.G. and Fisher, J. (1940) 'The affective value of English speech sounds.' *Quarterly Journal of Speech*, 26, part 4, pp.589–594.

61   Eisenson, J., Fisher, J. and Sucher, S. (1943) 'A second study in the affective value of speech sounds.' *Quarterly Journal of Speech*, 29, pp.457–464.

62   Kris, E. (1955) 'Laughter as an expressive process.' In *Psychoanalytic Explorations in Art*. New York: International University Press, pp.217–39.

63   Milner, M. (1956) 'The communication of primary sensual experience: the yell of joy.' *International Journal of Psycho-analysis*, 37, pp.278–81.

64 Maslow, A.H. (1937) 'Dominance-feeling, behaviour and status.' *Psychological Review*, 44, pp.404–429.

65 Bell, H.M. (1931) *Adjustment Inventory*. Stanford: Stanford University Press.

66 Bernreuter, R. (1931) *Personality Inventory*. Stanford: Stanford University Press.

67 Allport, G.W. and Cantril, H. (1931) *Study of Values: A Scale for Measuring the Dominant Interests in Personality*. Boston: Houghton Mifflin.

68 Vernon, P.E. and Allport, G.W. (1931) 'A test for personal values.' *Journal of Abnormal Social Psychology*, 26, pp.231–248.

69 Stagner, R. (1936) 'The Wisconsin scale of personality traits.' *Journal of Abnormal and Social Psychology*.

70 Hollingshead, A.B. (1957) *Two Factor Index of Status Position*. New Haven, pp.1–11.

71 McKelvey, D.P. (1953) 'Voice and personality.' *Western Speech*, 17, pp.91–94.

72 Tyler, L. (1953) 'Test review no. 77.' In O. Buros (ed) *The Fourth Mental Measurements*, ed. by . New Jersey: Gryphon Press.

73 Campbell, D.T. (1960) 'Recommendations for APA test standards regarding construct, trait, or discriminant validity.' *American Psychol.*, 15, pp.546–553.

74 Kramer, E. (1964) 'Personality stereotypes in voice: a reconsideration of the data.' *Journal of Social Psychology*, 62, pp.247–51.

75 Eisenberg, P. and Zalowitz, E. (1938) 'Judging expressive movement: iii. judgments of dominance-feeling from phonograph records of voice.' *Journal of Applied Psychology*, 22, pp.620–31, (p.629).

76 Sanford, F.H. (1942) 'Speech and personality.' *Psychological Bulletin*, 39, 1, pp.811–845.

77 Duncan, M.H. (1945) 'An Experimental study of some of the relationships between voice and personality among students of speech.' *Speech Monograph*, M107, 12, p.49 (p.47–60).

78 Henton, C. (1985) 'Breathiness in normal female speech: inefficiency versus desirability.' *Language and Communication*, 5, pp.221–27.

79 Montepare, J. and Vega, C. (1988) 'Women's vocal reaction to intimate and casual male friends.' *Personality and Social Psychology Bulletin*, 14, pp.103–13.

80 Zuckerman, M. and Driver, R. (1900) 'What sounds beautiful is good: the vocal attractiveness stereotype.' *Journal of Nonverbal Behaviour*, 14, pp.97–112.

81 Montepare, J. and Zebrowitz-McArthur, L. (1987) 'Perceptions of adults with child-like voices in two cultures.' *Journal of Experimental Social Psychology*, 23, pp.331–49.

82 Berry, D. (1900) 'Vocal attractiveness and vocal babyishness: effects on stranger, self, and friend impressions.' *Journal of Nonverbal Behaviour*, 14, pp.141–53.

83 Berry, D. (1992) 'Vocal types and stereotypes: joint effects of vocal attractiveness and vocal maturity on person perception.' *Journal of Nonverbal Behaviour*, 16, pp.41–54.

84 von Franz, M.L. (1970) *The Problem of the Puer Aeternus*. New York: Spring.

85 Hillman, J. ed., (1989) *Puer Papers*. Dallas: Spring.

86 Rodenburg, P. (1992) *The Right to Speak: Working with the Voice*. London: Methuen Drama, p.4.

87 Jenks, W.B. (1932) 'Speech training as a means of training maladjustments of personality.' Unpublished doctoral thesis, University of Chicago.

88 Duncan, M.H. (1945) 'An experimental study of some of the relationships between voice and personality among students of speech.' *Speech Monograph*, M107, 12, pp.47–60, (p.60).

89   Stagner, R. (1936) 'Judgments of voice and personality', *Journal of Educational Psychology*, 27, pp.272–277, (pp.276–277).

90   Haskell, J. (1987) 'Vocal self-perception: the other side of the equation.' *Journal of Voice*, 1, pp.172–79.

91   Haskell, J. (1991) 'Adjusting adolescents' vocal self-perception.' *Language, Speech and Hearing Services in Schools*, 22, pp.168–72.

92   Rodenburg, P. (1992) *The Right to Speak: Working with the Voice*. London: Methuen Drama, p.54.

93   Weiss, D.A. (1955) 'The psychological relations to one's own voice.' *Folia Phoniatrica*, 7, pp.209–222.

94   Heimann, P. (1950) 'On counter-transference.' *International Journal of Psychoanalysis* 31, pp.81–4, (p.81).

95   Freud, S. (1953–74) *Standard Edition of the Complete Psychological Works of Sigmund Freud*, vol. 7, James Strachey (ed) in collaboration with Anna Freud, assisted by Alix Strachey and Alan Tyson. London: Hogarth Press and the Institute of Psychoanalysis, p.116.

96   Racker, H. (1968) *Transference and Countertransference*. London: Maresfield reprint, p.133.

97   Racker, H. (1968) *Transference and Countertransference*. London: Maresfield reprint, p.133.

98   Naumberg, M. (1958) 'Art therapy: its scope and function.' In E. F. Hammer (ed) *Clinical Applications of Projective Drawings*. Springfield: C C Thomas, p.511.

99   Hillman, J. (1978) 'Further notes on images.' *Spring: A Journal of Archetypal Psychology and Jungian Thought*, pp.152–82, (p.162.).

100   Rudd, E. 'A phenomological approach to improvisation in music therapy: a research method.' Paper read at the Sixth World Congress of Music Therapy, Rio de Janero, 15–20 July, 1990.

101   Bright, R. (1993) 'Cultural aspects of music therapy.' In M. Heal and T. Wigram (eds) *Music Therapy in Health and Education*. London: Jessica Kingsley, pp.193–207.

102   Samuels, A. (1993) *The Political Psyche*. London: Routledge, p.313.

103   Zipes, J. (1994) *Fairy Tale as Myth, Myth as Fairy Tale*. Kentucky: University Press of Kentucky.

104   Zipes, J. (1983) *Fairy Tales and the Art of Subversion*. New York: Routledge.

105   Warner, W. (1995) from *The Beast to the Blonde: On Fairy Tales and their Tellers*. London: Vintage.

106   Wolf, N. (1992) *The Beauty Myth: How Images of Beauty are Used Against Women*. London: Doubleday.

107   Jung, C.G. (1953) *The Collected Works of C. G. Jung, vol. 8*. (Bollingen Series XX) H. Read, M. Fordham, G. Adler and W. McGuire (eds). Princeton, New Jersey: Princeton University Press and London: Routledge and Kegan Paul, pp.322–326.

108   Jung, C.G. (1953) *The Collected Works of C. G. Jung, vol. 11*. (Bollingen Series XX) H. Read, M. Fordham, G. Adler and W. McGuire (eds). Princeton, New Jersey: Princeton University Press and London: Routledge and Kegan Paul, p.544.

109   Jung, C.G. (1953) *The Collected Works of C. G. Jung, vol. 8*. (Bollingen Series XX) H. Read, M. Fordham, G. Adler and W. McGuire (eds). Princeton, New Jersey: Princeton University Press and London: Routledge and Kegan Paul, pp.325–26.

110   Jung, C.G. (1953) *The Collected Works of C. G. Jung, vol. 6*. (Bollingen Series XX) H. Read, M. Fordham, G. Adler and W. McGuire (eds). Princeton, New Jersey: Princeton University Press and London: Routledge and Kegan Paul, p.63.

111   Winnicott, D.W. (1988) *Playing and Reality*. Harmondsworth: Penguin, p.44.

112 Case, C. and Dalley, (1992) *The Handbook of Art Therapy*. London: Routledge.

113 Jacobsen, E. (1929) 'Electrical measurements of neuromuscular states during mental activities: imagination of movement involving skeletal muscle.' *American Journal of Physiology*, 91, pp.597–608.

114 (1978) 'Salivation: the significance of imagery in its voluntary control.' *Psychophysiology*, 15, 3, pp.196–203.

115 Schneider, J., Smith, C. and Whitcher, S. (1982–83) 'The relationship of mental imagery to white blood cell (neutrophil) function.' In 'Hypnosis and the Immune System: A Review with Implications for Cancer and the Psychology of Healing.' *Journal of Clinical Hypnosis*, 25, 2–3, pp.92–103.

116 Quarterly Journal of Biofeedback and Self Regulation.

117 Schultz, G. and Luthe, W. (1969) *Autogenic Training: A Physiological Approach to Psychotherapy*. New York: Grune and Stratton.

118 Achterberg, J. (1985) *Imagery in Healing: Shamanism and Modern Medicine*. Boston: Shambhala.

119 Sheikh, A. and Jordon, C. (1983) 'Clinical uses of mental imagery.' In *Imagery: Current Theory, Research and Application*. New York: Wiley.

120 Singer, J. and Pope, K. (1978) *The Power of Human Imagination: New Methods in Psychotherapy*. New York: Plenum.

121 Leuner, H. (1977) 'Guided affective imagery: An account of its development'. *Journal of Mental Imagery*, 1, pp. 73-92.

122 Janet, P. (1898) *Neuroses et Idées Fixes*. Paris: Alacan.

123 Reyher, J. (1977) 'Spontaneous visual imagery: implications for psychoanalysis, psychopathology, and psychotherapy.' *Journal of Mental Imagery*, 2, p.253.

124 Shorr, J. (1972) *Psycho-Imagination Therapy: The Integration of Phenomenology and Imagination*. Intercontinental Medical Book Corp.

125 Happich, C. (1932) 'Das bildbewusstsein als ansatzstelle psychischer behandling.' *Zbl. Psychotherapy*, 5, pp.663–67.

126 Singer, J. (1974) *Imagery and Daydream Methods in Psychotherapy and behaviour Modification*. New York: Academic.

127 Desoille, R. (1965) *The Directed Daydream*. New York: Psychosynthesis Research Foundation.

128 Gendlin, E. (1978) *Focussing*. Everest House.

129 Sheikh, A. (1978) 'Eidetic psychotherapy.' In J. Singer and K. Pope (ed) *The Power of Human Imagination: New methods in Psychotherapy*. New York: Plenum, pp.197–224.

130 Ashen, A. (1968) *Basic Concepts in Eidetic Psychotherapy*. New York: Brandon House.

131 Assagioli, E. (1990) *Psychosynthesis: A Manual of Principles and Techniques*. Wellingborough: Crucible.

132 Faulkner, W.B., Jnr., (1942) 'The effect of the emotions upon diaphragmatic function: observations in five patients.' *Psychosomatic Medicine*, 3, 2, 187–89, (p.189).

133 Jellineck, A. (1953) 'Observations on the therapeutic use of spontaneous imagery in speech therapy.' *Folia Phoniatrica*, 5, 1, pp.166–182, (p.173).

134 Jellineck, A. (1956) 'Treatment of vocal disorders with spontaneous imagery.' *Folia Phoniatrica*, 8, pp.70–84, (pp.70–71).

135   Rowland, J. (1984) *Inside Motion: An Anatomical Basis for Movement Education.* Amsterdam: John Roland, p.10.

136   Todd, M.E. (1937) *The Thinking Body: A Study of the Balancing Forces of Dynamic Man.* New York: Dance Horizons Inc.

137   Todd, M.E. (1929) *The Balancing of Forces in the Human Being: Its Application to Postural Patterns.* New York: Mabel Todd, p.49. Cited in L. E. Sweigard (1974) *Human Movement Potential: Its Ideokinetic Facilitation.* New York: Dodd, Mead and Co., p.6.

138   Clark, B. (1975) *Body Proportion Needs Depth.* Illinois: Barbara Clark.

139   Sweigard, L.E. (1974) *Human Movement Potential: Its Ideokinetic Facilitation.* New York: Dodd, Mead & Co.

140   Bonpensiere, L. (1953) *New Pathways to Piano Technique: A Study of the Relations Between Mind and Body with Special Reference to Piano Playing.* New York: Philosophical Library.

141   Fulkerson, M. (1981–82) *The Move to Stillness.* Dartington Theatre Papers, Fourth Series.

142   Newham, P. (1997) *Shouting for Jericho: The Work of Paul Newham on the Human Voice.* London: Tigers Eye Press/Class Productions.

143   Bless, D. (1991) 'Voice assessment: the need for standards.' Paper read at the British Voice Association International Symposium, University College, London, June 1991.

144   Juhan, D. (1987) *Job's Body: A Handbook for Bodywork.* New York: Station Hill, p.164.

145   Hollings. A. (1989) 'The aims of singing versus speech and the therapeutic potential.' Newsletter of the Voice Research Society (Now the British Voice Association) 4, 1, pp.6–14, (pp.6–7).

146   Joseph, A. (1988) 'The joy of singing.' Unpublished manuscript, p.5.

147   Joseph, A. (1990) 'Voice – a metaphor for life: pedagogical concepts for their application and implementation.' Unpublished manuscript, p.4.

148   Joseph, A. (1990) 'Voice – a metaphor for life: pedagogical concepts for their application and implementation.' Unpublished manuscript, p.5.

149   Joseph, A. (1988) 'The joy of singing.' Unpublished manuscript, p.1–2.

150   Gellhorn, E. (1964) 'Motion and emotion.' *Psychological Review,* 71, 6, pp.457–472.

151   Fonagy, I. (1981) 'Emotions, voice and music: research aspects on singing.' Publication of the Royal Swedish Academy of Music 33, pp.51–79.

Ethics and Guidelines

Naturally, Therapeutic Voicework is a medium which is both 'subtle and powerful' and clients can be catalysed into expressing deep psychic experience, intense emotion and, possibly, aspects of psychopathology. Thus the practitioner needs 'to approach the work thoughtfully',[1] recognising that there are those whose condition is such that Therapeutic Voicework is contraindicated and may be dangerous.

Furthermore, because the work can be so provocative and enlightening, disturbing and frightening, inspiring and liberating, the Therapeutic Voiceworker should, in my view, be trained to practice the work within a framework of ethical, responsible, contractual and professional parameters.

The training which I direct aims to offer the first comprehensive training for those wishing to practice the integrated methodology of Therapeutic Voicework, parts of which I have described in this book. This training is held in London, UK and in Boston, USA. In addition to covering the subjects outlined in this book, the training encourages students to experience placements where they can pursue what has been described as an essential opportunity for any trainee of a discipline which involves intimate contact with people to observe other relevant forms of professional practice in the workplace.[2] Upon graduation, practitioners are encouraged to enter into supervision with someone with whom he or she can discuss their case load – a process which is entirely necessary to help the practitioner,[3] providing an opportunity to 'reduce anxiety', 'explore fresh approaches, examine prejudices' and 'encourage the practitioner to think independently and self-critically about their work thereby improving the service to the client'.[4] Langs has provided a comprehensive investigation of the supervision process which is helpful in enabling prospective practitioners to know what they can expect from a supervisor.[5] Supervision can also help the practitioner in developing the ability to record case studies, which, for many people entering such a field, can be an anomaly, and Higgins has provided a useful book on the nature of case study for those new to the field.[6]

Supervision can also provide a forum within which to discuss issues such as touch for there is a long-established 'tradition in voice training which uses touch to make it easier for the client to understand how a muscle needs to work in order to create a certain sound'.[7] Indeed, in the method of Therapeutic Voicework which I have developed, touch is an integral part of the process not only because it can assist in voice production but because it can facilitate the exploration of the unconscious, as has been explored by McNeely.[8] There are now a number of psychotherapeutic modalities based on a body-orientated approach and the use of touch in psychotherapy is a complex issue which has been reviewed by Scheller.[9] In addition to discussing issues such as touch, supervision can help the practitioner develop strategies which assist in maintaining his or her own well-being in what can be a stressful and demanding role.

The training and supervision meetings which I have augmented constitute a concerted effort to respect Therapeutic Voicework as a discipline which can contribute to the ever-diversifying spectrum of creative, therapeutic and educational strategies of the modern age.

Training in Voice Movement Therapy

The training in Voice Movement Therapy provides an opportunity for trainees to explore both artistic and therapeutic processes and the contributory teachers to the programme come from both artistic and therapeutic backgrounds. The subjects covered are those which I have outlined in this book and there is a strong emphasis on the trainee's experience of his or her own personal journey of psychological discovery through the medium of voice. On the training, the practical exploration of song-writing, dance, theatre, singing, voice production, mask-making, breathwork, massage, musical improvisation and other relevant areas are combined with lectures on subjects which include physiology, psychotherapy, infant development, acoustics, philosophy and the arts. This ensures that graduating practitioners are able to work on the interface between artistic and therapeutic procedures with a specialised focus on the medium of vocal expression.

This training which I direct culminates in the Diploma in Voice Movement Therapy and permits membership of the *International Association for Voice Movement Therapy*. It is currently the only training in Voice Movement

Therapy and in fact the only qualifying accredited training in a therapeutic approach to Voicework. However, there are, of course, many individual practitioners drawing on a therapeutic approach to vocal work who do not have formal training because up until now, no training existed. Moreover, without such practitioners the notion of Therapeutic Voicework may not have been given shape. Indeed, in most new disciplines, the eventual training is implemented only after a period of practice by untrained innovators who initiate a fresh approach which eventually consolidates around a training programme. The work of innovators in the field of Voicework has been the inspiration for the formal training which I have implemented.

Though I have a great deal of respect for such pioneers, many of whom I have tried to acknowledge in this book, I also believe that there are dangers in the prolonged dissemination of Therapeutic Voicework without training; for we cannot rely on the hope that everyone who draws on Therapeutic Voicework will have the requisite skills and insights necessary to ensure safe, diligent and ethical application.

The training which I have designed is in the specific approach to Therapeutic Voicework which I have called Voice Movement Therapy. In addition, I also run a number of short courses in specific aspects of Therapeutic Voicework for professionals seeking training with a specific focus relevant to their field of work in therapy, education and the arts.

Meanwhile, some other Voiceworkers are currently beginning to extend the structure and nature of their voice workshops into a shape more comparable to a training which imparts to participants their own approach. Perhaps, in the future, there will be a number of trainings in different kinds of approaches to Therapeutic Voicework.

Personal Therapy, Personal Work, Personal Training

In the field of psychotherapy, probably the most important aspect of the practitioner's training is his or her own personal therapy. This is always conducted with a psychotherapist who is distinct and separate from the training course to ensure that the unfolding of the client's personal process is not judged in a way that may compromise the perception of his or her professional efficacy as a practitioner. In addition, the personal therapy of a trainee is usually conducted with a therapist of the same orientation and focus as the paradigm which the client is studying to practice.

Those people on the Voice Movement Therapy training work individually with Voice Movement Therapy practitioners so that they can experience the model as a client. However, because the work is new, it can occur that there is no practitioner in the vicinity of the trainee's place of residence and in such cases the trainee usually finds a therapist who works within a model that compliments the Voice Movement Therapy paradigm.

Association, Supervision and Sport

In my view, a thorough training in Therapeutic Voicework is not sufficient without experience of some kind of personal work on the self in a sealed container with a practitioner who is independent from the training process. However, this is not enough either. In addition, any professional dealing with human beings, particularly one working within a new field, needs to belong to a group of fellows who can support and challenge the practitioner's work.

In response to this, I set up the *International Association for Voice Movement Therapy* which provides a containing structure for graduate practitioners of this approach to Therapeutic Voicework.

Members of the Association meet regularly, sometimes with me and at other times with senior colleagues, to receive supervisory support. At such meetings, members present case studies, disclose problems, share ideas and partake in a forum which helps maintain continuity and fertilise the new work with the outcome of its dissemination in the real world.

In addition, members of the Association agree to be in supervision with an independent supervisor, with whom they can discuss their case-load in a context which is separate and distinct from their peers and trainers. This also means that the work is further enriched by diverse supervisory opinion, for members bring to the supervision meetings the opinions of their own supervisors, which prevents the work becoming incestuously founded on unchallenged internal principles.

The Code of Ethics

A further reason for implementing the *International Association for Voice Movement Therapy* was to ensure that practitioners of the work each abide by a common ethical code. The Association therefore has a detailed and comprehensive Code of Ethics which governs the way Voice Movement Therapy should and should not be disseminated. Agreeing to work within this code is a condition of membership.

Of course there may be persons in the future who claim to be administering Voice Movement Therapy who are not members and who have not properly completed the requirements for qualification and membership. Indeed, most new fields of work have encountered such a situation, the result being a dilution of the work and a weakening of the work's integrity. However, at least by having an Association and a qualification, those who have properly trained and qualified can be distinguished.

A Personal Note

I should say, finally, that the work which I have created and the way in which I have structured it is not the only way. There are many other practitioners working consistently with dedication and inspiration to bring the medium of the human voice more central to therapeutic enquiry. Indeed, the purpose of this book, as I outlined at the very beginning, has been as much to honour and acknowledge the work of others as it has been to introduce my own contribution. Therapeutic Voicework as a general field of enquiry is, I believe, here to stay, and Voice Movement Therapy, I hope, will sustain a positive contribution to such a field. I trust that this book has revealed that there is an immense breadth of work and an impressive volume of practitioners from different perspectives who have discovered that the voice can be a messenger for the soul. Providing it is remembered that the implications of such a discovery are truly deserving of serious respect, it might be that the forthcoming years of therapeutic investigation are enriched with a therapeutic use of singing to balance the well established therapeutic use of talking.

Notes

1   Moore Meigs, M. (1994) 'Therapeutic voicework.' In David Jones (ed) *Innovative Therapy: A Handbook*. Buckingham: Open University Press, 174–188 (p.181).

2   Teasdale, C. (1993) 'The role of clinical placement therapy training: toward consolidating our professional identity.' *The Arts in Psychotherapy*, 20, 205–212.

3   Edwards, D. (1993) 'Learning about feelings: the role of supervision in art therapy.' *The Arts in Psychotherapy*, 20, 213–222.

4   Edwards, D. (1993) 'Learning about feelings: the role of supervision in art therapy.' *The Arts in Psychotherapy*, 20, 213–222.

5   Langs, R. (1994) *Doing Supervision and Being Supervised*. London: Karnac.

6   Higgins, R. (1993) *Approaches to Case-Study: A Handbook for Those Entering the Therapeutic Field*. London: Jessica Kingsley.

7   Moore Meigs, M. (1994) 'Therapeutic voicework.' In David Jones (ed) *Innovative Therapy: A Handbook*. Buckingham: Open University Press, pp.174–188 (p.184).

8   McNeely, D. (1987) *Touching: Body Therapy and Depth Psychology*. Toronto: Inner City Books.

9   Scheller, M. (1992–93) 'To touch or not to touch: legal, ethical and clinical issues concern-
     ing incorporation of non-sexual touch into verbal psychotherapy.' *Somatics: Journal of Bodily
     Arts and Sciences, IX,* 1, p. 42–45.

The Newham/Jungr Voice Movement Therapy Notation System

These vocal components which constitute an integrated system have, for the purposes of notation, been translated into a graphic alphabet of signs by Barb Jungr as part of a research programme at Goldsmith's University, London. Jungr's work involves using the component system to plot the vocal characteristics which are identifiable in individual vocalists drawn from a multicultural context and representative of a spectrum of world singing styles. The system is known as the Newham/Jungr Notation System of Voice Movement Therapy.

The Three Arbitrary Vocal Tract Configurations
>< the flute configuration and timbre
<> the clarinet configuration and timbre
() the saxophone configuration and timbre

Oral/Sub-oral Part of the Tube
O oral part of the tube or vocal tract
SO sub-oral part of the tube or vocal tract
e.g. O >< denotes an oral tract in flute configuration
SO <> denotes a sub-oral tract in clarinet configuration

The Voice Registers

M　modal
F　falsetto
W　whistle
VF　vocal fry

Free Air

The degree of free air is indicated by placing a vertical line between the two symmetrical shapes which form the harmonic resonance sign. To indicate the amount of free air which is heard in a sound, the line is placed either in the centre, to the left or the right. A vertical line placed in the centre indicates a moderate amount of free air, a vertical line placed to the right indicates a maximum amount of free air and a vertical line placed to the left indicates just a minimal amount of free air.

>|< flute timbre, moderate amount of free air
<|> clarinet timbre, moderate amount of free air
(|) saxophone timbre, moderate amount of free air

>|< flute timbre, maximum amount of free air
<ᑫ clarinet timbre maximum amount of free air
(ᑫ saxophone timbre, maximum amount of free air

>|< flute timbre, minimum amount of free air
◀> clarinet timbre, minimum amount of free air
ᑫ) saxophone timbre, minimum amount of free air

The Pitch of the Voice

The pitch of the voice is denoted by a sign composed of two adjacent vertical lines, **II**, across which a horizontal line is placed to indicate height or depth of pitch. The higher the horizontal line is placed, the higher the pitch it designates.

H middle-pitched voice
Π high-pitched voice
Ш low-pitched voice

Volume

A voice perceived to be loud is indicated by placing a vertical, upwardly pointing arrow head ⌢ at the top of the pitch sign whilst a voice perceived to be quiet is indicated by placing a vertical, downwardly pointing arrow head ⌣ at the bottom of the pitch sign.

T̂Τ loud voice high in pitch
ΤΤ̬ quiet voice high in pitch
Ĥ loud middle-pitched voice
Η̬ quiet middle-pitched voice
L̂Ι loud voice low in pitch
LΙ̬ quiet voice low in pitch

Pitch Fluctuation

The pitch fluctuation is denoted by zigzag wave lines. The interval distance between the notes is denoted by the height of the points; the higher the point, the larger the interval distance. The speed of pitch fluctuation is denoted by the breadth between the points; the wider the breadth, the slower the speed.

⋀⋀ large pitch interval, very quick vocalisation
⋀⋀⋀ large pitch interval, very slow vocalisation
ᴟᴟ narrow pitch interval, very quick vocalisation
ᴧᴧᴧ narrow pitch interval, very slow vocalisation

Glottal Attack

The sign for glottal attack is comprised of a double-curve, ⊃, which is placed in relation to a vertical line, |.

ⴷ hard glottal attack
|ⴵ soft glottal attack

Disruption

The presence of disruption is indicated by a series of corrugated lines, with more lines indicating greater degree of disruption.

〰〰 mild disruption
〰〰〰 more extreme disruption

Violin

Finally, the quality of violin is indicated by an inverted triangle, ▼, and a vertical line, |

▼| maximum violin
|▼ minimal violin

Separation Sign

̓ entered before a new cluster of signs is recorded, when the voice changes pitch, for example.

The Newham/Jungr system of notation has a number of uses. First, for Therapeutic Voiceworkers, it provides a quick and convenient way of recording the major vocal transformations which occur in a session – which can be consulted as a reminder of what happened when discussing a case in supervision or in other professional contexts. Second, for ethnomusicologists and researchers working in the field, it provides an expedient way of recording the predominant vocal singing styles used in various cultures – enabling analytic work to be initiated by comparing the spectrum of sign clusters recorded.

Further Information

For a catalogue of currently available publications and audio-visual resources, a full training prospectus for the Diploma in Voice Movement Therapy, a list of Voice Movement Therapy practitioners who are members of the International Association for Voice Movement Therapy, or other information, please contact:

Voice Movement Therapy
International Head Office
PO Box 4218
London
SE22 OJE

Tel: (Int +44) (0)171 403 7375

Fax: (Int +44) (0)171 403 7385

E-mail: info@voicework.com

Information is also available on the Internet:
http://www.voicework.com

Bibliography

Achterberg, J. (1985) *Imagery in Healing: Shamanism and Modern Medicine.* Boston: Shambhala.

Adams, M. (1996) *The Multicultural Imagination: Race, Colour and the Unconscious.* London: Routledge.

Adams, B. *So Far So Good.* Cassette. A&M Records.

Addington, D. (1968) 'The relationship of selected vocal characteristics to personality perception.' *Speech Monographs,* 35.

Aitchison, J. 'A web of deceit: the origin of language.' The 1996 Reith Lectures: Lecture 2. Broadcast on BBC Radio 4, Tuesday 13 February 1996.

Aldridge-Morris, R. (1989) *Multiple Personality: An Exercise in Deception.* London: Erlbaum.

Alexander,F.M (1987), *The Use of the Self,* London:Victor Gollancz.

Allen, P. (1976) 'A depopulated manict community.' In M. Dimen and E. Friedl (ed) *Regional Variation in Modern Greece and Cyprus: Towards a Perspective on the Ethnohgraphy of Greece.* New York: Annals of the New York Academy of Sciences.

Allport, G.W. and Cantril, H. (1931) *Study of Values: A Scale for Measuring the Dominant Interests in Personality.* Boston: Houghton Mifflin.

Alvin, J. (1991) *Music Therapy.* London: Stainer and Bell.

American Psychiatric Association (1980) *American Psychiatric Association, Diagnostic Manual of Mental Disorders,* 3rd Edn. Washington DC: American Psychiatric Association.

Anderson Sutton, R. (1989) 'Identity and individuality in an ensemble tradition: the female vocalist in Java.' In E. Koskoff (ed) *Women and Music in Cross Cultural Perspective.* Illinois: University of Illinois Press.

Andrews, J. *Broadway: The Music of Richard Rodgers.* CD. Philips.

Andrews, T. (1994) *Sacred Sounds: Transformation through Music and Word.* St. Paul, MC: Llwellyn Publications.

Anhalt, I. (1984) *Alternative Voices: Essays on Contemporary Vocal and Choral Composition.* Toronto: University of Toronto Press.

Anzieu, D. (1976) 'L'enveloppe sonore due soi.' *Nouvelle Revue de Psychanalyse,* 13.

Anzieu, D. (1979) 'The sound image of the self.' *Int. Review of Psychanalyse.*

Apel, D. (1989) 'The interrelationship of psyche and soma in functional voice trading.' Masters Thesis submitted to Antioch University.

Apollonio, U. (ed) (1973) *Futurist Manifestos*. London.

Apple, W., Streeter, L. and Krauss, R. (1979) 'Effects of pitch and speech rate on personal attributions.' *Journal of Personality and Social Psychology*, 37.

Appleman, R. (1986) *The Science of Vocal Pedagogy*. Indiana: Indiana University Press.

Armatrading, J. *Joan Armatrading*. CD. A&M Records.

Armstrong, F. (1992) *As Far as the Eye Can Sing: An Autobiography*. London: The Women's Press.

Armstrong, F. (1996) Cited in M. Law 'Interviews with contemporary voice practitioners.' Unpublished research papers prepared for the International Association for Voicework.

Armstrong, F. (1995) Unpublished information leaflet on current voice teachers.

Armstrong, L. 'What a wonderful world.' In *Various Artists, The All Time Greatest Love Songs*. CD. Columbia Records.

Arnold, G. (1962) 'Vocal Nodules and Polyps: Laryngeal Tissue Reaction to Habitual Hyperkinetic Dysphonia.' *Journal of Speech Disorders*, 27.

Aronson, A. (1990) *Clinical Voice Disorders*. New York: Thieme.

Artaud, A. (1981) *The Theatre and Its Double*. Trans. by V. Corti. London: John Calder.

Arye, L. (1988) 'Music the messenger.' Unpublished Master's Thesis for Antioch University. Zurich, Switzerland.

Ashen, A. (1968) *Basic Concepts in Eidetic Psychotherapy*. New York: Brandon House.

Assagioli, R. (1990) *Psychosynthesis: A Manual of Principles and Techniques*. Wellingborough: Crucible.

Attali, J. (1989) *Noise: The Political Economy of Music*. Trans. by B. Massumi. Minneapolis: University of Minneapolis Press.

Auerbach, S. (1989) 'From singing to lamenting: women's musical role in a Greek village.' In E. Koskoff (ed) *Women and Music in Cross Cultural Perspective*. Illinois: University of Illinois Press.

Author unknown, 'The Art of Noise', *The Times*, 30 June 1913

Ayab, O. *African Voices: Songs of Life*. CD. Narada media.

Aznavour, C. *Greatest Golden Hits*. CD. EMI Music.

Bachelard, G. (1994) *The Poetics of Space*. Boston: Beacon Press.

Backes-Clement, C. 'Voice and madness; echo of the origin of man.' *Lettres Francaises*. Cited in 'Roy Hart Theatre.' Unpublished anthology of reviews, extracts from articles and other material, compiled by Barrie Coghlan with assistance from Noah Pikes in 1979.

Baez, J. *Hits/Greatest and Others*. CD. Vanguard Records.

Baibl, C. (1978) 'Programmation de l'ecoute (1).' *Cahiers du Cinema*, p.293.

Ball, H. (1974) *Flight Out of Time*. New York: Viking Press.

Bamberger, J. (1982) 'Revisiting children's drawings of simple rhythms: a function for reflection-in-action.' In S. Strauss and R. Stavy (ed) *U-Shaped Behavioural Growth*. New York: Academic Press, .

Barbeau, M. (1974) 'Tsimsyan Songs.' In E. Garfield (ed) *The Tsimshian: Their Arts and Music*. American Ethnological Society publication 18, 1974.

Barba, E. (1979) *The Floating Islands*. Holstebro: Odin Teatret Forlag.

Barba, E. (1995) *The Paper Canoe: A Guide to Theatre Anthropology* London: Routledge.

Barnwell, Y. (1996) Lecture given at Songs of Heaven and Earth Conference. Findhorn Foundation, Forres, 30 March–6 April .

Bartenieff, I. (1975) 'Dance therapy: a new profession of rediscovery of an ancient role of the dance?' In H. Chaiklin (ed) *Marian Chace: Her Papers*. Maryland: American Dance Therapy Association.

Barthes, R. (1990) 'The grain of the voice' in S. Frith and A. Goodwin (eds) *Rock, Pop and the Spoken Word*. London: Pantheon.

Bassey, S. *Four Decades of Song*. CD. EMI Records.

Bateson, C. (1975) 'Mother-infant exchanges: the epigenesis of conversational interaction.' In D. Aronson and R. Rieber (ed) *Developmental Psycholinguistics and Communication Disorders, Annals of the New York Academy of Sciences*, 263. New York: New York Academy of Sciences.

Bateson, G. (1987) *Steps to an Ecology of Mind*. USA: Aronson.

Baur, A. (1993) *Healing Sounds: Fundamentals of Chirophonetics*. Fair Oaks, California: Rudolf Steiner College Press.

Baylor, E. *The Live Experience*. CD. World Records.

Beaulieu, J. (1987) *Music and Sound in the Healing Arts: An Energy Approach*. New York: Station Hill Press.

Becker, J., Breedlove, M. and Crews, D. (eds) (1992) *Behavioural Endocrinology*. Cambridge: MIT Press.

Bell, H.M. (1931) *Adjustment Inventory*. Stanford: Stanford University Press.

Berberian, C. (1984) Cited in I. Anhalt *Alternative Voices: Essays on Contemporary Vocal and Choral Composition*. Toronto: University of Toronto Press.

Berendt, J.E. (1988) *Nada Brama: The World is Sound*. London: East West.

Berendt, J.E. (1992) *The Third Ear On Listening to the World*. New York: Holt.

Berndt, R.M. (1946–48) 'Wuradjeri magic and clever men.' *Oceania*, 17, pp.327–65 and p.18 (1947–48).

Bernhardt, P. (1991) *The Secret Music of the Soul*. Québec: Imagine.

Bernreuter, R. (1931) *Personality Inventory*. Stanford: Stanford University Press.

Berry, C. (1987) *The Actor and his Text*. London: Harrap.

Berry, C. (1973) *Voice and the Actor*. London: Harrap.

Berry, C. (1987) *Your Voice and How to Use it Successfully.* London: Harrap.

Berry, D. (1992) 'Vocal attractiveness and vocal babyishness: effects on stranger, self and friend impressions.' *Journal of Nonverbal Behaviour,* 16.

Berryman, J.C. with Hargreaves, D., Herbert, M. and Taylor, A. (1991) *Developmental Psychology and You.* London: British Psychological Society/Routledge.

The Bible

Bion, W. (1962) 'A theory of thinking.' *International Journal of Psychoanalysis,* 43.

Blacking, J. (1967) *Venda Children's Songs: Sociological Analysis.* Chicago: University of Chicago Press.

Bless, D. (1991) 'Voice assessment: the need for standards.' Paper read at the British Voice Association International Symposium, University College, London, June 1991.

Bliss, B. (1984) 'The singer and the voice.' Diploma Thesis for C.G. Jung Institute, Zurich.

Bloch, P. (1960) 'New limits of vocal analysis.' *Folia Phoniatrica,* 12.

Bloom, K. (1974) 'Eye contact as a setting event for infant learning.' *Journal of Experimental Child Psychology,* 17.

Bloom, K. (1990) 'Selectivity and early infant vocalisation.' In J. Enns (ed) *The Development of Attention: Research and Theory.* New York: Elsevier.

Blotcky, M. and Looney, J. (1980) 'A psychotherapeutic approach to silent children.' *American Journal of Psychotherapy,* 24.

Boal, A. (1993) *Theatre of the Oppressed,* trans. C. and M. London: Pluto.

Boal, A. (1990) *Méthode Boal de Théâtre et de Thérapie: l'Arc-en-ciel du Désir.* Paris: Ramsay.

Boal, A. (1995) *The Rainbow of Desire.* London: Routledge.

Bolton, M. *The One Thing.* Cassette. Sony Music.

Bon Jovi, J. *These Days.* CD. Polygram Records.

Bonaventura, M. (1935) 'Ausdruck der personlichkeit in der sprechtstimme und im photogramm.' *Arch. Gen. Psychol.,* 94.

Bonny, H. and Savary, L. (1990) *Music and your Mind.* New York: Station Hill Press.

Bonpensiere, L. (1953) *New Pathways to Piano Technique: A Study of the Relations Between Mind and Body with Special Reference to Piano Playing.* New York: Philosophical Library.

Boone, D. and McFarlane, S. In (1988) *The Voice and Voice Therapy.* New Jersey: Simon and Schuster.

Booth, M. (1995) 'Nineteenth century theatre.' In J. Brown (ed) *The Oxford Illustrated History of Theatre.* Oxford: Oxford University Press.

Bowra, C. (1962) *Primitive Song.* New York: World Publishing.

Boysen, G. and Boysen, M. (1987) *Biodynamik des Lebens: Die Gerda Boysen Methode.* Essen: Synthesis Verlag Gerken.

Boysen, G. (1987) *Über den Körper die Seele Heilen: Biodynamische Psychologie and Psychotherapie.* München: Kösel-Verlag.

Boysen, G. (1995) *Von der Lust am Heilen.* München: Kösel-Verlag.

Braddock, G. (1995) *Body Voices: Using the Power of Breath, Sound and Movement to Heal and Create New Boundaries.* Berkeley: Page Mill Press.

Bradley, D. (1992) *Hyper Ventilation Syndrome: A Handbook for Bad Breathers.* Berkeley, California: Celestial Arts.

Bragg, B. *Workers Playtime.* Cassette. Warner Communications.

Brazier, D. (1995) *Zen Therapy.* London: Constable.

Bright, R. (1993) 'Cultural aspects of music therapy.' In M. Heal and T. Wigram (eds) *Music Therapy in Health and Education.* London Jessica Kingsley.

Brodnitz, F.S. (1988) *Keep Your Voice Health.* USA: College Hill.

Brodnitz, F.S. (1954) 'One hundred years of laryngoscopy: to the memory of Garcia, Tuerck and Czemak.' *Transactions of the American Academy of Ophthalmology and Otolaryngology,* 53.

Brodnitz, F.S. (1962) 'The holistic study of the voice.' *Quarterly Journal of Speech,* 48, 3.

Brody, M.W. (1943) 'Neurotic manifestations of the voice.' *Psychoanalytical Quarterly,* 12.

Brook, P. (1988) *The Shifting Point: Forty Years of Theatrical Exploration.* London: Metheun.

Brookes, J. (1975) 'Producing Marat/Sade: theatre in a psychiatric hospital.' *Hospital and Community Pschiatry,* 26, 7.

Brown, J. *20 All Time Greatest Hits.* CD. Polygram Records.

Brownell, A. (1989) 'The voice and dance movement therapy.' Unpublished paper. Author's archives.

Brownell, A. and Lewis, P. (1990) 'The Kestenberg movement profile in assessment of vocalization.' In P. Lewis and S. Loman (eds) *The Kestenberg Movement Profile: Its Past, Present Applications and Future Directions.* Keene: Antioch New England Graduate School.

Brownell, A. (1987) 'The singing self.' Unpublished Masters Thesis, Lesley College, Cambridge, Mass.

Buhler, H. (1934) *Sprachtheorie.* Berlin: Jena.

Bunch, M. (1993) *Dynamics of the Singing Voice.* New York: Springer-Verlag Wien.

Bunch, M. (1989) *Speak with Confidence.* London: Kogan Page.

Bush, C. (1995) *Healing Imagery and Music.* Portland: Rudra Press.

Bush, K. *The Whole Story.* Cassette. EMI Music.

Butcher, P., Elias, A. and Raven, R. (1993) *Psychogenic Voice Disorders and Cognitive-Behaviour Therapy.* London: Whurr.

Buteyko, Dr. Unpublished papers.

Butterfield, S. (1968) 'An extended version of modification of sucking with auditory feedback.' Bureau of Child Research Laboratory, Children's Rehabilitation, MIT. Medical Centre. Working Paper 43.

Caesari, E.H. (1965) *The Alchemy of Voice.* London: Robert Hale.

Caesari, E.H. (1969) *Vocal Truth.* London: Hale.

Cale, J.J. *Naturally.* Cassette. Phonogram International.

Campbell, D. (1990) *The Roar of Silence: Healing Powers of Breath, Tone and Music.* Wheaton: Theosophical Publishing House.

Campbell, D. (1991) *Music: Physician for Times to Come.* Wheaton: Quest Books.

Campbell, D. (1992) *Music and Miracles.* Wheaton: Quest Books.

Campbell, D.T. (1960) 'Recommendations for APA test standards regarding construct, trait or discriminant validity.' *American Psychol.,* 15.

Candland, D. (1993) *Feral Children and Clever Animals.* Oxford: Oxford University Press.

Canner, N. (1968) *And a Time to Dance.* Boston: Plays Inc.

Canner, N. (1972) 'Stimulating sounds and vocalization through body movement and rhythm with hospitalized children.' In *Writings on Body Movement and Communication.* Columbia, MD: American Dance Therapy Association.

Cantonese Opera, *Red Mansion Dream.* (Sound Factory).

Carey, D. (1992) 'A course with a world wide reputation.' *Human Communication,* February 1992.

Carey, M. *Music Box.* CD. Columbia Records.

Carlson, N. (1991) *Physiology of Behaviour.* Boston: Allyn and Bacon.

Caruso, E. and Tetrazzini, L. (1975) *The Art of Singing.* New York: Dover.

Case, C. and Dalley, T. (1992) *The Handbook of Art Therapy.* London: Routledge.

Cassirer, E. (1953–59) *The Philosophy of Symbolic Forms 3 vols.* New Haven: Yale University Press.

Casteneda, C. (1968) *The Teachings of Don Juan: A Yaqui Way of Knowledge.* Berkeley: University of California Press.

Casteneda, C. (1971) *A Separate Reality: Further Conversatins with Don Juan.* New York: Simon and Schuster.

Casteneda, C. (1972) *Journey to Ixtlan: The Lessons of Don Juan.* New York: Simon and Schuster.

Casteneda, C. (1974) *Tales of Power.* New York: Simon and Schuster.

Cayce, E. (1972) 'Music as the bridge.' In S.R. Winston (ed) *Music as the Bridge.* Virginia: ARE Press.

Celletti, R. (1991) *A History of Bel Canto.* Oxford: Clarendon Press.

Chaitrow, L. (1988) *Soft-Tissue Manipulation.* Rochester: Healing Arts Press.

Chapman, T. *Tracy Chapman.* CD. Elektra Records.

Chethik, M. 'Amy: the intensive treatment of an elective mute.' In J. Macdermott and S. Harrison (ed) *Psychiatric Treatment of the Child.* New York: Aronson.

Chion, M. (1982) *La Voix au Cinéma.* Paris: Éditions de L'Etoile.

Chodorow, J. (1991) *Dance Therapy and Depth Psychology.* London: Routledge.

Choksy, L. (1988) *The Kodály Method.* New Jersey: Prentice Hall.

Christofellis, A. *Farinelli Et Son Temps.* CD. EMI Records.

Clark, B. (1975) *Body Proportion Needs Depth.* Illinois: Barbara Clark.

Clarkson, A. 'Creative listening: an archetypal attitude to musical experience'. Paper presented to the 13th World Congress of the International Society for Music Education, Ontario, 12–20 August 1978.

Clifford Turner, J. (1977) *Voice and Speech in the Theatre.* London: Pitman.

Cline, P. *Twelve Greatest Hits.* CD. MCA Records.

Cloutier, D. (1973) *Spirit, Spirit: Shaman Songs, Incantations.* Rhode Island: Copper Beech Press.

Cocteau Twins, *Milk and Kisses.* CD. Capitol Records.

Coger, L. (1952) 'A comparison for the oral interpreter of the teaching methods of Curry and Stanislavski'. Ph.D. dissertation, Northwestern University's School of Speech.

Cohn, M. *The Rainy Season.* CD. Atlantic Records.

Comins, J. (1996) 'Voice clinic: let's get physical.' *The Singer.* (Sept./Oct. 1996).

Connor, S. (1990) *Post-Modernist Culture: An Introduction to the Theories of the Contemporary.* Oxford: Blackwell.

Cooper, M. (1984) *Change Your Voice, Change Your Life.* New York: Macmillan.

Costanzo, F., Markel, N. and Costanzo, P. (1969) 'Voice quality profile and perceived emotion.' *Journal of Counselling Psychology,* 16.

Country Collection, vols. 1–3. CD. Hallmark.

Cousto, H. (1988) *The Cosmic Octave: Planets, Tones, Colours – The Power of Inherent Vibrations.* Trans. by C. Baker. California: Life Rhythm.

Crash Test Dummies, *God Shuffled His Feet.* CD. BMG Music.

Crowley, B. and Crowley, E. (1994) *Words of Power: Sacred Sounds of East and West.* St. Paul, Minnesota: Llewellyn.

Crystal, D. (1969) *Prosodic Systems and Intonation Systems in English.* Cambridge: Cambridge University Press.

Cymatics (1986) *The Healing Nature of Sound* (pts. 1, 2 and 3). Video produced by Jeff Volk. Brookline, MA: Macromedia.

Dalcroze, J. (1965) 'Les études musicales et l'education de l'oreille.' In *Le Rythme, la Musique et l'Education*. Lausanne: Foetische.

Dalcroze, J. (1965) 'L'initiation au rythme.' In *Le Rythme, la Musique et l'Education*. Lausanne: Foetische.

Daniélou, A. (1995) *Music and the Power of Sound: The Influence of Tuning and Interval on Consciousness*. Vermont: Inner Traditions.

David, W. (1980) *The Harmonics of Sound, Color and Vibration: A System for Self-Awareness and Soul Evolution*. Santa Monica: DeVorss.

Davidson, L. (1985) 'Tonal structures of children's early songs.' *Music Perception*, 2.

Davies, M.H. (1987) 'Drama therapy and psychodrama.' In S. Jennings (ed) *Dramatherapy: Theory and Practice for Teachers and Clinicians*. London: Routledge.

Davis, T. (1938) 'Sounds in language.' *Journal of Nervous and Mental Diseases*, 4. October 1938.

Davitz, J.R. and Davitz, L.J. (1959) 'The communication of feelings by content-free speech.' *Journal of Communication*, 9.

Day, D. *Doris Day*. CD. Telstar Records.

De Maria, L. (ed) (1968) *Opere di F. T. Marinetti*, vol. 2. Verona.

Deak, F. 'Robert Wilson.' *The Drama Review*, 18, June 1974.

Deason-Barrow, M. (1996) Lecture given at *Songs of Heaven and Earth Conference*. Findhorn Foundation Forres, 30 March–6 April.

Delwin Dusenbury and Knower, Franklin H. (1939) 'Experimental studies of the symbolism of action and voice II: a study of the specificity of meaning in abstract tonal symbols.' *Quarterly Journal of Speech*, 25, part 1.

Densmore, F. (1948) 'The use of music in the treatment of the sick by American Indians.' In D.M. Schullian and M. Schoen (ed) *Music and Medicine*. New York: Henry Schuman.

Derrida, J. (1967) *L'Ecriture et la Différence*. Paris: Seuil.

Desoille, R. (1965) *The Directed Daydream*. New York: Psychosynthesis Research Foundation.

Devereux, G. (1980) *Basic Problems of Ethnopsychiatry*. Chicago: University of Chicago Press.

Dewhurst-Maddock, O. (1993) *The Book of Sound Therapy: Heal Yourself with Music and Voice*. London: Gaia.

Di Franco, G. (1993) 'Music therapy: a methodological approach in the mental health field.' In M. Heal and T. Wigram (eds) *Music Therapy in Health and Education*. London: Jessica Kingsley.

Diamanda Galas, *The Divine Punishment*. CD. Mute Records.

Diehl, C.F. and McDonald, E.T. (1956) 'Effect of Voice Quality on Communication.' *Journal of Speech and Hearing Disorders*, 21, 2.

Dietrich, M. *The Great Marlene Dietrich*. CD. Intermusic.

Doane, J.J and Hodges,D. (1992) *From Klein to Kristeva: Psychoanalytic Feminism and the Search for the 'Good Enough' Mother.* Michigan: University of Michigan Press.

Diangelo, S. (1994) 'Resources of the Cosmos.' *Caduceus,* 23.

Douglas, A. (1993) *The Beast Within: Man, Myths and Werewolves.* London: Orion.

Dowling. W.J. (1982) 'Development of musical schemata in children's spontaneous singing.' In W.R. Crozier and A.J. Chapman (ed) *Cognitive Processes in the Perception of Art.* Amsterdam: Elsevier.

Drury, N. (1985) *Music for Inner Space: Techniques for Meditation and Visualisation.* Dorset: Prism.

Dylan, B. *Bob Dylan.* CD. CBS Records.

Eagleton, T. (1983) *Literary Theory: An Introduction.* Oxford: Blackwell.

Edwards, D. (1993) 'Learning about feelings: the role of supervision in art therapy.' *The Arts in Psychotherapy,* Vol. 20.

Edwards, S. (1982–93) 'Bio-acoustics: the potential to reverse disease using individual signature sounds.' In Sharry Edwards, *Signature Sound.* Published Papers.

Eisenberg, P. and Zalowitz, E. (1938) 'Judging expressive movement III: judgments of dominance-feeling from phonograph records of voice.' *Journal of Applied Psychology,* 22.

Eisenson, J., Fisher, J. and Sucher, S. (1943) 'A second study in the affective value of speech sounds.' *Quarterly Journal of Speech,* 29.

Eisenson, J., Sucher, S.G. and Fisher, J. (1940) 'The affective value of English speech sounds.' *Quarterly Journal of Speech,* 26, part 4.

Eldre, S.H. and Price, D.B. (1958) 'A linguistic evaluation of feeling states in psychotherapy.' *Psychiatry,* 21.

Eliade, M. (1989) *Shamanism: Archaic Technique of Ecstasy.* London: Penguin.

Ellis, G. (1993) *The Breath of Life: Mastering the Breathing Techniques of Pranayama and Qi Gong.* North Hollywood, California: Newcastle Publishing.

Engel, S. (1995) *The Stories Children Tell: Making Sense of the Narratives of Childhood.* New York: W.H. Freeman.

Enigma, *Enigma.* CD. Virgin Records.

Enya, *Watermark.* CD. WEA Records.

Esslin. M. (1991) 'Modernist drama: Wedekind to Brecht' In M. Bradbury and J. McFarlane (eds) *Modernism: A Guide to European Literature 1890–1930.* London: Penguin.

Estill, J. (1988) 'Belting and classic voice quality: some physiological differences.' *Medical Problems of Performing Artists,* 3.

Estill, J., Yanagisawa, E., Kmucha, S. and Leder, S. (1989) 'The contribution of aryepiglotic constriction to "ringing" voice quality: a video laryngoscopy study with acoustic analysis.' *Journal of Voice,* 4, 3.

Estill, J. (1986) 'An EMG study of two voice qualities: nasal twang and opera with *Squillo.'* In M. Hirano and S. Hibi (eds) *Proceedings of the International Conference on Voice.* Japan: Karume.

Fairbanks, G. and Pronovost, W. (1938) 'Vocal pitch during simulated emotion.' (Preliminary report), *Science,* 8.

Fairbanks, G. and Pronovost, W. (1939) 'An experimental study of the pitch characteristics of the voice during the expression of emotion.' *Speech Monograph,* M47, 6.

Faithfull, M. *Strange Weather.* CD. BMG Records.

Farmer, P. (1972) *Tarzan Alive: A Definitive Biography of Lord Greystoke.* New York: Doubleday.

Faulkner Jnr., W.B. (1942) 'The effect of the emotions upon diaghragmatic function: observations in five patients.' *Psychosomatic Medicine,* 3, 2.

Fawcus, M. (ed) (1991) *Voice Disorders and their Management.* London: Chapman and Hall.

Fay, P.J. and Middleton, W.C. (1939) 'Judgment of spranger personality types from the voice as transmitted over a public address system.' *Character and Personality,* 8.

Fay, P.J. and Middleton, W.C. (1940) 'Judgment of intelligence from the voice as transmitted over a public address system.' *Quarterly Journal of Speech,* 28, 2.

Fay, P.J. and Middleton, W.C. (1941) 'The ability to judge sociability from the voice as transmitted over a public Address System.' *Journal of Social Psychology,* 13.

Fay, P.J. and Middleton, W.C. (1941) 'The ability to judge truth-telling or lying from the voice as transmitted over a public address system.' *Journal of General Psychology,* 24.

Fay, P.J. and Middleton, W.C. (1942) 'Judgment of introversion from the transcribed voice as transmitted over a public address system.' *Quarterly Journal of Speech,* 28, 2.

Fay, P.J. and Middleton, W.C. (1943) 'Judgment of leadership from the transcribed voice.' *Journal of Social Psychology,* 17.

Feils, R. (1988) *Breathing Alive: A Guide to Conscious Living.* Shaftesbury: Element.

Feld, S. (1990) *Sound and Sentiment: Birds, Weeping, Poetics and Song in Kaluli Expression.* Philadelphia: University of Pennsylvania Press.

Fels, F.M. (1891) 'Die moderne.' *Moderne Rundschau,* IV.

Ferenczi, S. (1926) 'Psychogenic anomalies of voice production.' In *Further Contributions to the Theory and Technique of Psychoanalysis.* London: Hogarth Press.

Fernald, A., Taeschner, T., Dunn, J., Papousek, M.D., De Boysson, B., Bardies and Ikuko, F. (1989) 'A cross-language study of prosodic modifications in mothers' and fathers' speech to preverbal infants.' *Journal of Child Language,* 16.

Ferrein, A. (1741) 'De la formation de la voix de l'homme.' In *Memories de l'Académie Royale des Sciences*. Paris.

Fitzgerald, E. *The Classic Ella Fitzgerald*. CD. Charly Popular.

Fiumara, G. (1990) *The Other Side of Language: A Philosophy of Listening*. London: Routledge.

Flaszen, L. (1975) 'Akropolis – treatment of the text.' In J. Grotowski (ed) *Towards a Poor Theatre*. London: Methuen.

Flaszen, L. 'Studium o Hamlecie.' (Opole, March 1964). (1987) Cited in Jennifer Kumiega, *The Theatre of Grotowski*. London: Methuen.

Fleshman, B. and Fryrear, J. (1981) *The Arts in Therapy*. Chicago: Nelson-Hall.

Flint, R. (1972) *Marinetti: Selected Writings*. New York: Straus and Giroux.

Folkworks Vocal Chords Festival (1996) Programme notes Newcastle-upon-Tyne, 3–5 May, 1996 and London, 4–6 May.

Forrester, J. (1980) *Language and the Origins of Psychoanalysis*. London: Macmillan.

Fossey, D. (1983) *Gorillas in the Mist*. Boston: Houghton Mifflin.

Fraiberg, S. (1977) *Insights from the Blind*. New York: Basic Books.

Frank, J.D. (1961) *Persuasion and Healing*. Baltimore: Johns Hopkins Press.

Freid, R. (1990) *The Breath Connection: How to Reduce Psychosomatic and Stress-Related Disorders with Easy to do Breathing Exercises*. New York: Plenum Press.

Freud, A. (1965) *Normality and Pathology in Childhood: Assessment of Development*. New York: International 1 University Press.

Freud, S. (1953–74) *Standard Edition of the Complete Psychological Works of Sigmund Freud*. James Strachey (ed) in collaboration with Anna Freud, assisted by Alix Strachey and Alan Tyson. London: Hogarth Press and the Institute of Psychoanalysis.

Frey-Rohn, L. (1990) *From Freud to Jung: A Comparative Psychology of the Unconscious*. Boston: Shambhala

Fry, D. (1991) *The Physics of Speech*. Cambridge: Cambridge University Press.

Fulkerson, M. (1981–82) *The Move to Stillness*. Dartington Theatre Papers, Fourth Series.

Furst, P. (ed) (1972) *Flesh of the Gods: The Ritual Use of Hallucinogens*. New York: Praeger.

G. Rosolato, (1974) 'La voix: entre corps et langage.' *Revue Francaise de Psychanalyse*, 37, 1.

Gandrung Banyuwangi, *Songs Before Dawn*. CD. Smithsonian/Folkways.

Gardner, H. (1979) 'Developmental psychology after piaget: an approach in terms of symbolisation.' *Human Development*, 22.

Gardner, H. (1982) *Art, Mind and Brain: A Cognitive Approach to Creativity*. New York: Basic Books.

Gardner, H. (1993) *Multiple Intelligences: A Theory in Practice.* New York: Basic Books.

Gardner, H. (1994) *The Arts and Human Development.* New York: Basic Books.

Gardner, K. (1990) *Sounding the Inner Landscape.* Stonington, ME: Caduceus.

Gardner-Gordon, J. (1993) *The Healing Voice: Traditional and Contemporary Toning, Chanting and Singing.* Freedom, CA: Crossing Press.

Garfield, L.M. (1987) *Sound Medicine: Healing with Music, Voice and Song.* Berkeley: Celestial Arts.

Garfunkel, A. *Scissors Cut.* CD. Columbia Records.

Gatheru, R. (1960) 'The medicine man as psychotherapist.' In W. Goldschmidt (ed) *Exploring the Ways of Mankind.* New York: Holt, Rinehard and Winston.

Gellhorn, E. (1964) 'Motion and emotion.' *Psychological Review,* 71, 6.

Gendlin, E. (1978) *Focusing.* Everest House.

George, M. *Drink from the well.* Cassette. Sounds True Audio: Boulder, Colorado.

Gerber, R. (1988) *Vibrational Medicine: New Choices for Healing Ourselves.* Santa Fe: Bear and Co.

Gilligan, C. (1993) *In a Different Voice: Psychological Theory and Women's Development.* Cambridge: Harvard University Press.

Gindler, E. (1995) 'Gymnastik for people whose lives are full of activity.' In D. Johnson (ed) *Bone, Breath and Gesture: Practises of Embodiment.* Berkeley: North Atlantic Books.

Giving Voice (1993–96) Conference series notes and information leaflet to Giving Voice, four annual conferences held at Cardiff, Centre for Performance Research.

Glasgow, G.M. (1944) 'The effects of nasality on oral communication.' *Quarterly Journal of Speech,* 30.

Godwin, J. (1987) *Harmonies of Heaven and Earth The Spiritual Dimension of Music from Antiquity to the Avant-Garde.* London: Thames and Hudson.

Godwin, J. (1987) *Music, Mysticism and Magic: A Sourcebook.* London: Arkana.

Godwin, J. (1989) *Cosmic Music: Musical Keys to the Interpretation of Reality.* Rochester: Inner Traditions.

Godwin, J. (1993) *The Harmony of the Spheres: A Sourcebook of the Pythagorean Tradition in Music.* Rochester: Inner Traditions.

Goldberg, R. (1995) *Performance Art: From Futurism to the Present.* London: Thames and Hudson.

Goldman, J. (1992) *Healing Sounds: The Power of Harmonics.* Shaftesbury: Element.

Goll, K. (1979) 'Role structure and subculture in families of elective mutism.' *Family Proceedings,* 18.

Goodchild, C. (1989) 'A servant of voice and sound.' *Human Potential,* October 1989–May 1990.

Goodchild, C. (1993) *The Naked Voice*. London: Random House.

Goodman, N. (1976) *Languages of Art*. Indianapolis: Hackett.

Goodman, N. (1978) *Ways of Worldmaking*. Indianapolis: Hackett.

Grand Maitre Franco Luambo Makiadi, *Azda*. CD. (Sonodisc).

Greene, M. and Conway, J. (1963) *Learning to Talk: A Study in Sound of Infant Speech Development*. New York: Folkways Records.

Greene, M. and Mathieson, L. (1989) *The Voice and its Disorders*, 5th edn. London: Whurr.

Greene, M. and Mathieson, L. (1991) *The Voice and its Disorders*. London: Whurr.

Grof, S. (1975) *Realms of the Human Unconscious: Observations from LSD Research*. New York: Viking Press.

Grof, S. (1988) *The Adventure in Self-Discovery: Dimensions of Consciousness and New Perspectives in Psychotherapy and Inner Exploration*. New York: State University of New York.

Grof, S. (1985) *Beyond the Brain: Birth, Death and Transcendence in* Psychotherapy. *New York*: State University of New York Press.

Grof, S. (1993) *Realms of the Human Unconscious: Observations from LSD Research*. London: Souvenir Press.

Grof, S. and Halifax, J. (1978) *The Human Encounter with Death*. New York: Dutton.

Grotowski, J. (1987) 'Dziady jako model teatru nowoczesnego.' *Wspolczesnosc*, 21. Cited in L. Kumiega, *The Theatre of Grotowski*. London Methuen.

Grotowski, J. (1975) 'Theatre is an encounter.' In J. Grotowski (ed) *Towards a Poor Theatre*. London: Methuen.

Gruen, K. and Virato, S. (1992) 'An interview with Gabrielle Roth.' *New Frontier*. (February/March 1992).

Grunwell, P. (1982) *Clinical Phonology*. London: Croom Helm.

Guilbert, Y. (1929) *La Passante Emerveillée*. Paris: Bernard Grasset.

Gullan, M. (1929) *Speech Training in the School*. London: Evans Brothers.

Gunther, M. (1985) Interview with David Williams, Malerargues, France, February 1985, cited in 'The Roy Hart Theatre: Documentation and Interviews.' *Dartington Theatre Papers*, Fifth Series, No. 14, ed. by David Williams. Series ed. by Peter Hulton. Dartington College of Arts

Gunther, M. (1990) 'The human voice.' Paper read at the National Conference on Drama Therapy, Antioch University, San Francisco, November 1986. Published on audio tape by Roy Hart Theatre, Malerargues, France..

Gunther, M. (1990) 'The human voice: on Alfred Wolfsohn.' *Spring: A Journal of Archetype and Culture*, 50.

Gusinde, M. *Die Feurland Indianer*, 3 vols. Vienna, 1931–74, cited in H. Kalweit *Shamans, Healers and Medicine Men*. Boston: Shambhala, 1992.

Hát Chéo, *Traditional Folk Theatre of Vietnam*. CD. Unesco Collection.

Haberman, F. (1954) 'English sources of American elocution.' In K. Wallace (ed) *History of Speech Education in America.* New York: Appleton-Century-Crofts.

Hahn, R. (1920) *Du Chant.* Paris.

Hale, L. (1954) 'Dr James Rush,' 'English sources of American elocution.' In K. Wallace (ed) *History of Speech Education in America.* New York: Appleton-Century-Crofts.

Hale, L. (1949) 'Dr James Rush – Psychologist and Voice Scientist.' *Quarterly Journal of Speech*, 35, 4.

Hale, S. (1995) *Song and Silence: Voicing the Soul.* New Mexico: La Alameda Press.

Halifax, J. (1991) *Shamanic Voices: A Survey of Visionary Narratives.* London: Penguin.

Halpern, S. (1985) *Sound Health.* San Francisco: Harper and Row.

Hamel, P. (1986) *Through Music to the Self: How to Experience Music Anew.* Shaftesbury: Element.

Hamilton, V. (1982) *Narcissus and Oedipus: The Children of Psychoanalysis.* London: Karnac.

Happich, C. (1932) 'Das bildbewusstsein als ansatzstelle Psychischer Behandling.' *Zbl. Psychotherapy*, 5.

Hargreaves, D. (1992) *The Developmental Psychology of Music.* Cambridge: Cambridge University Press.

Harms, L.S. (1961) 'Listener judgments of status cues in speech.' *Quarterly Journal of Speech*, 47, 2.

Harner, M. (ed) (1973) *Hallucinogens and Shamanism.* Oxford: Oxford University Press.

Harner, M. (1990) *The Way of the Shaman.* New York: Harper Collins.

Harris, J. (1990) *Early Language Development: Implications for Clinical and Educational Practice.* London Routledge.

Hart, M. (1990) *Drumming at the Edge of Magic: A Journey into the Spirit of Percussion.* San Francisco: Harper Collins.

Hart, R. (1957–1960) Unpublished phonograph recordings.

Hart, R. (1968) 'Context.' Paper read at the Third International congress of Psychodrama, Vienna.

Hart, R. *et al.* (1985) 'An outline of the work of the Alfred Wolfsohn voice research centre'. Subsequently published in 'The Roy Hart theatre: documentation and interviews.' *Dartington Theatre papers, Fifth Series*, 14, David Williams (ed). Peter Hulton (series ed). Dartington College of Arts. ISSN 0309 - 8036.

Hart, R. (1967) 'How voice gave me a conscience.' Unpublished paper read at the Seventh International Congress for Psychotherapy, Wiesbaden. Repository: Roy Hart Theatre Archives, Malerargues, France.

Haskell, J. (1991) 'Adjusting adolescents: vocal self-perception.' *Language, Speech and Hearing Services in Schools*, 22.

Haskell, J. (1987) 'Vocal self-perception: the other side of the equation.' *Journal of Voice*, 1.

Hassan, I. (1987) *The Post-Modern Turn: Essays in Post-Modern Theory and Culture.* Ohio: Ohio State University.

Heather, S. (1996) Cited in M. Law, 'Interviews with contemporary voice practitioners'. Unpublished research papers prepared for the International Association for Voicework.

Heaver, L. 'Psychiatric observations on the personality structure of patients with habitual dysphonia.' *Logos* (1958). Cited in P. Bloch (1960) 'New Limits of Vocal Analysis.' *Folia Phoniatrica*, 12.

Heilpern, J. (1989) *Conference of the Birds: The Story of Peter Brook in Africa.* London: Methuen.

Heimann, P. (1950) 'On counter-transference.' *International Journal of Psychoanalysis*, 31.

Henton, C. (1985) 'Breathiness in normal female speech: inefficiency versus desirability.' *Language and Communication*, 5.

Herbenet, E. and Busnel, M. (eds) (1982) *L'Aube du Sens.* Paris: Stock.

Heron, A. and Myers M. (1983) *Intellectual Impairment: Battle Against Handicaps.* New York: Academic Press.

Higgins, R. (1993) *Approaches to Case-Study: A Handbook for Those Entering the Therapeutic Field.* London: Jessica Kingsley.

Hillman, J. (1977) 'An inquiry into image.' *Spring: A Journal of Archetypal Psychology and Jungian Thought*, pp.62-88.

Hillman, J. (1978) 'Further notes on images.' *Spring: A Journal of Archetypal Psychology and Jungian Thought.*

Hillman, J. (1977) *Re-Visioning Psychology.* New York: Harper and Row.

Hillman, J.(1971) 'The Feeling Function' in M.L. von Franz, *Lectures on Jung's Typology.* New York/Zurich: Spring Publications, pp74-150.

Hillman, J. (ed) (1989) *Puer Papers.* Dallas: Spring.

Hines, J. (1982) *Great Singers on Great Singing.* New York: Doubleday.

Hirano, M. and Bless D. (1993) *Video Stroboscopic Examination of the Larynx.* London: Whurr.

Hodgson, J. and Preston-Dunlop, V. (1990) *Rudolf Laban: An Introduction to his Work and Influence.* Plymouth: Northcote House.

Hoffman, L. and Hoffman-Ostwald, D. (1961) *Deutsches Arbeitertheatre 1918–1933.* Berlin: Henschelverlag.

Hollien, H. *et al.* 'On the nature of vocal fry.' *Journal of Speech and Hearing Research.*

Hollings, A. (1989) 'The aims of singing versus speech and the therapeutic potential.' *Newsletter of the Voice Research Society*, (now the British Voice Association), 4, 1.

Hollingshead, A.B. (1957) *Two Factor Index of Status Position*. New Haven.

Holman, E. *Unchained Melodies*. CD. Star Direct.

Homer, (1980) *The Odyssey*. Oxford: Oxford University Press.

Honikman, B. (1964) 'Articulatory settings' In D. Abercrombie, D. Fry, P. MacCarthy, N. Scott and J. Trim (eds) *In Honour of Daniel Jones*. London: Longmans.

Hortaçsu, N. and Ekinci, B. (1992) 'Children's reliance on situational and vocal expression of emotions: consistent and conflicting cues.' *Journal of Non-verbal Behaviour*, 16.

Hough, A. (1994) *Physiotherapy in Respiratory Care*. London: Chapman and Hall.

House, A. and Andrews, H. (1987) 'The psychiatric and social characteristics of patients with functional dysphonia.' *Journal of Psychosomatic Research*, 31, 4, pp. 483-90.

House, A. and Andrews, H. (1988) 'Life events and difficulties preceding the onset of functional dysphonia.' *Journal of Psychosomatic Research*, 32, 3, pp. 311-19.

Houseman, B. (1994) 'Voice and the release and exploration of emotion (from a theatre perspective).' *Dramatherapy*, 16, 2 and 3.

Huang, J. (1993) *The Primordial Breath: An Ancient Chinese Way of Prolonging Life Through Breath Control*, vols. 1 and 2. California: Original Books, Newcastle Publishing.

Hurd Duncan, M. (1945) 'An experimental study of some of the relationships between voice and personality among students of speech.' *Speech Monograph*, M107, 12.

Huxley, A. (1963) *The Doors of Perception and Heaven and Hell*. New York: Harper and Row.

Hyde, G. (1991) 'Russian futurism.' In M. Bradbury and J. McFarlane (eds) *Modernism: A Guide to European Literature 1890–1930*. London: Penguin.

Hymes, D. (1971) 'Competence and performance in linguistic theory.' In R. Huxley and E. Ingram (eds) *Language Acquisition: Models and Methods*. London: Academic Press.

Inayat Khan, H. (1983) *The Music of Life*. Lebanon: Omega.

Information leaflet, Rosehill Hospital, September 1996.

Ingram, T. (1972) 'Classification of speech and language disorders in young children.' In M. Rutter and J. Martin (eds) *The Child with Delayed Speech*. London: SIMP.

Innes, C. (1981) *Holy Theatre: Ritual and the Avant Garde*. Cambridge: Cambridge University Press.

Innes, C. (1993) *Avant Garde Theatre 1892–1992*. London: Routledge.

Isaak, C. *Wicked Game*. CD. WEA Records.

Jackson, J. *Stepping Out*. CD. A&M Records.

Jackson, M. *21 Songs of Faith and Inspiration*. CD. Music Collection International.

Jackson, M. *Thriller*. CD. Sony Music.

Jacobsen, E. (1929) 'Electrical measurements of neuromuscular states during mental activities: imagination of movement involving skeletal muscle.' *American Journal of Physiology*, 91.

James, C. (1993) 'I'd like to teach the world to sing.' *Kindred Spirit*, 22.

James, E. *Etta James*. CD. BMG Music.

James, H. (1891) 'On the occasion of *Hedda Gabler*.' *New Review*, June.

James, J. (1995) *The Music of the Spheres: Music, Science and the Natural Order of the Universe*. London: Abacus.

Janet, P. (1898) *Neuroses et Idees Fixes*. Paris: Alacan.

Jasraj, P. *Ragas: Triveni and Multani*. CD. Navras Records.

Jellineck, A. (1953) 'Observations on the therapeutic use of spontaneous imagery in speech therapy.' *Folia Phoniatrica*, 5, No. 1.

Jellineck, A. (1956) 'Treatment of vocal disorders with spontaneous imagery.' *Folia Phoniatrica*, 8.

Jenks, W.B. (1932) 'Speech training as a means of training maladjustments of personality.' Unpublished doctoral thesis, University of Chicago.

Jennings, S. (ed) (1987) *Dramatherapy: Theory and Practice for Teachers and Clinicians*. London: Routledge.

Jennings, S. (ed) (1992) *Dramatherapy: Theory and Practice 2*. London: Routledge.

Jenny, H. (1967/92) *Cymatics*, Vol. 1 and 2. Basel: Basilius press.

Jesperson, O. (1922) *Language: Its Nature, Development and Origin*.

Jochaim, H. (1969) *Die Welt*, 20 October 1969.

Jolson, A. *The Very Best of Al Jolson*. CD. MCA Records.

Jones, G. *Warm Leatherette*. CD. Island Records.

Jones, H.E. (1942) 'The analysis of voice records.' *Journal of Consulting Psychology*, 6.

Jones, H.E. (1943) *Development in Adolescence*. New York: Appleton-Century.

Joplin, J. *Greatest Hits*. Cassette. Columbia Records.

Joseph, A. (1988) 'The joy of singing'. Unpublished manuscript.

Joseph, A. (1990) 'Voice – a metaphor for life: pedagogical concepts for their application and implementation'. Unpublished manuscript.

Journal of the Arts in Psychotherapy. New York: Pergamon.

Juhan, D. (1987) *Job's Body: A Handbook for Bodywork*. New York: Station Hill.

Jung, C.G. (1953) *Collected Works of C.G. Jung.* (Bollingen Series XX). H. Read, M. Fordham, G. Adler and W. McGuire (eds). Princeton University Press and London: Routledge and Kegan Paul.

Jungr, B.(1997)'Three Singers in London'.Unpublished Master Thesis, Goldsmiths College, London.

Just, R. (1989) *Women in Athenian Law and Life.* London: Routledge.

Kalweit, H. (1992) *Shamans, Healers and Medicine Men.* Boston: Shambhala.

Kaplan, S. and Escott, P. (1973) 'Treatment of two silent adolescent girls.' *Journal of the American Academy of Child Psychiatry,* 12.

Kauffman, P.E. (1954) 'An investigation of some psychological stimulus properties of speech behaviour.' Unpublished doctoral thesis. University of Chicago.

Keleman, S. (1985) *Emotional Anatomy.* Berkeley: Center Press.

Kelerova, I. (1995–6), Publicity brochure of the International School of the Human Voice.

Kestenberg, J. (1995) *Sexuality, Body Movement and the Rhythms of Development.* Northvale, New Jersey.

Keyes, L.E. (1973) *Toning, The Creative Power of the Voice.* Santa Monica: DeVorss.

Khan, Nusrat Fateh Ali , *Shahen-Shah* CD. Real World Music.

Kilcoyne, A. (1991) 'Common sense: making use of the sense of touch.' *The British Journal of Visual Impairment,* 9, 2.

Killingmo, B. (1990) 'Beyoantics: a clinical study of isolation.' *International Journal of Psychoanalysis.*

Kindred Spirit, 2, 10.

Kindsley, C.F. (1934) 'The psycho-physical determinants of voice quality.' *Speech Monograph,* 1.

King, BB *Ain't Nobody Home: The Best of BB King.* Cassette. MCA Records.

Kings' Fund Centre (1980) 'An ordinary life: comprehensive locally based residential services for mentally handicapped people.' Project Paper 24. London: King Edward's Hospital Fund for London.

Kirby, M. (1971) *Futurist Performance.* New York: EP Dutton.

Kirchner-Bockholt, M. (1922) *Fundamental Principles of Curative Eurythmy.* London: Temple Lodge.

Klein, M. (1948) *Contributions to Psychoanalysis.* London: Hogarth Press.

Knill, P. (1978) *Intermodal Learning in Education and Therapy.* Unpublished manuscript.

Kofler, K. (1893) *The Art of Breathing as the Basis of Tone Production.* New York: Edgar S. Werner.

Kovel, J. (1991) *A Complete Guide to Therapy: From Psychoanalysis to Behaviour Modification.* London: Penguin.

Kramer, E. (1964) 'Personality stereotypes in voice: a reconsideration of the data.' *Journal of Social Psychology*, 62.

Kravitt, E. (1976) 'The joining of words and music in late romantic melodrama.' *Music Quarterly*, LXII.

Kretschmer, E. (1925) *Physique and Character*. New York: Harcourt and Brace.

Kretzmer, H. (1979) 'Stunning – this trip with the human voice.' *Daily Express*. Cited in 'Roy Hart Theatre.' Unpublished anthology of reviews, extracts from articles and other material, compiled by Barrie Coghlan with assistance from Noah Pikes.

Kris, E. (1955) 'Laughter as an expressive process.' In *Psychoanalytic Explorations in Art*. New York: International University Press.

Kristeva, J. (1980) *Desire in Language: A Semiotic Approach to Literature and Art*. New York: Columbia University Press.

Kristeva, J. (1987) *Tales of Love*. Trans. by L. Roudiez. New York: Columbia University Press.

Kroeber, A. (1940) 'Psychotic factors in shamanism.' *Character and Personality*, 8.

Kugler, P. (1978) 'Image and sound: an archetypal approach to language.' *Spring: A Journal of Archetypal Psychology and Jungian Thought*.

Kugler, P. (1979) 'The phonetic imagination.' *Spring: A Journal of Archetypal Psychology and Jungian Thought*.

Kumar, S. (1986) 'Sound in mind and body.' *Resurgence*, 115.

Kumiega, J. (1987) *The Theatre of Grotowski*. London: Methuen.

Kurth, E. (1931) *Musikpsychologie*. Berlin: M. Hesse.

Laban, R. (1960) *The Mastery of Movement*, 2nd edn. London: McDonald and Evans.

LaBarre, W. (1964) 'Confession as cathartic therapy in American Indian tribes.' In A. Kiev (ed) *Magic Faith and Healing*. New York: Free Press of Glencoe.

Ladefoged, P. (1996) *Elements of Acoustic Phonetics*. Chicago: University of Chicago press.

Laine, C. *Solitude*. CD. BMG Music.

Lamb, W. (1965) *Posture and Gesture: An Introduction to the Study of Physical Behaviour*. London: Duckworth.

Lamb, W. and Watson, E. (1987) *Body Code: The Meaning in Movement*. Princeton: Princeton.

Lane, D. (1994) *Music as Medicine*. Michigan: Zondervan.

Langer, S. (1953) *Feeling and Form*. London: Routledge and Kegan Paul.

Langer, S. (1963) *Philosophy in a New Key*, 3rd Edn. Cambridge, Massachusetts: Harvard University press.

Langs, R. (1994) *Doing Supervision and Being Supervised*. London: Karnac.

Laver, J. (1978) 'The concept of articulatory settings: an historical survey.' *Historiographia Linguistica*, 5.

Laver, J. (1980) *Phonetic Description of Voice.* Cambridge: Cambridge University Press.

Laver, J., Wirz, S., MacKenzie, J. and Hillier, S. (1981) 'A perceptual protocol for the analysis of vocal profiles.' Work in progress, Department of Linguistics, university of Edinburgh, 14.

Law, M. (1996) 'Interviews with contemporary voice practitioners.' Unpublished research papers prepared for the International Association of Voicework.

Law, M. (1996) 'The practice of voice: an investigation into the diversity of approaches to vocal work as exemplified by current practitioners.' Unpublished research project prepared for the International Association of Voicework.

Le Mée, K. (1994) *Chant: The Origins, Form, Practice and Healing Power of Gregorian Chant.* London: Random House.

Lebrun, Y. (1990) *Mutism.* London: Whurr.

Leeds, J. (1995) 'Revising the map of the musician's odyssey.' *Open Ear*, 3.

Lehmann, L. (1993) *How to Sing.* New York: Dover.

Lesser-Katz, M. (1986) 'Stranger reaction and elective mutism in children.' *American Journal of Orthopsychiatry*, 56.

Leuner, H.(1977), 'Guided affective imagery: An account of its development' *Journal of Mental Imagery*, 1, pp.73-92.

Lever, S. (1996), cited in M. Law 'Interviews with contemporary voice practitioners.' Unpublished research papers prepared for the International Association of Voicework.

Levine, E. (1995) *Tending the Fire: Studies in Art, Therapy and Creativity.* Toronto: Palmerston Press.

Levine, S. (1997) *Poesis: The Language of Psychology and the Speech of the Soul.* London: Jessica Kingsley.

Lewis, J. L. *The EP Collection.* CD. See for Miles Records.

Lewis, M.M. (1936) *Early Response to Speech and Babbling in Infant Speech.* London: Kegan Paul.

Lewis, P. (1994) 'The clinical interpretation of the Kestenberg movement profile'. Unpublished thesis.

Lewis, P. (1995) Personal communication with the author. Boston, November 1995.

Lewis, P. (1986) *Theoretical Approaches in Dance Movement Therapy*, 1 and 2. Dubque: Kendall Hunt.

Lingerman, H.A. (1983) *The Healing Energies of Music.* Wheaton, Il: Quest Books.

Linklater, K. (1976) *Freeing the Natural Voice.* New York: Drama Book.

Lisa Gerrard and the Victorian Philharmonic Orchestra, *The Mirror Pool*. CD. Beggars Banquet Music.

Lissau, R. (1987) *Rudolf Steiner: Life, Work, Inner Path and Social Initiatives*. Stroud: Hawthorn Press.

Lofting, H. (1950) *The Voyages of Dr. Doolittle*. Philadelphia: Lippincott.

Lomax, A. (1978) *A Folk Song Style and Culture*. New Jersey: Transaction Books.

Lonsdale, S. (1981) *Animals and the Origin of Dance*. London: Thames and Hudson.

Lord, A. (1960) *The Singer of Tales*. Cambridge: Harvard University Press.

Lorenz-Poschmann, A. (1982) *Breath, Speech and Therapy*. New York: Mercury Press.

Lotz, J. (1955) *Linguistics: Symbols Make Humans*. New York: Language and Communication Research Centre, Columbia University.

Lowen, A. (1976) *Bioenergetics*. London: Penguin.

Luchsinger, R. and Dubios, C.L. (1956) 'Phonetische und stroboskopische untersuchungen an einem stimmphanomen.' *Folia Phiatrica*, 8, 4.

Luchsinger, R. and Arnold, G. (eds.) (1965) *Voice, Speech and Language*. London: Constable.

Lynch, G.E. (1934) 'A phonophotographic study of trained and untrained voices reading factual and dramatic material.' *Archives of Speech*, 1.

Lynn Kittelson, M. (1996) *Sounding the Soul: The Art of Listening*. Einnsiedein: Daimon.

Lynn, V. *We'll Meet Again: Her Greatest Hits*. CD. Woodford Music.

Lyotard, J.F. (1984) *The Post-Modern Condition: A Report on Knowledge, Theory and History of Literature*, Volume 10. Manchester: Manchester University Press.

M People, *Bizarre Fruit*. CD. BMG Records.

Madonna, *Something to Remember*. CD. Warner Communications.

Mahl, G.F. (1956) 'Disturbances and silences in the patient's speech in psychotherapy.' *Journal of Abnormal Social Psychology* 53.

Mahler, M. (1968) *On Human Symbiosis and the Vicissitudes of Individuation*. New York: International University Press.

Makeba, M. *Welela*. CD. Polygram Records.

Malinowski, B. (127) 'Supplement' In C.K. Ogden and I.A. Richards (eds) *The Meaning of Meaning*. New York: Harcourt and Brace.

Manen, L. (1989) *Bel Canto: The Teaching of the Classical Italian Song-Schools, its Decline and Restoration*. Oxford: Oxford University Press.

Marafioti, P. (1981) *Caruso's Method of Voice Production: The Scientific Culture of the Voice*. New York: Dover.

Marinetti, F.T. (1960) *Teatro F.T. Marinetti*. Giovanni Calendoli (ed) 3 vols. Rome.

Marleau-Ponty (1970) cited in P. Lewis 'Marleau-Ponty and the phenomenology of language' In J. Ehrmann (ed) *Structuralism*. New York: Anchor Books.

Marshall, K. (ed.) (1993) *Rediscovering the Muses: Women's Musical Traditions*. Boston: Northeastern University Press.

Martin, D. *The Best of Dean Martin*. CD. EMI Music.

Martin, J. (1991) *Voice in Modern Theatre*. London and New York: Routledge.

Maslow, A.H. (1937) 'Dominance-feeling, behaviour and status.' *Psychological Review*, 44.

Masson, J. (1992) *The Assault on Truth: Freud and Child Sexual Abuse*. London: Harper Collins.

Mathieu, W. (1991) *The Listening Book: Discovering Your Own Music*. Boston: Shambhala.

Matthews, J. (1974) *Theatre in Dada and Surrealism*. Syracuse: Syracuse University Press.

Mayakovsky, V. (1970) *How are Verses Made?* trans. G. Hyde. London: Pluto Press.

Mayakovsky, V. *et al.* (1991) 'A slap in the face of public taste.' Cited in G. Hyde 'Russian Futurism.' In M. Bradbury and J. McFarlane (eds) *Modernism: A Guide to European Literature 1890–1930*. London: Penguin.

Mayland, E. (1995) 'The Rosen method.' In D. Johnson (ed) *Bone, Breath and Gesture: Practises of Embodiment*. Berkeley: North Atlantic Books.

McCallion, M. (1988) *The Voice Book*. London: Faber and Faber.

McClellan, R. (1991) *The Healing Force of Music: History, Theory and Practice*. Shaftesbury. Element.

McCloud, J. (1993) 'Spirituality for sale: plastic medicine men invade Europe.' *American Indian Community House Bulletin*, VIII, XIII.

McColl, E. (1992) cited in S. Richards *Sonic Harvest: Towards Musical Democracy*. Oxford: Amber Lane.

McGehee, F. (1937) 'The reliability of the identification of the human voice.' *Journal of General Psychology*, 17.

McKelvey, D.P. (1953) 'Voice and personality.' *Western Speech*, 17.

McNeely, D. (1987) *Touching: Body Therapy and Depth Psychology*. Toronto: Inner City Books.

McNiff, S. (1981) *The Arts in Psychotherapy*. Springfield, Ill: Charles C. Thomas.

McNiff, S. (1986) *Educating the Creative Arts Therapist: A Profile of the Profession*. Springfield, Ill: Charles C. Thomas.

McNiff, S. (1996) Interview with P. Newham at Endicott College, June 1996.

Meat Loaf. *Bat Out of Hell*. Cassette. Sony Music.

Meekums, B. (1992) 'Dance movement therapy in a family service unit' and 'Monika Steiner', Helen Payne (ed). London: Tavistock/Routledge.

Melanie, *The Four Sides of Melanie*. CD. Unidisc Productions.

Merman, E. *I Get a Kick out of You.* CD. Pavilion Records.

Merriam, A. (1980) *The Anthroplogy of Music.* Illinois: NorthWestern University Press.

Mettler, B. (1979) *Materials of Dance as a Creative Activity.* Tuscon, Arizona: Mettler Studios Inc.

Mettler, B. (1985) *Dance as an Element of Life.* Tuscon, Arizona: Mettler Studios Inc.

Michael, W. and Crawford, C.C. (1927) 'An experiment in judging intelligence by the voice.' *Journal of Educational Psychology,* 18.

Middendorf, I. (1990) *The Perceptible Breath: A Breathing Science.* Paderborn: Junfermann-Verlag.

Miller, R. (1986) *The Structure of Singing: System and Arts in Vocal Technique.* New York: Schirmer.

Milner, M. (1956) 'The communication of primary sensual experience: the yell of joy.' International Journal of Psycho-analysis, 37.

Minett, G. (1994) *Breath and Spirit: Rebirthing as a Healing Technique.* London: Harper Collins.

Minnelli, L. *Maybe this Time.* CD. Capitol Records.

Mitchell, J. *Reprise.* CD. Warner Communications.

Mitchell, S. (1992) 'Therapeutic theatre: a para-theatrical model of dramatherapy.' In Sue Jennings (ed) *Dramatherapy: Theory and Practice,* 2. London: Routledge.

Moi, T. (1985) *Sexual-Textual Politics: Feminist Literary Theory.* London: Routledge.

Moi, T. (ed)(1986) *The Kristeva Reader.* Oxford: Blackwell.

Monroe, M. *Born Free: Greatest Hits.* CD. EMI Records.

Montepare, J. and Vega, C. (1988) 'Women's vocal reaction to intimate and casual male friends.' *Personality and Social Psychology Bulletin,* 14.

Montepare, J. and Zebrowitz-McArthur, L. (1987) 'Perceptions of adults with child-like voices in two cultures.' *Journal of Experimental Social Psychology,* 23.

Moog, H. (1976) *The Musical Experience of the Preschool Child.* London: Schott.

Moolenaar-Biji, A.I. (1957) 'The laryngeal whistle.' *Folia Phoniatrica,* 9.

Moore Meigs, M. (1994) 'Voicework' In D. Jones (ed) *Innovative Therapy: A Handbook.* Buckingham: Open University Press.

Moore Meigs, M. (1992) 'Voicework.' *Self and Society,* XX, 1.

Moore Meigs, M. (1991) 'Introduction to music therapy.' *Self and Society,* XVIX, 1.

Moore, C.E. (1938) 'A preliminary study of the emotional effects of letter sounds.' *Quarterly Journal of Speech,* 24, 1.

Moreno, J.L. (1946) *Psychodrama,* 1 and 2. New York: Beacon House.

Moroney, P. (1980) 'Apples on a lilac tree: silence and song in the individuation process.' Diploma Thesis for C.G. Jung Institute, Zurich.

Morrant, J. (1981) 'The First Few Minutes.' *Canadian Journal of Psychiatry,* 26(6).

Morrison, M.D., Nichol, H. and Rammage, L.A. (1986) 'Diagnostic criteria in functional dysphonia.' *Laryngoscope*, 94.

Morrison, V. *Days Like This*. CD. Vanguard Records.

Moser, H.M., Dreher, J.J. and Adler, S. (1955) 'Comparison of hyponasality, hypernasality and normal voice quality on the intelligibility of two digit numbers.' *Jounral of Acoustical Society of America*, 27.

Moses, P.J. (1942) 'The study of voice records.' *Journal of Consulting Psychology*, 6.

Moses, P.J. (1953) 'Speech and voice therapy in otolaryngology.' *Eye, Ear, Nose and Throat Monthly*, 32, 7.

Moses, P.J. (1954) *The Voice of Neurosis*. New York: Grune and Stratton.

Moses, P.J. (1958) 'Reorientation of concepts and facts in phonetics.' *Logos*.

Moses, P.J. (1961) Letter to A. Wolfsohn, 16 April 1961. Repository: Alfred Wolfsohn Private Archives, Malerargues, France. ©Marita Gunther. Re-printed by permission.

Mothersole, A. (1920) 'La Rythmique est-elle une lubie?' *La Rythme*, 5.

Mukunda, V. (1996) Lecture given at *Songs of Heaven and Earth Conference*. Findhorn Foundation, Forres, 30 March–6 April 1996.

Murphy, J. (1964) 'Psychotherapeutic aspects of shamanism on St. Lawrence Island, Alaska.' In A. Kiev (ed) *Magic, Faith and Healing*. New York: Free Press of Glencoe.

Naumberg, M. (1958) 'Art Therapy: its scope and function.' In *Clinical Applications of Projective Drawings*, ed. by E.F. Hammer. Springfield: C.C. Thomas.

Needleham, J. (1983) 'Psychiatry and the sacred' In J. Welwood (ed) *Awakening the Heart: East / West Approaches to Psychotherapy and the Healing Relationship*. Boston: Shambhala.

Neumann, E. (1970) *The Origins and History of Consciousness*. Princeton: Princeton University Press. Bollingen Series XLII.

Newham, P. (1993) 'The singing cure: how voice movement therapy has evolved'. *Human Communication* 2, no. 2, February 1993 pp.6-8.

Newham, P. (1990) 'The voice and the shadow'. *Performance* 60, Spring 1990, pp. 37-47.

Newham, P. (1992) 'Jung and Alfred Wolfsohn: analytical psychology and the singing voice.' *Journal of Analytical Psychology*, 37, pp.323-336.

Newham, P. (1992) 'Singing and psyche: towards voice movement therapy'. *Voice: Journal of the British Voice Association*. 1, pp.75-102.

Newham, P. (1993) 'The psychology of voice and the founding of the Roy Hart Theatre'. *New Theatre Quarterly*, IX, no. 33, February 1993, pp.59-65.

Newham, P. (1993) 'Saying with sounds'. *Community Living* 6, no. 4, April 1993, pp.25-27.

Newham, P. (1993) The singing cure'. *Human Potential*. Summer 1993, pp. 6-8.

Newham, P. (1994) 'Voice movement therapy: towards an arts therapy for voice'. *Dramatherapy* 16, no. 2 & 3, pp. 28-33.

Newham, P. (1995) 'Animal magic: giving voice to the animal within'. *Human Potential.* Spring 1995, pp. 6-7.

Newham, P. (1995-1996) 'Making a song and dance: the musical voice of language'. Journal of the Imagination in Learning. III, pp. 28-33.

Newham, P. (1997) *'Shouting for Jericho': The Work of Paul Newham on the Human Voice.* London: Tigers Eye Press/Class Productions.

Newham, P.(1997) *'Prayers and Prophecies'.* London: Tigers Eye Press

Newham, P. (1998) *The Singing Cure: Liberating Self Expression through Voice Movement Therapy.* Boulder: Sounds True.

Newman, R. *Lonely at the Top.* CD. Warner Communications.

Nichols, M., (1996) cited in M. Law 'Interviews with contemporary voice practitioners'. Unpublished research papers prepared for the International Association of Voicework.

Noack, A. (1992) 'On a Jungian approach to dance movement therapy.' In H. Payne (ed) *Dance Movement Therapy: Theory and Practice.* London: Tavistock/ Routledge.

Nordoff, P. and Robbins, C. (1992) *Therapy in Music for Handicapped Children.* London: Victor Gollancz.

Nusrat Fateh Ali Khan, *Shahen-Shah* CD.(Real World Music).

Jesperson, O. (1922) *Language: Its Nature, Development and Origin.* London: Allen and Unwin.

Odetta, *The Essential Odetta.* CD. Vanguard Records.

O'Brien, B. (1996) 'Rehearsal, character, voice and self: the actor's experience of emotion and character when working through the voice'. Unpublished paper presented to the International Association for Voicework, October 1996.

O'Connor, S. *Am I Not Your Girl?.* Cassette. Ensign Records.

O'Shea, J. (1993) *Music and Medicine: Medical Profiles of Great Composers.* London: Dent.

Opie, I. and P. (1967) *Children's Games in Street and Playground.* Oxford: Oxford University Press.

Opie, I. and P. (1984) *The Lore and Language of Schoolchildren.* Oxford: Oxford University Press.

Opie, I. and P. (1988) *The Singing Game.* Oxford: Oxford Unity Press.

Opie, I. and P. (1959) *The Lore and Language of Schoolchildren.* Oxford University Press.

Orbison, R. *All-time Greatest Hits.* Cassette. Skyline Records.

Orr, L. and Ray, S. (1983) *Rebirthing in the New Age.* Berkeley: Celestial Arts.

Osbourne, O. *Bark at the Moon.* CD. Sony Music.

Ostwald, P. (1973) 'Linguistic contributions to the study of human sounds.' In *The Semiotics of Human Sound*. The Hague and Paris: Mouton.

Ostwald, P. (1960) 'Musical behaviour in early childhood.' *Developmental Medicine and Child Neurology*, 15, pp. 367-95.

Ostwald, P.F. (1960) 'Human sounds.' In D.A. Barbara (ed) *Psychological and Psychiatric Aspects of Speech and Hearing*. Springfield, Illinois: Charles C. Thomas.

Ostwald, P.F. (1973) *The Semiotics of Human Sound*. The Hague and Paris: Mouton.

Padel, R. (1992) *In and Out of Mind: Greek Images of the Tragic*. Princeton: Princeton University Press.

Panconcelli-Calzia, G. (1943) *Leonardo als Phonetiker*. Hamburg.

Papas, I. *Aphrodite's Child, 666*. CD. Polygram Records.

Pardo, E. (1984) 'Dis-membering dionysus: image and theatre.' *Spring: A Journal of Archetypal Psychology and Jungian Though*.

Parton, D. *Dolly Parton: Her Greatest Hits*. CD. Woodford Music.

Partridge, P. (1994) 'The voice as a clue.' *Dramatherapy*, 16, 2 and 3.

Passalacqua, L. (1995/96) 'Voice work in dramatherapy.' *Dramatherapy*, 17, 3.

Paxton, S. (1981–82) 'Contact improvisation.' *Dartington Theatre Papers, Fourth Series*.

Payne, H. (ed.) (1992) *Dance Movement Therapy: Theory and Practice*. London: Tavistock/Routledge.

Pear, T.H. (1927) *Radio Times*, 14 January.

Pear, T.H. (1931) *Voice and Personality*. New York: Wiley.

Pearl Jam, *Pearl Jam*. CD. Sony Music.

Pearson, J. (1996) *Discovering the Self Through Movement and Drama*. London: Jessica Kingsley.

Peri, J. (1952) 'Preface to Eurydice.' Translated by O. Strunk in *Source Readings in Music History*, London. Cited in part in C. Headington, R. Westbrook and T. Barfoot (1991) *Opera: A History*, London: Arrow Books.

Perls, F. (1969) *Gestalt Therapy Verbatim*. Utah: Real People Press.

Peters, L. (1978) 'Psychotherapy in Tamang shamanism.' *Ethnos*, 6, 2.

Pfaff, P.L. (1954) 'An experimental study of the communication of feeling without contextual material.' *Speech Monograph*. 21.

Phillips, K. *Teaching Kids to Sing*. New York: Schirmer Books, p.48.

Piaf, E. *The Legendary Edith Piaf*. CD. EMI Records.

Picken, L. (1957) 'The music of Far Eastern Asia 1: China.' In E. Wellwsz (ed) *The New Oxford History of Music, vol. 1. Ancient and Oriental Music*. London: Oxford University Press.

Pierce, J. (1992) *The Science of Musical Sound*. New York: Freeman and co.

Pierce, J. (1992) *The Science of Musical Sound*. New York: Freeman.

Pies, H. (1833) *Kasper Hauser*. London: Simpkin and Marshall.

Pikes, N. (1993) 'Giving voice to hell.' *Spring: A Journal of Archetype and Culture*, 55.

Pikes, N. (1994) *The Whole Voice – The Creative Voice Publicity Pamphlet*.

Pinker, S. (1994) *The Language Instinct*. London: Penguin.

Piontelli, A. (1992) *From Foetus to Child: An Observational and Psychoanalytic Study*. London: Tavistock/Routledge.

Pitney, G. *Greatest Hits*. Cassette. MAMC Music.

Pittam, J. (1994) 'Voice in social interaction: an interdisciplinary approach.' *Language and Language Behaviours*, 5. London: Sage.

Pittenger, R.E., Hocket, C.F. and Danehy, J.J. (1960) *The First Five Minutes*. Ithaca, New York: Paul Martineau.

Plato, *Laws*.

Plato, *Republic*.

Plutarch, *The Life of Solon*.

Plutchik, R. (1955) 'The emotions: facts, theories and a new model.' *Psychosomatic Medicine*.

Presley, Elvis, *From the Heart: His Greatest Love Songs*. Cassette. BMG Music.

Prince, *Greatest Hits*, vol. 1and2. CD. Warner Communications.

Purce, J. (1996) cited in M. Law (1996) 'Interviews with contemporary voice practitioners.' Unpublished research papers prepared for the International Association for Voicework.

Purce, J. (1996) Publicity leaflet for workshops.

Purna Das Baul, *Songs of Love and Ecstasy*. CD. Real World.

Quarterly Journal of Biofeedback and Self-Regulation.

Schechner, R. (1982) *The End of Humanism: Writings on Performance*. New York: Performance Arts Journal Press.

Racker, H. (1968) *Transference and Counter-Transference*. London: Maresfield.

Rakusen, J. (1996), cited in M. Law 'Interviews with contemporary voice practitioners.' Unpublished research papers prepared for the International Association for Voicework.

Rama, S., Bellentine, R. and Hymes, A. (1990) *The Science of Breath*. Pennsylvania: The Himalayan International Institute.

Ramacharaka, Y. (1905) *The Science of Breath: A Complete Manual of the Oriental Breathing Philosophy*. Chicago: Yogi Publication Society.

Ramacharaka, Y. (1905) *The Hindu-Yogi Breathing Exercises: A System of Physical, Mental and Soul Development*. Chicago: Yogi Publication Society.

Rasmussen, K. (1958) 'An Eskimo shaman purifies a sick person.' In Lessa and Vogt (ed) *Reader in Comparative Religion*. Evanston, Illinois: Row, Peterson.

Ray, J. *Remember Johnie Ray*. CD. Document Records.

Rayburn, W. (1982) 'Clinical applications of monitoring foetal activity.' *American Journal of Obstetrics and Gynaecology*, 144.

Redfearn, J. (1985) 'My self, my many selves.' *Library of Analytical Psychology*, vol. 6. London: Academic Press.

Reich, W. (1948) *Character Analysis.* London: Vision Press, 3rd edn.

Reich, W.(1961) *The Function of the Orgasm.* London: Panther.

Reid, C. (1971) *Bel Canto: Principles and Practices.* New York: Joseph Patelson Music House.

Relph, A. (1996), cited in M. Law 'Interviews with contemporary voice practitioners.' Unpublished research papers prepared for the International Association for Voicework.

Reyher, J. (1977) 'Spontaneous visual imagery: implications for psychoanalysis, psychopathology and psychotherapy.' *Journal of Mental Imagery*, 2.

Reznikoff, I. (1994) cited in 'Therapy of pure sound, reaching deep consciousness to heal: Iégor Reznikoff interviewed by Caduceus.' *Caduceus*, Issue 23.

Reznikoff, I. (1996) Lecture given at Songs of Heaven and Earth Conference. Findhorn Foundation, Forres, 30 March–6 April 1996.

Rheingold, H., Gerwirtz, J. and Ross (1959) 'Social conditioning of vocalisations in the infant.' *Journal of Comparative Physiological Psychology*, 52.

Richards, S. (1992) *Sonic Harvest: Towards Musical Democracy.* Oxford: Amber Lane.

Rieffert, J.B. (1931) 'Sprechtypen.' 12th Kongr. Ges. Pscyhol.

Riperton, Minnie, *The Best of Minnie Riperton.* CD. Capitol Records.

Robbins, A. (1986) *Expressive Therapy: A Creative Arts Approach to Depth-Orientated Treatment.* New York: Human Sciences Press, p.242.

Roberts, R. (1996) cited in M. Law 'Interviews with contemporary voice practitioners.' Unpublished research papers prepared for the International Association of Voicework.

Robeson, P. *Live in Concert from Tchaikovsky Hall, Moscow.* CD. Fenix Entertainment.

Roche, J. (1980) 'La voix d'enfant.' *Le Journal d'Audiophonologie.*

Rodenburg, P. (1992) *The Right to Speak: Working with the Voice.* London: Methuen Drama.

Rodenburg, P. (1993) *The Need for Words: Voice and the Text.* London: Methuen.

Rohmert, G. (1991) *Der Sänger auf dem Weg zum Klang.* Köln: Die Deutsche Bibliothek.

Rolf, I. (1990) *Rolfing and Physical Reality.* Rochester: Healing Arts Press.

Rolli, R. Workshop publicity, January 1996.

Rolling Stones. *Rolled Gold: The Very Best of the Rolling Stones.* Cassette. Decca.

Roose-Evans, J. (1989) *Experimental Theatre: From Stanislavski to peter Brook,* 4th edn. London: Routledge.

Rose, F., Whurr, R. and Wyke, M. (1993) *Aphasia*. London: Whurr.

Rosen, M. and Brenner, S. (1991) *The Rosen Method of Movement*. (Berkeley: North Atlantic Books.

Roth, G. (1990), cited in M. Albert 'Teachings of an urban shaman.' *Yoga Journal*, December.

Roth, G. (1990) *Maps to Ecstasy: Teachings of an Urban Shaman*. London: HarperCollins.

Rouget, G. (1985) *Music and Trance: A Theory of the Relations Between Music and Possession*. Chicago: University of Chicago Press.

Roussos, D. *The Story of Demis Roussos*. CD. BR Music.

Rowland, J. (1984) *Inside Motion: An Anatomical Basis for Movement Education*. Amsterdam: John Rowland.

Rubenfield, I. (1995) 'Interview with Irmgard Bartenieff.' In D. Johnson (ed) *Bone, Breath and Gesture: Practises of Embodiment*. Berkeley: North Atlantic Books.

Rudd, E. 'A phenomological approach to improvision in music therapy: a research method'. Paper read at the Sixth World Congress of Music Therapy, Rio de Janiero, 15–20 July 1990.

Ruesch, J. and Kees, W. *Nonverbal communication: Notes on the Visual Perception of Human Relations*. Berkeley and Los Angeles: University of California Press.

Rush, J. (1827) *The Philosophy of the Human Voice: Embracing its Physiological History; Together with a System of Principles, by which Criticism in the Art of Elocution may be Rendered Intelligible, and Instruction, Definite and Comprehensive, To which is Added a Brief Analysis of Song and Recitative*. Philadelphia.

Russell, J. (1864) 'A case of hysteric aphonia.' *British Medical Journal*, 2.

Russolo, L. (1967) *The Art of Noise*. New York.

Rutter, M., Tizard, J. and Whitmore, K. (1970) *Education, Health and Behaviour*. London: Longman.

Ruzicka, B. and Sackin, D. (1974) 'Elective mutism.' *Journal of the American Academy of Child Psychiatry*, 13.

Sachs, C. (1942) *The History of Musical Instruments*. London: Dent.

Sachs, C. (1943) *The Rise and Fall of Music in the Ancient World: East and West*. New York: Norton.

Sachs, C. (1958) *Our Musical Heritage*. New York: Prentice Hall.

Sachs, C. (1962) *The Wellsprings of Music*. The Hague: Martinus Nijhoff.

Sakata, H. (1989) 'Hazara women in afghanistan: innovators and preservers of musical tradition.' In E. Koskoff (ed) *Women and Music in Cross Cultural perspective*. Illinois: University of Illinois Press.

Salaman, E. (1989) *Unlocking Your Voice: Freedom to Sing*. London: Gollancz.

Samuels, A. (1985) *Jung and the Post-Jungians*. London: Routledge.

Samuels, A. (1993) *The Political Psyche*. London: Routledge.

Sanford, Fillmore H. (1942) 'Speech and personality.' *Psychological Bulletin*, 39, 10.

Sapir, E. (1921) *Language: An Introduction in the Study of Speech*. New York: Harcourt and Brace.

Sapir, E. (1927) 'Speech as a personality trait.' *American Journal of Sociology*, 32.

Sarno, L. (1993) *Song from the Forest: My Life Among the Ba-Benjellé Pygmies*. London: Penguin.

Saussure, F. (1916) *A Court in General Linguistics*. New York: McGraw-Hill.

Schafer, R. (1994) *The Soundscape: Our Sonic Environment and the Tuning of the World*. Vermont: Destiny.

Schattner, G. and Courtney, R. (eds) (1980) *Drama in Therapy*, 1 and 2. New York: Drama Book.

Schechner, R. (1985) *Between Theatre and Anthroplogy*. Philadelphia: University of Pennsylvania Press.

Schechner, R. (1994) *Performance Theory*. London: Routledge.

Schechner, R. (1995) *The Future of Ritual: Writings on Culture and Performance*. London: Routledge.

Scheller, M. (1992–93) 'To touch or not to touch: legal, ethical and clinical issues concerning incorporation of non-sexual touch into verbal psychotherapy.' *Somatics: Journal of Bodily Arts and Sciences*, IX, 1, pp. 42–45.

Schick, J. (1995) 'Interview with Charlotte Selver.' In D. Johnson (ed) *Bone, Breath and Gesture: Practises of Embodiment*. Berkeley: North Atlantic Books.

Schieffelin, B. (1990) *The Give and Take of Everyday Life: Language Socialization of Kaluli Children*. New York: Cambridge University Press.

Schlaf, J. (1906) *Maurice Maeterlink*. Berlin.

Schneider, J., Smith, C. and Whitcher, S. (1982–83) 'The relationship of mental imagery to white blood cell (neutrophil) function.' In 'Hypnosis and the immune system: a review with implications for cancer and the psychology of healing.' *Journal of Clinical Hypnosis*, 25, 2–3.

Schoop, T. and Mitchell, P. (1979) 'Reflections and projections: the Schoop approach to dance therapy.' In P. Bernstein (ed) *Eight Theoretical Approaches to Dance Movement Therapy*. Dubuque: Kendall Hunt.

D.M. Schullian and M. Schoen (eds) (1948) *Music and Medicine*. New York: Henry Schuman.

Schultz, G. and Luthe, W. (1969) *Autogenic Training: A Physiological Approach to Psychotherapy*. New York: Grune and Stratton.

Schutzman, M. and Cohen-Cruz, J. (eds) (1994) *Playing Boal: Theatre, Therapy, Activism*. London: Routledge.

Schweidlenka, R. (1993) 'Spirituality for sale: plastic medicine men invade Europe.' *American Indian Community House Bulletin*, VIII, XIII.

Screamin' Jay Hawkins, *Voodoo Jive*. CD. CBS Records.

Seagren, R. (1991) 'Overtones of health: an interview with Don Campbell.' *Open Ear Fall.*

Seal, *Seal.* CD. ZTT Records.

Sedaka, N. *Oh Carol: His Greatest Hits.* CD. Woodford Music.

Seymour, A. (1987) 'Revelations in Poland.' *Plays and Players,* 33–34. Cited in J. Kumiega, *The Theatre of Grotowski.* London: Methuen.

Shanghai Opera, *An Introduction to Chinese Opera,* vol. 4. CD. Marco Polo.

Sharpe, E. (1940) 'Psychophysical problems revealed in language.' *International Journal of Psychoanalysis,* 21.

Shaw, C. (1995) 'A theft of spirit?' *Kindred Spirit,* July/August.

Shawn, T. (1954) *Every Little Movement.* New York: Whitmark and Sons.

Shehan, V. (1989) 'Balkan women as preservers of traditional music and culture.' In E. Koskoff (ed) *Women and Music in Cross Cultural Perspective.* Illinois: University of Illinois Press.

Sheikh, A. (1978) 'Eidetic psychotherapy.' In J. Singer and K. Pope (eds) *The Power of Human Imagination: New Methods in Psychotherapy.* New York: Plenum.

Sheikh, A. and Jordon, C. (1983) 'Clinical uses of mental imagery.' In *Imagery: Current Theory, Research and Application.* New York: Wiley.

Sheppard, L. (1964) 'An empirical therapy based on an extension of vocal range and expression in singing and drama.' Unpublished paper read at the Sixth International Congress of Psychotherapy, London, August 1964.

Sheridan, T. (1968) cited in R.C. Alston (ed) *Thomas Sheridan: A Course of Lectures on Elocution 1762.* Menston: Scolar Press.

Shewell, C. (1991) 'A lack of understanding about two professions.' *Human Communication,* November 1991.

Shklovsky, V. (1974) *Mayakovsky and his Circle.* London: Pluto Press.

Shorr, J. (1972) *Psycho-Imagination Therapy: The Integration of Phenomenology and Imagination.* Intercontinental Medical Book Corp.

Showalter, E. (1987) *The Female Malady: Women, Madness and Culture 1830–1980.* London: Virago Press.

Shu-De, *Voices from the Distance Steppe.* CD. Real World Music.

Shyer, L. (1989) *Robert Wilson and his Collaborators.* New York: Theatre Communications.

Silverman, H. (ed) (1990) *Post-Modernism – Philosophy and the Arts.* London: Routledge.

Silverman, J. (1967) 'Shamanism and acute schizophrenia.' *American Anthropologist,* 69.

Silverman, K. (1988) *The Acoustic Mirror: The Female Voice in Psychoanalysis and Cinema.* Bloomington and Indianapolis: Indiana University Press.

Simmer, B. (1976) 'Robert Wilson and therapy.' *Drama Review,* T69, 21, 1.

Simone, N. *Lady Blue.* CD. Charly Popular.

Sinason, V. (1992) *Mental Handicap and the Human Condition: New Approaches from the Tavistock.* London: Free Association Press.

Singer, J. (1974) *Imagery and Daydream Methods in Psychotherapy and Behaviour Modification.* New York: Academic.

Singer, J. and Pope, K. (1978) *The Power of Human Imagination: New Methods in Psychotherapy.* New York: Plenum.

Siouxsie and the Banshees,*Once Upon a Time and Twice upon a Time.*CD(Polydor/Geffen)

Skinner, B.F. (1957) *Verbal Behaviour.* New York: Appleton-Century-Crofts.

Skinner, E. R. (1935) 'A calibrated recording and analysis of the pitch, force and quality of vocal tones expressing happiness and sadness.' *Speech Monograph,* MIZ, vol. 2.

Skinner, R. (1993) 'Traditional Mongolian medicine – a resurgence.' *International Journal of Alternative and Complimentary Medicine,* 11, 5.

Sky, M. (1990) *Breathing: Expanding Your Power and Energy.* New Mexico: Bear and Company.

Smith, J. (1973) *Melodrama.* London: Methuen.

Smith, W. (1996) *'Voice, psychotherapy and feminism.'* Paper presented to the International Association for Voicework, London, October 1996.

Soskin, W.F. (1953) 'Some aspects of communication and interpretation in psychotherapy'. Paper read at American Psychological Association, Panel on Communication in the Counselling Situation. Cleveland, September 1953.

Soskin, W.F. and Kauffman, P.E. (1961) 'Judgment of emotion in word-free voice samples.' *Journal of Communication,* 11, 2.

Speads, C. (1992) *Ways to Better Breathing.* Vermont: Healing Arts Press.

Spencer, H. (1922) 'Essay on the origin of music', cited in O. Jesperson, *Language: Its Nature, Development and Origin.* London: Allen and Unwin.

Spranger, E. (1928) *Types of Men.* Halle (Saale): Niemeyer.

Springsteen, B. *Greatest Hits.* Cassette. Sony Music.

Stack, Sullivan, H. (1955) *The Psychiatric Interview.* London: Tavistock.

Stagner, R. (1936) 'Judgments of voice and personality.' *Journal of Educational Psychology,* 27.

Stagner, R. (1936) 'The Wisconsin scale of personality traits.' *Journal of Abnormal and Social Psychology.*

Stanford, W.B. (1983) *Greek Tragedy and the Emotions.* London: Routledge and Kegan Paul.

Stanislavski, C. (1979) *Building a Character,* trans. by E. Hapgood. London: Methuen.

Stanislavski, C. (1983) *Creating a Role.* Trans. by E. Hapgood. London: Methuen.

Stark, R.E. and Nathanson, S. (1975) 'Unusual features of crying in an infant dying suddenly and unexpectedly.' In J. Bosma and J. Showacre (ed) *Development of Upper Respiratory Anatomy and Function: Implications for SID*. Washington: U.S. Department of Health Education.

Starkweather, J.A. (1956) 'Content-free speech as a source of information about the speaker.' *Journal of Abnormal Psychology*, 52.

Starkweather, J.A. (1956) 'The communication value of content-free speech.' *American Journal of Psychology*, 69.

Steiner, R. (1983) *Curative Eurythmy*. London: Rudolf Steiner Press.

Steiner, R. (1987) 'Some thoughts on "la vive voix" by Ivan Fonagy.' *International Review of Psycho-Analysis*, 14.

Steiner, R. and Wegman, I., *Fundamentals of Therapy*.

Steinke, G. (1967) *The Life and Work of Hugo Ball*. The Hague: Mouton.

Stern, D. *et al.* (1982) 'Intonation contours as signal in maternal speech to pre-linguistic infants.' *Developmental Psychology*, 18.

Stewart, R. *The Best of Rod Stewart*. Cassette. Warner Communications.

Stockhausen, K. (1989) *Towards a Cosmic Music*. Trans. by T. Nevill. Dorset: Element.

Stoehr, S. (1983) *Eurythmy: An Art of Movement for Our Time*. Stourbridge: Robinswood Press.

Storr, A. (1992) *Music and the Mind*. London: Harper Collins.

Stowell, G. (1920) (ed) *The Book of Knowledge*, 5. London: Waverly.

Streisand, Barbra. *Greatest Hits* vol. 1 & 2. CD. (CBS).

Strindberg, A. (1990) *Introduction to Miss Julie in the Plays of Strindberg*, 1, Intro. and Trans. by M. Meyer. London: Methuen.

Sullivan, H.S. (1954) *The Psychiatric Interview*. New York: Norton.

Sumac, Y. *Fuego del Ande*. CD. The Right Stuff.

Sundberg, J. (1987) *The Science of the Singing Voice*. Illinois: Northern Illinois University Press.

Sutton, J. (1993) 'The guitar doesn't know this song: an investigation into parallel development in speech/language and music therapy.' In M. Heal and T. Wigram (ed) *Music Therapy in Health and Education*. by. London: Jessica Kingsley.

Svenska, D. (1991) (July 1982) cited in J. Martin, *The Voice in Modern Theatre*. London: Routledge.

Sweet Honey in the Rock, (1992) *All for Freedom*. Cassette. Warner Bros. Records Inc.

Sweigard, L.E. (1974) *Human Movement Potential: Its Ideokinetic Facilitation*. New York: Dodd, Mead and Co.

Szönyi, E. (1990) *Kodály's Principles in Practice*. Budapest: Corvina.

Talking in Tune (1996) Publicity leaflet for *Talking in Tune* workshops.

Taylor, H.C. (1934) 'Social agreement on personality traits as judged from speech.' *Journal of Social Psychology*, 5.

Teasdale, C. (1993) 'The role of clinical placement therapy training: toward consolidating our professional identity.' *The Arts in Psychotherapy*, 20, pp. 205–212.

The Beach Boys, *Twenty Golden Greats*. CD. EMI Records.

The Carpenters, *25th Anniversary Celebration*. CD. A&M Records.

The Cranberries, *Everybody Else is Doing It, so Why Can't We?* CD. Island Records.

The Voices Foundation (1996) '*Developing Children Through Singing*'. Publicity brochure.

This, B. (1982) 'Foetologie.' In E. Herbenet and M. Busne (ed) *L'Aube du Sens*. Paris: Stock.

Timmins, M. *The Cowboy Junkies, The Trinity Session*. BMG Music.

Tiramakhan Ensemble, *Songs from the Gambia*. CD. Sounds of the World.

Todd, M.E. (1937) *The Thinking Body: A Study of the Balancing Forces of Dynamic Man*. New York: Dance Horizons Inc.

Todd, M.E. (1974) *The Balancing of Forces in the Human Being: Its Application to Postural Patterns*. New York: Mabel Todd. Cited in L.E. Sweigard, *Human Movement Potential: Its Ideokinetic Facilitation*. New York: Dodd, Mead and Co.

Tom Robinson Band, *Power in the Darkness*. CD. EMI Records.

Tomatis, A. (1991) *The Conscious Ear: My Life of Transformation Through Listening*. New York: Station Hill Press.

Tong, R. (1989) *Feminist Though: A Comprehensive Introduction*. London: Routledge.

Torrey, E.F. (1969) 'The case for the indigenous therapist.' *Archive of General Psychiatry*, 20.

Trager, G.L. (1958) 'Paralanguage: a first approximation.' *Studies in Linguistics*, 13.

Trilling, O. 'Robert Wilson's Ka Mountain and Guardenia Terrace.' *Drama Review*, T58, 17.

Trojan, F. (1959) 'Die ausdruckstheorie der sprechtstimme.' *Phonetica*, 4.

Turner, Tina. *Simply the Best*. Cassette. Capitol Records.

Tyler, Bonnie. *The Collection*. Cassette. Capitol Records.

Tyler, L. (1953) 'Test review no. 77' In O. Buros (ed) *The Fourth Mental Measurements*. New Jersey: Gryphon Press.

Valéry, P. (1958) *The Art of Poetry*. New York: Princeton, Bollingen Series, Volume VII.

Various Artists, *Melodies of Love: Timeless Love Songs*. GTV.

Various Artists, *Punk: The Worst of Total Anarchy*. Disky Records.

Various Artists, *The Singing Cowboys*. CD. K-Tel.

Various Artists, *Yodelling Songs of the Alps*. CD. Legacy International.

Vaughan, Sarah. *The Best*. CD. BMG Music.

Vedder, E. and Nusrat Fateh Ali Khan, *The Long Road*. CD. Sony Music.

Vega, S. *Solitude Standing*. A&M Records.

Vernon, P.E. and Allport, G.W. (1931) 'A test for personal values.' *Journal of Abnormal Social Psychology*, 26.

von Franz, M.L. (1970) *The Problem of the Puer Aeternus*. New York: Spring.

Wagoner, L.C. (1925) 'Speech as an indication of temperamental traits.' *Quarterly Journal of Speech Education*, 2.

Waits, T. *Rain Dogs*. CD. Island Records.

Walker, D. *Becoming a Profession: The History of Art Therapy in Britain 1940–82*. London: Tavistock/Routledge (1991) and J. Alvin, *Music Therapy*. London: Stainer and Bell. (1991).

Walker-Andrews, A. and Lennon, E. (1991) 'Infants' discrimination of vocal expressions: contributions of auditory and visual information.' *Infant Behaviour and Development*, 14.

Wallace, M. (1987) *The Silent Twins*. London: Penguin.

Ward-Jones, T. (1992) *Journal for South Asian Dance*, 16. Publicity leaflets dated 1996. Interview May 1996.

Warner, M. (1994) *From the Beast to the Blonde: On Fairy Tales and Their Tellers*. London: Chatto and Windus.

Warner, M. (1995) *From the Beast to the Blonde: On Fairy Tales and Their Tellers*. London: Vintage.

Warren, B. (1993) *Using the Creative Arts in Therapy: A Practical Introduction*. London: Routledge.

Watson, A. and Drury, N. (1989) *Healing Music: The Path to Inner Wholeness*. Bridport: Prism.

Watson, I. (1993) 'Towards a third theatre.' *Eugenio Barber and the Third Theatre*. London: Routledge.

Watson, L. (1995) *Dark Nature*. London: Hodder and Stoughton.

Weisberg, P. (1963) 'Social and non-social conditioning of infant vocalization.' *Child Development*, 34.

Weiser, E. (1955) 'Stimme ohne fessel.' *Die Weltwoche*, 30 September 1955.

Weiss, D.A. (1955) 'The psychological relations to one's own voice.' *Folia Phoniatrica*, 7.

Welwood, J. (ed.) (1983) *Awakening the Heart: East/West Approaches to Psychotherapy and the Healing Relationship*. Boston: Shambhala.

Werbeck-Svärdström, V. (1985) *Uncovering the Voice*. London: Rudolf Steiner Press.

Werner Wolff, (1950) 'Voice and personality.' In *The Expression of Personality*. New York: Hermitage House.

Wethered, A. (1973) *Drama and Movement in Therapy*. London: MacDonald and Evans.

Whitcher, D. (1978) '*Animal Empathy.*' Unpublished graduating thesis for the Jung Institute, Zurich.

White, B. *The Collection*. Cassette. Polygram Records.

Whitehouse, M.S. (1979) 'C. G. Jung and dance therapy: two major principles.' In P.L. Bernstein (ed) *Eight Theoretical Approaches in Dance-Movement Therapy*, Vol.1. Dubuque: Kendall/Hunt.

Wilbur Moore, E. (1939) 'Personality traits and voice quality deficiencies.' *Journal of Speech Disorders*, 4.

Wilma, L. *et al.* (1942) *Analysis and Interpretation of the Creative Work of John Sanders*. Institute of Child Welfare, Study of Adolescence: University of California.

Wilson, R. (1994) cited in S. Brecht *The Theatre of Visions: Robert Wilson*. London: Methuen.

Wilson, R. Production notes to *The King of Spain*, cited in F. Deak 'Robert Wilson.' *The Drama Review*, 18.

Winner, E. (1982) *Invented Worlds: The Psychology of the Arts*. Cambridge, Massachusetts: Harvard University Press.

Winnicott, D. (1971) *Playing and Reality*. London: Routledge.

Winnicott, D. (1975) *Playing and Reality*. London: Tavistock.

Winnicott, D. (1988) *Playing and Reality*. Harmondsworth: Penguin.

Winstadt, R. (1951) *The Malay Magician*. London: Routledge and Kegan Paul.

Withers, B. *Greatest Hits*. CD. Sony Music.

Wolf, N. (1992) *The Beauty Myth: How Images of Beauty are Used Against Women*. London: Doubleday.

Wolff, W. (1930) 'Ueber faktoren characterologischen urteilsbildung.' *Zsch. F. Angrew. Psychol.*, 35.

Wolfsohn, A. cited in E. Weiser (1955) 'Stimme ohne fessel.' *Die Weltwoche*, 30. Trans. by I. Halcrow.

Wolfsohn, A. (1949) 'Notes on Orpheus.' Supplement to 'Orpheus or the way to a mask.' London. Posthumously published in *Spring: A Journal of Archetype and Culture*, 50, 1990.

Wolfsohn, A. 'Orpheus or the way to a mask.' Trans. by M. Gunther (unpublished manuscript written Berlin, 1936–38). Repository: Alfred Wolfsohn Private Archives, Malerargues, France. ©M. Gunther. Reprinted by permission.

Wolfsohn, A. 'The biography of an idea.' Trans. by M. Gunther. Unpublished hand-written fragment written in Germany, undated. Repository: Alfred Wolfsohn Private Archives, Malerargues, France. ©Marita Gunther. Reprinted by permission.

Wright, C. (1995) 'The resurrection of Gregorian chant.' *Open Ear*, Winter.

Wright, H., Millder D., Cook, M. and Littman, J. (1985) 'Early identification and intervention with children who refuse to speak.' *Journal of the American Academy of Child Psychiatry*, 24.

Wright, K. (1991) *Vision and Separation Between Mother and Baby*. London: Free Association Press.

Wright, P. (1996), cited in M. Law 'Interviews with contemporary voice practitioners.' Unpublished research papers prepared for the International Association for Voicework.

Wright, P. and Priestly, M. (1975) *Music Therapy in Action*. London: Constable.

Young, N. *After the Gold Rush*. CD. Warner Communications.

Youngerman, J. (1979) 'The syntax of silence: electively mute therapy.' International Review of Psychoanalysis, 6.

Zeldin, T. (1994) *An Intimate History of Humanity*. London: Sinclair-Stevenson.

Zi, N. (1994) *The Art of Breathing: A Course of Six Simple Lessons to Improve Performance and Well-Being*. Glendale, California: Vivi Coo.

Zipes, J. (1983) *Fairy Tales and the Art of Subversion*. New York: Routledge.

Zipes, J. (1994) *Fairy Tale as Myth, Myth as Fairy Tale*. Kentucky: University Press of Kentucky.

Zuckerman, M. and Driver, R. (1990) 'What sounds beautiful is good: the vocal attractiveness stereotype.' *Journal of NonVerbal Behaviour*, 14.

Zweig, C. and Abrams, J. (eds.) (1991) *Meeting the Shadow: The Hidden Power of the Dark Side of Human Nature*. Los Angeles: Jeremy P. Tarcher.

Subject Index

References in italic indicate figures.

Name Index

Milton Keynes UK
Ingram Content Group UK Ltd.
UKHW032020121024
449584UK00006B/118